ANAESTHESIA

ANAESTHESIA

EDITED BY

WALTER S. NIMMO

BSc, MD, FRCP, FFARCS
University Department of Anaesthesia
University of Sheffield Medical School
Beech Hill Road
Sheffield S10 2RX

GRAHAM SMITH

BSc, MD, FFARCS
University Department of Anaesthesia
Leicester Royal Infirmary
Leicester LE1 5WW

IN TWO VOLUMES
VOLUME 2

BLACKWELL SCIENTIFIC PUBLICATIONS

OXFORD LONDON EDINBURGH

BOSTON MELBOURNE

© 1989 by
Blackwell Scientific Publications
Editorial offices:
Osney Mead, Oxford OX2 0EL
   (*Orders*: Tel. 0865 240201)
8 John Street, London WC1N 2ES
23 Ainslie Place, Edinburgh EH3 6AJ
3 Cambridge Center, Suite 208
   Cambridge, Massachusetts 02142, USA
107 Barry Street, Carlton
   Victoria 3053, Australia

First published 1989

Set by Macmillan India Ltd.
Printed and bound in Great Britain
by Butler & Tanner Ltd
Frome and London

DISTRIBUTORS

USA
   Year Book Medical Publishers
   200 North LaSalle Street
   Chicago, Illinois 60601
   (*Orders*: Tel. 312 726–9733)

Canada
   The C. V. Mosby Company
   5240 Finch Avenue East
   Scarborough, Ontario
   (*Orders*: Tel. 416–298–1588)

Australia
   Blackwell Scientific Publications
   (Australia) Pty Ltd
   107 Barry Street
   Carlton, Victoria 3053
   (*Orders*: Tel. (03) 347 0300)

British Library
Cataloguing in Publication Data

Anaesthesia.
   1. Medicine. Anaesthesia & analgesia
   I. Nimmo, W. S. (Walter S.)   II. Smith, G.
   (Graham), 1941–
   617′. 96

   ISBN 0–632–02257–4

Contents

List of Contributors

A. P. ADAMS MB, PhD, FFARCS, *Professor of Anaesthesia, Guy's Hospital, London SE1 9RT*

A. R. AITKENHEAD MD, FFARCS, *Professor of Anaesthesia, University Department of Anaesthesia, Queen's Medical Centre, Clifton Boulevard, Nottingham NG7 2UH*

E. N. ARMITAGE FFARCS, *Consultant Anaesthetist, Brighton General Hospital and Royal Hospital for Sick Children, Brighton*

P. J. F. BASKETT MB, FFARCS, *Consultant Anaesthetist, Frenchay Hospital, Bristol BS16 1LE*

D. R. BEVAN MA, MB, MRCP, FFARCS, *Anaesthetist in Chief, Royal Victoria Hospital, 687 Pine Avenue West, Montreal, Quebec, Canada H3A 1A1*

D. G. BJORAKER MD, *Assistant Professor, Department of Anesthesiology, University of Florida, College of Medicine, Gainesville, Florida 32610, USA*

C. E. BLOGG MB, BS, FFARCS, *Consultant Anaesthetist, Nuffield Department of Anaesthetics, Radcliffe Infirmary, Oxford OX2 6HE*

J. B. BOWES MB, FFARCS, *Consultant Anaesthetist, Sir Humphry Davy Department of Anaesthesia, Bristol Royal Infirmary, Bristol BS2 8HW*

W. C. BOWMAN BPharm, PhD, DSc, FIBiol, FPS, FRAC, FFARCS, *Professor, Department of Physiology and Pharmacology, University of Strathclyde, Glasgow G1 1XW, Scotland*

D. P. BRAID MB, ChB, FFARCS, *Consultant Anaesthetist, Glasgow Western Infirmary, Glasgow G11 6NT*

B. R. BROWN JR, MD, PhD, FFARCS, *Head of the Department of Anesthesiology, University of Arizona College of Medicine, Tuscon, Arizona, USA*

F. P. BUCKLEY MB, FFARCS, *Department of Anesthesiology, University of Washington School of Medicine, Seattle, WA 98195, USA*

K. BUDD MB, ChB, FFARCS, *Consultant Anaesthetist, Bradford Royal Infirmary, Duckworth Lane, Bradford, W Yorks, BD9 6RJ*

T. N. CALVEY PhD, *Senior Lecturer, Department of Pharmacology and Therapeutics, University of Liverpool, New Medical Building, Ashton Street, PO Box 147, Liverpool*

I. T. CAMPBELL MD, FFARCS, *Senior Lecturer, University Department of Anaesthesia, Royal Liverpool Hospital, PO Box 147, Liverpool L69 3BX*

G. R. D. CATTO MD, DSc, FRCP, *Professor of Medicine and Therapeutics, Department of Medicine, University of Aberdeen, Fosterhill, Aberdeen AB9 2ZB*

W. A. CHAMBERS MD, FFARCS, *Consultant Anaesthetist, Department of Anaesthetics, Royal Infirmary of Edinburgh, Lauriston Place, Edinburgh*

C. R. CHAPMAN PhD, *Professor of Anesthesiology, Department of Anesthesiology, University of Washington. School of Medicine, Seattle, WA 98195, USA*

J. E. CHARLTON MB, BS, FFARCS, DObst RCOG, *Consultant Anaesthetist, Royal Victoria Infirmary, Newcastle Upon Tyne NE1 4LP*

M. J. COUSINS MB, BS, FFARACS, FFARCS, MD, *Professor and Chairman, Department of Anaesthesia and Intensive Care, Flinders Medical Centre, Bedford Park, Adelaide, SA 5042, Australia*

B. G. COVINO PhD MD, *Professor of Anesthesia, Department of Anesthesia, Brigham and Women's Hospital, Harvard Medical School, 75 Francis Street, Boston, Massachusetts 02115, USA*

R. H. CRUICKSHANK MB, BS, FFARCS, *Senior Registrar in Anaesthesia, Department of Anaesthesia, University of Sheffield Medical School, Beech Hill Road, Sheffield S10 2RX*

J. M. DAVIES MSc, MD, FRCPC, *Associate Professor, Department of Anaesthesia, Foothills Hospital at the University of Calgary, 1403 29th Street NW, Calgary, Alberta, Canada T2N 2T9*

G. DOLAN MB, ChB, MRCP, *Senior Registrar, Department of Haematology, Royal Hallamshire Hospital, Sheffield S10 2JF*

D. J. R. DUTHIE MB, ChB, FFARCS, *Lecturer, University Department of Anaesthesia, University of Sheffield Medical School, Beech Hill Road, Sheffield S10 2RX*

F. R. ELLIS PhD, MB, ChB, FFARCS, *Reader in Anaesthesia, University Department of Anaesthesia, St James's University Hospital, Leeds LS9 7TF*

THE LATE J. V. FARMAN FFARCS, *Formerly Consultant Anaesthetist, Addenbrooke's Hospital, Hills Road, Cambridge CB2 2QQ*

D. FELL MB, ChB, FFARCS, *Senior Lecturer, University Department of Anaesthesia, Leicester Royal Infirmary, Leicester LE1 5WW*

W. FITCH BSc, MB, ChB, PhD, FFARCS, MRCP, *Professor of Anaesthesia, University Department of Anaesthesia, Glasgow Royal Infirmary, 8–16 Alexandra Parade, Glasgow G31 2ER*

P. FOËX MD, FFARCS, *Clinical Reader in Anaesthesia, Nuffield Department of Anaesthetics, The Radcliffe Infirmary, Oxford OX2 6HE*

C. D. FORBES DSc, MD, FRCP, *Professor of Medicine, Ninewells Hospital, Dundee*

A. H. GIESECKE MD, *Jenkins Professor and Chairman, Department of Anesthesiology, University of Texas, Southwestern Medical School, Dallas, Texas, USA*

I. S. GRANT MB, ChB, MRCP, FRCP (Edin. & Glas.), FFARCS, *Consultant Anaesthetist and Medical Director, Intensive Therapy Unit, Western General Hospital, Edinburgh EH4 2XU*

G. M. HALL PhD, FFARCS, *Reader and Honorary Consultant, Department of Anaesthetics, Royal Postgraduate Medical School, Hammersmith Hospital, Du Cane Road, London W12 OHS*

M. J. HALSEY BSc, PhD, *Head of Section of Metabolism, Division of Anaesthesia, Clinical Research Centre, Watford Road, Harrow, Middlesex HA1 3UJ*

C. D. HANNING BSc, MB, BS, FFARCS, *Senior Lecturer, Department of Anaesthesia, The General Hospital, Gwendolen Road, Leicester LE5 4PW*

D. J. HATCH MB, BS, FFARCS, *Consultant in Anaesthesia and Respiratory Measurement, Hospital for Sick Children, Great Ormond Street, London*

T. E. J. HEALY MD FFARCS, *Professor of Anaesthesia, Department of Anaesthetics, University Hospital of Manchester, Withington Hospital, Manchester M20 8LR*

D. E. HOLLAND MRCP, FFARCS, *Senior Registrar in Anaesthetics, Nuffield Department of Anaesthetics, John Radcliffe Hospital, Oxford OX3 9DU*

J. N. HORTON MB, BS, FFARCS, *Consultant Anaesthetist, Department of Anaesthetics, University Hospital of Wales, Heath Park, Cardiff CF4 4XW*

K. HOUGHTON MB, ChB, DRCOG, FFARCS, *Senior Registrar in Anaesthesia, Sir Humphry Davy Department of Anaesthesia, Bristol Royal Infirmary, Bristol BS2 8HW*

C. J. HULL MB, ChB, FFARCS, *Professor of Anaesthesia, Department of Anaesthesia, Royal Victoria Infirmary, Newcastle Upon Tyne NE1 4LP*

J. E. HUNSLEY MB, ChB, FFARCS, *Consultant Anaesthetist, Department of Anaesthetics, Northern General Hospital, Sheffield S5 7AU*

A. INNES MB, ChB, MRCP, *Senior Registrar in Renal and General Medicine, City Hospital, Nottingham NG5 1PB*

J. L. JENKINSON MB, ChB, FFARCS, *Consultant Anaesthetist, Western General Hospital and Royal Infirmary Hospital, Edinburgh, and Part-time Senior Lecturer, The University of Edinburgh*

M. J. JONES FFARCS, MRCP, *Lecturer, University Department of Anaesthesia, Leicester Royal Infirmary, Leicester LE1 5WW*

R. M. JONES MB, ChB, FFARCS, *Senior Lecturer, Department of Anaesthesia, Guy's Hospital, London SE1 9R7*

S. W. KRECHEL MD, *Associate Professor, Department of Anesthesiology, University of Missouri, Columbia School of Medicine, 3N15 Health Sciences Centre, Columbia, Missouri 65212, USA*

I. McA. LEDINGHAM MB, ChB, MD, FRCS, FRCP, FIBiol, FRSE, *Professor and Chairman, Department of Emergency and Critical Care Medicine, The United Arab Emirates University, Faculty of Medicine and Health Sciences, PO Box 1551—AL Ain, United Arab Emirates*

E. S. LIN *Lecturer in Anaesthesia, University Department of Anaesthesia, Leicester Royal Infirmary, Leicester LE1 5WW*

L. LOH FFARCS, *Consultant Anaesthetist, Nuffield Department of Anaesthetics, Radcliffe Infirmary, Oxford OX2 6HE*

J. N. LUNN MD, FFARCS, *Reader in Anaesthetics, University College of Wales, College of Medicine, Heath Park, Cardiff CF4 4XN*

D. B. L. McCLELLAND MB, ChB, PhD, FRCP, *Director, South-east Regional Scottish National Blood Transfusion Service, Royal Infirmary of Edinburgh, Lauriston Place, Edinburgh EH3 9HB*

P. J. McKENZIE MB, ChB, MD, FFARCS, *Consultant in Anaesthesia, Nuffield Department of Anaesthetics, Radcliffe Infirmary, Oxford OX2 6HE*

H. J. McQUAY MD, FFARCS, *Clinical Reader in Pain Relief, Oxford Regional Pain Relief Unit, Abingdon Hospital Abingdon, Oxon OX14 1AG*

W. R. MacRAE MB, ChB, FFARCS, *Consultant Anaesthetist, Royal Infirmary of Edinburgh, Lauriston Place, Edinburgh EH3 9HB*

D. T. MANGANO MD, PhD, *Professor of Anesthesiology and Vice-Chairman, Department of Anesthesiology, Veterans Administration Medical Center, San Francisco, California, USA*

B. E. MARSHALL MD, FRCP, FFARCS, *Professor of Anesthesia, Department of Anesthesia, University of Pennsylvania, 3400 Spruce Street, Philadelphia 19104-4283, USA*

L. E. MATHER PhD, FFARCS, *Professor of Anaesthesia, Department of Anaesthesia and Intensive Care, Flinders Medical Centre, Bedford Park, Adelaide SA 5042, Australia*

M. MORGAN MB, BS, DA, FFARCS, *Senior Lecturer and Honorary Consultant, Department of Anaesthetics, Royal Postgraduate Medical School, Hammersmith Hospital, Du Cane Road, London W12 OHS*

R. S. NEILL MD, FFARCS (I), *Consultant Anaesthetist, Royal Infirmary, Glasgow G31 4ER*

W. S. NIMMO BSc, MD, FRCP, FFARCS, *Professor of Anaesthesia, University Department of Anaesthesia, University of Sheffield Medical School, Beech Hill Road, Sheffield S10 2RX*

I. OSWALD MA, MD, DSc, FRCPsych, *Professor of Psychiatry, University Department of Psychiatry, Royal Edinburgh Hospital, Edinburgh EH10 5HF*

H. OWEN FFARCS, *Staff Specialist/Lecturer, Department of Anaesthesia and Intensive Care, Flinders Medical Centre, Bedford Park, Adelaide SA 5042, Australia*

E. G. PAVLIN, *Professor of Anesthesiology, Department of Anesthesiology, University of Washington School of Medicine, Seattle, WA 98195, USA*

J. E. PEACOCK MB, ChB, FFARCS, *Lecturer, University Department of Anaesthesia, University of Sheffield Medical School, Beech Hill Road, Sheffield S10 2RX*

B. J. POLLARD MD, FFARCS, *Senior Lecturer in Anaesthesia, Department of Anaesthetics, University Hospital of Manchester, Withington Hospital, Manchester M20 8LR*

L. F. PRESCOTT MD, FRCPE, *Professor of Clinical Pharmacology, University Department of Clinical Pharmacology, Royal Infirmary, Lauriston Place, Edinburgh EH3 9YW*

D. S. PROUGH MD, *Associate Professor, Department of Anaesthesia and Neurology, Head of the Section of Critical Care, Bowman Gray School of Medicine, 300 South Hawthorne Road, Winston-Salem, North Carolina 27103, USA*

C. S. REILLY MB, ChB, FFARCS, *Senior Lecturer, University Department of Anaesthesia, University of Sheffield Medical School, Beech Hill Road, Sheffield, S10 2RX*

S. REIZ MD, PhD, *Professor of Anaesthesiology, Department of Anaesthesiology, University of Umeå, Umeå, Sweden*

D. J. ROWBOTHAM MB, ChB, MRCP, FFARCS, *Lecturer, University Department of Anaesthesia, University of Sheffield Medical School, Beech Hill Road, Sheffield S10 2RX*

D. ROYSTON FFARCS, *Senior Lecturer, Royal Postgraduate Medical School, Hammersmith Hospital, Du Cane Road, London W12 OHS*

W. B. RUNCIMAN BSc, MBBCh, FFARCS, PhD, *Professor and Head, Department of Anaesthesia and Intensive Care, Royal Adelaide Hospital, Adelaide, Australia*

J. W. SEAR MA, BSc, PhD, FFARCS, *Clinical Reader in Anaesthesia, Nuffield Department of Anaesthetics, John Radcliffe Hospital, Oxford OX3 9DU*

J. F. SEARLE MB, BS, FFARCS, *Consultant Anaesthetist, Royal Devon and Exeter Hospital, Barrack Road, Exeter EX2 5DW*

P. S. SEBEL MB, BS, PhD, FFARCSI, *Associate Professor of Anesthesiology, Department of Anesthesiology, Emory University School of Medicine, Atlanta, Georgia, USA*

K. H. SIMPSON MB, ChB, FFARCS, *Senior Lecturer, Department of Anaesthesia, St James' University Hospital, Leeds LS9 7TF*

P. J. SIMPSON MD, FFARCS, *Consultant Anaesthetist, Frenchay Hospital, Bristol, and Senior Clinical Lecturer in Anaesthetics, University of Bristol.*

G. SMITH BSc, MD, FFARCS, *Professor of Anaesthesia, University Department of Anaesthesia, Leicester Royal Infirmary, Leicester LE1 5WW*

A. A. SPENCE MD, FRCP FFARCS, *Professor of Anaesthesia, Department of Anaesthetics, Royal Infirmary of Edinburgh, Lauriston Place, Edinburgh EH3 9YW*

G. T. TUCKER PhD, *Professor of Pharmacology, University Department of Pharmacology and Therapeutics, Royal Hallamshire Hospital, Sheffield S10 2JF*

D. A. B. TURNER MB, BS, FFARCS, *Consultant Anaesthetist, Intensive Therapy Unit, Leicester Royal Infirmary, Leicester LE1 5WW*

R. G. TWYCROSS MA, DM, FRCP, *Consultant Physician, Sir Michael Sobell House, The Churchill Hospital, Headington, Oxford OX3 7LJ*

M. URQUHART MD, *Attending Anesthesiologist, Overlake Hospital Medical Center, Bellevue, WA 98004, USA*

J. WATKINS PhD, *Principal Scientific Officer, Department of Immunology, Royal Hallamshire Hospital, Sheffield S10 2JF*

D. WEATHERILL BSc, MB, ChB, PhD, FFARCS, *Senior Lecturer, Department of Anaesthetics, Royal Infirmary of Edinburgh, Lauriston Place, Edinburgh EH3 9YW*

G. A. WESTON MB, ChB, FFARCS, *Consultant Anaesthetist, Department of Anaesthetics, Northern General Hospital, Sheffield S5 7AU*

D. C. WHITE FFARCS, *Consultant Anaesthetist, Northwick Park Hospital, Watford Road, Harrow, Middlesex*

P. F. WHITE PhD, MD, *Professor and Director of Clinical Research, Department of Anesthesiology, University of Washington, School of Medicine, Seattle, WA 98195, USA*

J. A. W. WILDSMITH MD, FFARCS, *Consultant Anaesthetist, Department of Anaesthetics, Royal Infirmary of Edinburgh, Lauriston Place, Edinburgh EH3 9YW*

S. M. WILLATTS FRCP, FFARCS, *Consultant Anaesthetist, Department of Anaesthetics, Bristol Royal Infirmary, Bristol BS2 8HW*

I. H. WRIGHT MB, BS, MRCP, FFARCS, *Senior Registrar in Anaesthetics, South Western Regional Training Scheme, Bristol Royal Infirmary, Bristol*

M. WOOD MB, ChB, FFARCS, *Professor of Anesthesiology, Vanderbilt University, Nashville, Tennessee 3732, USA*

Preface

Over the past decade there have been dramatic changes in the practice of anaesthesia. This is manifest not only in the practical administration of anaesthetics, but also by the progressive migration of anaesthetists into areas of medical practice outside the immediate operating room environment. Thus, the provision of obstetric analgesic services has been extended, involvement of anaesthetists in intensive care continues to expand steadily and there has emerged a new specialty of intractable pain, in which anaesthetists play a predominant role. In addition, in some countries, and especially in the United Kingdom, there has been a renaissance in local analgesic techniques which has stimulated research into this area.

As may be expected, these changes have been associated with alterations in training requirements. There has been an accompanying change in format of postgraduate examinations, at least in those conducted by the Faculty of Anaesthetists of the Royal College of Surgeons of England.

This book was conceived at a time, we believe, when there was no single major textbook of anaesthesia which reflected these developments in anaesthetic practice and which provided a broad and balanced account appropriate for the new examinations.

This text was designed primarily therefore for anaesthetists preparing for the new final part of the FFARCS examination. Our aim was to provide for the first time, within a single work, virtually all the anaesthetic information required by a candidate with a sound knowledge of medicine and surgery. In attempting to achieve this objective, it follows that the text should be valuable also for all tutors and supervisors of trainee anaesthetists, and established consultants requiring a comprehensive and readily available source of reference.

Anaesthesia teaching has standards which are judged on a world stage and this work is intended to fill a gap in available texts for trainees in other English speaking nations—a glance at the list of contributors illustrates our attempts to recruit a truly international team.

The text is in five main sections for ease of reference. Section I, *The Application of Scientific Principles to Clinical Practice*, serves as a reminder to trainees of their basic science knowledge and is intended to place this information into clinical perspective. Section II is the largest section and is devoted to all aspects of *General Anaesthesia* including the design of operating rooms, and current recommendations in 1989 on handling patients with AIDS or hepatitis. This is a core section for examination preparation and it is divided into 33 chapters for ease of reading, study or reference. *Local Anaesthesia* is described in detail in Section III; this comprehensive review of all relevant aspects of the subject is unique in this type of textbook. Section IV is devoted to the management of *Acute and Chronic Pain* and once again the subject matter is detailed and comprehensive with practical—in addition to theoretical—advice. The last section contains 11 chapters describing *Intensive Care* and includes medical, surgical and anaesthetic aspects of this important field of knowledge.

The text has been prepared by a team of experts, many of whom are international authorities. Some contributors are drawn from non-anaesthetic disciplines and many are practising currently outside the UK. The majority of our authors are from the UK, but in their writing they reflect the best of practice in all countries of the world. We are grateful for the excellence of their contributions and the timely return of their chapters so that the book appears very soon after submission of manuscripts in an attempt to be as contemporary as possible. For the rapid typesetting, we are grateful to our publishers and in particular to Peter Saugman, Edward Wates and Emmie Williamson at Blackwell Scientific Publications. We are also grateful to Drs Sue Coley, Rhian Lewis, Boyd Meiklejohn, Robin Mitchell and Malcolm Parsloe for proof reading.

The text is offered by the editors as an attempt to facilitate preparation for examinations, teaching, ward rounds or theatre sessions, or simply for the caring anaesthetist to remain contemporary in his knowl-edge. It represents a major effort of organization and study and also some satisfaction obtained by collabor-ation with distinguished men and women. If the contributors think the effort worthwhile and the reader finds the text as useful as the editors have found the project stimulating, all will be well.

WALTER S. NIMMO
GRAHAM SMITH
Sheffield and Leicester
1988

SECTION III
LOCAL ANAESTHESIA

56

Local Anaesthetic Drugs—
Mode of Action and Pharmacokinetics

G. T. TUCKER

Local anaesthetics cause reversible blockade of the conduction of impulses in the peripheral nervous system. An understanding of the principles involved in the movement of these compounds to and from their sites of action in nerves, their interaction with the axonal membrane, and the factors controlling their eventual removal from the body is essential to the practice of effective and safe regional anaesthesia. This chapter will consider the inter-relationships between the chemical structure and physico-chemical properties of these drugs and their mechanism of action and pharmacokinetic characteristics.

Chemical structure

A variety of chemicals are capable of blocking nerve conduction. Most of the clinically useful local anaesthetics conform to a structural sequence consisting of an aromatic ring linked by a carbonyl-containing moiety through a carbon chain to a substituted amino group (Table 56.1). The total length of the molecules is about 1.5 nm, and they are amphipathic in nature i.e. partly lipophilic and partly hydrophilic.

For the purpose of classifying the different agents the most important feature is the nature of the carbonyl-containing linkage group. Thus, the ester-type agents include cocaine, benzocaine, procaine, 2-chloroprocaine and amethocaine, whilst the amides include lignocaine, prilocaine, mepivacaine, bupivacaine and etidocaine. Cinchocaine is also an amide but with the group inserted the other way round, as a carbamoyl linkage. Unlike the amides, the esters are hydrolysed readily, especially on repeated autoclaving and under alkaline conditions. Rapid enzymatic hy-drolysis takes place also once they are in the blood-stream. This is promoted by the addition to procaine of a chlorine atom at the 2 position (chloroprocaine), whereas the addition of a butyl group to the aromatic nitrogen (amethocaine) has the opposite effect.

In procaine and its analogues the aromatic moiety is incorporated into a para-aminobenzoic acid nucleus whereas in lignocaine and its analogues the aromatic system is typically 2,6-xylidine. Prilocaine differs in being based upon o-toluidine, thereby lacking one of the aromatic methyl groups shielding the amide link.

The carbon chain consists of either one or two methylene groups as in lignocaine and procaine, respectively; it may also be branched as in prilocaine and etidocaine or incorporated into a heterocyclic ring as in mepivacaine and bupivacaine. The latter two arrangements allow for the presence of an asymmetric carbon atom. This gives rise to stereo-isomeric forms with different anaesthetic, vasoactive and toxic proper-ties. However, only the racemates of prilocaine, mepiv-acaine, bupivacaine and etidocaine are used clinically. Ropivacaine, a new addition to the amide series undergoing evaluation in man, has been developed as a single enantiomer.

The terminal subunit is typically a tertiary amine group. Exceptions are found in prilocaine, which has a secondary amino group, and benzocaine, which has no amino group at all. Thus, benzocaine apart, all of the clinically used local anaesthetics are weak bases, existing in solution as both un-ionized (free-base) and ionized (cation) forms.

Differences in the chemical structure of the various compounds are expressed in their physico-chemical properties which in turn relate to anaesthetic and kinetic properties.

	Aromatic ring	Linkage group	Carbon chain	Amino group

Table 56.1 Chemical structures of clinically important local anaesthetic agents. (From Tucker, 1983)

Esters
Cocaine

Benzocaine

Procaine (Novocaine)

2—Chloroprocaine (Nesacaine)

Amethocaine (Tetracaine, Pontocaine, Decicaine)

Amides
Cinchocaine (Dibucaine, Nupercaine)

Prilocaine (Citanest)

Lignocaine (Lidocaine, Xylocaine)

Mepivacaine (Carbocaine)

Bupivacaine (Marcain)

Etidocaine (Duranest)

* Indicates an asymmetric carbon atom and therefore the existence of stereo-isomers. Ropivacaine, the N-propyl homologue of mepivacaine and bupivacaine, is currently under development as a single enantiomer.

Physico-chemical properties

Some physico-chemical properties of the esters and the amides are shown in Table 56.2.

Molecular weight

Molecular weights of the agents span a relatively small range from 220 to 288. This indicates that differences in their aqueous diffusion coefficients will also be small as these values are related to the inverse of the square root of the molecular weight.

Dural permeability is claimed to be more dependent on molecular weight than lipophilicity, but the relationship is unconvincing within a series of opioids having physico-chemical properties similar to the amide local anaesthetics (Moore *et al.*, 1982). On the other hand, molecular weight might be relevant to the movement of local anaesthetics in the sodium channel of the nerve membrane (see below).

Lipid-solubility

Heptane:buffer distribution coefficients reflect the relative lipid-solubility of local anaesthetics (Table 56.2), showing good rank–order correlation with *in vitro* partition into rat sciatic nerve and human extradural and subcutaneous fat (Rosenberg *et al.*, 1986).

Increases in lipid-solubility are achieved by modifications at either end of the molecules. In the ester series the lipophilicity of procaine is enhanced by addition of a chlorine atom to the aromatic ring to give 2-chloroprocaine and by butyl substitution on the aromatic amine group as in amethocaine. In the amide series a similar effect is achieved mainly by alkyl substitution on the terminal aliphatic amine group. For example, replacement of the methyl group in mepivacaine by a butyl group gives bupivacaine, a much more lipidsoluble agent. Net lipid-solubility is independent of ester or amide grouping. Thus, amethocaine is highly lipophilic, as are bupivacaine and etidocaine.

A high lipid-solubility would be expected to promote diffusion through membranes, thereby speeding the onset of action, and to enhance interaction with hydrophobic components of axonal receptor sites, thereby increasing potency and duration of effect (see below). Increased sequestration by non-specific tissue components and fat near the site of action exert also a modulating effect on the anaesthetic profile.

Ionization

The esters have higher pKa values (8.5–8.9) than the amides (7.6–8.1) and will, therefore, be more ionized at physiological pH. The effect on pKa values of differences in structure within the two main types of agents is

Table 56.2 Physico-chemical properties of local anaesthetics. (From Tucker & Mather, 1980)

Agent	Mol.wt	pKa (25 °C)	Distribution coefficient*	Protein binding (%)	Aqueous solubility† (mg HCl/ml; pH 7.37, 37 °C)	Lipid diffusion index‡
Esters						
Procaine	236	8.9	0.02	5.8**	—	1
Chloroprocaine	271	8.7	0.14	—	—	—
Amethocaine	264	8.5	4.1	76**	1.4	51
Amides						
Prilocaine	220	7.9	0.9	55††	—	21
Lignocaine	234	7.9	2.9	64††	24	55
Mepivacaine	246	7.6	0.8	77††	15	10
Bupivacaine	288	8.1	27.5	95††	0.83	72
Etidocaine	276	7.7	141	94††	—	445

* *N*-heptane; pH 7.4, buffer.

† Dudziak and Uihlein (1978).

‡ Calculated from the product of the fraction un-ionized × fraction unbound to protein × the partition coefficient of the un-ionized base (Hull, 1985) and expressed relative to the value for procaine.

** Nerve homogenate binding.

†† Plasma protein binding, 2 μg/ml.

complex, involving steric factors as well as the inductive effects of alkyl substituents on the amine nitrogen. For example, the greater pKa of bupivacaine compared with mepivacaine is explained by the effect of greater alkyl substitution making the nitrogen atom more negative. In contrast, the lower pKa of etidocaine relative to lignocaine seems to reflect the effect of bulkier substituents in decreasing cation stabilization by hydration.

By promoting ionization, a higher pKa would be expected to delay diffusion, thereby prolonging onset of action. This may account also, in part, for the relatively poor penetrance of the esters compared with the amides. The influence of pKa on onset of action is considered in more detail in the section on the dynamics of nerve block.

Ionization is relevant also to the stability, solubility, and activity of local anaesthetics and their equilibrium distribution in various body compartments.

To ensure the stability of the ester-type agents, they must be dispensed in quite acidic solutions such that they exist predominantly in the more stable and soluble ionized form. Hence the pH of plain solutions of the esters may be as low as 2.8 compared with 4.4–6.4 for those of the amides. In turn, the lower pH of ester solutions means that less (un-ionized) drug will be available initially to diffuse to sites of action, thereby contributing to delay in blocking the nerve. Since instability is not a problem with the amides, further decreasing their ionization by alkalinization of the injected solution would be expected to shorten the latency of blockade (see below).

Protein binding

Besides being more lipid-soluble, the more potent and longer-acting local anaesthetics are bound also more extensively to plasma and tissue proteins (Table 56.2). This suggests that the forces attracting these compounds to non-specific sites and to axonal receptors have a large hydrophobic component. Binding to non-specific proteins near the site of action may delay onset of action by lowering the concentration gradient of diffusible drug (see below).

Aqueous solubility

The aqueous solubility of a local anaesthetic is related directly to its extent of ionization (and therefore decreases as pH is raised) and related inversely to its lipid solubility (Table 56.2).

Benzocaine, which lacks an amino group attached to the carbon chain, is almost insoluble in water. For this reason, its use is confined to topical anaesthesia, although it has been injected for prolonged intercostal nerve block after solubilization with dextran.

A low aqueous solubility may be a limiting factor when selecting an agent for subarachnoid block. Thus, there has been concern over the possible neurotoxicity of 1% solutions of bupivacaine HCl as they become opalescent on mixing with cerebrospinal fluid (CSF) *in vitro* (Dudziak & Uihlein, 1978). However, whether or not precipitation of the compound occurs *in vivo* is debatable (Meyer & Nolte, 1978; Starke & Nolte, 1978; Dennhardt & Ammon, 1980), and animal studies indicate that morphological effects on the spinal cord of the less water-soluble agents are apparent only after intrathecal injection of concentrations greater than 2% (Adams *et al.*, 1974, 1977).

Mechanism of action

Electrophysiological effects

The transmission of an electrical impulse down a nerve can be likened to knocking over a sequence of dominoes. Removal of one of the dominoes in the chain is analogous to the application of a local anaesthetic. The primary electrophysiological effect of these compounds is to cause a local decrease in the rate and degree of depolarization of the nerve membrane such that the threshold potential for transmission is not achieved and the electrical impulse is not propagated down the nerve (Fig. 56.1). There is no effect on the resting or threshold potentials, but prolongation of the repolarization phase and refractory period may also play a role in anaesthetic action (Covino, 1980).

Effect on ionic fluxes

Evidence from studies in which sodium ion concentration was varied and others in which its flux was measured directly have shown that the primary effect of local anaesthetics on depolarization and repolarization of the nerve membrane is mediated by their ability to impair membrane permeability of sodium ions. Metabolic inhibition of the sodium pump may be discounted (Covino, 1980).

Although some anaesthetics, particularly procaine and cocaine, impair potassium ion flux also, the effect is much less than that on sodium transport and is probably not involved in conduction blockade (Covino,

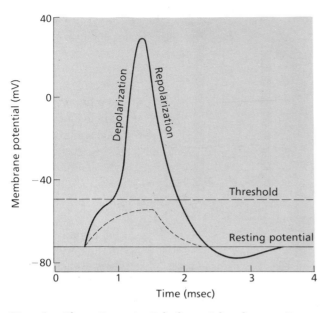

Fig. 56.1 The action potential of a peripheral nerve. On exposure to a local anaesthetic the rate and degree of depolarization are decreased (dashed line), such that the threshold potential is not attained and the impulse is not propagated down the nerve.

1980). Nevertheless, this has prompted investigations into the possibility of using potassium chloride to lower resting membrane potential, thereby potentiating the effects of local anaesthetics. Earlier clinical studies did show some advantage of the combination, albeit using potentially toxic doses of potassium (Bromage & Burfoot, 1966; Aldrete *et al.*, 1969). More recent studies using lower doses found no effect on intravenous regional anaesthesia and brachial plexus block with prilocaine but faster onset of sensory block with bupivacaine injected into the brachial plexus (McKeown & Scott, 1984; Parris & Chambers, 1986).

Raising and lowering calcium ion concentration around a nerve antagonizes and enhances local anaesthetic block respectively, and it has been suggested that local anaesthetics compete with membrane-bound calcium. Whether this action relates directly to the opening and closing of sodium channels and therefore conduction blockade remains controversial (Covino, 1980; Saito *et al.*, 1984).

Marked circadian variation in the duration of action of local anaesthetics when used for dental surgery may reflect circadian variation in the membrane permeability of ions (Pollmann, 1981).

Site of action of local anaesthetics

Three distinct sites have been proposed where local anaesthetics might exert their effect on sodium conductance across the nerve membrane (Ritchie, 1975). These are:

1 On the membrane surface, involving alteration of the fixed negative charge and hence transmembrane potential, without change in resting intracellular potential.

2 Within the membrane matrix, involving its lateral expansion, thereby causing distortion of the sodium channel.

3 Specific receptors within the sodium channel.

Although these possibilities are not mutually exclusive in that different agents may act at different sites, only the specific receptor theory is compatible with all of the following experimental observations (Covino, 1980):

1 Completely un-ionized drugs, such as benzocaine, are active.

2 Ionized forms act on the internal surface of the axonal membrane (evidence based upon internal and external perfusion of the giant squid axon with solutions of tertiary amine and quaternary analogues of lignocaine).

3 Optical isomers of some local anaesthetics show differential activity.

4 Local anaesthesia can be modulated by varying the frequency of nerve stimulation.

Thus, Hille (1977) has developed a model for a single receptor in the sodium channel that accommodates the actions of all clinically used local anaesthetics but which proposes different routes of access for ionized and un-ionized species. Three different conformational states of the sodium channel are postulated (Fig. 56.2):

1 A resting state (R), in which sodium activation and inactivation gates (m and h respectively) are closed and which predominates before nerve stimulation.

2 An open state (O), in which both gates are open, allowing passage of sodium ions during stimulation. This state is present during depolarization of the membrane.

3 An inactive state (I), in which the m-gate remains open but the h-gate is closed immediately following stimulation. This state is associated with the initial phase of repolarization and the refractory period. The rest of the repolarization phase is associated with an increase in potassium ion conductance and efflux from the internal side of the membrane.

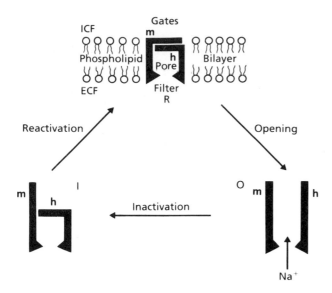

Fig. 56.2 The functional components and possible conformational states of a sodium channel. R = resting state; O = open state, allowing sodium influx; I = inactive state; ICF = intracellular fluid; ECF = extracellular fluid. (Redrawn from Wildsmith, 1986.)

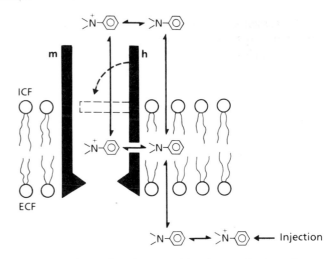

Fig. 56.3 The paths of access of local anaesthetic to the 'local anaesthetic receptor' in the neuronal sodium channel. Un-ionized and ionized forms can reach the binding site from the intracellular fluid (ICF) if activation (m) and inactivation (h) gates are both open. The un-ionized form can also reach the receptor through the membrane phase. The binding site has an important hydrophobic component and closure of the h-gate enhances the hydrophobic interaction. (Redrawn from Wildsmith, 1986.)

Local anaesthetics bind to the receptor in all three channel states and prevent electrical conduction during the O-state. Furthermore, closure of the h-gate enhances drug–receptor interaction and promotes channel inactivation. Movement of un-ionized, lipophilic species to and from the receptor is possible in all three states via diffusion through the membrane matrix, whereas movement of ionized, hydrophilic species is only possible through the open h-gate when the channel is in the O-state (Fig. 56.3).

Although the single-site theory has aesthetic appeal, Mrose & Ritchie (1978) have presented experimental data more compatible with a two-site model. Thus, when solutions of lignocaine (partially ionized) and benzocaine (un-ionized) were chosen such that each produced separately a given equilibrium response on an isolated frog sciatic nerve preparation, mixtures of the two solutions did not reproduce that same response.

The effect of pH

It is clear that both ionized and un-ionized molecules can produce conduction blockade. However, the question as to which species contributes most to the action of partially ionized agents has not been resolved satisfactorily.

Earlier studies showed that, whereas a high external pH potentiated the effect of local anaesthetics on nerves with intact sheaths, the drugs were more effective in neutral or acidic solution when desheathed nerves were used (Ritchie et al., 1965; Strobel & Bianchi, 1970). This has been rationalized by assuming that equilibrium blockade was not achieved with the sheathed preparations and that alkalinization promoted diffusion of free base to the receptor. Diffusional delays being minimal in the desheathed preparations, a greater drug potency in acidic solution signified that the cation is the active species (Covino, 1986). However, although some recent data obtained using sheathed rabbit vagus support this interpretation (Gissen et al., 1986), other data obtained using sheathed and unsheathed frog sciatic nerve do not (Bokesch et al., 1987). Thus, the first of these groups showed that the rate of blockade with bupivacaine occurs slowly and is potentiated by alkalinization. On the other hand, Bokesch et al. (1987) concluded that acidification (with hydrochloric acid) lowers the potency of lignocaine irrespective of whether the perineurium is present or not, and state that diffusional delays are insufficient to explain potentiation of block under alkaline conditions.

There is agreement that acidification with carbon dioxide increases local anaesthetic potency (Catchlove,

1972; Gissen *et al.*, 1985; Bokesch *et al.*, 1987) and that this may be mediated by its rapid diffusion across the membrane to cause a lowering of intracellular pH. This effect would be consistent with the cationic forms of local anaesthetics being the dominant active species. In addition, whereas Bokesch *et al.* (1987) do not exclude a direct action of carbon dioxide itself on the membrane but do discount any effect on extracellular pH, Gissen *et al.* (1985) conclude that carbonation is without effect on membrane sensitivity but does increase extracellular pH.

Frequency-dependent block

An increase in the frequency of nerve stimulation has been shown to enhance the effect of local anaesthetics on sodium conductance and action potential (Strichartz, 1973; Courtney, 1975).

Thus, if an *in vitro* nerve preparation is stimulated at a very low frequency and exposed to a low concentration of a local anaesthetic, a constant decrease in impulse transmission develops (tonic or 'resting' block). Increasing the stimulus frequency with the same concentration of anaesthetic will increase the degree of block until a new steady state is reached (phasic, 'use-', or 'frequency-dependent' block). After a period of rest, the original level of conduction will return.

This phenomenon may be explained on the basis of Hille's 'modulated receptor' (Hille, 1977). As shown in Fig. 56.4, the drug binds to sodium channels in the O- and I-states but has a very low affinity for channels in the R-state. After a long rest, all channels are in a relative drug-free state, but binding to open and inactivated channels develops during the action potential. If dissociation from these sites is fast relative to the frequency of stimulus there is no accumulation of blockade beyond the first stimulus (Fig. 56.4A). However, more rapid stimulation allows the h- and m-gates to remain open for longer periods of time, thereby maximizing access of drug to the receptor. The drug binds more tightly, dissociation is incomplete before the next stimulus is applied, and the block deepens (Fig. 56.4B). The conditions of membrane potential that favour the open-channel state enhance also the rates at which block develops and reverses.

The relevance of frequency-dependent block to clinical anaesthesia has not been established. However, somatic motor fibres have no frequency threshold whereas sensory fibres do with respect to the transmission of nociceptive stimuli. Therefore, variability in the

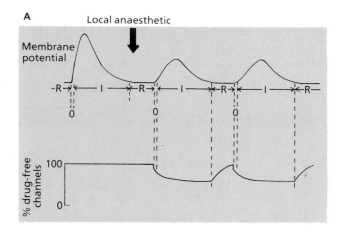

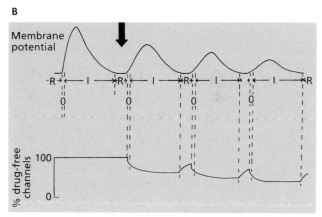

Fig. 56.4 Changes in sodium channel states and block of sodium channels associated with the nerve action potential in the presence of a local anaesthetic.
A The effect of infrequent stimulation, leading to a tonic block.
B The effect of frequent stimulation, leading to a phasic or 'frequency-dependent' block. The drug binds to sodium channels in open (O) and inactivated (I) states but has a very low affinity in the rested (R) state. Drug dissociation is time dependent and becomes incomplete during frequent stimulation, resulting in an accumulation of drug-associated (blocked) channels with successive impulses. (Redrawn from Clarkson & Hondeghem, 1985.)

ability of different agents to produce frequency-dependent and differential block may be related (Scurlock *et al.*, 1978). In the treatment of chronic pain it has been suggested that onset and depth of anaesthesia might be augmented by combining the use of local anaesthetics and nerve stimulators (Covino, 1980).

Although the implications of frequency-dependence for clinical nerve block are unclear, there is good reason to believe that this phenomenon contributes to the relative cardiotoxicity of some local anaesthetics. Thus, the antiarrhythmic effect of lignocaine and the greater risk of cardiac depression and arrhythmogenesis with bupivacaine are accounted for by observations suggesting that whereas lignocaine blocks sodium channels in the myocardium in a 'fast-in, fast-out' manner, bupivacaine is fast-in and slow-out (Clarkson & Hondeghem, 1985).

Structure–activity relationships

Studies of the relationships between structure and local anaesthetic activity are complicated by the need to distinguish between the relative potencies of cationic and free-base forms and between tonic and phasic block.

With regard to tonic block there is general agreement that potency increases with lipid-solubility (Courtney, 1980; Wildsmith *et al.*, 1987) of both neutral and protonated species (Bokesch *et al.*, 1986). However, blockade does not depend uniquely on hydrophobicity as predicted if lipid partitioning alone determines potency i.e. simple Meyer–Overton theory does not apply—equal blockade is not produced by equal membrane concentrations of either base or cation in a series of compounds. Similarly, neither molecular size nor the concentration of the ionized species in solution explain the experimental observations for tonic blockade. Therefore, specific structural features as well as physico-chemical properties seem to contribute to anaesthetic potency (Bokesch *et al.*, 1986). Suggestions that esters are more potent than amides at similar lipid-solubility depend on correlations using the partition coefficient of un-ionized base (Courtney, 1980; Wildsmith *et al.*, 1987). However, the esters have higher pKa values and if distribution coefficients (which are based on measurements of the sum of neutral and charged species in the aqueous phase) are used the differences tend to disappear.

According to Hille's 'modulated receptor theory', the extent and rate of frequency-dependent block are predicted to correlate inversely with lipid-solubility. Thus, ionized, hydrophilic species, which can only come and go through the open gates, should exhibit greater phasic block than un-ionized, lipophilic species whose movement through the membrane is independent of gate opening. This was supported by experiments with completely ionized (quaternary) and completely un-ionized agents (Hille, 1977). It was an anomaly, therefore, that very lipid-soluble agents such as bupivacaine were found to produce marked frequency dependence at low rates of channel activation (Courtney *et al.*, 1978). Subsequent studies suggested

that molecular size is important, rapid receptor-binding and unbinding of molecules like bupivacaine being impeded by their bulk (Courtney, 1980). However, further investigations with lignocaine homologues have indicated that the ability to produce frequency-dependent block is neither a simple function of molecular weight nor of partition coefficient or pKa (Bokesch *et al.*, 1986). These findings emphasized also that the molecular features for optimal tonic and phasic block are not the same, suggesting that perhaps two distinct binding sites are involved (Strichartz, 1985).

Whatever the finer details of the topography of the interaction between local anaesthetics and their axonal 'receptor(s)' eventually turn out to be, the clinical potency of these drugs is related broadly to their lipid-solubility. Thus, etidocaine, bupivacaine and amethocaine are effective in lower doses than lignocaine, prilocaine and mepivacaine, while chloroprocaine and procaine are even less potent. To some extent, this order is determined also by vasoactive properties and non-specific tissue sequestration. For example, a greater intrinsic potency of lignocaine compared with prilocaine appears to be offset by its greater vasodilating effect resulting in faster systemic uptake from the site of injection. A lower potency of etidocaine with respect to bupivacaine for sensory blockade after extradural injection may reflect its greater solubility in adipose tissue within the extradural space.

The dynamics of nerve block

Factors affecting the onset and spread of neural blockade include dispersion by bulk flow of the injected solution and diffusion of the local anaesthetic agent. Duration of effect is determined by the rate of diffusion of drug away from the nerve as well as by its vascular uptake. The latter process will be considered later in the context of systemic absorption. Neural and perineural breakdown of local anaesthetics appears to be negligible and does not influence the time-course of anaesthesia (Tucker & Mather, 1980).

Bulk flow

This can be assessed using marker dyes or radiocontrast media. Spread of analgesia is only partially dependent on bulk flow of the injected solution.

SUBARACHNOID BLOCK

Hydrodynamic considerations are more important following subarachnoid injection than any other regional anaesthetic procedure. The outcome depends on a complex interplay of baricity, posture and volume and has been reviewed in detail by Greene (1985) and Wildsmith and Rocco (1985).

EXTRADURAL BLOCK

Studies using radiopaque markers have shown that increasing the volume of injectate causes a disproportionately small increase in cephalad spread (Burn *et al.*, 1973). This may reflect greater spillage into the paravertebral spaces with larger volumes and is consistent with spread of analgesia relationships (Grundy *et al.*, 1978). Below a limiting volume (constant dose), the spread and intensity of block become independent of volume, indicating that factors other than bulk flow are more important for the ultimate dispersion of the local anaesthetic.

In general, altering the speed of injection has been found to have little influence on spread of either solution or analgesia, although confounding factors include the drug used, the age of the patient and the direction of the needle bevel (Erdemir *et al.*, 1966; Husemeyer & White, 1980; Rosenberg *et al.*, 1981; Cohen *et al.*, 1984). Extremely rapid injection of bupivacaine (over 5 sec) was shown to hasten onset of block and to enhance perineal anaesthesia (Griffiths *et al.*, 1987).

Changes in posture have a minimal effect on the dynamics of extradural block, although a decrease in cephalad spread of analgesia in the sitting position has been observed in obese patients (Hodgkinson & Husain, 1981).

Increases in the longitudinal spread and duration of extradural anaesthesia with increasing age have been assigned to reduced lateral leakage of solution, owing to progressive sclerotic closure of the paravertebral foramina (Bromage, 1975). Partial support for this comes from studies with radioactive markers (Nishimura *et al.*, 1959; Burn *et al.*, 1973). However, more recent work indicates that the relationship between decline in dose requirement and age is more complex than proposed originally (Grundy *et al.*, 1978; Sharrock, 1978; Park *et al.*, 1980).

INTERCOSTAL BLOCK

There has been considerable debate as to the extent of spread of solutions injected into the intercostal groove. Using cadavers, radiopaque dyes, or computed tomography, some groups have concluded that the solution spreads via an extrapleural route into intercostal spaces adjacent to the one injected (Nunn & Slavin, 1980; Crossley & Hosie, 1987), whereas others found no such spread (Moore, 1981; Johansson *et al.*, 1985). The clinical significance of this relates to the practice of multiple or continuous administration of local anaesthetics into one intercostal space to provide prolonged analgesia over an extensive field (O'Kelly & Garry, 1981; Murphy, 1983).

BRACHIAL PLEXUS BLOCK

Winnie *et al.* (1979) used a mixture of bupivacaine and radiopaque dye to document the spread of solution following injection into the brachial plexus sheath, and have made recommendations designed to improve the flow in the desired direction. These were based on the concept of a continuous, single fascial compartment surrounding the brachial plexus. Thompson and Rorie (1983) have challenged this view, however, with evidence from dissections and computed tomography for the presence of individual fascial compartments around each of the major branches of the plexus. They concluded that connective tissue septa interfere with circumferential spread of local anaesthetic, explaining the occasional occurrence of incomplete sensory blockade. Subsequently, Vester-Andersen *et al.* (1986), using gelatine injections, found no evidence for septa. Lack of contact between some of the nerves and the gelatine was accounted for by obstruction of circumferential spread of solution owing to the position of the arm during injection.

Diffusion

Once the local anaesthetic has been deposited and spread physically in the extraneural fluids it diffuses to the nerve membrane.

SUBARACHNOID BLOCK

After subarachnoid injection, the relatively high lipid-solubility of local anaesthetics promotes local cord uptake rather than extensive cephalad spread via CSF flow. Thus, drug concentrations in the CSF decline in both directions from the point of injection and exponentially at the site of injection as uptake proceeds (Koster *et al.*, 1936; Meyer & Nolte, 1978; Post *et al.*, 1985). Direct diffusion along the concentration gradient from CSF through the pia mater directly into the cord delivers drug to superficial parts of the structure.

Access to deeper areas is effected by diffusion in the CSF contained in the spaces of Virchow–Robin which connect with perineural clefts surrounding the bodies of nerve cells within the cord (Greene, 1983). Further penetration of drug into the cord may occur also through uptake into spinal radicular arteries (Fig. 56.5).

The pattern of drug distribution within the cord is a complex function of accessibility by diffusion from the CSF, the relative myelin (lipid) content of various tracts, and the rate of drug removal by local perfusion. Studies in animals using radiolabelled local anaesthetics have shown their accumulation along the posterior and lateral aspects of the cord as well as in the spinal nerve roots, with less in the dorsal root ganglion and the centre of the cord. Uptake of drug was higher in the grey matter than in the white matter and posterior nerve roots had higher concentrations than anterior roots (Howarth, 1949; Bromage et al., 1963; Cohen, 1968; Post et al., 1985).

EXTRADURAL BLOCK

Local anaesthetics appear rapidly in the CSF after extradural injection (Wilkinson & Lund, 1970) in sufficient concentrations to block spinal nerve roots. By 30 min, high drug concentrations are achieved also in the peripheral cord and in the spinal nerves in the paravertebral space (Bromage et al., 1963).

Apart from direct diffusion of drug across the dura, access to the cord, particularly the dorsal horn region, may be mediated by diffusion and bulk flow through the arachnoid villi at the dural root sleeves, by uptake into the posterior branch of spinal segmental arteries and by centripetal subneural and subpial spread from the remote paravertebral nerve trunks (Fig. 56.5) (Bromage, 1967, 1975). These suggestions are consistent with clinical observations of the distribution of analgesia during induction and regression of block. A segmental pattern of analgesia during onset may relate to the initial diffusion into spinal nerves and roots, with subsequent non-segmental regression resulting from ultimate diffusion to structures within the cord (Urban, 1973).

Studies with implanted electrodes in monkeys indicate that the depth of penetration of the cord increases with the concentration and lipid-solubility of the local anaesthetic (Cusick et al., 1980, 1982). A marked effect of etidocaine on lower limb reflexes after thoracic extradurals in humans is consistent with blockade of relatively deep motor tracts within the cord (Bromage, 1974).

Much of an extradural dose of local anaesthetic may be sequestered temporarily in extraneural tissues at the site of injection. Prolonged storage in extradural

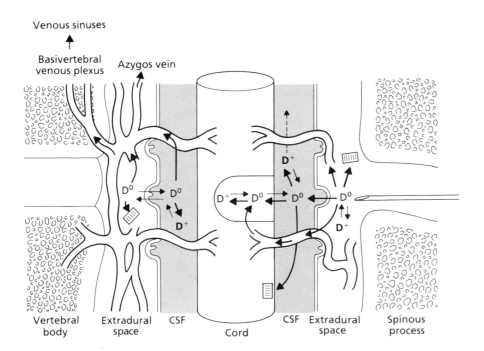

Fig. 56.5 The pathways of local distribution and systemic uptake of a local anaesthetic in the extradural and subarachnoid spaces. A needle is shown delivering drug into the extradural space, followed by attachment to non-specific lipid binding sites (shaded squares) and transfer across the dura. In the spinal cord, interaction with spinal receptors as well as non-specific lipid sites is shown. Deeper penetration of the cord is indicated via uptake into spinal arteries. Extradural veins, in close proximity to arachnoid granulations, are depicted as the major route of vascular clearance after both extradural and spinal injection. Two alternative routes of drainage, via the azygos veins or the basivertebral venous plexus, are shown. (Redrawn from Cousins & Mather, 1984).

fat, particularly of more lipid-soluble agents, has been shown in sheep (Tucker & Mather, 1980).

BRACHIAL PLEXUS BLOCK

Progression of blockade from upper arm to hand and then to fingers is explained by more rapid diffusion of local anaesthetic into mantle fibres that innervate more proximal regions than do core fibres (DeJong, 1977). To explain why the onset of motor block often precedes that of sensory loss, Winnie *et al.* (1977a) have suggested that this is due to the more peripheral location of motor fibres in the median nerve. According to the classical view, the sequence of recovery should be the same as that of onset: arm first, then hand and fingers (DeJong, 1977). This follows if the concentration gradient within the nerve now becomes reversed, decreasing from core to mantle. However, this has been challenged by Winnie *et al.* (1977b) who observed the reverse order of recovery with significant motor block that outlasted analgesia. To account for this, it was proposed that a more rapid vascular uptake occurs near the more distally innervating sensory fibres located in the core of the nerve. As intraneural blood vessels pass from mantle to core they become increasingly branched, thereby offering a larger surface area for drug absorption.

DIFFERENTIAL BLOCK

As discussed with reference to extradural and brachial plexus block, the anatomical location of nerve fibres and their accessibility by diffusion may influence their susceptibility to local anaesthetic effect. In addition, there are intrinsic differences in the ability to block various types of nerve fibre subserving different functional modalities. Thus, the sequence of clinical observations after injection of a local anaesthetic for major nerve block is generally:

1 Elevation of skin temperature (B-block).
2 Loss of pain–temperature sensation (Aδ- and C-block).
3 Loss of proprioception (Aγ-block).
4 Loss of touch and pressure sensation (Aβ-block).
5 Loss of motor function (Aα-block).

Classically, this order is explained by increases in fibre diameter and extent of myelinization raising the intrinsic margin of safety for conduction (The anomalous position of unmyelinated C-fibres with respect to the larger B-fibres may reflect their grouping in Remak bundles). If a critical number of nodes of Ranvier must be blocked to ensure complete inhibition of impulse propagation, a lower concentration of drug should be necessary to block smaller fibres since the number of nodes is inversely proportional to fibre size. Contrary to this view, however, recent re-evaluation of the differential sensitivity of mammalian nerve fibres indicates that the facility of equilibrium blockade decreases in the order A-, B- and C-fibres (Gissen *et al.*, 1980, 1982a, b). The apparent disparity between these *in vitro* findings and the sequence of clinical block was explained by the absence of equilibrium under the latter conditions. Thus, less drug reaches the larger fibres owing to the delaying effect of their diffusion barriers and attrition by vascular uptake. Some support for Gissen's conclusion is provided by other electrophysiological studies (Palmer *et al.*, 1983; Rosenberg & Heinonen, 1983; Ford *et al.*, 1984), but Fink and Cairns (1984) discount diffusion within a nerve as a contributory factor to differential block. They argue also that differential block is probably unrelated to fibre-size differences in susceptibility.

DRUG-RELATED FACTORS

Concentration

An increase in local anaesthetic concentration or dose will shorten the latency of block and increase its duration. However, the gains are disproportionate, as a simple diffusion model and some experimental data indicate that duration and the reciprocal of onset time are related logarithmically to dose (Tucker & Mather, 1980).

Physico-chemical properties

It has been suggested that the onset of conduction block in isolated nerves is determined primarily by the pKa of the individual agents (Covino, 1986). However, diffusion is determined not only by the fraction of un-ionized drug but also by the lipid-solubility of this form. Additionally, *in vivo*, non-specific binding or solubility in tissue along the diffusion pathway will modulate the rate at which local anaesthetic molecules reach their receptor sites on the nerve membrane. Therefore, a more rigorous predictor of onset of anaesthesia should be the lipid diffusion index, the product of un-ionized fraction, the partition coefficient of the free base and the fraction unbound to protein (Hull, 1985). Estimates of this index are given in Table 56.2. Procaine is predicted to have a slow onset followed by mepivacaine, prilocaine, then amethocaine and lignocaine, with bupivacaine and particularly etidocaine having very fast onset. Clinically, this order is modified by the dosage used. Thus, bupivacaine is relatively slow in onset when used as a 0.25% solution but latency decreases significantly on going to 0.75%. Two-chloroprocaine would be expected to have a low diffusion potential and onset, but this is overcome by its use in high concentration (3%).

Differences in diffusion index seem also to account for differences in differential block between agents. For example, on this basis Gissen *et al.* (1982b) have explained the clinical observation that, whereas in low doses bupivacaine produces good sensory analgesia with minimum motor loss, etidocaine produces profound motor blockade. Thus, differences in the relative rates of onset of C(pain)- and A(motor)-fibre block for the two drugs were reproduced in an *in vitro* preparation (Fig. 56.6).

Duration of anaesthesia, like potency, is related to the lipid-solubility and binding affinity of local anaesthetics and is influenced also by their intrinsic vasoactivity.

EFFECTS OF pH

If diffusion of local anaesthetics to the axonal membrane is rate limiting and rapid tissue buffering does not occur, increasing the pH of the injected solution should shorten the latency of action. This is borne out by some clinical studies showing faster onset and longer dur-

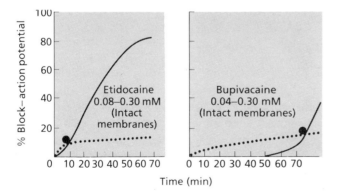

Fig. 56.6 Effects of etidocaine and bupivacaine on the onset of blockade of the compound action potential of the sheathed rabbit vagus nerve at 22 °C. Dashed line: C-fibre response; solid line: A-fibre response. The cross-over points (closed circles), when A-block exceeds C-block, is much later with bupivacaine. (Redrawn from Gissen *et al.*, 1982b.)

ation after adding sodium bicarbonate to bupivacaine solutions immediately before extradural or brachial plexus injection (Galindo, 1983; Hilgier, 1985; DiFazio *et al.*, 1986; McMorland *et al.*, 1986). However, other investigators found no effect of alkalinization on peripheral nerve blocks (Smith *et al.*, 1986; Bedder *et al.*, 1987).

The use of carbonated (CO_2) solutions of local anaesthetics might be expected to have a similar effect on latency as those to which bicarbonate is added. However, the results of controlled clinical studies are again equivocal (Brown *et al.*, 1980; McClure & Scott, 1981; Martin *et al.*, 1981; Morison, 1981; Nickel *et al.*, 1986). Dissipation of the effect of carbon dioxide on intracellular pH may be too rapid *in vivo*, and its vasodilating effect might promote systemic absorption of local anaesthetic.

Cohen *et al.* (1968) have suggested that tachyphylaxis on repeated injection of local anaesthetics could be explained by the pH-lowering effect of their usually acidic solutions. A progressive lowering of CSF pH has been noted after subarachnoid injections (Cohen *et al.*, 1968; Tucker & Mather, 1980) but rapid buffering seems to occur in the extradural space (Wurst & Stanton-Hicks, 1983). More peripheral injections cause sustained lowering of tissue pH, especially when adrenaline is added to the solution, but this acidosis does not appear to influence duration of block (Wennberg *et al.*, 1982; Buckley *et al.*, 1985). Tachyphylaxis is not explained adequately by pH effects alone (Mather, 1986).

Systemic absorption

A knowledge of the rates of systemic absorption of local anaesthetics helps to set confidence limits on the likelihood of systemic toxic reactions after the various block procedures. Indirectly, these rates suggest also the relationship between blockade and the amount of drug remaining at the site of injection.

In man, measurement of drug concentration–time profiles in the peripheral circulation has been used widely to assess systemic uptake of the different agents. Because these profiles are the net result of both systemic absorption and disposition, they are of value mainly to determine relative changes in drug uptake. Variables affecting absorption are assumed usually not to influence disposition. To assess safety margins, vascular drug concentrations after perineural injection are compared with estimates of threshold values associated with the onset of significant CNS toxicity.

These range from 5 to 10 μg/ml for lignocaine and from 2 to 4 μg/ml for bupivacaine and etidocaine. Although these values are useful guidelines, they refer to the mythical 'average subject' and must be interpreted in the light of a number of considerations. These include whether measurements are made of plasma or blood, total or unbound drug, ionized or un-ionized species, optical isomers, and active drug metabolites. The site of blood sampling (artery or vein) may be critical also when drug concentrations are changing rapidly (Tucker, 1986).

If blood drug concentration–time profiles are available also after intravenous administration, it becomes possible to calculate drug absorption rates using more sophisticated techniques of pharmacokinetic analysis such as deconvolution (Tucker, 1986).

Because local anaesthetics are relatively lipid-soluble compounds, their diffusion across the capillary epithelium is not likely to be rate limiting. Hence their absorption rates will primarily be related directly to blood flow and inversely to local tissue binding.

Important determinants of systemic absorption include the physico-chemical and vasoactive properties of the agent, the site of injection, dosage factors, the presence of additives such as vasoconstrictors, factors related to nerve block, and pathophysiological features of the patient.

Agent

The extensive data on peak blood and plasma concentrations of the amide local anaesthetics and the times of their occurrence after various routes of injection have been tabulated elsewhere (Tucker & Mather, 1979, 1980, 1987). For example, after extradural injection of plain solutions, the increment in peak whole-blood drug concentration per 100 mg of dose is about 0.9–1.0 μg/ml for lignocaine and mepivacaine, slightly less for prilocaine, and approximately 50% as much for bupivacaine and etidocaine. Although differences in disposition kinetics contribute to this order (see below), it appears that, despite similar peak times, net absorption of the long-acting, more lipid-soluble agents is slower. This is consistent with data on residual concentrations of the agents in extradural fat after injection into sheep (Tucker & Mather, 1980) and is confirmed by pharmacokinetic calculations of the time-course of drug absorption in man (Tucker & Mather, 1979; Burm, 1985). The latter show that systemic uptake after extradural injection is a biphasic process, the contribution of the initial rapid phase being greater for

lignocaine than for the long-acting analogues (Table 56.3; Fig. 56.7). This slower net absorption of the latter adds to their systemic safety margin after accurate injection.

Differences in the absorption rates of the various agents have implications for their accumulation during repeated and continuous administration. Whereas systemic accumulation is most marked with the short-acting amides, extensive local accumulation is predicted for bupivacaine and etidocaine, despite their longer dosage intervals (Tucker & Mather, 1975; Tucker et al., 1977; Inoue et al., 1985).

Observations of relatively low blood concentrations of prilocaine with respect to the toxic threshold, particularly after brachial plexus block (Fig. 56.8) and intravenous regional anaesthesia, support the claim that this compound should be the agent of choice for such single-dose procedures (Wildsmith et al., 1977). In this case, however, a high systemic clearance, rather than slow absorption, is mainly responsible for the low blood drug concentrations.

Although the rate of systemic absorption of local anaesthetics is controlled largely by the extent of local binding, their intrinsic vasoactive properties could also modulate local perfusion and hence uptake (Blair, 1975; Aps & Reynolds, 1976, 1978; Fairley &

Table 56.3 Mean dose fractions (F) and half-lives characterizing the absorption of lignocaine and bupivacaine after subarachnoid and extradural injection in man (Burm, 1985). The data were obtained after deconvolution of plasma drug concentration–time profiles measured after simultaneous intravenous injection of deuterated drug and spinal/extradural injection of non-labelled drug. The time-course of unabsorbed bupivacaine was described by a bi-exponential function after both subarachnoid and extradural injection, whereas that of lignocaine was mono-exponential after subarachnoid and bi-exponential after extradural injection. F = total systemic availability compared with the intravenous injection.

| | Lignocaine | | Bupivacaine | |
	Sub-arachnoid	Extra-dural	Sub-arachnoid	Extra-dural
F_1	—	0.38	0.35	0.29
$t_{\frac{1}{2}}$, abs$_1$ (min)	—	9.3	50	8
F_2	—	0.58	0.61	0.64
$t_{\frac{1}{2}}$, abs$_2$ (min)	71	82	408	371
F	1.03	0.96	0.96	0.91

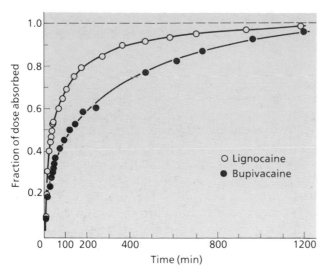

Fig. 56.7 Fraction of local anaesthetic dose absorbed into the general circulation as a function of time after extradural injection. The data points represent values determined by deconvolution of the measured plasma drug concentrations in representative subjects against the intravenous unit impulse curve in each subject. The curves represent biexponential functions fitted to the data points by non-linear regression. (Redrawn from Tucker, 1986.)

Reynolds, 1981; Jones *et al.*, 1985). However, the contribution of these phenomena to the relative absorption of drugs after peripheral and central nerve blocks is difficult to evaluate. Some studies of spinal cord blood flow in animals indicate greater vasodilatation with amethocaine compared with amide agents (Dohi *et al.*, 1984; Kozody *et al.*, 1985).

Site of injection

Vascularity and the presence of tissue and fat that can bind local anaesthetics are primary influences on their rate of removal from specific sites of injection. In general, and independent of the agent used, absorption rate decreases in the order: intercostal block > caudal block > extradural block > brachial plexus block > sciatic and femoral nerve block (Tucker & Mather, 1980, 1987).

INTERCOSTAL BLOCK

Maximum circulating concentrations of the agents after intercostal blocks using plain solutions may exceed the toxic threshold, but effects are obtunded presumably by light general anaesthesia and premedication.

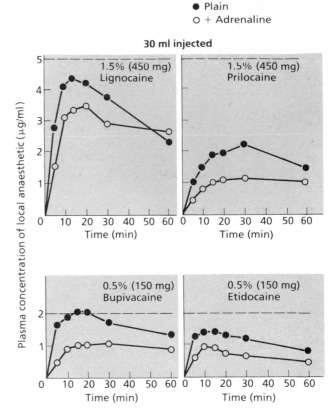

Fig. 56.8 Mean plasma concentrations of amide-type local anaesthetics after interscalene brachial plexus block. Thirty ml of agent, with (open circles) or without (closed circles) adrenaline, were injected. The broken lines indicate the putative toxic thresholds. (Redrawn from Tucker, 1986.)

EXTRADURAL BLOCK

The role of fat deposits within the extradural space in delaying the absorption of local anaesthetics has been discussed already. Vascular uptake will take place into the extradural veins and thence to the azygos vein. In the presence of raised intrathoracic pressure, however, absorbed drug could be redirected also up the internal vertebral venous system to cerebral sinuses (Fig. 56.5).

Vascular absorption of local anaesthetic from different regions of the extradural space (cervical, lumbar, thoracic) appears to be similar (Mayumi *et al.*, 1983).

BRACHIAL PLEXUS BLOCK

The various techniques for blocking the brachial plexus are not associated with significant differences in local anaesthetic absorption rate (Vester-Andersen *et al.*, 1981; Maclean *et al.*, 1988).

SUBARACHNOID BLOCK

Systemic uptake after subarachnoid injection is believed to occur predominantly after passage of drug across the dura into the more vascular extradural space (Cohen, 1968), as well as from blood vessels within the spinal space, in the pia mater, and the cord itself (Fig. 56.5). Extensive diffusion into the extradural space would be expected to result in sequestration in fat, thereby retarding the absorption of the longer-acting agents to a greater extent than the short-acting ones. Pharmacokinetic analysis shows that there are differences in the pattern of systemic absorption after subarachnoid and extradural injection, and confirms that there is a slower net absorption of bupivacaine compared to lignocaine (Table 56.3). The slower initial uptake from the subarachnoid space may reflect dural diffusion. The similarity of the slower uptake phase for subarachnoid bupivacaine and the overall mono-exponential uptake of subarachnoid lignocaine with the corresponding slow phases of uptake after extra-dural injection suggest a common rate-limiting removal from extradural fat.

INTRAVENOUS REGIONAL ANAESTHESIA

A pharmacokinetic analysis of plasma lignocaine concentrations measured after intravenous regional anaesthesia has shown that, if the cuff is inflated correctly for at least 10 min after injection, only about 20–30% of the dose enters the systemic circulation during the first minute after cuff release. The rest emerges rather slowly, with approximately 50% of the dose still in the arm after 30 min (Tucker & Boas, 1971). Direct experimental support for this comes from observations of sustained high concentrations of local anaesthetic in the venous drainage from the blocked arm (Evans et al., 1974). Longer application of the cuff delays wash-out of drug from the arm (Tucker & Boas, 1971).

TRACHEAL ADMINISTRATION

Doses of lignocaine up to 400 mg produce peak plasma drug concentrations usually within 10–15 min well below the toxic threshold (Tucker & Mather, 1980, 1987). The concentrations are significantly lower in spontaneously breathing patients than in paralysed patients since the former are more likely to swallow some of the dose, which then undergoes first-pass hepatic metabolism following absorption from the gut (Scott et al., 1976). Application only to areas below the vocal cords may result in excessive plasma drug concentrations because of less transfer to the gut (Curran et al., 1975).

Dosage factors

Differences in absorption rates as a function of concentration and volume of injectate (constant dose) (Tucker & Mather, 1980, 1987; Denson et al., 1983) and speed of injection (Scott et al., 1972; Rosenberg et al., 1981; Vester-Andersen et al., 1984) are small. There is some evidence for a disproportionate increase in peak plasma drug concentration with increasing dose (Bridenbaugh et al., 1974; Lund et al., 1975), but again the changes are probably not of clinical significance.

Adrenaline

The degree to which adrenaline decreases the systemic absorption rate of local anaesthetic is a complex function of the type, dose and concentration of local anaesthetic and of the characteristics of the injection site (Tucker & Mather, 1980, 1987).

Although the peak plasma concentrations of local anaesthetics after most of the common regional blocks are lowered by adrenaline, it does not always prolong the time to peak (Tucker & Mather, 1979, 1980, 1987). In general, the greatest effects are seen after intercostal blocks and with short-acting rather than long-acting agents. This suggests that the greater local binding of the latter and their vasodilatory effects tend to offset the vasoconstriction caused by adrenaline. Differences in the effect of adrenaline on the systemic uptake of different local anaesthetics are reflected broadly in its effect on duration of block (Covino, 1986).

Physical and pathophysiological factors

AGE AND WEIGHT

In adults, plasma concentrations of local anaesthetics after extradural and other nerve blocks are correlated poorly with age and weight (Scott et al., 1972; Tucker et al., 1972; Moore et al., 1976a,b). Studies designed specifically to compare groups of young and elderly patients suggest a trend to more rapid absorption in the latter after extradural and caudal injections (Rosenberg et al., 1981; Finucane & Hammonds, 1984; Freund et al., 1984). Limited data are available in children which indicate somewhat faster absorption than in adults (Eyres *et al.*, 1978, 1983; Ecoffey *et al.*, 1984; Takasaki, 1984; Rothstein *et al.*, 1986).

PREGNANCY

Although engorgement of vertebral veins and a hyperkinetic circulation might be expected to enhance absorption of local anaesthetics after extradural block, plasma drug concentration–time profiles appear to be similar in pregnant and non-pregnant women (Morgan *et al.*, 1977).

DISEASE AND SURGERY

Changes in local perfusion associated with altered haemodynamics as a result of disease or surgery may modify absorption of local anaesthetics and hence duration of anaesthesia. For example, acute hypovolaemia slows lignocaine absorption after extradural injection in dogs (Morikawa *et al.*, 1974) and prolongs anaesthesia in patients undergoing thoracotomy with regional block (Quimby, 1965). Conversely, a decreased duration of brachial plexus block in patients with chronic renal failure may reflect a hyperkinetic circulation and enhanced systemic uptake of local anaesthetic (Bromage & Gertel, 1972; Strasser *et al.*, 1981).

Systemic disposition

After systemic absorption local anaesthetics are distributed by the bloodstream to the organs and tissues of the body and cleared, mostly by metabolism and to a small extent by renal excretion. In pregnant women a proportion of the dose also crosses the placenta into the baby.

The role of the lung

The first capillary bed to be exposed to local anaesthetic once it has entered the systemic circulation is that in the lung. This structure acts as a capacitor, sequestering temporarily a large quantity of drug because of a high lung:blood partition coefficient. Hence, after rapid intravenous input, the arterial blood drug concentration which hits the target organs for toxicity, the brain and the heart (via the coronary circulation), is attenuated considerably compared with the drug concentration in the pulmonary artery (Tucker & Boas, 1971; Lofstrom, 1978; Jorfeldt *et al.*, 1979).

Arthur (1981) has shown that lung uptake of

prilocaine in man exceeds that of lignocaine and contributes to its greater systemic safety margin. The rank order of uptake in rat lung slices was found to be bupivacaine > etidocaine > lignocaine (Post *et al.*, 1979). The extravascular pH of the lung is low relative to plasma pH and this encourages ion-trapping of local anaesthetic (Post & Eriksdotter-Behm, 1982). Other basic drugs e.g. propranolol, may compete with local anaesthetics for pulmonary binding sites, thereby decreasing their first-pass extraction (Rothstein *et al.*, 1987). On the other hand, general anaesthesia and severe respiratory deficiency do not appear to have a marked effect (Jorfeldt *et al.*, 1983).

Local anaesthetic drugs injected into patients with intracardiac right–left shunts (Bokesch *et al.*, 1985) or injected inadvertently into the carotid or vertebral artery during attempted stellate ganglion block, bypass the lung, resulting in a high probability of CNS toxicity. Furthermore, Aldrete *et al.* (1977, 1978) have shown that the introduction of local anaesthetics, under pressure, into the lingual, brachial, or femoral artery of baboons and the facial artery of dogs can produce a retrograde flow facilitating direct access of high concentrations of drug to the cerebral circulation.

Blood binding

The long-acting amides are bound in plasma to a greater extent than the short-acting ones (Table 56.4). There are two classes of binding sites: a high-affinity, low-capacity site on α_1-acid glycoprotein and a quantitatively less important low-affinity, high-capacity site on albumin (Tucker *et al.*, 1970a; Mather *et al.*, 1971; Mather & Thomas, 1978; Piafsky & Knoppert, 1979; Routledge *et al.*, 1980; Denson *et al.*, 1984; Kraus *et al.*, 1986).

The extent of binding varies with the plasma concentration of α_1-acid glycoprotein, and both are elevated considerably in patients with cancer (Jackson *et al.*, 1982), chronic pain (Fukui *et al.*, 1984), trauma (Edwards *et al.*, 1982), inflammatory disease (Bruguerolle *et al.*, 1985) and uraemia (Grossman *et al.*, 1982), and in postoperative (Hasselstrom *et al.*, 1985) and postmyocardial infarction patients (Barchowsky *et al.*, 1981). Low plasma concentrations of α_1-acid glycoprotein in neonates are associated with much lower binding of local anaesthetics compared with that in adult plasma (Tucker *et al.*, 1970b; Petersen *et al.*, 1981; Wood & Wood, 1981; Piafsky & Woolner, 1982). Binding decreases as pH decreases (Burney *et al.*, 1978; McNamara *et al.*, 1981; Coyle *et al.*, 1984).

Table 56.4 Pharmacokinetic parameters describing the disposition kinetics of amide-type local anaesthetics in adult males. (From Tucker, 1986)

	Prilocaine	Lignocaine	Mepivacaine	Ropivacaine	Bupivacaine	Etidocaine
$K_{B/P}$	1.1	0.8	0.9	0.7	0.6	0.6
F_U	0.45	0.30	0.20	0.06	0.05	0.05
V_{SS}* (litre)	191	91	84	61	73	134
V_{USS}* (litre)	320	253	382	742	1028	1478
Cl* (litre/min)	2.37	0.95	0.78	0.73	0.58	1.11
E_H	?	0.65	0.52	0.49	0.38	0.74
$t_{\frac{1}{2},z}$ (hr)	1.6	1.6	1.9	1.9	2.7	2.7
MBRT (hr)	1.3	1.6	1.8	1.4	2.1	2.0

* Specified with respect to arterial blood drug concentration, with the exception of prilocaine and ropivacaine data which are specified with respect to peripheral venous blood drug concentration. Note, with the exception of lignocaine and ropivacaine, all data refer to racemic drug.

$K_{B/P}$ = blood/plasma drug concentration ratio.

V_{SS} = volume of distribution at steady state based on total blood drug concentration.

V_{USS} = volume of distribution at steady state based on unbound drug concentration in plasma water.

Cl = systemic clearance.

F_U = fraction unbound in plasma (at 2 μg/ml total concentration).

E_H = estimated hepatic extraction ratio.

$t_{\frac{1}{2},z}$ = terminal elimination half-life.

MBRT = mean body residence time.

Attachment of the agents to binding sites in or on erythrocytes is of similar order to plasma binding (Tucker *et al.*, 1970a). However, in the presence of plasma proteins, plasma binding competes with binding to the red cells. Hence, blood:plasma drug concentration ratios are related inversely to plasma binding (Table 56.4).

The role of plasma binding in the toxicity of local anaesthetics has been discussed by Tucker (1986).

Thus, it is important to allow for this phenomenon when interpreting measurements of plasma drug concentrations. For example, marked accumulation of total plasma drug concentrations postoperatively may not signify a risk of toxicity (Richter *et al.*, 1984). This change reflects the postoperative increase in α_1-acid glycoprotein and therefore plasma drug binding. Unbound (active) drug concentrations, which are likely to be a better index of effect, are similar before and after surgery (Fig. 56.9). When systemic drug input is gradual, as after perineural injection, distribution of the dose is spread over time and a large extravascular distribution space and extensive tissue binding (see below) ensures that only a small percentage remains in the blood at any time. Under these conditions, any changes in plasma binding are buffered effectively by a high volume of distribution. Also, for drugs like bupivacaine, with relatively low hepatic extraction ratios, any increase in free-drug concentration will be compensated by a faster elimination.

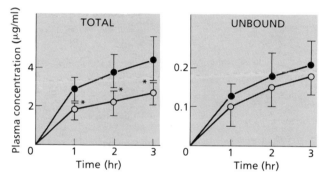

Fig. 56.9 Mean total and free plasma concentrations of bupivacaine during intravenous infusions of bupivacaine HCl 2 mg/min in seven cholecystectomy patients studied 3 hr before surgery (open circles) and 72 hr after operation (closed circles). *Statistically significant difference. (Redrawn from Tucker, 1986.)

There is a theoretical possibility that plasma binding may limit the initial uptake of local anaesthetics into the brain and myocardium following rapid, inadvertent, intravenous injection, thereby modulating toxicity. However, it is probable that a toxic dose would produce sufficiently high blood drug concentrations to overwhelm the blood binding capacity on first-pass through the brain and heart. Furthermore, studies of the initial brain uptake of local anaesthetics in rats indicate that there is an enhanced dissociation from plasma binding sites in the microcirculation (Terasaki *et al.*, 1986) (Fig. 56.10).

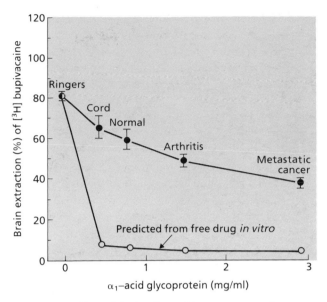

Fig. 56.10 Effect of the binding of bupivacaine to human serum on its first-pass brain uptake in rats. The closed circles represent the brain extraction of bupivacaine after carotid injection of drug ($1 \mu g/ml$) mixed in Ringer's solution or in umbilical cord, normal, arthritis or metastatic cancer human serum. Each point represents the mean $\pm$ SE for five to six experiments. The open circles represent the theoretical extraction predicted using free percentages measured *in vitro*. (Redrawn from Terasaki *et al.*, 1986.)

Tissue distribution

In the amide series of local anaesthetics, a greater extent of plasma binding is accompanied by a parallel increase in affinity for tissue components. Thus, steady-state volumes of distribution based on unbound drug (V_{USS}), which reflect net tissue binding, vary over a five-fold range, being greatest for the more lipid-soluble agents (Table 56.4). Distribution volumes based on total drug concentration in blood vary only two-fold, reflecting the balance between blood and tissue binding.

The toxicity of local anaesthetic is increased significantly by acidosis and hypercapnia (Englesson & Grevsten, 1974; Englesson, 1974). In theory, an increased brain and myocardial concentration of free ionized drug could account for this through haemo-dynamic changes and ion trapping. However, the latter possibility seems unlikely, as animal studies have shown that the partition coefficients of local anaesthetics between whole brain or myocardium and blood are similar (Simon *et al.*, 1984) or reduced (Nancarrow, 1986) during metabolic acidosis of the type associated with convulsions. This is because the

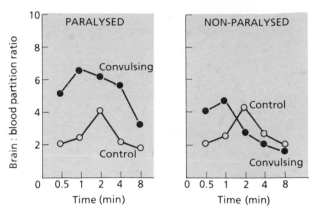

Fig. 56.11 Brain:blood partition ratios of lignocaine after intravenous injection into convulsing (closed circles) and non-convulsing (open circles) rats. The left-hand panel shows data for rats paralysed with gallamine and ventilated with nitrous oxide/oxygen; the right-hand panel shows data for non-paralysed animals. (Redrawn from Simon *et al.*, 1984.)

lowering of blood pH is similar to, or greater than, the lowering of tissue pH. On the other hand, Simon *et al.* (1984) have hypothesized that treatment of convulsions by paralysis and artificial ventilation will tend to exacerbate entry of local anaesthetic into the brain, because prevention of the systemic acidosis, but not the cerebral acidosis, promotes ion trapping of drug in the organ (Fig. 56.11). This does not imply that ventilation with oxygen is deleterious, but it may require the use of anticonvulsants for continuation of ventilation until the drug is cleared from the brain.

Excretion

Renal excretion of unchanged local anaesthetics is a minor route of elimination, accounting for less than 1–6% of the dose under normal conditions (Tucker & Mather, 1979). Depending on the agent, acidification of the urine increases this proportion to 5–20%, which is consistent with less tubular reabsorption as a result of greater ionization. However, this increase is insufficient to warrant the use of a forced acid diuresis in treating toxicity.

Metabolism

ESTERS

These are cleared in both the blood and the liver. *In vitro* half-lives in plasma reflect the action of pseudo-cholinesterase and in normal adults they vary from

10–20 sec for chloroprocaine (O'Brien et al., 1979; Kuhnert et al., 1986), 40 sec for procaine (Reidenberg et al., 1972; DuSouich & Erill, 1977), to several minutes for amethocaine (Foldes et al., 1965). Red cell esterases contribute also to blood clearance (Calvo et al., 1980).

In vitro half-lives are longer than those measured *in vivo* e.g. that of chloroprocaine after extradural injection is about 3 min (Kuhnert et al., 1986). However, this value probably reflects rate-limiting absorption rather than metabolic clearance. After high intravenous doses of procaine, clearances of 0.04–0.08 litre $\cdot$ min^{-1} $\cdot$ kg^{-1} and elimination half-lives of 7–8 min have been observed, probably reflecting some saturation of the enzyme systems (Seifen et al., 1979).

The clinical implication of the rapid clearance of the esters is that if a toxic concentration is attained after inadvertent intravenous injection, the ensuing reaction should be relatively short-lived. *In vitro* plasma half-lives are prolonged by about two to four times in patients with renal and liver disease (Reidenberg et al., 1972; DuSouich & Erill, 1977). However, normal esterase activity is preserved in their erythrocytes, suggesting that they may not be significantly more susceptible to toxicity (Calvo et al., 1980).

The hydrolysis products of procaine and chloroprocaine have been measured in human plasma but appear to be inactive pharmacologically (Brodie et al., 1948; O'Brien et al., 1979; Kuhnert et al., 1980; Krogh & Jellum, 1981), although the aminobenzoic acids may contribute to the rare allergic reaction.

AMIDES

The amide linkage is stable in blood, and most of the clearance of these agents occurs in the liver. Mean values vary in the order: bupivacaine < ropivacaine < mepivacaine (reflecting the size of the N-methyl substituent in this homologous series) < lignocaine < etidocaine < prilocaine (Table 56.4). Over the whole series, there is no relationship to anaesthetic potency or to lipid-solubility–protein binding. Etidocaine clearance is dependent mostly on liver perfusion, whereas that of bupivacaine should be more sensitive to changes in intrinsic hepatic enzyme function (Tucker, 1986). Although clearance of the former is double that of the latter and they are intrinsically equitoxic, any advantage this might offer for etidocaine is offset by the fact that twice the dose is needed to establish the same quality of sensory block as that produced by bupivac-

aine. The blood clearance of prilocaine exceeds liver blood flow indicating that some extrahepatic metabolism of this drug occurs.

Terminal elimination half-lives and mean body residence times are between 1.5 and 3 hr for all of the agents, reflecting a balance between their distribution and clearance characteristics (Table 56.4).

Identification of the biotransformation products of the amides in human urine indicates three major sites of metabolic attack, namely aromatic hydroxylation, N-dealkylation and amide hydrolysis (Tucker & Mather, 1980, 1987). Monoethylglycinexylidide, glycinexylidide and the 4-hydroxy product formed from lignocaine, pipecolylxylidide from mepivacaine and bupivacaine, and the mono-dealkylated derivatives of etidocaine have all been measured in human plasma. There is only evidence that the first of these contributes to the effects of the parent drug. On continuous infusion, unbound plasma concentrations of monoethylglycinexylidide are 70% of those of lignocaine (Drayer et al., 1983), and studies in rodents indicate that it is about 70% as toxic (Blumer et al., 1973). Metabolism of prilocaine to o-toluidine and subsequent hydroxylation of this product is responsible for methaemoglobinaemia at doses above 600 mg (Hjelm & Holmdahl, 1965). Other amides are hydrolysed to 2,6-xylidine which does not produce this problem (McLean et al., 1969).

EFFECTS OF PATIENT VARIABLES AND OTHER DRUGS

Most of the information on likely effects of patient variables and other drug therapy on the kinetics of local anaesthetics has been obtained from studies with intravenous lignocaine, and it may not be possible always to extrapolate the findings to patients receiving regional anaesthesia. This is a problem especially when haemodynamic factors are involved, since the cardiovascular effects of sympathetic nerve block may complicate the issue, and changes in drug elimination may be offset by opposite changes in drug absorption (Tucker, 1984). For example, although hypovolaemia decreases lignocaine clearance (Benowitz et al., 1974), plasma drug concentrations are lower following extradural block in the presence of blood loss as a result of an impaired absorption rate (Morikawa et al., 1974).

A summary of variables which have been studied with respect to the pharmacokinetics of the amide local anaesthetics is given in Table 56.5. Of these, the evidence suggests that old age (uncomplicated by disease), weight, sex, race, pregnancy and renal disease are of relatively minor impact, whereas cardiovascular disease and liver cirrhosis are associated with clinically more significant alterations in kinetics. Elimination half-lives are prolonged two- to three-fold in neonates, reflecting increased volumes of distribution or decreased clearance or both. Along with suggestions that absorption is faster in children than in adults, their unbound clearance (corrected for body weight) appears to be similar (lignocaine) or greater (bupivacaine). Corresponding volumes of distribution tend to be similar or higher, such that half-lives are comparable with those in adults.

Table 56.5 The influence of some patient variables and other drugs on the pharmacokinetics of local anaesthetic agents

Variable	Agent	Route	Change	Reference
Age				
Elderly	B	Exd	$\uparrow C_{max}$, $\downarrow T_{max}$?	Rosenberg *et al.* (1981)
	L, B	Caud	$\leftrightarrow C_{max}$, $\leftrightarrow$AUC	Freund *et al.* (1984)
	L	Exd	$\downarrow T_{max}$	Finucane and Hammonds (1984)
	L	i.v.	$\downarrow Cl$, $\leftrightarrow V$, $\uparrow t_{\frac{1}{2}}$ (♂) $\leftrightarrow Cl$, V, $t_{\frac{1}{2}}$ (♀)	Abernethy and Greenblatt (1984a)
	L	i.v.	$\leftrightarrow Cl$, $\uparrow V$, $\uparrow t_{\frac{1}{2}}$	Nation *et al.* (1977)
	L	i.v.	$\leftrightarrow Cl$, $\leftrightarrow V$, $\uparrow t_{\frac{1}{2}}$, $\downarrow F_U$	Cusack *et al.* (1985)
	L	i.v.	$\downarrow Cl$	Cusson *et al.* (1985)
Children	B	IC	$\uparrow Cl$,* V,* $\leftrightarrow t_{\frac{1}{2}}$, $\downarrow T_{max}$	Rothstein *et al.* (1986)
	L	i.v.	$\leftrightarrow Cl$,* V,* $t_{\frac{1}{2}}$	Finholt *et al.* (1986)
	L	Caud	$\leftrightarrow Cl$*	Ecoffey *et al.* (1984)
	B	Caud	$\uparrow Cl$,* V?*	Ecoffey *et al.* (1985)
Neonates	L	s.c.	$\leftrightarrow Cl$,* $\uparrow V$,* $\uparrow t_{\frac{1}{2}}$	Mihaly *et al.* (1978)
	M	s.c.	$\downarrow Cl$,* $\uparrow V$,* $\uparrow t_{\frac{1}{2}}$	Moore *et al.* (1978)
	B	Exd (mother)	$\uparrow t_{\frac{1}{2}}$	Magno *et al.* (1976); Caldwell *et al.* (1977)
	E	Exd (mother)	$\uparrow t_{\frac{1}{2}}$	Morgan *et al.* (1978)
Weight	L, M, B	Exd, Caud, IC, Periph	$\leftrightarrow C$–T	Scott *et al.* (1972); Tucker *et al.* (1972); Moore *et al.* (1976a, b)
	L	i.v.	$\leftrightarrow Cl$, $\uparrow V$, $\uparrow t_{\frac{1}{2}}$ (obesity)	Abernethy and Greenblatt (1984b)
	L	i.v.	$\uparrow Cl$	Cusson *et al.* (1985)
Sex	L	i.v.	$\leftrightarrow Cl$, $\uparrow V$(♀)	Abernethy and Greenblatt (1984a)
	L	i.v.	$\leftrightarrow Cl$, $\uparrow V$, $\uparrow t_{\frac{1}{2}}$, $\leftrightarrow F_U$(♀)	Wing *et al.* (1984)
Race	L	i.v.	$\leftrightarrow Cl$, V, $t_{\frac{1}{2}}$, F_U (Caucasian, Oriental, Black)	Goldberg *et al.* (1982)
Pregnancy	E	Exd	$\leftrightarrow C$–T	Morgan *et al.* (1977)
	L	Exd	$\leftrightarrow C_{max}$, T_{max}, $\downarrow Cl$, $\leftrightarrow F_U$ (pre-eclampsia vs. normal)	Ramanathan *et al.* (1986); Bottorff *et al.* (1987)
	L	i.v.	$\leftrightarrow Cl$,* $\uparrow V$,* $\uparrow t_{\frac{1}{2}}$ (sheep)	Bloedow *et al.* (1980)
	L	i.v.	$\uparrow Cl$,* $\leftrightarrow V$, *$\leftrightarrow t_{\frac{1}{2}}$ (sheep)	Arthur *et al.* (1985)
Disease				
Heart failure	L	i.v.	$\downarrow Cl$, $\downarrow V$, $\leftrightarrow t_{\frac{1}{2}}$	Thomson *et al.* (1973)
Orthostatic hypotension	L	i.v.	$\downarrow Cl$, $\downarrow V$, $\leftrightarrow t_{\frac{1}{2}}$, $\leftrightarrow F_U$ (sitting vs. supine)	Feely *et al.* (1982a)
Cardiopulmonary resuscitation	L	i.v.	$\downarrow Cl$, $\downarrow V$, $\leftrightarrow t_{\frac{1}{2}}$	Chow *et al.* (1981, 1983)
Cirrhosis	L	i.v.	$\downarrow Cl$, $\uparrow V$, $\uparrow t_{\frac{1}{2}}$	Thomson *et al.* (1973); Huet and Villeneuve (1983)

Table 56.5 (*continued*)

Variable	Agent	Route	Change	Reference
Chronic hepatitis	L	i.v.	$\uparrow Cl$, $\uparrow V$	Huet and LeLorier (1980)
Acute viral hepatitis	L	i.v.	$\downarrow Cl$, $\uparrow V$, $\uparrow t_{\frac{1}{2}}$	Williams *et al.* (1976)
Renal failure	L	i.v.	$\leftrightarrow Cl$, V, $t_{\frac{1}{2}}$	Thomson *et al.* (1973)
			$(\uparrow GX)$	Collinsworth *et al.* (1975)
Other drugs				
Halothane	L	i.v.	$\downarrow Cl$, $\uparrow V$, $\uparrow t_{\frac{1}{2}}$	Bentley *et al.* (1983)
	L	i.v.	$\downarrow Cl$	Mather *et al.* (1986)
Diazepam	B, E	Exd	$\uparrow C_{max}$?	Giasi *et al.* (1980)
	B	i.v., Exd	$\leftrightarrow Cl$, V, $t_{\frac{1}{2}}$	Thompson *et al.* (1986)
			$\leftrightarrow C{-}T$	
			(monkey)	
Noradrenaline	L	i.v.	$\downarrow Cl$, $\downarrow V$, $\uparrow t_{\frac{1}{2}}$	Benowitz *et al.* (1974)
			(monkey)	
Isoprenaline	L	i.v.	$\uparrow Cl$, $\uparrow V$, $\downarrow t_{\frac{1}{2}}$	Benowitz *et al.* (1974)
			(monkey)	
Ephedrine	L	i.v.	$\uparrow Cl$	Wiklund *et al.* (1977)
Propranolol	L	i.v., p.o.	$\downarrow Cl$, $\leftrightarrow F_U$	Tucker *et al.* (1984);
				Bax *et al.* (1985)
	B	i.v.	$\downarrow Cl$, $\leftrightarrow V$, $\uparrow t_{\frac{1}{2}}$	Bowdle *et al.* (1987)
Verapamil	L	i.v.	$\leftrightarrow Cl$, V, $t_{\frac{1}{2}}$	Chelly *et al.* (1987)
			(dog)	
Cimetidine	L	i.v.	$\downarrow Cl$, $\downarrow V$, $\leftrightarrow t_{\frac{1}{2}}$, $\uparrow F_U$	Feely *et al.* (1982b)
	L	i.v.	$\downarrow Cl$, $\downarrow V$, $\leftrightarrow t_{\frac{1}{2}}$, $\leftrightarrow F_U$	Wing *et al.* (1984)
	L	i.v.	$\downarrow Cl$, $\leftrightarrow V$, $\uparrow t_{\frac{1}{2}}$	Bauer *et al.* (1984)
	L	i.v.	$\downarrow Cl$, $\downarrow V$, $\leftrightarrow t_{\frac{1}{2}}$	Jackson *et al.* (1985)
	L	Exd, Axill	$\leftrightarrow C_{max}$, $\uparrow t_{\frac{1}{2}}$	Webb and Ward (1983)
	L	Exd	$\uparrow C_{max}$	Dailey *et al.* (1985)
	B	i.v.	$\downarrow Cl$	Noble *et al.* (1987)
Ranitidine	L	i.v.	$\leftrightarrow Cl$, V, $t_{\frac{1}{2}}$, F_U	Feely and Guy (1983)
	L	i.v.	$\downarrow Cl$, $\downarrow V$, $\leftrightarrow t_{\frac{1}{2}}$	Robson *et al.* (1985)
	L	i.v.	$\leftrightarrow Cl$, V, $t_{\frac{1}{2}}$	Jackson *et al.* (1985)
	L	Exd	$\leftrightarrow C_{max}$	Dailey *et al.* (1985)
	B	Exd	$\uparrow C{-}T$?	Moore *et al.* (1987)
	B	i.v.	$\leftrightarrow Cl$	Noble *et al.* (1987)
Phenytoin	L	i.v.	$\uparrow Cl$, $\leftrightarrow V$, $\leftrightarrow t_{\frac{1}{2}}$, $\downarrow F_U$	Perucca and Richens (1979);
				Routledge *et al.* (1981)

L = lignocaine; M = mepivacaine; B = bupivacaine; E = etidocaine.

Exd = extradural; Caud = caudal; IC = intercostal; Periph = peripheral nerve block; Axill = axillary block.

Cl = clearance; V = volume of distribution (mostly derived for steady state).

$t_{\frac{1}{2}}$ = terminal elimination half-life; C_{max} = maximum plasma drug concentration; $C{-}T$ = plasma drug concentration–time profile; T_{max} = time of C_{max}; AUC = area under plasma drug concentration–time curve; F_U = free fraction in plasma; GX = plasma glycinexylidide.

* Standardized to body weight.

$\uparrow\downarrow$ Trend only.

A number of drugs (notably halothane, cimetidine and propranolol) have been shown to lower the clearance of local anaesthetics, mainly by direct inhibition of mixed function oxidase activity, with a smaller contribution from decreased hepatic blood flow (Table 56.5). Several *in vitro* studies showing decreased plasma binding of local anaesthetic drugs in the presence of other drugs have been described. However, the clinical significance of these observations is questionable in view of the high concentrations used and because altered free fractions do not necessarily imply significant increases in free-drug concentrations *in vivo*.

Placental transfer

ESTERS

After maternal injection, 2-chloroprocaine appears in both maternal and cord plasma in very low concentrations (Kuhnert *et al.*, 1980; Abboud *et al.*, 1983, 1984). Thus, even though elimination half-lives of chloroprocaine and procaine are twice as long in cord plasma as in maternal plasma and pregnancy is associated with a decrease in pseudocholinesterase activity (Reidenberg *et al.*, 1972; O'Brien *et al.*, 1979; Kuhnert *et al.*, 1980), the absolute rate of hydrolysis in the mother remains fast and helps to reduce placental transfer and the risk of fetal intoxication.

AMIDES

At delivery, mean values of cord:maternal plasma concentration ratios of the amides decrease in the order: prilocaine (1.0–1.1), lignocaine (0.5–0.7), mepivacaine (0.7), bupivacaine (0.2–0.4) and etidocaine (0.2–0.3) (Tucker & Mather, 1979). These differences reflect differential maternal and fetal plasma binding of the drugs owing to relatively low fetal concentrations of α_1-acid glycoprotein. Although some discrepancy has been noted with bupivacaine using once-through perfusions of the rabbit placenta (Hamshaw-Thomas *et al.*, 1985), equilibrium ratios of the agents are predicted in humans and sheep from plasma-binding data, with allowance for ion trapping due to fetal acidosis (Tucker *et al.*, 1970b; Thomas *et al.*, 1976; Kennedy *et al.*, 1986). As such, therefore, these ratios are not direct predictors of relative fetal toxicity, as corresponding ratios of unbound (active) drug across the placenta are probably close to unity irrespective of the drug. (Negative followed by positive deviations from unity are expected with time as the transplacental concentration gradient reverses during the rise and fall of maternal drug concentrations.) Nevertheless, theory predicts that a high maternal:fetal binding ratio should delay equilibration of drug in fetal tissues, despite rapid equilibration across the placenta (Dawes, 1973). On the other hand, similar umbilical artery:umbilical vein concentration ratios observed for the various agents argue against large differences in their equilibration rates in the fetus (Tucker *et al.*, 1970b).

Finster and Pedersen (1979) and Kuhnert *et al.* (1981) have suggested that relatively low cord:maternal ratios of bupivacaine, based on total plasma drug concentrations, are due to more extensive uptake of this drug by the fetal tissues. Such an explanation is kinetically unsound and certainly cannot explain low umbilical venous:maternal ratios.

In the event of inadvertent maternal intravascular injection of local anaesthetic, it is advisable either to effect the delivery immediately before maximum fetal uptake occurs or, providing that maternal and fetal circulations remain adequate, to delay until significant back-transfer of drug to and clearance by the mother has taken place (Gupta *et al.*, 1986). An intermediate window will exist in which the body burden to the newborn, whose capacity to eliminate the drug may be impaired, is relatively high.

References

Abboud T.K., Afrasiabi A., Sarkis F., Daftarian, Nagappala S., Noueihed R., Kuhnert B.R. & Miller F. (1984) Continuous infusion epidural analgesia in parturients receiving bupivacaine, chloroprocaine or lidocaine—maternal, fetal and neonatal effects. *Anesthesia and Analgesia* **63**, 421–8.

Abboud T.K., Kim K.C., Nouehed R., Kuhnert B.R., DerMardirossian N., Moumdjian J., Sarkis F. & Nagappala S. (1983) Epidural bupivacaine, chloroprocaine, or lidocaine for Cesarian section—maternal and neonatal effects. *Anesthesia and Analgesia* **62**, 914–19.

Abernethy D.R. & Greenblatt D.J. (1984a) Impairment of lidocaine clearance in elderly male subjects. *Journal of Cardiovascular Pharmacology* **5**, 1093–6.

Abernethy D.R. & Greenblatt D.J. (1984b) Lidocaine disposition in obesity. *American Journal of Cardiology* **53**, 1183–6.

Adams H.J., Mastri A.R. & Doherty J. (1977) Bupivacaine: morphological effects on spinal cords of cats and durations of spinal anesthesia in sheep. *Pharmacology Research Communications* **9**, 847–55.

Adams H.J., Mastri A.R., Eicholzer A.W. & Kilpatrick G. (1974) Morphological effects of intrathecal etidocaine and tetracaine on the rabbit spinal cord. *Anesthesiology* **53**, 904–8.

Aldrete J.A., Barnes D.R. & Sigon M.A. (1969) Studies on effects of addition of potassium chloride to lidocaine. *Anesthesia and Analgesia* **48**, 269–76.

Aldrete J.A., Nicholson J., Sada T., Davidson W. & Garastasu G. (1977) Caphalic kinetics of intra-arterially injected lidocaine. *Oral Surgery* **44**, 167–72.

Aldrete J.A., Romo-Salas F., Arora S., Wilson R. & Rutherford R. (1978) Reverse arterial blood flow as a pathway for central nervous system toxic response following injection of local anesthetics. *Anesthesia and Analgesia* **57**, 428–33.

Aps C. & Reynolds F. (1976) The effect of concentration on vasoactivity of bupivacaine and lignocaine. *British Journal of Anaesthesia* **48**, 1171–4.

Aps C. & Reynolds F. (1978) An intradermal study of the local anaesthetic and vascular effects of the isomers of bupivacaine. *British Journal of Clinical Pharmacology* **6**, 63–8.

Arthur G.R. (1981) *Distribution and Elimination of Local Anaesthetic Agents: The Role of Lung, Liver and Kidney*. PhD Thesis, University of Edinburgh.

Arthur G.R., Morishima H.O., Finster M., Pedersen H. & Covino B.G. (1985) Effect of pregnancy on lidocaine pharmacokinetics in sheep. *Anesthesiology* **63**, A229.

Barchowsky A., Stargel W.W., Shand D.G. & Routledge P.A. (1981) On the role of alpha$_1$-acid glycoprotein in lignocaine accumulation following myocardial infarction. *British Journal of Clinical Pharmacology* **13**, 411–15.

Bauer L.A., Edwards W.A.D., Randolph F.P. & Blouin R.A. (1984) Cimetidine-induced decrease in lidocaine metabolism. *American Heart Journal* **108**, 413–15.

Bax N.D.S., Tucker G.T., Lennard M.S. & Woods H.F. (1985) The impairment of lignocaine clearance by propranolol—major contribution from enzyme inhibition. *British Journal of Clinical Pharmacology* **19**, 597–603.

Bedder M.D., Kozody R. & Craig D.B. (1987) A comparison of bupivacaine and alkalinized bupivacaine in brachial plexus anesthesia. *Anesthesia and Analgesia* **66**, S9.

Benowitz N., Forsyth R.P., Melmon K.L. & Rowland M. (1974) Lidocaine disposition kinetics in monkey and man. II: Effects of hemorrhage and sympathomimetic drug administration. *Clinical Pharmacology and Therapeutics* **16**, 99–109.

Bentley J.B., Glass S. & Gandolfi A.J. (1983) The influence of halothane on lidocaine pharmacokinetics in man. *Anesthesiology* **59**, A246.

Blair M.R. (1975) Cardiovascular pharmacology of local anaesthetics. *British Journal of Anaesthesia* **47**, 247–52.

Bloedow D.C., Ralston D.H. & Hargrove J.C. (1980) Lidocaine pharmacokinetics in pregnant and non-pregnant sheep. *Journal of Pharmacological Science* **69**, 32–7.

Blumer J., Strong J.M. & Atkinson A.J. (1973) The convulsant potency of lidocaine and its N-dealkylated metabolites. *Journal of Pharmacology and Experimental Therapeutics* **186**, 31–6.

Bokesch P.M., Post C. & Strichartz G. (1986) Structure–activity relationship of lidocaine homologs producing tonic and frequency-dependent impulse blockade in nerve. *Journal of Pharmacology and Experimental Therapeutics* **237**, 773–81.

Bokesch P.M., Raymond S.A. & Strichartz G. (1987) Dependence of lidocaine potency on pH and Pco_2. *Anesthesia and Analgesia* **66**, 9–17.

Bokesch P.M., Ziemer G., Castaneda A.R. & Arthur G.R. (1985) Arterial lidocaine concentrations in intracardiac right-to-left shunts. *Anesthesiology* **63**, A468.

Bottorff M.B., Pieper J.A., Boucher B.A., Hoon T.J., Ramanathan J. & Sibai B.M. (1987) Lidocaine protein binding in preeclampsia. *European Journal of Clinical Pharmacology* **31**, 719–22.

Bowdle T.A., Freund P.R. & Slattery J.T. (1987) Propranolol reduces bupivacaine clearance. *Anesthesiology* **66**, 36–8.

Bridenbaugh P.O., Tucker G.T., Moore D.C., Bridenbaugh L.D. & Thomspon G.E. (1974) Preliminary clinical evaluation of etidocaine (Duranest): a new long-acting local anesthetic agent. *Acta Anaesthesiologica Scandinavica* **18**, 165–71.

Brodie B.B., Lief P.A. & Poet R. (1948) The fate of procaine in man following its intravenous administration and methods for the estimation of procaine and diethylaminoethanol. *Journal of Pharmacology and Experimental Therapeutics* **94**, 359–95.

Bromage P.R. (1967) Physiology and pharmacology of epidural analgesia. *Anesthesiology* **28**, 592–622.

Bromage P.R. (1974) Lower limb reflex changes in segmental epidural analgesia. *British Journal of Anaesthesia* **46**, 504–8.

Bromage P.R. (1975) Mechanisms of action of extradural analgesia. *British Journal of Anaesthesia* **47**, 199–211.

Bromage P.R. & Burfoot M.F. (1966) Quality of epidural blockade. II. Influence of physicochemical factors, hyaluronidase and potassium. *British Journal of Anaesthesia* **38**, 857–65.

Bromage P.R. & Gertel M. (1972) Brachial plexus anesthesia in chronic renal failure. *Anesthesiology* **36**, 488–93.

Bromage P.R., Joyal A.C. & Binney J.C. (1963) Local anesthetic drugs: penetration from the spinal extradural space into the neuraxis. *Science* **140**, 392–3.

Brown D.T., Morison D.H., Covino B.G. & Scott D.B. (1980) Comparison of carbonated bupivacaine and bupivacaine hydrochloride for extradural anaesthesia. *British Journal of Anaesthesia* **52**, 419–22.

Bruguerolle B., Philip-Joet F., Arnaud C. & Arnaud A. (1985) Consequences of inflammatory processes on lignocaine protein binding during anaesthesia in fibreoptic bronchoscopy. *British Journal of Clinical Pharmacology* **20**, 180–1.

Buckley P., Neto G.D. & Fink B.R. (1985) Acid and alkaline solutions of local anesthetics: duration of nerve block and tissue pH. *Anesthesia and Analgesia* **64**, 477–82.

Burm A.G. (1985) *Pharmacokinetics and Clinical Effects of Lidocaine and Bupivacaine Following Epidural and Subarachnoid Administration in Man*. PhD Thesis, University of Leiden.

Burn J.M., Guyer P.B. & Langdon L. (1973) The spread of solutions into the epidural space. A study using epidurograms in patients with the lumbosciatic syndrome. *British Journal of Anaesthesia* **45**, 338–44.

Burney R.G., Difazio C.A. & Foster J.H. (1978) Effects of pH on protein binding of lidocaine. *Anesthesia and Analgesia* **57**, 478–80.

Caldwell J., Moffatt J.R., Smith R.L., Lieberman A.B., Beard R.W., Sneddon W. & Wilson B.W. (1977) Determination of bupivacaine in human fetal and neonatal blood samples by gas liquid chromatography mass spectrometry. *Biomedical Mass Spectrometry* **4**, 322–5.

Calvo R., Carlos R. & Erill S. (1980) Effects of disease and acetazolamide on procaine hydrolysis by red cell enzymes. *Clinical Pharmacology and Therapeutics* **27**, 175–83.

Catchlove R.F.H. (1972) The influence of CO_2 and pH on local anesthetic action. *Journal of Pharmacology and Experimental Therapeutics* **181**, 298–309.

Chelly J.E., Hill D.C., Merin R.G., Dlewati A. & Abernethy D.R. (1987) Effect of verapamil on lidocaine pharmacokinetics and dynamics in conscious dogs. *Anesthesia and Analgesia* **66**, S25.

Chow M.S.S., Ronfeld R.A., Hamilton R.A., Helmink R. & Fieldman A. (1983) Effect of external cardiopulmonary resuscitation on lidocaine pharmacokinetics in dogs. *Journal of Pharmacology and Experimental Therapeutics* **224**, 531–7.

Chow M.S.S., Ronfeld R.A., Ruffett D. & Fieldman A. (1981) Lidocaine pharmacokinetics during cardiac arrest and external cardiopulmonary resuscitation. *American Heart Journal* **102**, 799–801.

Clarkson C.W. & Hondeghem L.M. (1985) Mechanism for bupivacaine depression of cardiac conduction: fast block of sodium channels during the action potential with slow recovery from block during diastole. *Anesthesiology* **62**, 396–405.

Cohen E.N. (1968) Distribution of local anesthetic agents in the neuraxis of the dog. *Anesthesiology* **29**, 1002–5.

Cohen E.N., Levine D.A., Colliss J.E. & Gunther R.E. (1968) The role of pH in the development of tachyphylaxis to local anesthetic agents. *Anesthesiology* **29**, 994–1001.

Cohen S., Luykx W.M. & Marx G.F. (1984) High versus low flow rates during lumbar epidural block. *Regional Anesthesia* **9**, 8–11.

Collinsworth K.A., Strong J.M., Atkinson A.J., Winkle R.A., Periroth F. & Harrison D.C. (1975) Pharmacokinetics and metabolism of lidocaine in patients with renal failure. *Clinical Pharmacology and Therapeutics* **18**, 59–64.

Courtney K.R. (1975) Mechanism of frequency-dependent inhibition of sodium currents in frog myelinated nerve by the lidocaine derivative GEA 968. *Journal of Pharmacology and Experimental Therapeutics* **195**, 225–36.

Courtney K.R. (1980) Structure–activity relations for frequency-dependent sodium channel block in nerve by local anesthetics. *Journal of Pharmacology and Experimental Therapeutics* **213**, 114–19.

Courtney K.R., Kendig J.J. & Cohen E.N. (1978) The rates of interaction of local anaesthetics with sodium channels in nerve. *Journal of Pharmacology and Experimental Therapeutics* **207**, 594–604.

Cousins M.J. & Mather L.E. (1984) Intrathecal and epidural administration of opioids. *Anesthesiology* **61**, 276–310.

Covino B.G. (1980) The mechanism of local anaesthesia. In *Topical Reviews in Anaesthesia*, vol. 1 (Eds Norman J. & Whitwam J.) pp. 85–134. J. Wright & Sons, Bristol.

Covino B.G. (1986) Pharmacology of local anaesthetic agents. *British Journal of Anaesthesia* **58**, 701–16.

Covino B.G. (1987) Local anaesthetics. In *Drugs in Anaesthesia: Mechanism of Action* (Eds Feldman S.A., Scurr C.F. & Paton W.) pp. 261–91. Edward Arnold, London.

Coyle D.E., Denson D.D., Thompson G.A., Myers G.A., Arthur G.R. & Bridenbaugh P.O. (1984) The influence of lactic acid on the serum protein binding of bupivacaine: species differences. *Anesthesiology* **61**, 127–33.

Crossley A.W.A. & Hosie H.E. (1987) Radiographic study of intercostal nerve blockade in healthy volunteers. *British Journal of Anaesthesia* **59**, 149–54.

Curran J., Hamilton C. & Taylor T. (1975) Topical analgesia before tracheal intubation. *Anaesthesia* **30**, 765–8.

Cusack B., O'Malley K., Lavan J., Noel J. & Kelly J.G. (1985) Protein binding and disposition of lignocaine in the elderly. *European Journal of Clinical Pharmacology* **29**, 323–9.

Cusick J.F., Myklebust J.B. & Abram S.E. (1980) Differential neural effects of epidural anesthetics. *Anesthesiology* **53**, 299–306.

Cusick J.F., Myklebust J.B., Abram S.E. & Davidson A. (1982) Altered neural conduction with epidural bupivacaine. *Anesthesiology* **57**, 31–6.

Cusson J., Nattel S., Matthews C., Talajic M. & Lawand S. (1985) Age-dependent lidocaine disposition in patients with acute myocardial infarction. *Clinical Pharmacology and Therapeutics* **37**, 381–6.

Dailey P.A., Hughes S.C., Rosen M.A., Healy K., Cheek D.B.C., Pytka S., Fisher D.M. & Shnider S.M. (1985) Lidocaine levels during Cesarian section after pretreatment with ranitidine or cimetidine. *Anesthesiology* **63**, A444.

Dawes G.S. (1973) A theoretical analysis of fetal drug equilibration. In *Fetal Pharmacology* (Ed. Boreus L.) pp. 381–99. Raven Press, New York.

DeJong R.H. (1977) *Local Anesthetics* 2nd edn. pp. 63–83. Charles Thomas, Springfield.

Dennhardt R. & Ammon K. (1980) Untersuchungen zur Loslichkeit von Bupivacain im Liquor cerebrospinalis. *Der Anaesthesist* **29**, 10–13.

Denson D.D., Bridenbaugh P.O., Turner P.A. & Phero J.C. (1983) Comparison of neural blockade and pharmacokinetics after subarachnoid lidocaine in the rhesus monkey. II: Effects of volume, osmolality, and baricity. *Anesthesia and Analgesia* **62**, 995–1001.

Denson D.D., Coyle D.E., Thompson G.A. & Myers J.A. (1984) Alpha$_1$-acid glycoprotein and albumin in human serum bupivacaine binding. *Clinical Pharmacology and Therapeutics* **35**, 409–15.

DiFazio C.A., Carron H., Grosslight K.R., Moscicki J.C., Bolding W.R. & Johns R.A. (1986) Comparison of pH-adjusted lidocaine solutions for epidural anesthesia. *Anesthesia and Analgesia* **65**, 760–4.

Dohi S., Matsumiya N., Takeshima R. & Naito H. (1984) The effects of subarachnoid lidocaine and phenylephrine on spinal cord and cerebral blood flow in dogs. *Anesthesiology* **61**, 238–44.

Drayer D.E., Lorenzo B., Werns S. & Reidenberg M.M. (1983) Plasma levels, protein binding, and elimination data of lidocaine and active metabolites in cardiac patients of various ages. *Clinical Pharmacology and Therapeutics* **34**, 14–22.

Dudziak R. & Uihlein M. (1978) Loslichkeit von Lokalanaesthetika im Liquor cerebrospinalis und ihre Abhangigkeit von der Wasserstoffionenkonzentration. *Der Anaesthesist* **27**, 32–7.

DuSouich P. & Erill S. (1977) Altered metabolism of procainamide and procaine in patients with pulmonary and cardiac diseases. *Clinical Pharmacology and Therapeutics* **21**, 101–2.

Ecoffey C., Desparmet J., Berdeaux A., Maury M., Giudicelli J.F. & Saint-Maurice C. (1984) Pharmacokinetics of lignocaine in children following caudal anaesthesia. *British Journal of Anaesthesia* **56**, 1399–401.

Ecoffey C., Desparmet J., Maury M., Berdeaux A., Giudicelli J.F. & Saint-Maurice C. (1985) Bupivacaine in children: pharmacokinetics following caudal anesthesia. *Anesthesiology* **63**, 447–8.

Edwards D.J., Lalka D., Cerra F. & Slaughter R.L. (1982) Alpha$_1$-acid glycoprotein concentration and protein binding in trauma. *Clinical Pharmacology and Therapeutics* **31**, 62–7.

Englesson S. (1974) The influence of acid–base changes on central nervous system toxicity of local anaesthetic agents. I. *Acta Anaesthesiologica Scandinavica* **18**, 79–87.

Englesson S. & Grevsten S. (1974) The influence of acid–base changes on central nervous system toxicity of local anaesthetic agents. II. *Acta Anaesthesiologica Scandinavica* **18**, 88–103.

Erdemir H.A., Soper L.E. & Sweet R.E. (1966) Studies of factors affecting peridural anesthesia. *Anesthesia and Analgesia* **44**, 400–4.

Evans C.J., Dewar J.A., Boyes R.N. & Scott D.B. (1974) Residual nerve block following intravenous regional anaesthesia. *British Journal of Anaesthesia* **46**, 668–70.

Eyres R.L., Bishop W., Oppenheim R.C. & Brown T.C.K. (1983) Plasma bupivacaine concentrations in children during caudal epidural analgesia. *Anaesthesia and Intensive Care* **11**, 20–2.

Eyres R.L., Kidd J., Oppenheim R.C. & Brown T.C.K. (1978) Local anaesthetic plasma levels in children. *Anaesthesia and Intensive Care* **6**, 243–7.

Fairley J.W. & Reynolds F. (1981) An intradermal study of the local anaesthetic and vascular effects of the isomers of mepivacaine. *British Journal of Anaesthesia* **53**, 1211–16.

Feely J. & Guy E. (1983) Lack of effect of ranitidine on the disposition of lignocaine. *British Journal of Clinical Pharmacology* **15**, 378–9.

Feely J., Wade D., McAllister C.B., Wilkinson G.R. & Robertson D. (1982a) Effect of hypotension on liver blood flow and lidocaine disposition. *New England Journal of Medicine* **307**, 866–9.

Feely J., Wilkinson G.R., McAllister C.B. & Wood, A.J.J. (1982b) Increased toxicity and reduced clearance of lidocaine by cimetidine. *Annals of Internal Medicine* **96**, 592–4.

Finholt D.A., Stirt J.A., DiFazio C.A. & Moscicki, J.C. (1986) Lidocaine pharmacokinetics in children. *Anesthesia and Analgesia* **65**, 279–82.

Fink B.R. & Cairns A.M. (1984) Diffusional delay in local anesthetic block *in vitro*. *Anesthesiology* **61**, 555–7.

Fink B.R. & Cairns A.M. (1985) Differential slowing and block of conduction by lidocaine in individual afferent myelinated and unmyelinated axons. *Anesthesiology* **60**, 111–20.

Finster M. & Pedersen H. (1979) Placental transfer and fetal uptake of drugs. *British Journal of Anaesthesia* **51**, 25S–28S.

Finucane B.T. & Hammonds W.D. (1984) Influence of age on vascular absorption of lidocaine injected epidurally in man. *Regional Anesthesia* **9**, 36–7.

Foldes F.F., Davidson G.N., Duncalf D. & Kuwabarra S. (1965) The intravenous toxicity of local anesthetic agents in man. *Clinical Pharmacology and Therapeutics* **6**, 328–35.

Ford D.J., Prithvi Raj P., Singh P., Regan K.M. & Ohlweiler D. (1984) Differential peripheral nerve block by local anesthetics in the cat. *Anesthesiology* **60**, 28–33.

Freund P.R., Bowdle T.A., Slattery J.T. & Bell L.E. (1984) Caudal anesthesia with lidocaine or bupivacaine: plasma local anesthetic concentration and extent of sensory spread in old and young patients. *Anesthesia and Analgesia* **63**, 1017–20.

Fukui T., Hameroff S.R. & Gandolfi A.J. (1984) Alpha$_1$-acid glycoprotein and beta-endorphin alterations in chronic pain patients. *Anesthesiology* **60**, 494–6.

Galindo A. (1983) pH adjusted local anesthetics: clinical experience. *Regional Anesthesia* **8**, 35–6.

Giasi R.M., D'Agostino E. & Covino B.G. (1980) Interaction of diazepam and epidurally administered local anesthetic agents. *Regional Anesthesia* **3**, 8–11.

Gissen A.J., Covino B.G. & Gregus J. (1980) Differential sensitivities of mammalian nerve fibers to local anesthetic agents. *Anesthesiology* **53**, 467–74.

Gissen A.J., Covino B.G. & Gregus J. (1982a) Differential sensitivity of fast and slow fibers in mammalian nerve. II. Margin of safety for nerve transmission. *Anesthesia and Analgesia* **61**, 561–9.

Gissen A.J., Covino B.G. & Gregus J. (1982b) Differential sensitivity of fast and slow fibers in mammalian nerve. III. Effect of etidocaine and bupivacaine on fast/slow fibers. *Anesthesia and Analgesia* **61**, 570–5.

Gissen A.J., Covino B.G. & Gregus J. (1985) Differential sensitivity of fast and slow fibers in mammalian nerve. IV. Effect of carbonation of local anesthetics. *Regional Anesthesia* **10**, 68–75.

Gissen A.J., Covino B.G. & Gregus J. (1986) Differential sensitivity of fast and slow fibers in mammalian nerve. VI. Effect of pH on blocking action of local anesthetics. *Regional Anesthesia* **11**, 132–8.

Goldberg M.J., Spector R. & Johnson G.F. (1982) Racial background and lidocaine pharmacokinetics. *Journal of Clinical Pharmacology* **22**, 391–4.

Greene N.M. (1983) Uptake and elimination of local anesthetics during spinal anesthesia. *Anesthesia and Analgesia* **62**, 1013–24.

Greene N.M. (1985) Distribution of local anesthetic solutions within the subarachnoid space. *Anesthesia and Analgesia* **64**, 715–30.

Griffiths R.B., Horton W.A., Jones I.G. & Blake D. (1987) Speed of injection and spread of bupivacaine in the epidural space. *Anaesthesia* **42**, 160–3.

Grossman S.H., Davis D., Kitchell B.B., Shand D.G. & Routledge P.A. (1982) Diazepam and lidocaine plasma protein binding in renal disease. *Clinical Pharmacology and Therapeutics* **31**, 350–7.

Grundy E.M., Ramamurthy S., Patel K.P., Mani M. & Winnie A.P. (1978) Extradural analgesia revisited. *British Journal of Anaesthesia* **50**, 805–9.

Gupta N., Kennedy R.L., Vicinie A., Seifert R., Edelmann C., Mandel M., Tyler I.L., Kupke K., Miller R.P. & de Sousa H. (1986) Fetal uptake of bupivacaine following bolus intravenous injection. *Anesthesiology* **65**, A382.

Hamshaw-Thomas A., Rogerson N. & Reynolds F. (1985) Transfer of bupivacaine, lignocaine and pethidine across the rabbit placenta: influence of maternal protein binding and fetal flow. *Placenta* **5**, 61–70.

Hasselstrom L., Nortved-Sorensen J., Kehlet H., Juel-Christiansen N., Brynjolff I., Munck O. & Tucker G.T. (1985) The influence of systemically administered bupivacaine on cardiovascular function in cholecystectomised patients. *Acta Anaesthesiologica Scandinavica* **29**, 76.

Hilgier M. (1985) Alkalinization of bupivacaine for brachial plexus block. *Regional Anesthesia* **8**, 59–61.

Hille B. (1977) Local anesthetics: hydrophilic and hydrophobic pathways for the drug–receptor reaction. *Journal of General Physiology* **69**, 497–515.

Hjelm M. & Holmdahl M.H. (1965) Biochemical effects of aromatic amines. II. Cyanosis, methaemoglobinaemia and Heinz-body formation induced by a local anaesthetic agent (prilocaine). *Acta Anaesthesiologica Scandinavica* **9**, 99–120.

Hodgkinson R. & Husain F.J. (1981) Obesity, gravity and spread of epidural anesthesia. *Anesthesia and Analgesia* **60**, 421–4.

Howarth F. (1949) Studies with a radioactive spinal anaesthetic. *British Journal of Pharmacology* **4**, 333–47.

Huet P-M. & LeLorier J. (1980) Effects of smoking and chronic hepatitis B on lidocaine and indocyanine green kinetics. *Clinical Pharmacology and Therapeutics* **28**, 208–14.

Huet P-M. & Villeneuve J-P. (1983) Determinants of drug disposition in patients with cirrhosis. *Hepatology* **3**, 913–18.

Hull C.J. (1985) The pharmacokinetics of opioid analgesics, with special reference to patient-controlled administration. In *Patient-Controlled Analgesia* (Eds Hamer M., Rosen M. & Vickers M.D.) pp. 7–17. Blackwell Scientific Publications, Oxford.

Husemeyer R.P. & White D.C. (1980) Lumbar extradural injection pressures in pregnant women. An investigation of relationships between rate of injection, injection pressures and extent of analgesia. *British Journal of Anaesthesia* **52**, 55–60.

Inoue R., Suganuma T., Echizen H., Ishizaki T., Kushida K. & Tomono Y. (1985) Plasma concentrations of lidocaine and its principal metabolites during intermittent epidural anesthesia. *Anesthesiology* **63**, 304–10.

Jackson J.E., Bentley J.B., Glass S.J., Fukui T., Gandolfi A.J. & Plachetka J.R. (1985) Effects of histamine-2 receptor blockade on lidocaine kinetics. *Clinical Pharmacology and Therapeutics* **37**, 544–8.

Jackson P.R., Tucker G.T. & Woods H.F. (1982) Altered plasma binding in cancer: role of alpha$_1$-acid glycoprotein and albumin. *Clinical Pharmacology and Therapeutics* **32**, 295–302.

Johansson A., Renck H., Aspelin P. & Jacobsen H. (1985) Multiple intercostal blocks by a single injection? A clinical and radiological investigation. *Acta Anaesthesiologica Scandinavica* **29**, 524–8.

Jones R.A., DiFazio C.A. & Longnecker D.E. (1985) Lidocaine constricts or dilates rat arterioles in a dose-dependent manner. *Anesthesiology* **62**, 141–4.

Jorfeldt L., Lewis D.H., Lofstrom B. & Post C. (1979) Lung uptake of lidocaine in healthy volunteers. *Acta Anaesthesiologica Scandinavica* **23**, 567–74.

Jorfeldt L., Lewis D.H., Lofstrom B. & Post C. (1983) Lung uptake of lidocaine in man as influenced by anaesthesia, mepivacaine infusion or lung insufficiency. *Acta Anaesthesiologica Scandinavica* **27**, 5–9.

Kennedy R.L., Miller R.P., Bell J.U., Doshi D., de Sousa H., Kennedy M., Heald D.L. & David Y. (1986) Uptake and distribution of bupivacaine in fetal lambs. *Anesthesiology* **65**, 247–53.

Koster H., Shapiro A. & Leikensohn A. (1936) Procaine concentration changes at the site of injection in subarachnoid anesthesia. *American Journal of Surgery* **33**, 245–8.

Kozody R., Swartz J., Palahniuk R.J., Biehl D.R. & Wade J.G. (1985) Spinal cord blood flow following subarachnoid lidocaine. *Canadian Anaesthetists' Society Journal* **32**, 472–8.

Kraus E., Polnaszek C.F., Scheeler D.A., Halsall H.B., Eckfeldt J.H. & Holtzman J.L. (1986) Interaction between human serum albumin and alpha$_1$-acid glycoprotein in the binding of lidocaine to purified protein fractions and sera. *Journal of Pharmacology and Experimental Therapeutics* **239**, 754–9.

Krogh K. & Jellum E. (1981) Urinary metabolites of chloroprocaine studied by combined gas chromatography–mass spectrometry. *Anesthesiology* **54**, 329–32.

Kuhnert B.R., Kuhnert P.M., Philipson E.H., Syracuse C.D., Kaine C.J. & Chang-hyon Y. (1986) The half-life of 2-chloroprocaine. *Anesthesia and Analgesia* **65**, 273–8.

Kuhnert B.R., Kuhnert P.M., Prochaska A.L. & Gross T.L. (1980) Plasma levels of 2-chloroprocaine in obstetric patients and their neonates after epidural anesthesia. *Anesthesiology* **53**, 21–5.

Kuhnert P.M., Kuhnert B.R., Stitts J.M. & Gross T.L. (1981) The use of a selected ion monitoring technique to study the disposition of bupivacaine in mother, fetus and neonate following epidural anesthesia for Cesarian section. *Anesthesiology* **55**, 611–17.

Lofstrom B. (1978) Tissue distribution of local anesthetics with special reference to the lung. *International Anesthesiology Clinics* **16**, 53–72.

Lund P.C., Bush D.F. & Covino B.G. (1975) Determinants of etidocaine concentrations in the blood. *Anesthesiology* **42**, 497–503.

McClure J.H. & Scott D.B. (1981) Comparison of bupivacaine hydrochloride and carbonated bupivacaine in brachial plexus block interscalene technique. *British Journal of Anaesthesia* **53**, 523–6.

McKeown D.W. & Scott D.B. (1984) Influence of the addition of potassium to 0.5% prilocaine solution during i.v. regional anaesthesia. *British Journal of Anaesthesia* **56**, 1167–70.

Maclean D., Chambers W.A., Tucker G.T. & Wildsmith J.A.W. (1988) Plasma prilocaine concentrations after three techniques of brachial plexus blockade. *British Journal of Anaesthesia* **60**, 136–9.

McLean S., Starmer G.A. & Thomas J. (1969) Methaemoglobin formation by aromatic amines. *Journal of Pharmacy and Pharmacology* **21**, 441–50.

McMorland G.H., Douglas M.J., Jeffery W.K., Ross P.L.E., Axelson J.E., Kim J.H.K., Gambling D.R. & Robertson K. (1986) Effect of pH-adjustment of bupivacaine on onset and duration of epidural analgesia in parturients. *Canadian Anaesthetists' Society Journal* **33**, 537–41.

McNamara P.J., Slaughter R.L., Pieper J.A., Wyman M.G. & Lalka D. (1981) Factors influencing serum protein binding of lidocaine in humans. *Anesthesia and Analgesia* **60**, 395–400.

Magno R., Berlin A., Karlsson K. & Kjellmer I. (1976) Anesthesia for Cesarian section. IV: Placental transfer and neonatal elimination of bupivacaine following epidural analgesia for elective Cesarian section. *Acta Anaesthesiologica Scandinavica* **20**, 141–6.

Martin R., Lamarche Y. & Tetreault L. (1981) Comparison of the clinical effectiveness of lidocaine hydrocarbonate and lidocaine hydrochloride with and without epinephrine in epidural anaesthesia. *Canadian Anaesthetists' Society Journal* **28**, 217–23.

Mather L.E. (1986) Tachyphylaxis in regional anaesthesia: can we reconcile clinical observation and laboratory measurements? In *New Aspects in Regional Anaesthesia*, number 4 (Eds Wust H.J. & Stanton-Hicks M.) pp. 3–8. Springer, Heidelberg.

Mather L.E., Long G.J. & Thomas J. (1971) The binding of bupivacaine to maternal and foetal plasma proteins. *Journal of Pharmacy and Pharmacology* **23**, 359–65.

Mather L.E., Runciman W.B., Carapetis R.J., Ilsley A.H. & Upton R.N. (1986) Hepatic and renal clearances of lidocaine in conscious and anesthetised sheep. *Anesthesia and Analgesia* **65**, 943–9.

Mather L.E. & Thomas J. (1978) Bupivacaine binding to plasma protein fractions. *Journal of Pharmacy and Pharamacology* **30**, 653–4.

Mayumi T., Dohi S. & Takahashi T. (1983) Plasma concentrations of lidocaine associated with cervical, thoracic, and lumbar epidural anesthesia. *Anesthesia and Analgesia* **62**, 578–80.

Meyer J. & Nolte H. (1978) Liquorkonzentration von Bupivacain nach subduraler Applikation. *Regional Anaesthesie* **1**, 38–40.

Mihaly G.W., Moore R.G., Thomas J., Triggs E.J., Thomas D. & Shanks C.H. (1978) The pharmacokinetics of the anilide local anaesthetics in neonates. I: Lignocaine. *European Journal of Clinical Pharmacology* **13**, 143–52.

Moore D.C. (1981) Intercostal nerve block: spread of india ink injected to the rib's costal groove. *British Journal of Anaesthesia* **53**, 325–9.

Moore R.A., Bullingham R.E.S., McQuay H.J., Hand C.W., Aspel J.B., Allen M.C. & Thomas D. (1982) Dural permeability to narcotics: *in vitro* determination and application to extradural administration. *British Journal of Anaesthesia* **54**, 1117–28.

Moore J., Flynn R.J., Wilson C.M., Fee J.P.H., McClean E. & Dundee J.W. (1987) The effect of H₂ receptor blockers on bupivacaine disposition. *Anesthesia and Analgesia* **66**, S122.

Moore D.C., Mather L.E., Bridenbaugh P.O., Balfour R.I., Lysons D.F. & Horton W.G. (1976a) Arterial and venous plasma levels of bupivacaine following peripheral nerve blocks. *Anesthesia and Analgesia* **55**, 763–8.

Moore D.C., Mather L.E., Bridenbaugh L.D., Balfour R.I., Lysons D.F. & Horton W.G. (1976b) Arterial and venous plasma levels of bupivacaine (Marcaine) following epidural and intercostal nerve blocks. *Anesthesiology* **45**, 39–45.

Moore R.G., Thomas J., Triggs E.J., Thomas B.D., Burnard E.D. & Shanks C.H. (1978) The pharmacokinetics and metabolism of the anilide local anaesthetics in neonates. III: Mepivacaine. *European Journal of Clinical Pharmacology* **14**, 203–12.

Morgan D.H., Cousins M.J., McQuillan D. & Thomas J. (1977) Disposition and placental transfer of etidocaine in pregnancy. *European Journal of Clinical Pharmacology* **12**, 359–65.

Morgan D.H., McQuillan D. & Thomas J. (1978) Pharmacokinetics and metabolism of the anilide local anaesthetics in neonates. II: Etidocaine. *European Journal of Clinical Pharmacology* **13**, 365–71.

Morikawa K.I., Bonica J.J., Tucker G.T. & Murphy T.M. (1974) Effects of acute hypovolaemia on lignocaine absorption and cardiovascular response following epidural block in dogs. *British Journal of Anaesthesia* **46**, 631–5.

Morison D.H. (1981) A double-blind comparison of carbonated lidocaine and lidocaine hydrochloride in epidural anaesthesia. *Canadian Anaesthetists' Society Journal* **28**, 387–9.

Mrose H.E. & Ritchie J.M. (1978) Local anesthetics: do benzocaine and lidocaine act at the same single site? *Journal of General Physiology* **71**, 223–5.

Murphy D.F. (1983) Continuous intercostal nerve blockade for pain relief after cholecystectomy. *British Journal of Anaesthesia* **55**, 521–4.

Nancarrow C. (1986) *Acute Toxicity of Lignocaine and Bupivacaine.* PhD Thesis. Flinders University of South Australia.

Nation R.L., Triggs E.J. & Selig M. (1977) Lignocaine kinetics in cardiac patients and aged subjects. *British Journal of Clinical Pharmacology* **4**, 439–48.

Nickel P.M., Bromage P.R. & Sherrill D.L. (1986) Comparison of hydrochloride and carbonated salts of lidocaine for epidural analgesia. *Regional Anesthesia* **11**, 62–7.

Nishimura N., Kitahara T. & Kusakabo T. (1959) The spread of lidocaine and I-131 solution in the epidural space. *Anesthesiology* **20**, 785–8.

Noble D.W., Smith K.J. & Dundas C.R. (1987) The effects of H₂ antagonists on the elimination of bupivacaine. *British Journal of Anaesthesia* **59**, 735–7.

Nunn J.F. & Slavin G. (1980) Posterior intercostal nerve block for pain relief after cholecystectomy. *British Journal of Anaesthesia* **52**, 253–9.

O'Brien J.E., Abbey V., Hinsvark O., Perel J. & Finster M. (1979) Metabolism and measurement of chloroprocaine, an ester-type local anesthetic. *Journal of Pharmaceutical Science* **68**, 75–8.

O'Kelly E. & Garry B. (1981) Continuous pain relief for multiple fractured ribs. *British Journal of Anaesthesia* **53**, 989–91.

Palmer S.K., Bosnjak Z.J., Hopp F., von Colditz J.H. & Kampine J.P. (1983) Lidocaine and bupivacaine differential nerve blockade of isolated canine nerves. *Anesthesia and Analgesia* **62**, 754–7.

Park W.Y., Massengale M., Kin S-I, Poon K.C. & MacNamara T.E. (1980) Age and the spread of local anesthetic solutions in the epidural space. *Anesthesia and Analgesia* **59**, 768–71.

Parris M.R. & Chambers W.A. (1986) Effects of the addition of potassium to prilocaine or bupivacaine. Studies on brachial plexus blockade. *British Journal of Anaesthesia* **58**, 297–300.

Perucca E. & Richens A. (1979) Reduction of oral bioavailability of lignocaine by induction of first-pass metabolism in epileptic patients. *British Journal of Clinical Pharmacology* **8**, 21–31.

Petersen M.C., Moore R.G., Nation R.L. & McMeniman W. (1981) Relationship between the transplacental gradients of bupivacaine and alpha₁-acid glycoprotein. *British Journal of Clinical Pharmacology* **12**, 859–62.

Piafsky K.M. & Knoppert D. (1979) Binding of local anesthetics to alpha₁-acid glycoprotein. *Clinical Research* **26**, 836A.

Piafsky K.M. & Woolner E.A. (1982) The binding of basic drugs to alpha₁-acid glycoprotein in cord serum. *Journal of Pediatrics* **5**, 820–2.

Pollmann L. (1981) Circadian changes in the duration of local anaesthesia. *Journal of Interdisciplinary Cycle Research* **12**, 187–92.

Post C., Andersson R.G.G., Ryrfeldt A. & Nilsson E. (1979) Physico-chemical modification of lidocaine uptake in rat lung tissue. *Acta Pharmacologica et Toxicologica* **44**, 103–9.

Post C. & Eriksdotter-Behm K. (1982) Dependence of lung uptake of lidocaine *in vivo* on blood pH. *Acta Pharmacologica et Toxicologica* **51**, 136–40.

Post C., Freedman J., Ramsay C-H. & Bonneviei A. (1985) Redistribution of lidocaine and bupivacaine after intrathecal injection in mice. *Anesthesiology* **63**, 410–17.

Quimby C.W. (1965) Influence of blood loss on the duration of regional anesthesia. *Anesthesia and Analgesia* **44**, 387–90.

Ramanathan J., Bottorff M., Jeter J.N., Khalil M. & Sibai B.M. (1986) The pharmacokinetics and maternal and neonatal effects of epidural lidocaine in preeclampsia. *Anesthesia and Analgesia* **65**, 120–6.

Reidenberg M.M., James M. & Dring L.G. (1972) The rate of procaine hydrolysis in serum of normal subjects and diseased patients. *Clinical Pharmacology and Therapeutics* **13**, 279–84.

Richter O., Klein K., Abel J., Ohnesorge F.K., Wust H.J. & Thiessen F.M.M. (1984) The kinetics of bupivacaine (Carbostesin) plasma concentrations during epidural anesthesia following intraoperative bolus injection and subsequent continuous infusion. *International Journal of Clinical Pharmacology, Therapy, and Toxicology* **22**, 611–17.

Ritchie J.M. (1975) Mechanism of action of local anaesthetic agents and biotoxins. *British Journal of Anaesthesia* **47**, 191–8.

Ritchie J.M., Ritchie B. & Greengard P. (1965) The active structure of local anesthetics. *Journal of Pharmacology and Experimental Therapeutics* **150**, 152–9.

Robson R.A., Wing L.M.H., Miners J.O., Lillywhite K.J. & Birkett D.J. (1985) The effect of ranitidine on the disposition of lignocaine. *British Journal of Clinical Pharmacology* **20**, 170–3.

Rosenberg P.H. & Heinonen E. (1983) Differential sensitivity of A and C nerve fibres to long-acting amide local anaesthetics. *British Journal of Anaesthesia* **55**, 163–7.

Rosenberg P.H., Kytta J. & Alila A. (1986) Absorption of bupivacaine, etidocaine, lignocaine and ropivacaine into n-heptane, rat sciatic nerve, and human extradural and subcutaneous fat. *British Journal of Anaesthesia* **58**, 310–14.

Rosenberg P.H., Saramies L. & Alila A. (1981) Lumbar epidural anaesthesia with bupivacaine in old patients: effect of speed and direction of injection. *Acta Anaesthesiologica Scandinavica* **25**, 270–4.

Ross R.A., Clarke J.E. & Armitage E.N. (1980) Postoperative pain prevention by continuous epidural infusion. *Anaesthesia* **35**, 663–8.

Rothstein P., Arthur G.R., Feldman H., Kopf G. & Covino B.G. (1986) Bupivacaine for intercostal nerve blocks in children: blood concentrations and pharmacokinetics. *Anesthesia and Analgesia* **65**, 625–32.

Rothstein P., Cole J.S. & Pitt B.R. (1987) Pulmonary extraction of (3H) bupivacaine: modification by dose, propranolol and interaction with (14C) 5-hydroxytryptamine. *Journal of Pharmacology and Experimental Therapeutics* **240**, 410–14.

Routledge P.A., Barchowsky A., Bjornsson T.D., Kitchell B.B. & Shand D.G. (1980) Lidocaine plasma protein binding. *Clinical Pharmacology and Therapeutics* **27**, 347–51.

Routledge P.A., Stargel W.W., Finn A.L., Barchowsky A. & Shand D.G. (1981) Lignocaine disposition in blood in epilepsy. *British Journal of Clinical Pharmacology* **12**, 663–6.

Saito H., Akutagawa T., Kitahata L.M., Stagg D., Collins J.G. & Scurlock J.E. (1984) Interactions of lidocaine and calcium in blocking the compound action potential of frog sciatic nerve. *Anesthesiology* **60**, 205–8.

Scott D.B., Jebsen P.J.R., Braid D.P., Ortengren B. & Frisch P. (1972) Factors affecting plasma levels of lignocaine and prilocaine. *British Journal of Anaesthesia* **44**, 1040–8.

Scott D.B., Littlewood D.G., Covino B.G. & Drummond G.B. (1976) Plasma lignocaine concentrations following endotracheal spraying with an aerosol. *British Journal of Anaesthesia* **48**, 899–901.

Scurlock J.E., Meymaris E. & Gregus J. (1978) The clinical character of local anesthetics: a function of frequency-dependent conduction block. *Acta Anaesthesiologica Scandinavica* **22**, 601–8.

Seifen A.B., Ferrari A.A., Seifen A.A., Thompson D.S. & Chapman J. (1979) Pharmacokinetics of intravenous procaine infusion in humans. *Anesthesia and Analgesia* **58**, 382–6.

Sharrock N.E. (1978) Epidural anaesthetic dose response in patients 20 to 80 years old. *Anesthesiology* **47**, 307–8.

Simon P., Benowitz N.L. & Culala S. (1984) Motor paralysis increases brain uptake of lidocaine during status epilepticus. *Neurology* **34**, 384–7.

Smith S.L., Albin M.S., Watson W.A., Pantoja G. & Bunegin L. (1983) Spinal cord and cerebral blood flow responses to intrathecal local anesthetics with and without epinephrine. *Anesthesiology* **59**, A312.

Smith S., Ramamurthy S. & Walsh N. (1986) Effect of sodium bicarbonate on the onset of blockade by bupivacaine. *Regional Anesthesia* **11**, 48.

Starke P. & Nolte H. (1978) pH des Liquor spinalis wahrend subduraler Blockade. *Der Anaesthesist* **27**, 41–3.

Strasser K., Abel J., Breulmann M. & Schumacher I. (1981) Plasmakonzentration von Etidocain in der ersten zwei Studen nach axillarer Blockade bei Gesunden und bei Patienten mit Niereninsuffizienz. *Regional Anaesthesie* **4**, 14–17.

Strichartz G.R. (1973) The inhibition of sodium currents in myelinated nerve by quaternary derivatives of lidocaine. *Journal of General Physiology* **62**, 37–57.

Strichartz G.R. (1985) Interactions of local anesthetics with neuronal sodium channels. In *Effects of Anesthesia* (Eds Covino B.G., Fozzard H.A., Rehder K. & Strichartz G.R.) pp. 39–52. American Physiological Society, Bethesda.

Strobel G.F. & Bianchi C.P. (1970) The effect of pH gradients on the action of procaine and lidocaine in intact and desheathed sciatic nerves. *Journal of Pharmacology and Experimental Therapeutics* **172**, 1–17.

Takasaki M. (1984) Blood concentrations of lidocaine, mepivacaine and bupivacaine during caudal analgesia in children. *Acta Anaesthesiologica Scandinavica* **28**, 211–14.

Terasaki T., Pardridge W.M. & Denson D.D. (1986) Differential effect of plasma protein binding of bupivacaine on its *in vivo* transfer into the brain and salivary gland of rats. *Journal of Pharmacology and Experimental Therapeutics* **239**, 724–9.

Thomas J., Long G., Moore G. & Morgan D. (1976) Plasma protein binding and placental transfer of bupivacaine. *Clinical Pharmacology and Therapeutics* **19**, 426–34.

Thompson G.A., Turner P.A., Bridenbaugh P.O., Stuebing R.C. & Denson D.D. (1986) The influence of diazepam on the pharmacokinetics of intravenous and epidural bupivacaine in the rhesus monkey. *Anesthesia and Analgesia* **65**, 151–5.

Thompson G.E. & Rorie D.H. (1983) Functional anatomy of the brachial plexus sheaths. *Anesthesiology* **59**, 117–19.

Thomson P.D., Melmon K.L., Richardson J.A., Cohn K., Steinbrunn W., Cudihee R. & Rowland M. (1973) Lidocaine pharmacokinetics in advanced heart failure, liver disease and renal disease in humans. *Annals of Internal Medicine* **78**, 499–508.

Tucker G.T. (1983) Chemistry and pharmacology of local anaesthetic drugs. In *Practical Regional Anaesthesia* (Eds Henderson J.J. & Nimmo W.S.) pp. 1–21. Blackwell Scientific Publications, Oxford.

Tucker G.T. (1984) Absorption and disposition of local anaesthetics in relation to regional blood flow changes. In *Current Concepts in Regional Anaesthesia* (Eds Van Kleek J.W., Burm A.G.L. & Spierdijk J.) pp. 192–202. Martinus Nijhoff, Boston and The Hague.

Tucker G.T. (1986) Pharmacokinetics of local anaesthetics. *British Journal of Anaesthesia* **58**, 717–31.

Tucker G.T., Bax N.D.S., Lennard M.S., Al-Asady S., Bharaj H.S. & Woods H.F. (1984) Effects of beta-adrenoceptor antagonists on the pharmacokinetics of lignocaine. *British Journal of Clinical Pharmacology* **17**, 21S–28S.

Tucker G.T. & Boas R.A. (1971) Pharmacokinetic aspects of intravenous regional anesthesia. *Anesthesiology* **34**, 538–49.

Tucker G.T., Boyes R.N., Bridenbaugh P.O. & Moore D.C. (1970a) Binding of anilide-type local anesthetics in human plasma. I: Relationships between binding, physicochemical properties and anesthetic activity. *Anesthesiology* **33**, 287–303.

Tucker G.T., Boyes R.N., Bridenbaugh P.O. & Moore D.C. (1970b) Binding of anilide-type local anesthetics in human Plasma. II: Implications *in vivo* with special reference to transplacental disposition. *Anesthesiology* **33**, 304–14.

Tucker G.T., Cooper S., Littlewood D., Buckley S.P., Covino B.G. & Scott D.B. (1977) Observed and predicted accumulation of local anaesthetic agents during continuous extradural analgesia. *British Journal of Anaesthesia* **49**, 237–42.

Tucker G.T. & Mather L.E. (1975) Pharmacokinetics of local anaesthetic agents. *British Journal of Anaesthesia* **47**, 213–24.

Tucker G.T. & Mather L.E. (1979) Clinical pharmacokinetics of local anaesthetic agents. *Clinical Pharmacokinetics* **4**, 241–78.

Tucker G.T. & Mather L.E. (1980) Absorption and disposition of local anesthetics: pharmacokinetics. In *Neural Blockade in Clinical Anesthesia and Management of Pain* (Eds Cousins M.J. & Bridenbaugh P.O.) pp. 45–85. Lippincott, Philadelphia.

Tucker G.T. & Mather L.E. (1987) Physicochemical properties, absorption and disposition of local anesthetic agents. In *Neural Blockade in Clinical Anesthesia and Management of Pain* 2nd edn. (Eds Cousins M.J. & Bridenbaugh P.O.) pp. 47–110. Lippincott, Philadelphia.

Tucker G.T., Moore D.C., Bridenbaugh P.O., Bridenbaugh L.D. & Thompson G.E. (1972) Systemic absorption of mepivacaine in commonly used regional block procedures. *Anesthesiology* **37**, 277–87.

Urban B.J. (1973) Clinical observations suggesting a changing site of action during induction and recession of spinal and epidural anesthesia. *Anesthesiology* **39**, 496–503.

Vester-Andersen T., Broby-Johansen U. & Bro-Rasmussen F. (1986) Perivascular axillary block. VI: The distribution of gelatine solution injected into the axillary neurovascular sheath of cadavers. *Acta Anaesthesiologica Scandinavica* **30**, 18–22.

Vester-Andersen T., Christiansen C., Hansen A., Sorensen M. & Meisler C. (1981) Interscalene brachial plexus block: area of analgesia, complications and blood concentrations of local anesthetics. *Acta Anaesthesiologica Scandinavica* **25**, 81–4.

Vester-Andersen T., Husum B., Lindeburg T., Borrits L. & Gothgen I. (1984) Perivascular axillary block V: Blockade following 60 ml of mepivacaine 1% injected as a bolus or as 30 + 30 ml with a 20-min interval. *Acta Anaesthesiologica Scandinavica* **28**, 612–16.

Webb T.D. & Ward D.S. (1983) Elimination of lidocaine following regional block is inhibited by cimetidine. *Anesthesiology* **59**, A213.

Wennberg E., Haljamae H., Edwall G. & Dhuner K-G. (1982) Effects of commercial (pH 3.5) and freshly prepared (pH 6.5) lidocaine–adrenaline solutions on tissue pH. *Acta Anaesthesiologica Scandinavica* **26**, 524–7.

Wiklund L., Tucker G.T. & Engberg G. (1977) Influence of intravenously administered ephedrine on splanchnic haemodynamics and clearance of lidocaine. *Acta Anaesthesiologica Scandinavica* **21**, 275–81.

Wildsmith J.A.W. (1986) Peripheral nerve and local anaesthetic drugs. *British Journal of Anaesthesia* **58**, 692–700.

Wildsmith J.A.W., Gissen A.J., Takman B. & Covino B.G. (1987) Differential nerve blockade: esters vs amides and the influence of pKa. *British Journal of Anaesthesia* **59**, 379–84.

Wildsmith J.A.W. & Rocco A.G. (1985) Current concepts in spinal anesthesia. *Regional Anesthesia* **10**, 119–24.

Wildsmith J.A.W., Tucker G.T., Cooper S., Scott D.B. & Covino B.G. (1977) Plasma concentrations of local anaesthetics after interscalene brachial plexus block. *British Journal of Anaesthesia* **49**, 461–6.

Wilkinson G.R. & Lund P.C. (1970) Bupivacaine levels in plasma and cerebrospinal fluid following peridural administration. *Anesthesiology* **33**, 482–6.

Williams R.L., Blaschke T.F., Meffin P.L., Melmon K.L. & Rowland M. (1976) Influence of viral hepatitis on the disposition of two compounds with high hepatic clearance: lidocaine and indocyanine green. *Clinical Pharmacology and Therapeutics* **20**, 290–9.

Wing L.M.H., Miners J.O., Birkett D.J., Foenander T., Lillywhite K. & Wanwimolruk S. (1984) Lidocaine disposition—sex differences and effects of cimetidine. *Clinical Pharmacology and Therapeutics* **35**, 695–701.

Winnie A.P., La Vallee D.A., Sosa B.P. & Masud K.Z. (1977a) Clinical pharmacokinetics of local anesthetics. *Canadian Anaesthetists' Society Journal* **24**, 252–62.

Winnie A.P., Radonjic R., Akkineni S.R. & Durrani Z. (1979) Factors influencing distribution of local anesthetic injected into the brachial plexus sheath. *Anesthesia and Analgesia* **58**, 225–34.

Winnie A.P., Tay C-H., Patel K.P., Ramamurthy S. & Durrani Z. (1977b) Pharmacokinetics of local anesthetics during plexus blocks. *Anesthesia and Analgesia* **56**, 852–61.

Wood M. & Wood A.J.J. (1981) Changes in plasma drug binding and alpha$_1$-acid glycoprotein in mother and newborn infant. *Clinical Pharmacology and Therapeutics* **29**, 522–6.

Wurst H.J. & Stanton-Hicks M.d'A. (1983) Changes of pH in epidural and spinal space and plasma levels of bupivacaine during acute and chronic epidurals in dogs. *Regional Anesthesia* **8**, 35–9.

General Considerations, Toxicity and Complications of Local Anaesthesia

B. G. COVINO

Chemical compounds that demonstrate local anaesthetic activity possess usually an aromatic and an amine group separated by an intermediate chain (Table 57.1). The clinically useful local anaesthetic agents fall essentially into one of two chemically distinct groups. Those agents which possess an ester link between the aromatic portion and the intermediate chain are referred to as amino esters and include procaine, chloroprocaine and amethocaine (tetracaine—USP). Local anaesthetics with an amide link between the aromatic end and the intermediate chain are referred to as amino amides and include lignocaine (lidocaine—USP), mepivacaine, prilocaine, bupivacaine and etidocaine. The ester and amide compounds differ in terms of their chemical stability, metabolic site and allergic potential. Amides are extremely stable agents whilst esters are relatively unstable in solution. The amino esters are hydrolysed in plasma by the enzyme cholinesterase, whereas the amide compounds undergo enzymatic degradation in the liver. Para-aminobenzoic acid is one of the metabolites of ester-type compounds which can induce allergic-type reactions in a small percentage of patients. The amino amides are not metabolized to para-aminobenzoic acid and reports of allergic reactions to these agents are extremely rare.

General considerations

The properties of the various local anaesthetic agents which are clinically important include potency, speed of onset, duration of anaesthetic activity and differential sensory/motor blockade. The clinical profile of the individual agents is determined essentially by the physico-chemical characteristics of the various compounds, which in turn are dependent on their chemical

structure. The physico-chemical properties which influence anaesthetic activity are lipid-solubility, protein binding and pKa. Minor changes in molecular structure have dramatic effects on these properties (Table 57.1).

Anaesthetic potency

Lipid-solubility appears to be the primary determinant of intrinsic anaesthetic potency. The nerve membrane is basically a lipoprotein matrix. The axolemma consists of 90% lipids and 10% proteins. As a result, chemical compounds which are highly lipophilic tend to penetrate the nerve membrane more easily, such that fewer molecules are required for conduction blockade resulting in enhanced potency. *In vitro* studies on isolated nerves show a correlation between the partition coefficient of local anaesthetics and the minimum concentration (C_{min}) required for conduction blockade (Gissen *et al.*, 1980; Wildsmith *et al.*, 1985). For example, among the amino amides, mepivacaine and prilocaine are the least lipid-soluble and weakest amide agents, while etidocaine is the most lipophilic and the most potent local anaesthetic (Fig. 57.1). A similar relationship between lipid-solubility and potency exists among the ester-type drugs. Procaine is the least lipid-soluble and the weakest agent, whilst amethocaine is the most lipophilic and the most potent ester-type drug.

Factors other than lipid-solubility may influence anaesthetic potency also. A comparison of the partition coefficient values of the base form of ester and amide agents and their relative anaesthetic potencies indicates that the potency of the amino esters is greater than that of amino amides at similar coefficient values. It has been suggested that the amino esters may

Table 57.1 Chemical structure, physico-chemical properties and pharmacological properties of local anaesthetic agents

Agent	Chemical configuration			Physico-chemical properties				Pharmacological properties		
	Aromatic lipophilic	Intermediate chain	Amine hydrophilic	Molecular weight (base)	pKa (25°C)	Partition coefficient	Percent protein binding	Onset	Relative potency	Duration
Esters										
Procaine	H₂N—C₆H₄—	—COOCH₂CH₂—	—N(C₂H₅)₂	236	8.9	0.02	6	Slow	1	Short
Amethocaine	H₉C₄N(H)—C₆H₄—	—COOCH₂CH₂—	—N(CH₃)₂	264	8.5	4.1	76	Slow	8	Long
Chloroprocaine	H₂N—C₆H₃(Cl)—	—COOCH₂CH₂—	—N(C₂H₅)₂	271	8.7	0.14	—	Fast	1	Short
Amides										
Prilocaine	CH₃—C₆H₄—	—NHCOCH(CH₃)—	—NH—C₃H₇	220	7.9	0.9	55	Fast	2	Moderate
Lignocaine	(CH₃)₂C₆H₃—	—NHCOCH₂—	—N(C₂H₅)₂	234	7.9	2.9	64	Fast	2	Moderate
Mepivacaine	(CH₃)₂C₆H₃—	—NHCO—	piperidine N—CH₃	246	7.6	0.8	78	Fast	2	Moderate
Bupivacaine	(CH₃)₂C₆H₃—	—NHCO—	piperidine N—C₄H₉	288	8.1	27.5	96	Moderate	8	Long
Etidocaine	(CH₃)₂C₆H₃—	—NHCOCH(C₂H₅)—	—N(C₂H₅)(C₃H₇)	276	7.7	141	94	Fast	6	Long

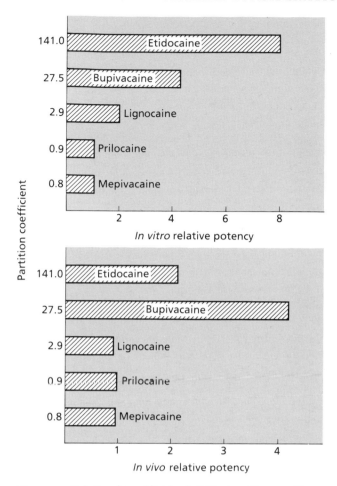

Fig. 57.1 Relationship of lipid-solubility (partition coefficient) to *in vitro* and *in vivo* anaesthetic potency.

interact with a greater number of local anaesthetic receptor sites which may explain their inherently greater potency (Wildsmith *et al.*, 1987).

In vivo studies in man indicate that the correlation between lipid-solubility and anaesthetic potency is not as precise as in an isolated nerve (Fig. 57.1). Lignocaine is approximately twice as potent as prilocaine and mepivacaine in an isolated preparation, but in man little difference in anaesthetic potency is apparent between these three agents. Similarly, etidocaine is more potent than bupivacaine in an isolated nerve while etidocaine is actually less active clinically than bupivacaine. The difference between *in vitro* and *in vivo* results is believed to be related to the vasodilator or tissue redistribution properties of the various local anaesthetics. For example, lignocaine causes a greater degree of vasodilatation than either mepivacaine or prilocaine, resulting in a more rapid vascular absorption of lignocaine such that fewer lignocaine molecules are available for neural blockade *in vivo*. The extremely

high lipid-solubility of etidocaine results in a greater uptake of this agent by adipose tissue such as in the extradural space which again results in fewer etidocaine molecules available for neural blockade compared with bupivacaine.

Duration of action

The duration of anaesthesia is related primarily to the degree of protein binding of the various local anaesthetics. Local anaesthetics are believed to combine with a protein receptor located within the sodium channel of the nerve membrane. Chemical compounds which possess a greater affinity for and bind more firmly to the receptor site remain within the channel for a longer period of time, resulting in a prolonged duration of conduction blockade. Most of the information regarding the protein binding of local anaesthetics has been obtained from studies involving the binding of these agents to plasma proteins. It is assumed that a relationship exists between the plasma protein binding of local anaesthetics and the degree of binding to membrane proteins.

In vitro studies have demonstrated that agents such as procaine which are poorly protein bound are washed out rapidly from isolated nerves whereas drugs such as amethocaine, bupivacaine and etidocaine are removed at an extremely slow rate. *In vivo* studies, including clinical investigations in man, have confirmed the relationship between protein binding of local anaesthetics and their duration of action (Covino, 1986a). For example, procaine produces a duration of brachial plexus blockade of 30–60 min while approximately 10 hr of anaesthesia have been reported following the use of bupivacaine or etidocaine for brachial plexus blockade (Fig. 57.2).

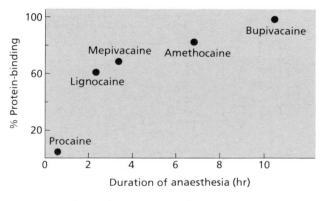

Fig. 57.2 Relationship of protein binding of various local anaesthetics to the duration of brachial plexus blockade.

In man, the duration of anaesthesia is influenced markedly by the peripheral vascular effects of the local anaesthetic agents. All local anaesthetics except cocaine tend to have a biphasic effect on vascular smooth muscle. At low concentrations, these agents tend to cause vasoconstriction whereas at clinically employed concentrations local anaesthetics cause vasodilatation (Johns *et al.*, 1985, 1986). However, differences exist in the degree of vasodilator activity produced by the various drugs. For example, lignocaine is a more potent vasodilator than mepivacaine or prilocaine. Although little difference in the duration of conduction block is apparent between these agents in an isolated nerve, *in vivo* the duration of anaesthesia produced by lignocaine is shorter than that of mepivacaine or prilocaine. Addition of a vasoconstrictor drug to these three local anaesthetics results in a similar duration of action.

Onset of action

The onset of conduction block in isolated nerves is determined primarily by the pKa of the individual agents. The pKa of a chemical compound is the pH at which the ionized and non-ionized forms are present in equal amounts. The uncharged form of the local anaesthetic agent is primarily responsible for diffusion across the nerve sheath and nerve membrane and therefore the onset of action is related directly to the amount of drug which exists in the base form (Fig. 57.3). The percentage of a specific local anaesthetic drug, which is present in the base form when injected into tissue at pH 7.4, is inversely proportional to the pKa of that agent. For example, mepivacaine,

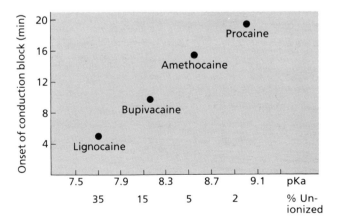

Fig. 57.3 Relationship of onset of anaesthesia of various local anaesthetic agents to their pKa and percentage of drug in un-ionized form.

lignocaine, prilocaine and etidocaine possess a pKa of approximately 7.7. When these agents are injected into tissue at a pH of 7.4, approximately 65% of these drugs exists in the ionized form and 35% in the non-ionized base form. On the other hand, amethocaine possesses a pKa of 8.6 and only 5% is present in the non-ionized form at a tissue pH of 7.4, while 95% exists in the charged cationic form. The pKa of bupivacaine is 8.1, which indicates that 15% of this agent is present in the non-ionized form at a tissue pH of 7.4, and 85% exists in the charged cationic form. Therefore, lignocaine, mepivacaine, prilocaine and etidocaine show a rapid onset of action, whereas procaine and amethocaine, with a high pKa, have a slow onset time (Fig. 57.3). Bupivacaine occupies an intermediate position in terms of pKa and latency of block.

The onset of conduction blockade *in vivo* is dependent in part on other miscellaneous considerations. The onset of action may be altered by the rate of diffusion through non-nervous tissue. For example, lignocaine and prilocaine possess a similar pKa and similar onset of action in an isolated nerve. However, *in vivo* prilocaine may be somewhat slower in onset than lignocaine. This difference may be related to an enhanced ability of lignocaine to diffuse through non-nervous tissue. More important, however, is the concentration of local anaesthetic agent employed. For example, bupivacaine 0.25% possesses a rather slow onset of action. However, increasing the concentration to 0.75% results in a significant decrease in the latency of anaesthetic activity. The rapid onset time of chloroprocaine *in vivo* may be related in part to improved diffusion through non-nervous tissue, but also to the use of a 3% concentration of this agent. The pKa of chloroprocaine is approximately 9 and its onset of action in isolated nerves is relatively slow (Rosenberg *et al.*, 1980). However, the low systemic toxicity of this agent allows the use of high concentrations. Therefore, the rapid onset time *in vivo* of chloroprocaine may be related simply to the large number of molecules placed in the vicinity of peripheral nerves.

Differential sensory/motor blockade

One other important clinical consideration is the ability of local anaesthetic agents to cause a differential blockade of sensory and motor fibres. The intrathecal administration of varying concentrations of procaine has been employed to provide a differential blockade of sensory, sympathetic and motor fibres. However, it has been extremely difficult to produce sensory anaesthesia sufficient for surgery without a significant impairment of motor function. Bupivacaine was the first agent which showed a relative specificity for sensory fibres such that adequate sensory analgesia without profound inhibition of motor fibres could be achieved for surgical, obstetrical and acute and chronic pain therapy regardless of the regional anaesthetic technique employed. Bupivacaine and etidocaine provide an interesting contrast in terms of their differential sensory/motor blocking activity, although they are both potent, long-acting anaesthetic agents (Fig. 57.4). For example, bupivacaine is used widely extradurally for both surgical and obstetrical procedures and relief of pain postoperatively due to its ability to provide adequate sensory analgesia with minimal blockade of motor fibres, particularly when used as an 0.25 or 0.5% solution. Thus, the patient in labour can be rendered pain-free and still be able to move her legs which is one of the primary reasons why this agent has enjoyed popularity for continuous extradural blockade during labour. Increasing the concentration of bupivacaine to 0.75% increases the depth of both sensory and motor blockade while shortening also latency and producing a more prolonged duration of anaesthesia (Scott et al., 1980). Etidocaine, on the other hand, shows little separation between sensory and motor blockade. In order to achieve adequate extradural sensory anaesthesia, 1.5% concentrations of etidocaine are required usually. At these concentrations, etidocaine has an extremely rapid onset of action and a prolonged duration of anaesthesia. However, sensory anaesthesia is associated with a profound degree of motor blockade. Thus, etidocaine is a valuable agent,

particularly for extradural blockade in surgical situations where optimum muscle relaxation is desirable, as it combines a rapid onset, prolonged duration and satisfactory quality of anaesthesia combined with profound motor blockade. However, this marked effect on motor function renders etidocaine of limited value for obstetric analgesia and postoperative pain relief.

The factors responsible for the differential sensory/motor separation associated with bupivacaine are not known precisely. Studies on isolated nerves have shown that at low concentrations, bupivacaine blocks initially unmyelinated C-fibres followed at a later time by a block of myelinated A-fibres (Gissen et al., 1982). On the other hand, etidocaine blocks both A- and C-fibres at approximately the same rate. The slow blockade of A-fibres by bupivacaine is believed to be a result of the relatively high pKa of this agent such that fewer uncharged molecules are available to penetrate the diffusion barriers surrounding large A-fibres. In vivo, the combination of the slow diffusion of bupivacaine and its absorption by the vasculature in the region of drug administration may result in a situation in which the number of bupivacaine molecules which penetrate ultimately the membrane of the large, motor A-fibres is insufficient to cause conduction blockade. The lack of diffusion barriers around the small sensory C-fibres allows a sufficient number of bupivacaine molecules to reach the receptor sites in the C-fibre membrane to cause sensory anaesthesia. Thus, bupivacaine may possess the optimal pKa and lipid-solubility characteristics required for differential sensory/motor blockade.

In summary, the pharmacological activity of local anaesthetic agents is related primarily to their physico-chemical properties. However, the activity of these agents in vivo may be altered by other actions which are unrelated essentially to their physico-chemical properties. On the basis of anaesthetic activity in man, the various agents may be classified as follows:
1 Agents of low anaesthetic potency and short duration of action: procaine and chloroprocaine.
2 Agents of intermediate anaesthetic potency and duration of action: lignocaine, mepivacaine and prilocaine.
3 Agents of high anaesthetic potency and prolonged duration of action: amethocaine, bupivacaine and etidocaine.

In terms of latency, chloroprocaine, lignocaine, mepivacaine, prilocaine and etidocaine possess a relatively rapid onset of action. Bupivacaine is intermediate

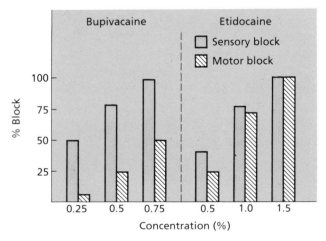

Fig. 57.4 Comparative sensory/motor blockade of bupivacaine and etidocaine following extradural administration.

in terms of onset of anaesthesia, whilst procaine and amethocaine demonstrate a long latency period.

Factors influencing anaesthetic activity

Although the inherent pharmacological properties of the various local anaesthetic agents determine basically their anaesthetic profile, other factors may influence the quality of regional anaesthesia also. These include:

1 Dosage of local anaesthetic administered.
2 Addition of a vasoconstrictor to the local anaesthetic solution.
3 Site of administration.
4 Carbonation or pH adjustment of local anaesthetic solutions.
5 Additives.
6 Mixtures of local anaesthetics.
7 Pregnancy.

Dosage of local anaesthetic solutions

The mass of drug administered influences the onset, depth and duration of anaesthesia (Fig. 57.5). As the dose of local anaesthetic is increased, the frequency of satisfactory anaesthesia and the duration of anaesthesia increase and the speed of onset of anaesthesia decreases. In general, the dosage of local anaesthetic administered can be increased by either administering a larger volume or a more concentrated solution. However, in clinical practice, an increase in dosage is achieved usually by employing a more concentrated solution of the specific agent. For example, increasing the concentration of extradurally administered bupivacaine from 0.125 to 0.5% whilst maintaining the same volume of injectate (10 ml) resulted in a decreased latency, improved incidence of satisfactory analgesia and an increased duration of sensory analgesia. Similarly, an increase in the concentration of extradural bupivacaine in surgical patients from 0.5% to 0.75% with a concomitant increase in dosage from approximately 100 mg to 150 mg produced a more rapid onset and prolonged duration of sensory anaesthesia, a greater frequency of satisfactory sensory anaesthesia and an enhanced depth of motor blockade (Scott *et al.*, 1980). Prilocaine (600 mg) administered extradurally either as 30 ml of a 2% solution or 20 ml of 3% solution showed no difference in onset, adequacy or duration of anaesthesia and onset, depth and duration of motor blockade which indicates that dosage rather than volume or concentration of anaesthetic solution is the primary determinant of anaesthetic activity. The volume of anaesthetic solution may influence the spread of anaesthesia. For example, 30 ml of lignocaine 1% administered into the extradural space produced a level of anaesthesia which was 4.3 dermatomes higher than that achieved when 10 ml of lignocaine 3% was employed. Thus, except for the possible effect on the spread of anaesthesia, the primary qualities of regional anaesthesia, namely, onset, depth and duration of blockade, are related to the mass of drug injected i.e. the product of volume and concentration.

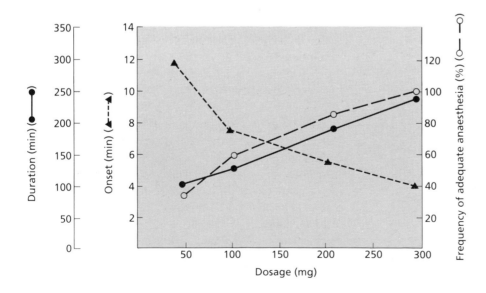

Fig. 57.5 Effect of dose of extradural etidocaine on onset, frequency and duration of anaesthesia.

Addition of a vasoconstrictor to local anaesthetic solutions

Vasoconstrictors, particularly adrenaline (epinephrine–USP), are added to local anaesthetic solutions frequently to decrease the rate of vascular absorption which allows more anaesthetic molecules to reach the nerve membrane and thereby improve the depth and duration of anaesthesia. Local anaesthetic solutions contain usually a 1/200 000 (5 µg/ml) concentration of adrenaline. This concentration of adrenaline has been reported to provide an optimal degree of vasoconstriction when employed with lignocaine for extradural or intercostal use. Other vasoconstrictor agents such as noradrenaline (norepinephrine—USP) and phenylephrine have been added also to solutions of local anaesthetics. Equipotent concentrations of adrenaline and phenylephrine appear to prolong the duration of spinal anaesthesia produced by amethocaine to a similar extent (Concepcion et al., 1984) (Fig. 57.6).

The effect of adrenaline on prolonging the duration of anaesthesia varies depending on the local anaesthetic employed and the site of injection. For example, the duration of action of all agents is prolonged by the addition of adrenaline when used for infiltration anaesthesia and peripheral nerve blocks. Adrenaline increases also the duration of extradural anaesthesia when added to procaine, mepivacaine and lignocaine but does not alter markedly the duration of action of extradurally administered prilocaine, bupivacaine or etidocaine. The decreased vasodilator action of prilocaine compared with lignocaine is believed responsible for the reduced effect of added adrenaline to solutions of prilocaine. The high lipid-solubility of bupivacaine and etidocaine may be responsible for the diminished effect of adrenaline. These agents are taken up substantially by extradural fat and then released slowly, which contributes to their prolonged duration of action. However, the interaction of adrenaline and the long-acting agents such as bupivacaine is dependent on the concentration of drug employed. For example, in extradural blockade for labour, the frequency and duration of adequate analgesia was improved when adrenaline 1/200 000 was added to bupivacaine 0.125% and 0.25%. However, the addition of adrenaline to 0.5 and bupivacaine 0.75% did not improve the adequacy or prolong the initial regression of extradural sensory anaesthesia in obstetrical or surgical patients. The profoundness but not the duration of motor blockade is enhanced following the extradural administration of adrenaline containing solutions of bupivacaine and etidocaine. In the subarachnoid space, adrenaline extends significantly the duration of action of amethocaine (Concepcion et al., 1984). Two or four segment regression of anaesthesia is not enhanced markedly when solutions of lignocaine or bupivacaine with adrenaline are administered intrathecally. However, anaesthesia in the lower thoracic and lumbosacral areas is prolonged. Thus, adrenaline added to spinal solutions of lignocaine and bupivacaine may not prolong significantly the duration of effective surgical anaesthesia in the abdominal area but provides an extended duration of anaesthesia in the lower limbs.

Site of injection

Although local anaesthetics are classified frequently as agents of short, moderate or long duration with a slow or rapid onset of action, these general properties are influenced by the type of anaesthetic procedure performed. In general, the most rapid onset but the shortest duration of action occurs following the intrathecal or subcutaneous administration of local anaesthetics, whilst the slowest onset times and the longest durations are observed during the performance of brachial plexus blocks. For example, an agent such as bupivacaine demonstrates an onset time of approximately 5 min and a duration of action of approximately 3–4 hr when administered into the subarachnoid space. However, when bupivacaine is administered for brachial plexus blockade, the onset time is approximately 20–30 min, whilst the duration of anaesthesia averages 10 hr. Differences in the onset and duration of

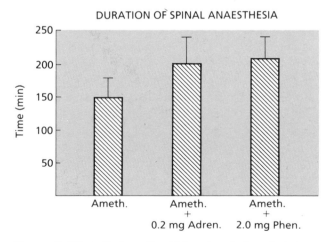

Fig. 57.6 Effect of adrenaline (Adren.) and phenylephrine (Phen.) on the duration of spinal anaesthesia produced by amethocaine (Ameth.).

anaesthesia depending on the site of injection result in part from the particular anatomy of the area of injection, the variation in the rate of vascular absorption, and the amount of drug employed for various types of regional anaesthesia. In the case of spinal anaesthesia, the lack of a nerve sheath around the spinal cord and deposition of the local anaesthetic solution in the immediate vicinity of the spinal cord is responsible for the rapid onset of action. On the other hand, the relatively small amount of drug employed for spinal anaesthesia accounts probably for the relatively short duration of action associated with this particular technique. In the case of brachial plexus blockade, the onset of anaesthesia is slow because the anaesthetic agent is deposited usually at some distance from the nerve roots, and the drug must diffuse through various tissue barriers before reaching the nerve membrane. The long duration of brachial plexus blockade is related probably to the decreased rate of vascular absorption from that site, and also the larger doses of drug employed commonly for this regional anaesthetic technique.

Carbonation and pH adjustment of local anaesthetics

In isolated nerve preparations, carbon dioxide enhances the diffusion of local anaesthetics through nerve sheaths resulting in a more rapid onset (Fig. 57.7) and a decrease in the minimum concentration (C_{min}) of local anaesthetic required for conduction blockade (Gissen & Covino, 1985). The enhanced onset and depth of conduction blockade is believed to result from the diffusion of carbon dioxide through the nerve membrane and a decrease in the axoplasmic pH. The lower pH increases the intracellular concentration of the active cationic form of the local anaesthetic which binds to a receptor in the sodium channel. In addition, the local anaesthetic cation does not diffuse readily through membranes such that the drug remains entrapped within the axoplasm, a situation referred to as ion trapping. Several investigations in man have demonstrated that lignocaine carbonate solutions produce a more rapid onset of brachial plexus and extradural blockade compared with the use of lignocaine hydrochloride solutions (Bromage, 1965, 1970). However, other studies have failed to demonstrate a significantly more rapid onset of action when lignocaine carbonate was compared with lignocaine hydrochloride for extradural blockade (Morrison, 1981). Similarly, it has been reported that bupivacaine–CO_2 is associated with a more rapid onset of action in man. However, double-blind studies in which bupivacaine carbonate was compared with bupivacaine hydrochloride for brachial plexus or extradural blockade, have failed to confirm these earlier reports of a significantly shorter onset of action of the carbonated solution (Brown et al., 1980; McClure & Scott, 1981). It is not certain if carbonation of local anaesthetic solutions decreases consistently the latency of conduction blockade in a clinical situation. However, it does appear that carbonated solutions do improve the profoundness of sensory anaesthesia and motor blockade when administered into the extradural space. The major advantage of these solutions may be in brachial plexus blocks where a more complete inhibition of conduction in the radial, median and ulnar nerves has been demonstrated.

Alkalinization of local anaesthetic solutions has also been employed in order to decrease the onset of conduction blockade. The addition of sodium bicarbonate increases the pH of the local anaesthetic solution which in turn increases the amount of drug in the uncharged base form. Thus, the rate of diffusion across the nerve sheath and nerve membrane should be enhanced, resulting in a more rapid onset of anaesthesia. Several clinical studies have been carried out in which the addition of sodium bicarbonate to solutions of bupivacaine or lignocaine did appear to produce a significant decrease in the latency of brachial plexus and extradural blockade. In addition, it has been

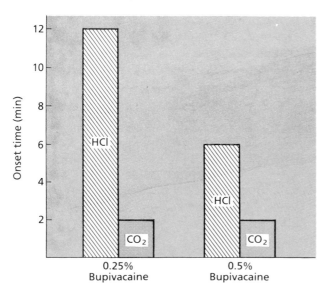

Fig. 57.7 Onset time of conduction block in an isolated nerve following exposure to bupivacaine–HCl and bupivacaine–CO_2.

reported also that the duration of brachial plexus block was prolonged by increasing the pH of bupivacaine (Hilgier, 1985).

Additives

Various attempts have been made to prolong the duration of anaesthesia by incorporating substances such as dextran into local anaesthetic solutions (Loder, 1960). Discrepancies exist with regard to the effectiveness of dextran, in prolonging the duration of regional anaesthesia. In one controlled clinical study, prolonged durations of anaesthesia were observed in some individual patients but the mean duration of intercostal nerve blockade was not altered significantly when solutions of bupivacaine with and without dextran were compared (Bridenbaugh, 1978).

It has been suggested that the difference in results obtained by various investigators may be related to the pH of the dextran solution employed. Dextran solutions with a pH of 8.0 prolonged significantly the duration of bupivacaine-induced coccygeal nerve blocks in rats, whereas the duration of block was not altered when dextran with a pH of 4.5–5.5 was added to bupivacaine. These results indicate that alkalinization of the anaesthetic solution may be responsible for prolonged conduction blockade rather than the dextran itself.

Mixtures of local anaesthetics

The use of mixtures of local anaesthetics for regional anaesthesia has become relatively popular in recent years. The basis for this practice is to compensate for the short duration of action of certain agents such as chloroprocaine or lignocaine and the long latency of other agents such as amethocaine and bupivacaine.

Theoretically, mixtures of chloroprocaine and bupivacaine should offer significant clinical advantages from the rapid onset and low systemic toxicity of chloroprocaine and the long duration of action of bupivacaine. It was reported originally that a mixture of chloroprocaine and bupivacaine did result in a short latency and prolonged duration of brachial plexus blockade. However, subsequent studies indicated that the duration of extradural anaesthesia produced by a mixture of chloroprocaine and bupivacaine was significantly shorter than that obtained with solutions of bupivacaine alone. Data from isolated nerve studies suggest that a metabolite of chloroprocaine may inhibit the binding of bupivacaine to membrane receptor sites (Corke et al., 1984). At present there do not appear to

be any clinically significant advantages to the use of mixtures of local anaesthetic agents. Etidocaine and bupivacaine provide clinically acceptable onsets of action and prolonged durations of anaesthesia. In addition, the use of catheter techniques for extradural anaesthesia and also for brachial plexus blockade makes it possible to administer repeated injection of the rapidly acting agents such as chloroprocaine or lignocaine which provide an anaesthetic duration of indefinite length.

Pregnancy

It is well known that the spread of extradural or spinal anaesthesia is greater in pregnant patients compared with non-pregnant subjects. This exaggerated spread has been attributed to mechanical factors associated with pregnancy i.e. dilated extradural veins tend to decrease the diameter of the extradural and subarachnoid space which results in a more extensive longitudinal spread of local anaesthetic solution. Recent studies have suggested that physiological alterations associated with pregnancy may play a role also in the apparent increase in local anaesthetic sensitivity during pregnancy. For example, the spread of extradural anaesthesia is similar in patients during the first trimester of pregnancy and in term patients which indicates that mechanical factors alone cannot explain the enhanced spread of anaesthesia in parturients (Fagraeus et al., 1983). Isolated nerve studies have shown a more rapid onset and an increased sensitivity to local anaesthetic-induced conduction blockade in vagus nerves obtained from pregnant rabbits (Datta et al., 1983). These results suggest that hormonal changes associated with pregnancy may alter the basic responsiveness of the nerve membrane to local anaesthetics. Thus, the drug dosage for any regional anaesthetic procedure probably should be reduced in patients during all stages of pregnancy.

Specific local anaesthetic agents (Table 57.2)

Amino ester agents

COCAINE

This compound, which was isolated from the Erythroxylin coca bush, was the first agent employed successfully for the production of clinical local anaesthesia. The relatively high potential for systemic toxicity and

Table 57.2 Clinical use of local anaesthetic agents

Agents	Primary clinical uses	Comments
Amino esters		
Cocaine	Topical	Limited use due to addictive potential
Procaine	Infiltration Spinal	Limited use due to: Slow onset Short duration Allergic potential
Chloroprocaine	Peripheral nerve blocks Obstetrical extradural blocks	Fast onset Short duration Low systemic toxicity
Amethocaine	Spinal anaesthesia	Limited use except for spinal anaesthesia due to: Slow onset High systemic toxicity
Amino amides		
Lignocaine	Infiltration i.v. regional anaesthesia Peripheral nerve block Surgical and obstetrical extradural blocks Spinal anaesthesia Topical	Most versatile agent
Mepivacaine	Infiltration Peripheral nerve blocks Surgical extradural blocks	Similar to lignocaine
Prilocaine	Infiltration i.v. regional anaesthesia Peripheral nerve blocks Surgical extradural blocks	Met-haemoglobinaemia at high doses Least systemic toxicity of amide agents
Bupivacaine	Infiltration Peripheral nerve blocks Obstetrical and surgical extradural blocks Spinal anaesthesia	Sensory/motor separation
Etidocaine	Infiltration Peripheral nerve blocks Surgical extradural blocks	Profound motor block
Miscellaneous		
Nupercaine	Spinal anaesthesia	Use limited to spinal and topical anaesthesia
Benzocaine	Topical	Use limited to topical anaesthesia

the addiction liabilities associated with its use resulted in the abandonment of this agent for most regional anaesthetic techniques. However, cocaine is an excellent topical anaesthetic agent and is the only local anaesthetic that produces vasoconstriction at clinically useful concentrations. As a result, it is still employed to anaesthetize and constrict the nasal mucosa prior to nasotracheal intubation. It is also employed frequently by otolaryngologists during nasal surgery because of its topical anaesthetic and vasoconstrictor properties.

PROCAINE

This was the first synthetic local anaesthetic agent introduced into clinical practice. Procaine is a relatively weak local anaesthetic with a slow onset and short duration of action. The relatively low potency and rapid plasma hydrolysis of this agent are responsible for the low systemic toxicity of procaine. However, procaine is hydrolysed to para-aminobenzoic acid which is responsible for the allergic reactions associated with the repeated use of this drug. At present, procaine is used primarily for infiltration anaesthesia, diagnostic differential spinal blocks in certain pain states and obstetrical spinal anaesthesia.

CHLOROPROCAINE

This agent is characterized by a rapid onset of action, a short duration and low systemic toxicity. Chloroprocaine is employed primarily for extradural analgesia and anaesthesia in obstetrics because of its rapid onset and low systemic toxicity in mother and fetus. However, frequent injections are required in order to provide adequate pain relief during labour. Often extradural analgesia is established in the pregnant patient with chloroprocaine followed by the use of a longer-acting agent such as bupivacaine. Chloroprocaine has also proven of value for various regional anaesthetic procedures performed in ambulatory surgical patients in whom the duration of surgery is not expected to exceed 30–60 min. Some concern exists regarding the potential neurotoxicity of chloroprocaine solutions following reports of prolonged sensory/motor deficits after the accidental intrathecal injection of large doses. These local irritant effects are believed to be related to the low pH and presence of sodium bisulphite in chloroprocaine solutions.

AMETHOCAINE

This agent is used primarily for spinal anaesthesia. Amethocaine may be employed as an isobaric, hypobaric or hyperbaric solution for spinal blockade although hyperbaric solutions of amethocaine are probably employed most commonly. Amethocaine provides a relatively rapid onset of spinal anaesthesia, excellent qualities of sensory anaesthesia and a profound block of motor function. Plain solutions of amethocaine provide an average duration of spinal anaesthesia of 2–3 hr while the addition of adrenaline can extend the duration of anaesthesia to 4–6 hr.

Amethocaine is used rarely for other forms of regional anaesthesia because of its extremely slow onset of action and the potential for systemic toxic reactions when larger doses are employed. Amethocaine possesses also excellent topical anaesthetic properties, and solutions of this agent have been employed for endotracheal surface anaesthesia. The absorption of amethocaine from the tracheobronchial area is extremely rapid, and several fatalities have been reported following the use of an endotracheal aerosol of this drug.

Amino amide agents

LIGNOCAINE

Lignocaine was the first drug of the amino amide type to be introduced into clinical practice. This agent remains the most versatile and most commonly used local anaesthetic because of its inherent potency, rapid onset, moderate duration of action and topical anaesthetic activity. Solutions of lignocaine are available for infiltration, peripheral nerve blocks and extradural anaesthesia. In addition, hyperbaric lignocaine 5% is useful for spinal anaesthesia of 30–60 min duration. Lignocaine is used also in ointment, jelly, viscous and aerosol preparations for a variety of topical anaesthetic procedures.

Intravenous lignocaine has also proven of value for certain non-anaesthetic indications. This agent has gained wide acceptance as an intravenous drug for the treatment of ventricular arrhythmias. In addition, lignocaine has been employed intravenously as an antiepileptic agent, as an analgesic for certain chronic pain states and as a supplement to general anaesthesia.

MEPIVACAINE

This agent is similar to lignocaine in its anaesthetic profile. Mepivacaine can produce a profound depth of anaesthesia with a relatively rapid onset and a moderate duration of action. This agent may be used for infiltration, peripheral nerve blocks and extradural anaesthesia, and in some countries, 4% hyperbaric solutions of mepivacaine are available also for spinal anaesthesia.

Mepivacaine is not effective as a topical anaesthetic agent and so is less versatile than lignocaine. In addition, the metabolism of mepivacaine is prolonged markedly in the fetus and newborn such that this agent is not employed usually for obstetrical anaesthesia. However, in adults, mepivacaine appears to be somewhat less toxic than lignocaine. In addition, the vasodilator activity of mepivacaine is less than that of lignocaine. Thus, mepivacaine provides a somewhat longer duration of anaesthesia than lignocaine when the two agents are used without adrenaline.

PRILOCAINE

The clinical profile of prilocaine is also similar to that of lignocaine. Prilocaine has a relatively rapid onset of action, whilst providing a moderate duration of anaesthesia and a profound depth of conduction blockade. This agent causes significantly less vasodilatation than lignocaine and so can be used without adrenaline. In general, the duration of prilocaine without adrenaline is similar to that of lignocaine with adrenaline. Thus, prilocaine is particularly useful in patients in whom adrenaline may be contra-indicated. Prilocaine is useful for infiltration, peripheral nerve blockade and extradural anaesthesia.

Prilocaine is the least toxic of the amino amide local anaesthetics. Thus, this agent is particularly useful for intravenous regional anaesthesia as CNS toxic effects are seen rarely following tourniquet deflation even when early accidental release of the tourniquet may occur.

Met-haemoglobinaemia may occur following the use of relatively large doses of prilocaine. This unusual side-effect has essentially eliminated the use of this drug in obstetrics, although prilocaine has not been reported to cause any significant adverse effects in mother, fetus or newborn. However, the cyanotic appearance of newborns delivered to mothers who have received prilocaine for extradural anaesthesia during labour results in sufficient confusion concerning the aetiology of the cyanosis such that the obstetrical use of this potentially valuable drug has been virtually abandoned.

BUPIVACAINE

Bupivacaine was the first local anaesthetic that combined the properties of an acceptable onset, long duration of action, profound conduction blockade and significant separation of sensory anaesthesia and motor blockade. This agent is used for various regional anaesthetic procedures, including infiltration, peripheral nerve blocks, extradural and spinal anaesthe-

sia. The average duration of surgical anaesthesia of bupivacaine varies from approximately 3 to 10 hr. Its longest duration of action occurs when major peripheral nerve blocks such as brachial plexus blockade are performed.

The major advantage of bupivacaine appears to be in the area of extradural obstetrical analgesia for labour where satisfactory pain relief of 2–3 hr duration is achieved which significantly decreases the need for repeated injections in the pregnant patient. Moreover, adequate analgesia is achieved usually without significant motor blockade such that the patient in labour is able to move her legs. This differential blockade of sensory and motor fibres is also the basis for the widespread use of bupivacaine for postoperative extradural analgesia and for certain chronic pain states.

ETIDOCAINE

This agent is characterized by very rapid onset, prolonged duration of action, and profound sensory and motor blockade. Etidocaine may be used for infiltration, peripheral nerve blockade and extradural anaesthesia. Etidocaine has a significantly more rapid onset of action than bupivacaine. Concentrations of etidocaine which are required for adequate sensory anaesthesia produce profound motor blockade. As a result, etidocaine is useful primarily as an anaesthetic for surgical procedures in which muscle relaxation is required. Thus, this agent is of limited use for obstetrical extradural analgesia and for postoperative pain relief because it does not provide a differential blockade of sensory and motor fibres.

Miscellaneous

NUPERCAINE (DIBUCAINE—USP)

This agent is used for spinal and topical anaesthesia. It is available in isobaric, hypobaric and hyperbaric solutions for spinal anaesthesia. Nupercaine is more potent than amethocaine whilst the onset of action of the two agents is similar. The duration of spinal anaesthesia is slightly longer with nupercaine. The degree of hypotension and the profoundness of motor blockade appear to be less in patients receiving intrathecal nupercaine compared with subjects in whom amethocaine was administered into the subarachnoid space, although the spread of sensory anaesthesia was similar in the two groups.

BENZOCAINE

This local anaesthetic is used exclusively for topical anaesthesia. It is available in a variety of proprietary and non-proprietary preparations. The most common forms used in an operating room setting are as aerosol solutions for endotracheal administration and an ointment for lubrication of endotracheal tubes.

Toxicity of local anaesthetic agents

Local anaesthetic agents are relatively free from side-effects if they are administered in an appropriate dosage and in the appropriate anatomical location. However, systemic and localized toxic reactions may occur, usually from the accidental intravascular or intrathecal injection or the administration of an excessive dose of local anaesthetic agent. In addition, specific adverse effects are associated with the use of certain agents such as allergic reactions to the amino ester or procaine-like drugs, and met-haemoglobinaemia following the use of prilocaine.

Systemic toxicity

Systemic reactions to local anaesthetics involve primarily the CNS and the cardiovascular system. In general, the CNS is more susceptible to the systemic actions of local anaesthetic agents than the cardiovascular system. The dose and blood concentration of local anaesthetic required to produce CNS toxicity is usually lower than that which results in circulatory collapse. Although local anaesthetic-induced cardiovascular depression occurs less frequently than CNS reactions, adverse effects involving the cardiovascular system tend to be more serious and more difficult to manage.

CENTRAL NERVOUS SYSTEM TOXICITY

The initial symptoms of local anaesthetic-induced CNS toxicity involve feelings of light-headedness and dizziness followed frequently by visual and auditory disturbances such as difficulty in focusing and tinnitus. Other subjective CNS symptoms include disorientation and occasional feelings of drowsiness. Objective signs of CNS toxicity are usually excitatory in nature and include shivering, muscular twitching and tremors involving initially muscles of the face and distal parts of the extremities. Ultimately, generalized convulsions of a tonic–clonic nature occur. If a sufficiently large dose

or a rapid intravenous injection of a local anaesthetic agent is administered, the initial signs of CNS excitation are followed rapidly by a state of generalized CNS depression. Seizure activity ceases and respiratory depression and ultimately respiratory arrest may occur. In some patients CNS depression without a preceding excitatory phase is seen, particularly if other CNS-depressant drugs have been administered.

Central nervous system excitation is believed to be the result of an initial blockade of inhibitory pathways in the cerebral cortex by local anaesthetic drugs (DeJong, 1977). The blockade of inhibitory pathways allows facilitatory neurons to function in an unopposed fashion which results in an increase in excitatory activity leading to convulsions. An increase in the dose of local anaesthetic administered leads to an inhibition of conduction in both inhibitory and facilitatory pathways resulting in a generalized state of CNS depression.

In general, a correlation exists between anaesthetic potency and intravenous CNS toxicity of various agents (Englesson, 1974). For example, in cats, the dose of procaine required to cause convulsions is approximately seven times greater than the convulsion dose of bupivacaine. However, bupivacaine is also approximately eight times more potent than procaine as a local anaesthetic agent. A similar study in dogs indicated that the relative CNS toxicity of bupivacaine etidocaine and lignocaine is 4:2:1 which is similar to the relative potency of these agents for the production of regional anaesthesia in man (Liu et al., 1983). Intravenous infusion studies in human volunteers have demonstrated also a relationship between the intrinsic anaesthetic potency of various agents and the dosage required to induce CNS toxicity.

The rate of injection and rapidity with which a particular blood concentration is achieved alters the toxicity of local anaesthetic agents. For example, in human volunteers an average dose of 236 mg of etidocaine and a venous blood concentration of 3.0 μg/ml were required before the onset of CNS symptoms occurred when an infusion rate of 10 mg/min was employed (Scott, 1981). When the infusion rate was increased to 20 mg/min, an average dose of 161 mg of etidocaine, which produced a venous plasma concentration of approximately 2 μg/ml, resulted in symptoms of CNS toxicity.

The acid–base status of animals and patients can affect markedly the CNS activity of local anaesthetic agents. In cats, the convulsive threshold of various local anaesthetics was related inversely to the arterial

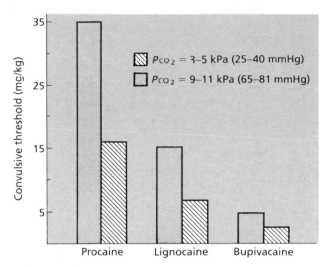

Fig. 57.8 Effect of hypercapnia on the convulsive threshold of procaine, lignocaine and bupivacaine.

P_{CO_2} level. (Fig. 57.8). For example, when the P_{CO_2} was elevated from 3.3–5.3 kPa (25–40 mmHg) to 8.7–10.8 kPa (65–81 mmHg) the convulsive threshold of procaine, mepivacaine, prilocaine, lignocaine and bupivacaine was decreased by approximately 50%. A decrease in arterial pH decreases also the convulsive threshold of these agents. In fact, pH exerts probably a greater influence on CNS toxicity of local anaesthetics than does P_{CO_2}. Respiratory acidosis with a resultant increase in P_{CO_2} and a decrease in arterial pH decrease consistently the convulsant threshold of local anaesthetic agents. However, an increase in P_{CO_2} in response to an elevated arterial pH (as may occur during metabolic alkalosis) exerts less of a potentiating effect on the CNS activity of local anaesthetic agents.

This potentiating effect of acidosis and/or hypercapnia may be a result of several factors. An elevation of P_{CO_2} enhances cerebral blood flow so that more anaesthetic agent is delivered to the brain. In addition, in the presence of hypercapnia, diffusion of carbon dioxide across the nerve membrane may result in a reduction in intracellular pH. Intracellular acidosis augments the conversion of the base form of local anaesthetic agents to the cationic form, resulting in an increase in the intraneuronal concentration of the active form of the local anaesthetic agent. The cationic form does not diffuse well across the nerve membrane so that ionic trapping occurs, which increases also the apparent CNS toxicity of local anaesthetic agents.

Hypercapnia and/or acidosis decrease also the plasma protein binding of local anaesthetic agents. Therefore, an elevation in P_{CO_2} or decrease in pH increases the proportion of free drug available for diffusion into the brain. On the other hand, acidosis increases the cationic form of the local anaesthetic which should decrease the rate of diffusion.

In summary, local anaesthetic agents can exert marked effects on the CNS. In general, signs of CNS excitation leading to frank convulsions are the most common manifestation of systemic anaesthetic toxicity. Excessive doses or rapid intravenous administration of these drugs may lead also to CNS depression and respiratory arrest. In general, the potential CNS toxicity of local anaesthetics is correlated with the inherent anaesthetic potency of the various agents but the toxicity of these agents can be altered by factors such as rate of injection, hypercapnia and acidosis.

CARDIOVASCULAR SYSTEM TOXICITY

Local anaesthetic agents can exert a direct action both on the heart and peripheral blood vessels.

Direct cardiac effects

The primary cardiac electrophysiological effect of local anaesthetics is a decrease in the maximum rate of depolarization in Purkinje fibres and ventricular muscle. This reduction in the maximum rate of depolarization is believed to result from a decrease in sodium conductance in the fast sodium channels in cardiac membranes.

Action potential duration and the effective refractory period are decreased also by local anaesthetics. However, the ratio of effective refractory period to action potential duration is increased both in Purkinje fibres and in ventricular muscle.

Qualitative differences may exist between the electrophysiological effects of various agents. Bupivacaine depresses the rapid phase of depolarization (V_{max}) in Purkinje fibres and ventricular muscle to a greater extent than lignocaine (Clarkson & Hohdeghem, 1985). In addition, the rate of recovery from a steady-state block is slower in bupivacaine-treated papillary muscles as compared with lignocaine. This slow rate of recovery results in an incomplete restoration of V_{max} between action potentials particularly at high heart rates. In contrast, recovery from lignocaine is complete, even at rapid heart rates. These differential effects of lignocaine and bupivacaine may explain the anti-arrhythmic properties of lignocaine and the arrhythmogenic potential of bupivacaine.

Electrophysiological studies in intact dogs and in man reflect essentially the findings observed in isolated cardiac tissue. As the dose and blood concentrations of lignocaine increase, a prolongation of conduction time through various parts of the heart occurs. These are reflected in the ECG as an increase in the PR interval and QRS duration. Extremely high concentrations of local anaesthetics depress spontaneous pacemaker activity in the sinus node resulting in sinus bradycardia and sinus arrest.

Local anaesthetic agents exert also profound effects on the mechanical activity of cardiac muscle. All local anaesthetics exert a dose-dependent, negative inotropic action on isolated cardiac tissue. This depression of cardiac contractility is proportional to the conduction-blocking potency of the various agents in isolated nerves (Block & Covino, 1982). Thus, the more potent local anaesthetics depress cardiac contractility at lower concentrations than the less potent drugs (Table 57.3). In general, local anaesthetics can be allocated into three groups in terms of their myocardial-depressant effect. The more potent agents, bupivacaine, amethocaine and etidocaine, depress cardiac contractility at the lowest concentrations. The agents of moderate anaesthetic potency i.e. lignocaine, mepivacaine, prilocaine, chloroprocaine form an intermediate group of compounds in terms of myocardial depression. Finally, procaine and chloroprocaine, which are the least potent of local anaesthetics, require the highest concentration to decrease cardiac contractility.

Studies in intact dogs in which a strain gauge arch was sutured to the right ventricle, revealed that all local anaesthetic agents evaluated exerted a negative inotropic action (Stewart et al., 1963). As in the isolated cardiac tissue studies, a relationship existed between the local anaesthetic potency of various agents and their relative myocardial-depressant effect (Fig. 57.9). For example, amethocaine, which is approximately 8–10 times more potent than procaine as

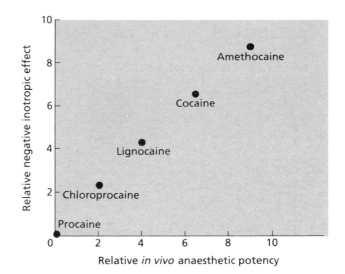

Fig. 57.9 Relationship between myocardial-depressant effect and relative anaesthetic potency of various local anaesthetics.

a local anaesthetic, was approximately eight times more potent as a depressant of myocardial contractility than procaine. Haemodynamic studies in closed-chest, anaesthetized dogs have shown that amethocaine, etidocaine and bupivacaine caused a 50% decrease in cardiac output at doses of 10–20 mg/kg, whilst 30–40 mg/kg of lignocaine, mepivacaine, prilocaine and chloroprocaine were required for a similar decrease in cardiac output. A dose of 100 mg/kg of procaine was needed to reduce cardiac output by 50%.

The mechanism by which local anaesthetics depress myocardial contractility is not known precisely but may involve an interaction with calcium. Both procaine and amethocaine can increase the release of calcium from isolated skeletal muscle preparations. The relative potency of amethocaine and procaine in terms of their ability to increase the rate of calcium

Table 57.3 Comparative effect of various local anaesthetic agents on cardiac contractility and cardiac output

Agent	Relative anaesthetic potency	Contractility of isolated guinea pig heart (50% ↓) μg/ml	Cardiac output in dogs (50% ↓) mg/kg
Procaine	1	277	100
Chloroprocaine	1	102	30
Cocaine	2	56	—
Lignocaine	2	67	30
Prilocaine	2	42	40
Mepivacaine	2	55	40
Etidocaine	6	—	20
Bupivacaine	8	6	10
Amethocaine	8	6	20

efflux from sartorius muscle was proportional to their local anaesthetic activity. A similar displacement of calcium from cardiac muscle should result in a decrease in myocardial contractility. However, studies in the isolated guinea pig heart indicated that an increase in the extracellular concentration of calcium failed to reverse the negative inotropic action of bupivacaine or lignocaine.

Direct peripheral vascular effects

Local anaesthetic agents appear to exert a biphasic effect on peripheral vascular smooth muscle. Direct measurements of the arteriolar diameter in the cremaster muscle of rats revealed that concentrations of lignocaine varying from 10^0 to 10^3 μg/ml produced a dose-related state of vasoconstriction varying from 88 to 60% of the control vascular diameter (Johns *et al.*, 1985). An increase in the concentration of lignocaine to 10^4 μg/ml produced approximately a 27% increase in arteriolar diameter indicative of a significant degree of vasodilatation. Isolated rat portal vein studies have demonstrated also that local anaesthetic drugs stimulate spontaneous myogenic contractions and augment basal tone at low concentrations but inhibit myogenic activity at higher concentrations.

In vivo studies have confirmed also the biphasic effect of local anaesthetics on the peripheral vasculature. Blood flow investigations in animal and man have demonstrated that lower doses of local anaesthetics may decrease peripheral arterial flow without any change in systemic arterial pressure, which is indicative of an increase in peripheral vascular resistance. Higher doses of local anaesthetics result in an increased blood flow in peripheral arteries indicating a state of vasodilatation. Cocaine is the only local anaesthetic that causes vasoconstriction consistently because of its ability to inhibit the uptake of noradrenaline by storage granules. The excess concentration of free circulating noradrenaline is responsible for the vasoconstriction associated with the use of cocaine. A comparison of the peripheral vascular effects of various local anaesthetic agents has failed to demonstrate a good correlation between the relative anaesthetic potency of these agents and their ability to cause peripheral vasodilatation. However, a correlation does appear to exist between the duration of action of these agents as local anaesthetics and their duration of vasodilatation. Thus, lignocaine, mepivacaine and prilocaine cause a duration of peripheral vasodilatation of approximately 5 min following intra-arterial injection into the femoral artery of dogs. On the other hand, agents such as bupivacaine, etidocaine and amethocaine, which are long-acting local anaesthetics, produce a prolonged period of vasodilatation.

The pulmonary vasculature appears to be particularly sensitive to the stimulatory effects of local anaesthetics. Procaine increased pulmonary vascular resistance markedly in a Starling heart–lung preparation. Studies in intact anaesthetized dogs employing pulmonary artery catheters showed also that both the ester and amide agents can cause marked increases in pulmonary artery pressure and pulmonary vascular resistance. Relatively large intravenous doses of procaine, chloroprocaine and amethocaine caused increases in pulmonary vascular resistance of approximately 300%. Increases of 100–200% in pulmonary vascular resistance were observed after the administration of 3 mg/kg of bupivacaine and etidocaine. The administration of 10 mg/kg doses of mepivacaine, lignocaine and procaine resulted in increases in pulmonary vascular resistance of approximately 50–100%. At doses of local anaesthetics which approached lethal levels, decreases in pulmonary artery pressure and pulmonary vascular resistance were seen with both the ester- and amide-type local anaesthetic agents.

The biphasic peripheral vascular effect of local anaesthetic agents may be related to changes in smooth muscle concentrations of calcium. A competitive antagonism exists between local anaesthetic drugs and calcium ions in smooth muscle. Local anaesthetic compounds may displace calcium from membrane binding sites, resulting in diffusion of this ion into the smooth muscle cytoplasm. Such an increase in cytoplasmic calcium concentration should stimulate the interaction between contractile proteins leading to an increase in myogenic tone which would produce a state of vasoconstriction. However, as the concentration of local anaesthetic agent at the smooth muscle membrane is increased, the displacement of calcium by these agents decreases ultimately both the cytoplasmic calcium concentration and the interaction between the contractile protein elements of smooth muscle, which then results in a state of muscle relaxation leading to vasodilatation.

Comparative cardiovascular toxicity of local anaesthetics

In general, a direct relationship exists between the anaesthetic potency and cardiovascular depressant potential of the various agents. In recent years, the more potent drugs i.e. bupivacaine and etidocaine, have been reported to cause rapid and profound cardiovascular depression in some patients following an accidental intravascular injection. Severe cardiac arrhythmias were observed and the cardiac depression appeared resistant to various therapeutic modalities. Thus, it has been suggested that the more potent and highly lipid-soluble drugs such as bupivacaine and etidocaine may be relatively more cardiotoxic than the less potent and less lipid-soluble agents, such as lignocaine.

The cardiotoxicity of the more potent agents such as bupivacaine appears to differ from that of lignocaine in the following manner:

1 The ratio of the dosage required for irreversible cardiovascular collapse and the dosage which produces CNS toxicity (convulsions) i.e. the CC:CNS ratio, is lower for bupivacaine and etidocaine compared with lignocaine.

2 Ventricular arrhythmias and fatal ventricular fibrillation may occur following the rapid intravenous administration of a large dose of bupivacaine but not lignocaine.

3 The pregnant animal or patient may be more sensitive to the cardiotoxic effects of bupivacaine than the non-pregnant animal or patient.

4 Cardiac resuscitation is more difficult following bupivacaine-induced cardiovascular collapse.

5 Acidosis and hypoxia potentiates markedly the cardiotoxicity of bupivacaine.

CC:CNS ratio

The ratio of the dosage and blood concentrations of bupivacaine and etidocaine associated with the development of convulsive activity and cardiovascular collapse has been reported to be lower in adult sheep than that of lignocaine (Morishima *et al.*, 1985). For example, a CC:CNS dose ratio of 7.1 ± 1.1 existed for lignocaine indicating that seven times as much drug was required to induce irreversible cardiovascular collapse as was needed for the production of convulsions (Fig. 57.10). On the other hand, the CC:CNS ratio for bupivacaine was 3.7 ± 0.5 and for etidocaine 4.4 ± 0.9. Although the CNS was more sensitive to the toxic effects of all three agents, a smaller difference did exist between the dose of bupivacaine and etidocaine that caused convulsions and that which led to irreversible cardiovascular collapse as compared with lignocaine. An examination of arterial drug concentrations associated with CNS and cardiovascular toxicity re-

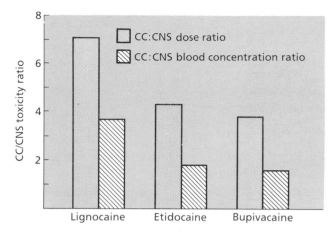

Fig. 57.10 CC:CNS dose and blood level ratio of lignocaine, etidocaine and bupivacaine in sheep.

vealed that lignocaine possessed a CC:CNS blood level ratio of 3.6 ± 0.3 compared with values of 1.6 to 1.7 for bupivacaine and etidocaine (Fig. 57.10). At the time of cardiovascular collapse, higher concentrations of bupivacaine and etidocaine were present in the myocardium compared with lignocaine. Thus, the enhanced sensitivity of the myocardium to these more potent agents appears to result from greater myocardial uptake.

Ventricular arrhythmias

A number of investigators have reported the development of ventricular arrhythmias in animals exposed to toxic doses of bupivacaine (Reiz & Nath, 1986) (Table 57.4). The incidence of ventricular fibrillation has been determined in dogs in which convulsant and supraconvulsant doses of various local anaesthetics were administered intravenously. Ventricular fibrillation did not occur in lignocaine-, mepivacaine- or amethocaine-treated dogs while approximately 20% of animals receiving etidocaine and 50% of those receiving bupivacaine developed ventricular fibrillation. The results suggest that the occurrence of ventricular fibrillation is not related to the basic piperidine ring structure of bupivacaine as mepivacaine, which contains the piperidine moiety, failed to cause these cardiac abnormalities. In addition, a precise correlation does not appear to exist between the frequency of ventricular arrhythmias and the lipid-solubility and protein binding of local anaesthetics. Large doses of etidocaine, which is more lipid-soluble than bupivacaine and equally protein bound, may cause ventricular arrhyth-

Animal model	Ventricular arrhythmias	
	Lignocaine	Bupivacaine
Unanaesthetized, paralysed cat	6% PVC	100% PVC
Anaesthetized dog	0	0
Unanaesthetized dog	0	40% VT, VF
Unanaesthetized sheep	0	80–100% PVC, VT
Hypoxic, acidotic sheep	0	17–50% VT, VF
Isolated guinea pig heart	0	30–50% PVC
		Bigeminy, trigeminy
Intracoronary injection in anaesthetized pigs	VF at 64 mg	VF at 4 mg
Intracranial injections in cats	17% VT	100% VT
Intracranial injections in rats	55% VT	55% VT
	No deaths	50% deaths

Table 57.4 Ventricular arrhythmias following the use of lignocaine and bupivacaine in various animal preparations

PVC = premature ventricular contractions.
VT = ventricular tachycardia.
VF = ventricular fibrillation.

mias and fibrillation but the incidence appears to be lower than that observed with bupivacaine.

It is not certain if the cardiac arrhythmias observed in bupivacaine-treated animals is related to a direct cardiac effect or is secondary to a CNS action or both. Isolated guinea pig hearts perfused with a bupivacaine solution revealed evidence of conduction block and bigeminy and trigeminy, but did not when perfused with lignocaine. In addition, ventricular fibrillation occurred in intact pigs in which bupivacaine was injected directly into the left anterior descending coronary artery. These results suggest that the ventricular arrhythmias are the result of a direct action on the heart. On the other hand, it has been shown that the injection of bupivacaine directly into certain regions of the brain resulted in the development of cardiac arrhythmias. Moreover, bupivacaine did not cause cardiac arrhythmias in dogs anaesthetized with pentobarbitone which may be indicative of a relationship between the CNS and cardiotoxic effects of bupivacaine.

Enhanced cardiotoxicity in pregnancy

Several of the cardiotoxic reactions reported following the use of bupivacaine have occurred in pregnant patients. As a result, the 0.75% solution is no longer recommended for use in obstetrical anaesthesia in the USA or UK. Studies in pregnant and non-pregnant sheep have shown that the CC:CNS dosage ratio of bupivacaine decreased from 3.7 ± 0.5 in non-pregnant sheep to 2.7 ± 0.4 in pregnant animals (Morishima et al., 1985). However, little difference was observed in the CC:CNS blood concentration ratio which varied from 1.6 ± 0.1 in non-pregnant animals to 1.4 ± 0.1 in pregnant ewes. However, the blood concentration of bupivacaine at which circulatory collapse occurred was lower in pregnant animals. No difference in the myocardial uptake of bupivacaine in pregnant and non-pregnant sheep was observed at the time of cardiovascular collapse. Thus, if the pregnant patient is more susceptible to the cardiotoxic effects of bupivacaine, it is not apparently related to a greater myocardial uptake of drug.

Cardiac resuscitation

Cardiopulmonary resuscitation may be difficult in patients in whom cardiotoxicity has occurred following the administration of a toxic dose of bupivacaine. Studies in acidotic and hypoxic sheep have indicated also that cardiac resuscitation following bupivacaine-induced toxicity is difficult (Covino, 1986b). Recent studies in cats and hypoxic dogs rendered toxic with bupivacaine indicate that resuscitation is possible if massive doses of adrenaline and atropine are employed. In addition, it has been shown that bretylium but not lignocaine could reverse the cardiodepressant effects of bupivacaine in dogs and also raise the threshold for ventricular tachycardia.

Effect of acidosis and hypoxia

Changes in acid–base status alter the potential cardiovascular toxicity of local anaesthetic agents (Covino, 1986). Isolated atrial tissue studies have shown that hypercapnia, acidosis and hypoxia tend to potentiate the negative chronotropic and inotropic action of lignocaine and bupivacaine. In particular, the combination of hypoxia and acidosis appears to potentiate markedly the cardiodepressant effects of bupivacaine. Hypoxia and acidosis increased markedly the frequency of cardiac arrhythmias and the mortality rate in sheep following the intravenous administration of bupivacaine. Enhanced toxicity in the presence of acidosis does not appear related to a greater myocardial tissue uptake of local anaesthetic because investigations in rabbits demonstrated a decreased cardiac concentration of bupivacaine in the presence of acidosis. Marked hypercapnia, acidosis and hypoxia occur very rapidly in some patients following seizure activity after the rapid accidental intravascular injection of local anaesthetic agents. Thus, the rapid cardiovascular depression observed in some patients following the accidental intravenous injection of bupivacaine may be related in part to the severe acid–base changes that occur during toxic reactions to these agents.

MISCELLANEOUS SYSTEMIC EFFECTS

A variety of miscellaneous systemic actions has been ascribed to local anaesthetic drugs, most of which are related to the generalized membrane-stabilizing property of this class of drugs. For example, local anaesthetics have been reported to possess neuromuscular blocking, ganglionic-blocking and anticholinergic activity. There is little evidence to suggest that any of these miscellaneous effects are clinically significant under normal conditions.

A unique systemic side-effect associated with a specific local anaesthetic agent is the formation of met-haemoglobinaemia following the administration of large doses of prilocaine. A dose–response relationship exists between the amount of prilocaine administered extradurally and the degree of met-haemoglobinaemia. In general, doses of prilocaine of 600 mg are required for the development of clinically significant levels of met-haemoglobinaemia. The formation of met-haemoglobinaemia is believed to be related to the chemical structure of prilocaine. This agent lacks a methyl group in the benzene ring. The metabolism of prilocaine in the liver results in the formation of *o*-toluidine which is responsible for the oxidation of haemoglobin to met-haemoglobin. The met-haemoglobinaemia associated with the use of prilocaine is reversible spontaneously or may be treated by the intravenous administration of methylene blue.

ALLERGIC EFFECTS

The amino ester agents such as procaine have been shown to produce allergic-type reactions. These agents are derivatives of para-aminobenzoic acid which is known to be allergenic in nature. The amino amide local anaesthetics are not derivatives of para-aminobenzoic acid and allergic reactions to the amino amides are extremely rare. Intradermal injections of both amino ester and amino amide local anaesthetics have been made in patients with and without a presumptive history of local anaesthetic allergy. Positive skin reactions were observed in 25 of 60 patients who did not describe any previous allergic symptomatology. In all cases, the cutaneous reactions occurred following the injection of an amino ester type of agent such as procaine, amethocaine and chloroprocaine. No cutaneous reactions occurred following the use of the amino amide agents, namely lignocaine, mepivacaine or prilocaine. Eleven patients were studied with a history of alleged local anaesthetic allergy. Eight of these patients showed a positive skin reaction to procaine, amethocaine or chloroprocaine. However, no positive cutaneous response was seen following the administration of lignocaine, mepivacaine or prilocaine. No signs of systemic anaphylaxis occurred in any of the subjects. It should be remembered that although the amino amide agents appear to be relatively free from allergic-type reactions, solutions of these agents may contain a preservative, methylparaben, whose chemical structure is similar to that para-aminobenzoic acid. It has been shown that patients in whom methylparaben was administered intradermally demonstrated a positive skin reaction.

Local tissue toxicity

Local anaesthetic agents which are employed clinically rarely produce localized nerve damage. Studies on isolated frog sciatic nerve revealed that concentrations of procaine, cocaine, amethocaine and nupercaine required to produce irreversible conduction blockade are far in excess of the concentration of these agents used clinically. A comparison of the intrathecal administration of lignocaine, amethocaine or etidocaine in

Type of study	Results
In vitro rabbit vagus nerve	Local irritation with 2-CP, but not lignocaine and bupivacaine
In vivo rat sciatic nerve	No irritation with 2-CP and lignocaine
In vitro rabbit vagus nerve	Irreversible block with commercial 2-CP and Na bisulphite but not with pure 2-CP
Spinal dog	Paralysis with 2-CP, but not with bupivacaine or low pH saline
Spinal rabbit	Paralysis with commercial 2-CP and Na bisulphite but not with pure 2-CP
Spinal sheep	Minimal toxicity with 2-CP, lignocaine, bupivacaine and control solution
Spinal monkey	Minimal toxicity with 2-CP and bupivacaine

Table 57.5 Animal studies concerning potential neurotoxicity of 2-chloroprocaine (2-CP) and other local anaesthetics

rabbits revealed histopathological spinal cord changes following the use of amethocaine 2% which is considerably greater than the maximum concentration of 1% employed for spinal anaesthesia in man. In recent years, prolonged sensory motor deficits have been reported in some patients following usually the extradural or subarachnoid injection of large doses of this particular drug (Ravindran *et al.*, 1980; Reisner *et al.*, 1980). Studies in animals have proven somewhat contradictory regarding the potential neurotoxicity of chloroprocaine (Table 57.5). The aetiology of the local neural irritation associated with the use of chloroprocaine solutions is believed to be related to the low pH and presence of the antioxidant, sodium bisulphite, in these solutions.

Paralysis was observed in rabbits in which intrathecal chloroprocaine solutions which contained sodium bisulphite were employed (Wang *et al.*, 1984). The use of pure solutions of chloroprocaine without sodium bisulphite did not cause paralysis, whereas the sodium bisulphite alone was associated with paralysis. A detailed study has been conducted on the isolated rabbit vagus nerve to investigate the neurotoxicity of the various components of commercial chloroprocaine solutions (Gissen *et al.*, 1984). Commercial solutions of chloroprocaine 3% contain the local anaesthetic agent itself, sodium bisulphite 0.2% and hydrogen ions which yield a pH of approximately 3.0. Application of commercial chloroprocaine 3% to isolated vagus nerves for 30 min resulted in irreversible conduction blockade. The use of a chloroprocaine 3% with sodium bisulphite solution buffered to a pH of 7.0 caused reversible conduction block. A chloroprocaine 3%

solution with a pH of 3.0 but without sodium bisulphite resulted also in reversible blockade. Application of an sodium bisulphite 0.2% solution at a pH of 3.0 resulted in irreversible conduction block whereas the use of a sodium bisulphite 0.2% solution with a pH of 7.0 caused no conduction block. The results of these studies suggest that the combination of a low pH and the presence of sodium bisulphite may be responsible for the neurotoxic reactions observed following the use of large amounts of chloroprocaine solution. Chloroprocaine, itself, does not appear to be neurotoxic.

Skeletal muscle appears to be more sensitive to the local irritant properties of local anaesthetic agents than other tissues. Skeletal muscle changes have been observed with most of the clinically used local anaesthetic agents such as lignocaine, mepivacaine, prilocaine, bupivacaine and etidocaine. In general, the more potent, longer-acting agents such as bupivacaine and etidocaine appear to cause a greater degree of localized skeletal muscle damage than the less potent, shorter-acting agents such as lignocaine and prilocaine. This effect on skeletal muscle is reversible, and muscle regeneration occurs rapidly and is complete within 2 weeks following injection of local anaesthetic agents. These changes in skeletal muscle have not been correlated with any overt clinical signs of local irritation.

Complications of regional anaesthesia

Certain regional anaesthetic techniques such as extradural or spinal anaesthesia are associated with sympathetic blockade that may result in profound hypotension. In general, the degree of hypotension is related to the extent of the sympathetic blockade.

Extradural anaesthesia

Cardiovascular alterations following extradural blockade are related to:
1 The level of block.
2 Drug dosage.
3 Specific local anaesthetic agent.
4 Addition of vasoconstrictors.
5 Blood volume status of the patient.

LEVEL OF BLOCK

Extradural blockade to the T5 dermatomal level or below is not accompanied usually by significant cardiovascular alterations (Bonica et al., 1970). As the level of anaesthesia extends from T5 to T1, a 20% fall in systemic arterial pressure has been observed. This hypotensive state is related almost exclusively to sympathetic inhibition and peripheral vasodilatation below the level of block which results in a significant decrease in systemic vascular resistance. At dermatomal levels of T1 and above, a reduction in heart rate and cardiac output may occur. The reduction in cardiac output may be related in part to the inhibition of myocardial sympathetic fibres resulting in a decreased cardiac contractility and also in a decrease in venous return from venodilatation and expansion of capacitance vessels.

DRUG DOSAGE

Relatively large amounts of local anaesthetic drug are required to achieve a satisfactory degree of extradural blockade. These local anaesthetic agents are absorbed rather rapidly and significant blood concentrations may be achieved. The absorbed local anaesthetic agent may produce systemic effects involving the cardiovascular system as discussed above. Blood concentrations of lignocaine of less than 4 μg/ml following extradural blockade resulted in a slight increase in arterial pressure produced by an increased cardiac output (Bonica et al., 1970). Doses of extradural lignocaine which produced blood concentrations in excess of 4 μg/ml caused hypotension resulting in part from the negative inotropic and the peripheral vasodilator actions of the drug.

SPECIFIC LOCAL ANAESTHETIC DRUG

Differences in the onset of extradural anaesthesia occur as a function of the specific agent employed. For example, drugs such as chloroprocaine, lignocaine and etidocaine produce a fairly rapid onset of anaesthesia, whilst bupivacaine has been shown to exert a significantly slower onset of action. The more rapidly acting agents produce a more profound degree of hypotension as a result of the more rapid blockade of sympathetic fibres. In addition, certain agents such as etidocaine can penetrate myelinated fibres more readily and again may be associated with a more profound degree of sympathetic blockade and hypotension.

ADDITION OF VASOCONSTRICTOR AGENTS

Adrenaline is added frequently to local anaesthetics intended for extradural use in order to decrease the rate of vascular absorption and prolong the duration of anaesthesia. Absorbed adrenaline itself may produce transient cardiovascular alterations. An exaggerated hypotensive effect has been reported following the use of adrenaline-containing local anaesthetics for extradural blockade (Bonica et al., 1972). The absorbed adrenaline is believed to stimulate β_2-adrenergic receptors in peripheral vascular beds leading to a state of vasodilatation and a reduction in diastolic arterial pressure. The β_1-adrenergic receptor stimulating effect of adrenaline results in an increase in heart rate and cardiac output which counteracts the peripheral vasodilator state to some extent. Although absorbed adrenaline may be responsible for the early cardiovascular changes observed following extradural blockade, the more prolonged hypotension seen after extradural anaesthesia with adrenaline-containing local anaesthetics is related probably to the achievement of a more profound degree of sympathetic blockade.

BLOOD VOLUME STATUS OF THE PATIENT

Cardiovascular depression is more severe and more dangerous following the production of extradural anaesthesia in hypovolaemic patients (Bonica et al., 1972). Extradural anaesthesia in hypovolaemic volunteers was associated with profound hypotension resulting from peripheral vasodilatation and a decrease in cardiac output and heart rate. The addition of adrenaline to the anaesthetic solution resulted in a less profound degree of hypotension in these subjects but was unable to prevent a significant reduction in systemic arterial pressure. The failure of adrenaline to increase cardiac output sufficiently in these subjects to prevent marked hypotension is obviously a result of the diminished circulating blood volume.

Spinal anaesthesia

In general, systemic hypotension occurs following the induction of spinal anaesthesia by blockade of sympathetic fibres. The degree of hypotension appears to be related almost exclusively to the extent of sensory and sympathetic blockade. Studies in man have shown that subarachnoid anaesthesia to the T5 level caused a decrease in stroke volume, cardiac output and peripheral vascular resistance (Ward *et al.*, 1965). The decrease in cardiac output and stroke volume following spinal anaesthesia which extends to the mid-thoracic level, is not believed to be related to a decrease in myocardial contractility but rather to a decrease in venous return. Placement of patients in a slightly head-down position or the infusion of crystalloid solutions are usually sufficient to reverse the hypotensive state. Studies have been carried out in monkeys in which the level of sensory anaesthesia following the intrathecal administration of amethocaine has been correlated with the degree of hypotension (Sivarajan *et al.*, 1975). Anaesthesia to the T10 dermatomal level resulted in a reduction in arterial pressure of approximately 15%. This hypotension was a result almost exclusively of a decrease in peripheral vascular resistance with little change in cardiac output. However, extension of the level of sympathetic and sensory block to the T1 dermatomal level was associated with a 35% decrease in arterial pressure. This exaggerated state of hypotension was caused in part by a decrease in peripheral vascular resistance but also by a significant reduction in cardiac output.

Conclusion

Local anaesthetics may be classified into three groups according to their potency and duration of action. Procaine and chloroprocaine are relatively weak agents of short duration. Lignocaine, mepivacaine and prilocaine are intermediate in terms of potency and duration. Amethocaine, bupivacaine and etidocaine are potent local anaesthetics with a prolonged duration of action. With regard to onset time, chloroprocaine, lignocaine, mepivacaine, prilocaine and etidocaine have a relatively rapid onset of action. Bupivacaine is intermediate whilst procaine and amethocaine demon-

strate a long latency period. Anaesthetic activity is determined primarily by physico-chemical factors such as pKa, lipid-solubility and protein binding. *In vivo* the anaesthetic properties of the various agents can be modified by the dosage administered, addition of vasoconstrictors, site of injection, carbonation and pH adjustment of solutions, use of additives or mixture of agents and the physiological status of the patient such as pregnancy.

The toxicity of local anaesthetics involves primarily the CNS and cardiovascular system. Central nervous system toxicity involves primarily excitation and convulsions. Large doses of local anaesthetics may lead to generalized CNS depression. The rapid intravenous administration or injection of large doses of local anaesthetics can cause hypotension, bradycardia and ultimately cardiac arrest. Certain agents such as bupivacaine may also produce ventricular arrhythmias. In general, the potential for CNS and cardiovascular toxicity is related to the anaesthetic potency of the various agents. Allergic reactions to local anaesthetic agents are limited primarily to the amino ester drugs by the metabolic formation of para-aminobenzoic acid. Met-haemoglobinaemia may occur following the administration of large doses of prilocaine.

Complications of regional anaesthesia are most frequent with extradural and spinal anaesthesia. Hypotension is the most common complication produced by sympathetic blockade associated with these regional anaesthetic procedures.

In general, local anaesthetic agents are very effective and relatively safe drugs when used correctly. However, as with any class of drugs, safe and effective regional anaesthesia requires a knowledge of the pharmacology and toxicity of the various agents, ability to perform regional anaesthesia correctly and a careful evaluation of the clinical status of the patient.

References

Block A. & Covino B.G. (1982) Effect of local anesthetic agents on cardiac conduction and contractility. *Regional Anesthesia* **6**, 55–61.

Bonica J.J., Berges P.V. & Morikawa K. (1970) Circulatory effects of peridural block. I. Effects of level of analgesia and dose of lidocaine. *Anesthesiology* **33**, 619–26.

Bonica J.J., Kennedy W.F., Akamatsu T.J. & Gerbershagen H.V. (1972) Circulatory effects of peridural block. III. Effects of acute blood loss. *Anesthesiology* **36**, 219–27.

Bridenbaugh L.D. (1978) Does the addition of low molecular weight dextran prolong the duration of action of bupivacaine? *Regional Anesthesia* **3**, 6.

Bromage P.R. (1965) A comparison of the hydrochloride and carbon dioxide salts of lidocaine and prilocaine in epidural analgesia. *Acta Anaesthesiologia Scandinavica* **16** (Suppl.), 55–69.

Bromage P.R. (1970) An evaluation of two new local anaesthetics for major conduction blockade. *Canadian Anaesthetists' Society Journal* **17**, 557–64.

Brown D.T., Morrison D.H., Covino B.G. & Scott D.B. (1980) Comparison of carbonated bupivacaine and bupivacaine hydrochloride for extradural anaesthesia. *British Journal of Anaesthesia* **52**, 419–27.

Clarkson C.W. & Hohdeghem L.M. (1985) Mechanism for bupivacaine depression of cardiac conduction: fast block of sodium channels during the action potential with slow recovery from block during diastole. *Anesthesiology* **62**, 396–405.

Concepcion M., Maddi R., Francis D., Rocco A.G., Murray E. & Covino B.G. (1984) Vasoconstrictors in spinal anesthesia with tetracaine. A comparison of epinephrine and phenylephrine. *Anesthesia and Analgesia* **63**, 134–8.

Corke B.G., Carlson C.G. & Dettbarn W.D. (1984) The influence of 2-chloroprocaine on the subsequent analgesic potency of bupivacaine. *Anesthesiology* **60**, 25–7.

Covino B.G. (1986a) Pharmacology of local anaesthetic agents. *British Journal of Anaesthesia* **58**, 701–16.

Covino B.G. (1986b) Toxicity of local anesthetics. *Advances in Anesthesia* **3**, 37–65.

Datta S., Lambert D.H., Gregus J., Gissen A.J. & Covino B.G. (1983) Differential sensitivities of mammalian nerve fibers during pregnancy. *Anesthesia and Analgesia* **62**, 1070–2.

DeJong R.H. (1977) *Physiology and Pharmacology of Local Anesthesia* 2nd edn. Charles C. Thomas, Springfield, Illinois.

Englesson S. (1974) The influence of acid–base changes on central nervous system toxicity of local anesthetic agents. I. An experimental study in cats. *Acta Anaesthesiologica Scandinavica* **18**, 79–87.

Fagraeus L., Urban B.J. & Bromage P.R. (1983) Spread of analgesia in early pregnancy. *Anesthesiology* **58**, 184–7.

Gissen A.J. & Covino B.G. (1985) Differential sensitivity of fast and slow fibres in mammalian nerve. IV. Effect of carbonation of local anesthetics. *Regional Anesthesia* **10**, 68–75.

Gissen A.J., Covino B.G. & Gregus J. (1980) Differential sensitivity of mammalian nerves to local anesthetic drugs. *Anesthesiology* **53**, 467–74.

Gissen A.J., Covino B.G. & Gregus J. (1982) Differential sensitivity of fast and slow fibres in mammalian nerve. III. Effect of etidocaine and bupivacaine on fast/slow fibres. *Anesthesia and Analgesia* **61**, 570–5.

Gissen A.J., Datta S. & Lambert D. (1984) The chloroprocaine controversy II. Is chloroprocaine neurotoxic? *Regional Anesthesia* **9**, 135–45.

Hilgier M. (1985) Alkalinization of bupivacaine for branchial plexus block. *Regional Anesthesia* **10**, 59–61.

Johns R.A., Di Fazio C.A. & Longnecker D.E. (1985) Lidocaine constricts or dilates rat arterioles in a dose-dependent manner. *Anesthesiology* **62**, 141–4.

Johns R.A., Seyde W.C., Di Fazio C.A. & Longnecker D.E. (1986) Dose-dependent effects of bupivacaine on rat muscle arterioles. *Anesthesiology* **65**, 186–91.

Liu P.L., Feldman H.S., Giasi R., Patterson M.K. & Covino B.G. (1983) Comparative CNS toxicity of lidocaine, etidocaine, bupivacaine and tetracaine in awake dogs following rapid IV administration. *Anesthesia and Analgesia* **62**, 375–9.

Loder R.E. (1960) A local anaesthetic solution with longer action. *Lancet* **2**, 346–7.

McClure J.H. & Scott D.B. (1981) Comparison of bupivacaine hydrochloride and carbonated bupivacaine in brachial plexus block by the inter-scalene technique. *British Journal of Anaesthesia* **53**, 523–6.

Morishima H.O., Pedersen H., Finster M., Feldman H.S. & Covino B.G. (1983) Etidocaine toxicity in the adult, newborn and fetal sheep. *Anesthesiology* **58**, 342–6.

Morishima H.O., Pedersen H., Finster M., Hiraoka H., Tsuji A., Feldman H., Arthur G.A. & Covino B.G. (1985) Bupivacaine toxicity in pregnant and nonpregnant ewes. *Anesthesiology* **63**, 134–9.

Morrison D.H. (1981) A double-blind comparison of carbonated lidocaine and lidocaine hydrochloride in epidural anaesthesia. *Canadian Anaesthetists' Society Journal* **28**, 387–9.

Ravindran R.S., Bond V.K., Tasch M.D., Gupta C.D. & Luerssen T.G. (1980) Prolonged neural blockade following regional analgesia with 2-chloroprocaine. *Anesthesia and Analgesia* **58**, 447–51.

Reisner L.S., Hochman B.N. & Plumer M.H. (1980) Persistent neurologic deficit and adhesive arachnoiditis following intrathecal 2-chloroprocaine injection. *Anesthesia and Analgesia* **58**, 452–4.

Reiz S. & Nath S. (1986) Cardiotoxicity of local anaesthetic agents. *British Journal of Anaesthesia* **38**, 736–46.

Rosenberg P.H., Heinowen E., Jansson S.E. & Gripenberg J. (1980) Differential nerve block by bupivacaine and 2-chloroprocaine. *British Journal of Anaesthesia* **52**, 1183–9.

Scott D.B. (1981) Toxicity caused by local anaesthetic drugs. *British Journal of Anaesthesia* **53**, 553–4.

Scott D.B., McClure J.H., Giasi R.M., Seo J. & Covino B.G. (1980) Effects of concentration of local anaesthetic drugs in extradural block. *British Journal of Anaesthesia* **52**, 1033–7.

Sivarajan M., Amory D.W., Lindbloom L.E. & Schwettmann R.S. (1975) Systemic and regional blood flow changes during spinal anesthesia in the Rhesus monkey. *Anesthesiology* **43**, 78–88.

Stewart D.M., Rogers W.P., Mahaffrey J.E., Witherspoon S. & Woods E.F. (1963) Effect of local anesthetics on the cardiovascular system in the dog. *Anesthesiology* **24**, 620–4.

Wang B.C., Hillman D.E., Spiedholz N.I. & Turndorf H. (1984) Chronic neurologic deficits and nesacaine-CE—an effect of the anesthetic, 2-chloroprocaine, or the antioxidant, sodium bisulfite? *Anesthesia and Analgesia* **63**, 445–7.

Ward R.J., Bonica J.J., Freund F.G., Akamatsu T., Danziger F. & Englesson S. (1965) Epidural and subarachnoid anesthesia: cardiovascular and respiratory effects. *Journal of the American Medical Association* **191**, 275–8.

Wildsmith J.A.W., Gissen A.J., Gregus J. & Covino B.G. (1985) Differential nerve blocking activity of amino-ester local anaesthetics. *British Journal of Anaesthesia* **57**, 612–19.

Wildsmith J.A.W., Gissen A.J., Takmon B. & Covino B.G. (1987) Differential nerve blockade: esters v amides and the influence of pKa. *British Journal of Anaesthesia* **59**, 379–89.

58

Subarachnoid and Extradural Anaesthesia

H. OWEN AND M. J. COUSINS

The temporary axonal blockade produced by subarachnoid injection of a local anaesthetic solution into the cerebrospinal fluid (CSF) is termed spinal subarachnoid anaesthesia. The injection is performed usually below the termination of the spinal cord (approximately L2 in adults) to avoid damage. A small volume of local anaesthetic blocks *all* sensation rapidly.

Between the spinal dura and the spinal periosteum lies the extradural space. Neural blockade produced by injecting a relatively large volume of local anaesthetic into this space is termed either extradural or epidural anaesthesia. Not all sensory modalities may be blocked even with complete block of nociception (i.e. analgesia not anaesthesia).

Spinal administration (i.e. subarachnoid or extradural) of opioids may produce selective analgesia (Cousins *et al.*, 1979). Their analgesic effects are mediated predominantly by an action on pre- and postsynaptic receptors on the dorsal horn neuron.

The techniques of subarachnoid anaesthesia in man are less than 100 yr old and have been taught widely only since the 1950s. Extradural anaesthesia was not described until after World War I and a systematic study began in the 1960s mainly as a result of the work of Bromage (1978). The important advances in the development of spinal subarachnoid and extradural anaesthesia are summarized in Table 58.1.

Cocaine was used initially to produce subarachnoid block, but because of its inherent toxicity and short duration of action, it was not until the introduction of safer synthetic local anaesthetics that the technique became popular. The importance of the curves of the vertebral column was realized by Barker (1908) and with the manufacture of hyperbaric and hypobaric solutions of local anaesthetics, spinal anaesthesia became controllable. The popularity of spinal anaes-

thesia increased after the introduction of local anaesthetics with longer durations of action. Greater duration of effect was obtained by the addition of adrenaline to the local anaesthetic solution or by using a continuous spinal technique. Tuohy's subarachnoid

Table 58.1 Important advances in the development of spinal subarachnoid and extradural anaesthesia

1764	Cerebrospinal fluid discovered by Catugno
1853	Invention of hypodermic syringe and needle by Alexander Wood
1860	Cocaine isolated from *Erythroxylen coca*
1884	Cocaine used for topical anaesthesia of eye by Koller
1885	First spinal anaesthetic by Corning
1886	Heat sterilization described
1891	Lumbar puncture standardized by Quincke as a simple clinical procedure
1898	First planned spinal anaesthetic for surgery performed by August Bier on 16 August
1903	Adrenaline used to increase duration and reduce toxicity of spinal anaesthesia
1905	Procaine introduced
1907	Hyperbaric solution of local anaesthetic introduced
1914	Hypobaric solution of local anaesthetic introduced
1921	Extradural anaesthesia for surgery described by Pagès
1927	Ephedrine used to maintain arterial pressure during spinal anaesthesia
1931	Extradural anaesthesia re-introduced by Dogliotti
1947	First clinical use of lignocaine by Gordh
1949	'Continuous' lumbar extradural analgesia introduced by Cleland
1954	Safety of spinal anaesthesia confirmed by Vandam and Dripps

needle was adapted for a continuous extradural technique with a ureteric catheter. In the 1950s, lumbar extradural anaesthesia was used first for obstetric pain relief and then for surgery and for postoperative pain relief. The use of caudal extradural anaesthesia waned at this time, as it was recognized that the technique required larger doses of local anaesthetic and was less predictable. Spinal anaesthesia was neglected also partly because of widely publicized neurological complications and consequent legal decisions, and partly because of introduction of new drugs and techniques for general anaesthesia.

In the last 20 yr, spinal anaesthesia has again become popular: rescued by the work of Dripps and Vandam (1954) which demonstrated how safe the technique can be. The realization that general anaesthesia also has risks and hazards has promoted the techniques of both spinal and extradural anaesthesia.

The technique and anatomy of spinal subarachnoid and extradural injection using the traditional midline approach

1 Arterial pressure is measured, heart rate recorded and continuous ECG monitoring instituted.

The patient is positioned and the midline of the spine and the appropriate interspace is found by inspection and palpation.

In an ideal position, the back of the patient is at the edge of the operating table and parallel to it. The knees are flexed and drawn up as much as possible to the abdomen and the head is brought down towards the knees. Special care is required to avoid rotation of hips and shoulders. The midline cannot be located reliably under the median crease for it may sag downwards (by many millimetres in the obese). The method of Labat i.e. grasping the spinous process between thumb and forefinger, is recommended (Fig. 58.1).

The easiest and safest extradural and spinal injections are made in the mid-lumbar region. Knowledge of the surface anatomy and landmarks is therefore crucial. The line drawn between the highest point of the two iliac crests passes usually through the spinous process of the fourth lumbar vertebra (Fig. 58.2). The interspinous space above this spinous process (L3–4) or one higher (L2–3) is the standard site of needle insertion for extradural block in adults, since the spinal cord ends usually at the lower border of vertebra L1. This is not the case in children and is one reason why the caudal route of entry is preferred to the lumbar route in young children. Also, the dural sac terminates

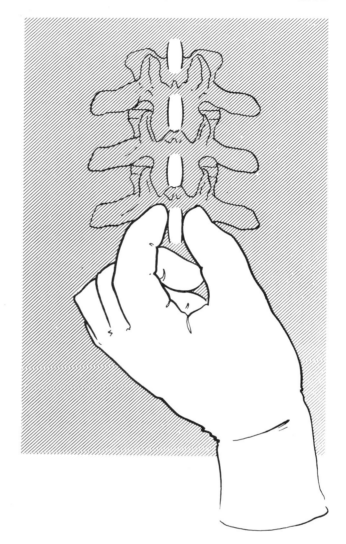

Fig. 58.1 Labat's method of checking the centre of the spinous processes uses the thumb and forefinger to grasp the spinous processes above and below the site of the needle puncture. (Reproduced from Cousins & Bridenbaugh, 1988.)

at the level of S2 in adults (S3 in small children): a line through the posterior superior iliac spines crosses this level. Attempts at puncture below L4 increases the difficulty of 'midline' extradural block because of the ill-defined interspinous ligament; also, puncture above L2 increases the risk of damage to the conus medullaris, so that the interspaces of L2–3 and L3–4 are both the safest and the easiest. Identification of L1 acts as a double check and confirms that the point of entry is safely below the conus medullaris. There is no difference in the potential danger of damaging the cord if one chooses the T12–L1 interspace or the C7–T1 interspace, both of which can often be technically easy;

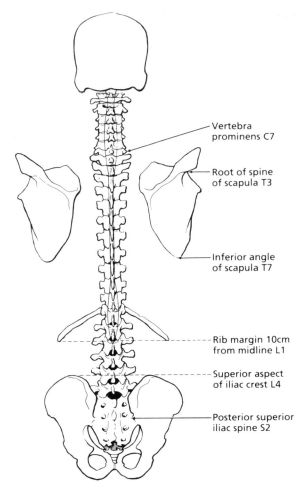

Fig. 58.2 Surface anatomy and landmarks for extradural blockade. The spinous process (vertebra prominens) at C7 is the most prominent spinous process when the neck is flexed. The spinous process at T3 lies opposite the roof of the spine of the scapula (arm by side). The spinous process at T7 lies opposite the inferior angle of the scapula (arm by side). For puncture between C7 and T1 there is direct access to the interlaminal space, but there are other hazards (see text). Puncture below T3 and above T7 is difficult because of angled spinous processes. Puncture below T7 becomes progressively similar to L2–3. Other hazards are the same as those for high puncture (see text). The spinous process at L1 (lower border) is noted by a line meeting the costal margin 10 cm from the midline. The spinous process at L4 (centre) lies at the top of the iliac crests. S2 is noted by the posterior superior iliac spines. Puncture is safest and easiest in the lumbar region. L2–3 and L3–4 are the preferred levels. (Reproduced from Cousins & Bridenbaugh, 1988.)

however, the spinal cord lies directly beneath the extradural space in both instances (Fig. 58.2). Thus, only anaesthetists experienced with extradural techniques require the anatomic landmarks above L1: the

inferior angle of scapula (T7), the root of the spine of the scapula (T3) and the vertebra prominens (C7).

Because of the extreme angulation of the spinous processes in the mid-thoracic region, midline puncture is difficult, and the paraspinous (paramedian) approach is preferable. In contrast, there is excellent access to the interlaminar space in the midline at C7–T1 and T1–2; the same applies in the low thoracic region. However, anatomical differences, such as a narrower extradural space, require greater technical skill at these levels and a technique somewhat different from that used usually for lumbar extradural block.

2 The anaesthetist scrubs and dons sterile gloves and gown. The patient is accompanied always by a nurse. A large area of the back around the chosen site is painted with antiseptic and the area draped with sterile towels. The extradural tray may be arranged whilst waiting for the antiseptic to become effective. The sterility control indicator on the tray is checked.

A small weal of anaesthetic solution is raised using a 25 or 27 gauge intradermal needle over the chosen interspace and the subcutaneous tissues are infiltrated also. A small incision in the skin is made using a scalpel blade or large needle. This prevents tough skin from gripping the needle and damping sensation, and also prevents a core of skin from being pushed into the deeper tissues.

3 The needle is pushed slowly forwards at right angles to the back in both planes. A thin flexible spinal needle (25 gauge) may require an introducer. The first resistance to advancing the needle is the supraspinous ligament (Fig. 58.3).

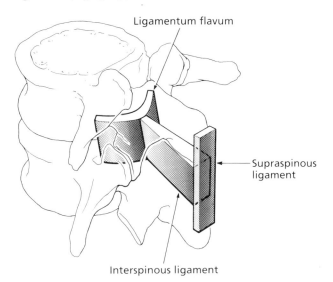

Fig. 58.3 Ligaments encountered during a midline puncture. (Reproduced from Cousins & Bridenbaugh, 1988.)

4 The supraspinous ligament is a strong fibrous cord that connects the apices of the spinous processes from the sacrum to C7, where it is continued upward to the external occipital protuberance as the ligamentum nuchae. It is thickest and broadest in the lumbar region and varies with patient age, sex and body build. In persons who engage in heavy physical activity and in labourers and the elderly, the ligament may become ossified, making midline puncture impossible.

The spinous processes are widest in the mid-lumbar region and have only a slight angulation, making insertion of the 16–18 gauge Tuohy needle into the centre of the supraspinous ligament relatively easy compared with elsewhere in the spine. The inferior border of the spinous process lies over the widest part of the interlaminar space (Fig. 58.4). The process becomes somewhat narrower superiorly, so that a needle may be guided by the lateral aspect of the spinous process to enter the mid-point of the ligamentum flavum (Fig. 58.4). In the mid-thoracic region, the spinous processes are much narrower, closer together and angulated sharply downward, thus obscuring the interlaminar space (Fig. 58.5). The inferior border of spinous processes in this region lies opposite the lamina of the vertebral body below. Insertion of an extradural needle may necessitate a paraspinous (paramedian) approach. If the needle is inserted beside the lower border of the spinous process *above* the interspace and angled upward at 130°, the lateral aspect of the process may again be used to guide the needle inward 25° towards the centre of the ligamentum flavum. In the cervical region, the spinous processes widen and become bifid with a wide supraspinous ligament. They are almost horizontal in the lower cervical region and permit easy access to the interlaminar space. The laminae and articular processes form the boundaries of the interlaminar foramen: in the lumbar region, the foramen is triangular when the lumbar spine is extended, with the base being formed by the upper borders of the laminae of the lower vertebra and the

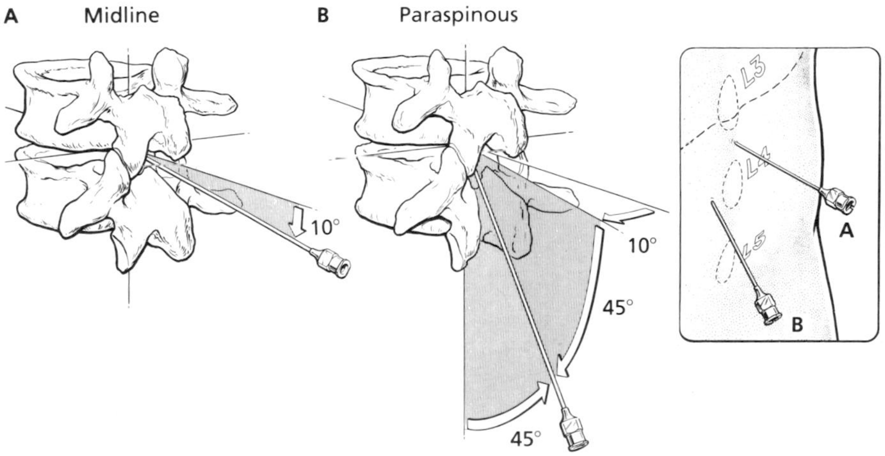

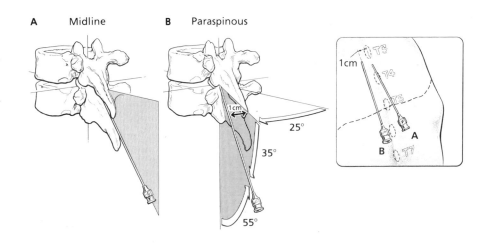

Fig. 58.4 Lumbar extradural.
A Midline. Note insertion closer to the superior spinous process and with a slight upward angulation.
B Paraspinous (paramedian). Note insertion beside caudad edge of 'inferior' spinous process, with 45° angulation to long axis of spine below. (Reproduced from Cousins & Bridenbaugh, 1988.)

Fig. 58.5 Thoracic extradural.
A Midline. Note extreme upward angulation required in mid-thoracic region. Therefore, a paraspinous approach may be easier.
B Paraspinous. Note needle insertion next to caudad tip of the spinous process above interspace of intended level of entry through ligamentum flavum. Upward angulation is 55° to long axis of spine below and inward angulation is 10° to 15°. (Reproduced from Cousins & Bridenbaugh, 1988.)

sides, by the medial aspects of the inferior articular processes of the vertebra above. However, if the lumbar spine is flexed, the inferior articular processes glide upward by means of the synovial joints between facets of articular processes, thus enlarging the interlaminar foramen to a diamond shape; borders of the superior articular process of the vertebra below now form the lower part of the lateral boundaries of the foramen (Fig. 58.2). It is worth noting that, in the lumbar region, the facets of the articular processes articulate at right angles to a circle with its centre in the middle of the vertebral body, so that rotation cannot take place; in contrast, in the thoracic region, the facets articulate in the same plane as such a horizontal circle, so that rotation of one vertebra on another occurs readily. This indicates further the potential increased difficulty of puncture in the thoracic compared with the lumbar region.

The lamina itself slopes down and back on its posterior surface, so that it may be contacted by a needle either superficially or deep. The lamina forms only the wide base of the interlaminar space; the remaining boundaries are formed laterally and superiorly by the articular processes (Fig. 58.4).

In the lumbar region, correct needle insertion takes full advantage of the fact that it is both easier and safer to insert the needle at the L2–3 or L3–4 interspace, with the needle entering the extradural space in the midline. The inferior aspects of the spinous processes, in the mid-lumbar region, lie opposite the line across the widest lateral extent of the interlaminar space. Thus, needle insertion should be close to the superior spinous process, since the upper border of the inferior spine lies over the lamina of its underlying vertebral body. A needle inserted with due regard to this requires very slight upward angulation to give an unobstructed approach to the interlaminar space (Fig. 58.4); this is in comparison with the angulation required to reach the extradural space in the thoracic region (Fig. 58.5). A surface anatomical aid that is often neglected involves checking that the needle is inserted in the centre of a line running through the middle of the superior and inferior aspects of the spinous processes: that is, in the centre of the supraspinous ligament. This is achieved best by grasping the spinous processes adjacent to the site of puncture between thumb and forefinger, while the needle is inserted through skin and subcutaneous tissue into the supraspinous ligament (Fig. 58.1). If this is done, the needle should sit firmly in the supraspinous ligament without angulation to one side. Obese subjects may require additional manoeuvres. Once pene-

trated, the supraspinous ligament supports the needle at right angles to the skin.

5 The needle is advanced further with the interspinous ligament offering continued resistance. The interspinous ligament runs obliquely between the spinous processes and is continuous anteriorly with the ligamentum flavum and posteriorly with the supraspinous ligament (Fig. 58.3). Its thickness is greatest above L4 in the lumbar region. Although it is a thin ligament, its fibres are attached along the entire superior and inferior surfaces of the spinous processes; thus, in the lumbar region, the ligament is rectangular and provides an identifiable resistance to injected air or solution.

6 An increase in resistance is felt when the needle enters the ligamentum flavum which is composed almost entirely of elastic fibres. Because of its tough elasticity and its thickness of several millimetres in the lumbar region, the ligament imparts a characteristic 'springy' resistance, particularly to a large-bore needle with an upturned end (Tuohy needle). The ligament runs from the anterior and inferior aspects of the lamina above to the posterior and superior aspects of the lamina below. Laterally, the ligament narrows as it blends with the capsule of the joint between the articular processes (Fig. 58.3). Because developmentally two laminae fuse at each level to form the root of the spinous process, two ligamenta flava meet in the median plane and here become continuous with the deep fibres of the interspinous ligament. Thus, an extradural needle advancing in the midline encounters continuing resistance that increases immediately as the needle passes into the ligamentum flavum. There is evidence from cadaver dissections that the ligamentum flavum may retain a midline cleft or sulcus in some cases.

7 After a few more millimetres advancement, a sudden loss of resistance occurs as the needle tip enters the extradural space. The distance to the extradural space from the skin varies widely. It is most commonly 4 cm (50%) and is 4–6 cm in 80% of the population according to detailed records of 3200 cases. In obese patients, however, this distance may be greater than 8 cm but is less than 3 cm in thin patients.

The ligamentum flavum should be entered in the centre of the interlaminar gap, regardless of where the needle enters the skin (midline or paraspinous). Even with midline puncture, failure to control the penetration of the ligament results in a second loss of resistance, signalling dural puncture. Entry at the lateral aspect of the interlaminar gap may result also in dural puncture, because the extradural space is narrow at this point; there is also an increased risk of puncturing an extradural vein with return of blood from the extradural needle. An aid to monitoring depth of insertion is Lee's modification of the Tuohy needle which is marked along its length in centimetre bands alternately polished and shaded.

The extradural space should permit easy injection of solution and easy threading of an extradural catheter. Uncontrolled entry or failure to fix the needle securely during subsequent injections or catheter insertions may result in pushing the needle tip forward until it touches the dura. This results in some resistance to injected local anaesthetic and may cause the extradural catheter to puncture the dura if undue force is used when catheter insertion becomes difficult. Many textbooks fail to explain why catheter insertion is impossible, and why further progress of the needle may sometimes be obstructed immediately after an otherwise impeccably correct loss of resistance through the ligamentum flavum. The explanation lies in the anatomy of the lamina and ligamentum flavum; the latter attaches to posterosuperior aspects of the lamina below. Thus, a needle piercing the ligamentum flavum at its extreme inferior aspect may be held up by the upper edge of the sloping lamina. Usually, re-insertion of the needle, more to the centre of the interlaminar space, is then necessary. Less commonly, a needle angled sharply upwards may undergo a clear-cut loss of resistance as its tip penetrates the ligamentum flavum, but attempts to pass a catheter meet with bony resistance. In this case, the recurved tip of an extradural needle still lies partially in the ligamentum flavum immediately adjacent to its attachment to the lamina above. If the extradural needle can be advanced without further resistance, and the catheter then threads easily without aspiration of CSF, this confirms a high entry through the interlaminar gap. However, recent evidence indicates that the extradural space narrows superiorly. More rarely, but of great importance, a needle angled acutely laterally may penetrate the ligamentum flavum close to a spinal nerve. Subsequent attempts to pass a catheter may lead to resistance and the immediate report of a unisegmental paraesthesia. This calls for repositioning of the needle, because persistence may lead to spinal nerve trauma.

It is unusual not to obtain a jet of CSF back through an 18 gauge (or larger) needle if it pierces the dura. Thus, the syringe should always be disconnected as soon as the loss of resistance through the ligamentum flavum is obtained, or if a subsequent second loss of

resistance is noted. The width of the posterior extradural space, beneath the ligamentum flavum, varies considerably, depending on the level of the bony spine at which it is approached and the horizontal point of needle entry; it is widest in the midline in the mid-lumbar region (5–6 mm) but narrows next to the articular processes. In the mid-thoracic region, it is 3–5 mm in the midline and very narrow laterally. In the lower cervical region, the distance between ligamentum flavum and dura is only 1.5–2 mm in the midline; however, this increases below C7 to 3–4 mm, particularly if the neck is flexed.

The extradural space extends from the base of the skull to the sacrococcygeal membrane and has complicated direct communications with the paravertebral space and indirect communications with the CSF. It leads also directly to the vascular system by way of its large extradural veins, which have no valves and connect with the basivertebral venous plexus, intracranial veins (if flow is reversed by high thoraco-abdominal pressure) and the azygos vein. These are potential direct routes to the brain and heart for drugs, air or other material injected inadvertently into an extradural vein. Within the cranium, there is no extradural space, as the meningeal dura and endosteal dura are closely adherent, except where they separate to form the venous sinuses. At the foramen magnum, these two layers separate; the former becomes the spinal dura, and the latter becomes the periosteum of the spinal canal.

Thus, although local anaesthetics cannot enter between the endosteal and meningeal layer of the cerebral dura, they may diffuse across the spinal dura at the base of the brain into the CSF, and thence to the brain. Between the spinal dura and the spinal periosteum lies the extradural space. The ligamentum flavum completes the posterior wall in direct continuity with the periosteum of the spinal canal. Because the spinal canal is approximately triangular in cross-section and the articular processes indent the triangle, the extradural space narrows posterolaterally and then widens again laterally towards the intervertebral foramina. The safest point of entry into the extradural space is therefore in the midline.

Although the extradural space is nearly circular at the cervical level, it becomes more triangular in the thoracic region and resin injection studies in cadavers have shown that the lumbar extradural space is divided into three compartments: one ventral and two dorsolateral. The dorsal extradural space may be subdivided further by a dorsomedian fold of dura mater (White, 1982).

The dorsal extradural space (studied with computed axial tomography) has a sawtooth shape, with the dorsal extradural space narrowest near the rostral lamina (1.3–1.6 mm) and widest near the caudad lamina (6.9–9.1 mm) of each interspace. This is in keeping with the attachment of ligamentum flavum to the anterior surface of the rostral lamina and the posterior surface of the caudad lamina. It emphasizes the desirability of not entering the extradural space close to the rostral lamina. In addition to nerve roots that traverse the extradural space, there are fat, areolar tissue, lymphatics, arteries, and the extensive internal vertebral venous plexus of Batson. The extradural veins are most prominent along the lateral walls of the spinal canal in the lateral position of the extradural space.

Extradural veins. The large valveless extradural veins are part of the internal vertebral venous plexus, which drains the neural tissue of spinal cord, the CSF and the bony spinal canal. The major portion of this plexus lies in the anterolateral part of the extradural space. The plexus has rich segmental connections at all levels within intervertebral foramina and extradural space, and within the body of the vertebrae (the basivertebral veins). Superiorly, the plexus communicates with venous sinuses within the cranium. Inferiorly, the sacral venous plexus link the vertebral plexus to uterine and iliac veins. By way of the intervertebral foramina at each level, the vertebral plexus communicates with thoracic and abdominal veins, so that pressure changes in these cavities are transmitted to the extradural veins but not to the supporting bony elements of the neural arch and the vertebral bodies. Thus, marked increases in intra-abdominal pressure may compress the inferior vena cava while distending the extradural veins and increasing flow up the vertebrobasilar plexus. This increased flow is accommodated mostly by means of the azygos vein, which ascends in the right chest over the root of the right lung into the superior vena cava (Fig. 58.6). However, it is also possible for a small dose of local anaesthetic injected rapidly into an extradural vein to be channelled directly up the basivertebral system to a cerebral venous sinus; this is most likely to occur in a pregnant woman in the supine position when the inferior vena cava is obstructed, and intrathoracic pressure increases during active bearing down, so that the azygos flow is temporarily increased. Clearly, local anaesthetic

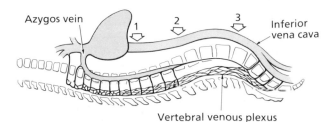

Fig. 58.6 Extradural veins (vertebral venous plexus) and their connections with inferior vena cava (IVC) and azygos vein. Extradural veins are protected from compression by the vertebral canal; thus, obstruction to IVC results in rerouting of venous return by way of extradural veins, and thence to the azygos vein above the level of obstruction. Some common sites of IVC obstruction are shown: (1) below the liver (e.g. severe ascites); (2) thoracolumbar junction (e.g. abdominal pressure) in prone position; (3) pelvic brim (e.g. pregnancy). (Redrawn from Bromage, 1978.)

should not be injected into the extradural space under such conditions. More likely, distension of extradural veins, produced by direct inferior vena caval obstruction (e.g. by the uterus) or by increased thoraco-abdominal pressure, diminishes also the effective volume of the extradural space, with the result that injected local anaesthetics spread more widely. In addition, the potential absorptive area of venules and capillaries is increased, with increased amounts of drug reaching the heart by way of the azygos vein.

There are three important points with regard to safety:

1 The extradural needle should pierce the ligamentum flavum in the midline to avoid the large laterally placed extradural veins.

2 Insertion of extradural needles or catheters, or injection of local anaesthetic should be avoided during episodes of marked increase in size of extradural veins, such as that which occurs with increased thoraco-abdominal pressure during straining.

3 The presence of vena caval obstruction calls for a reduction in dose, a decreased rate of injection, and increased care in aspirating for blood (see below) before injection.

An intriguing feature of the extradural veins is their importance in draining CSF and in the transfer of local anaesthetic to the CSF. In the region of the dural cuffs, bulbs of arachnoid mater protrude through the dura into the extradural space, where they often invaginate the walls of extradural veins that drain the spinal cord and nerve root area. Although the primary function of these arachnoid granulations is to drain CSF and remove debris from the CSF into the vascular system, they provide also a favourable site for transfer of local anaesthetic into the spinal fluid (Fig. 58.7).

8 From the description so far it is obvious that 'feel' is important in placing correctly the extradural (or spinal) needle. The extradural space may be identified positively by either 'loss of resistance to the injection' of fluid (air or saline) or by a negative pressure test (usually the 'hanging-drop' negative pressure test).

In the lumbar region, the major cause of generation of a negative pressure lies in 'coning' of the dura by the advancing needle point. The negative pressure increases as the needle advances across the extradural space towards the dura.

Blunt needles with side-openings produce the greatest negative pressure: they produce a good 'coning' effect on the dura without puncturing it and transmit the negative pressure well because of their side-opening.

Slow introduction of the needle produces the greatest negative pressure. Even if the needle is halted and the pressure equalized, further advances of the needle continue to produce a negative pressure until the dura is eventually punctured.

Greater negative pressure may be obtained if the dura is not distended (e.g. by gravity in the sitting position or by high abdominal or thoracic pressure).

The absence of an initial negative pressure after entering the extradural space in Bryce-Smith's studies (1950), and in at least 12% of the patients of Usubiaga

et al. (1967a) in the lying position suggests that negative pressure is an unreliable sign of initial entry into the lumbar extradural space. Further advancement of the needle in the extradural space may be able to demonstrate a negative pressure where it is initially absent. This appears to conflict with the optimal clinical technique of halting the extradural needle as soon as it enters the space. Techniques of lumbar extradural puncture that are based on 'loss of resistance' tests through ligamentum flavum with air-filled or fluid-filled syringes offer a more reliable means of achieving this optimal technique in the lumbar area (see below). If the anaesthetist finds it easier to use the two-handed grip in the 'hanging-drop' negative pressure test (Bromage, 1953), it is important to ensure that pressure in the lumbar extradural space is as low as possible by positioning the patient in the lateral position, with a slight head-down tilt, to lower intra-abdominal pressure.

In the thoracic region, the major determinant of negative pressure is the transmission of negative respiratory pressures from the thorax by way of the paravertebral space and intervertebral foramina to the extradural space.

The reliability of a 'hanging-drop' negative pressure sign in the thoracic region has led to the recommendation that this technique be used at least in the mid-thoracic region. The narrowness of the extradural space in this region and the excellent control afforded

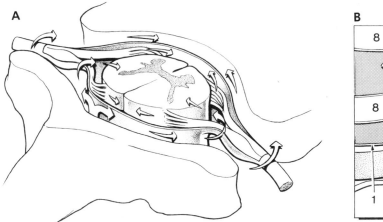
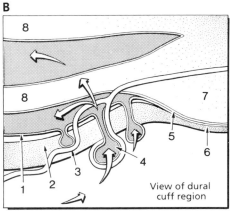

Fig. 58.7 A Horizontal spread of local anaesthetic in extradural space. Major spread posteriorly to the region of 'dural cuff' (root sleeve) region is shown, with subsequent entry to cerebrospinal fluid (CSF) and spinal cord. Minor spread into anterior extradural space is also shown.

B Enlarged view of dural cuff region shows rapid entry of local anaesthetic into CSF by way of arachnoid granulations: (**1**) arachnoid membrane; (**2**) dura; (**3**) extradural vein; (**4**) arachnoid 'granulation' protruding through dura and in contact with extradural vein; (**5**) perineural epithelium of spinal nerve in continuity with arachnoid; (**6**) epineurium of spinal nerve in continuity with dura; (**7**) dorsal root ganglion; (**8**) intradural spinal nerve roots. (Reproduced from Cousins & Bridenbaugh, 1988.)

by the two-handed grip of the winged 'hanging-drop' needle give support to this recommendation.

If one uses a negative pressure test routinely for extradural puncture, it is important to be aware of factors that result in marked changes in pressure.

In severe lung diseases such as emphysema, negative pressure may be abolished, particularly if the patient is lying down.

Any factor that increases abdominal pressure and/or occlusion of the inferior vena cava may distend the extradural veins (see above) and increase pressure in the lumbar space. This results in only slight changes in the thoracic extradural space, particularly if the patient is sitting.

During labour, baseline lumbar extradural pressures are higher in women in the supine position compared with those in the lateral position. As labour progresses, baseline pressures increase to as high as $+10$ cmH$_2$O at full dilatation. Also, there are peaks of pressure during each uterine contraction, with increases of $8-15$ cmH$_2$O.

Coughing or a Valsalva manoeuvre increases both intrathoracic and intra-abdominal pressure, so that pressures in both the thoracic and lumbar extradural spaces increase.

Changes in pressure in the extradural space have implications also for the ease of injection and spread of local anaesthetic solutions. Studies by Usubiaga et al. (1967b) have helped to explain why successful entry into the extradural space is followed sometimes by 'drip-back' when local anaesthetic is injected subsequently; classic pressure–volume compliance studies showed that compliance decreased with increasing age and that residual pressure after injection of 10 ml of solution at a standard rate had a positive correlation with age. Thus, some patients with a low compliance in the extradural space are unable to accommodate a large volume of solution if it is injected rapidly; 'drip-back' is less common in young patients if injection is made slowly because, although there was increased pressure in young patients, Usubiaga et al. found that pressure was essentially back to baseline in 30 sec.

As expected, Usubiaga et al. (1967b) found that spread of analgesia correlated positively with residual extradural pressure and with age. These studies tend to support radiological studies, in which 'periodurograms' with water-soluble contrast media showed a reduced longitudinal spread of injected solutions in young patients because of widely patent intervertebral foramina. In contrast, in elderly patients with relatively obstructed foramina, longitudinal spread was increased. More recent radiological studies have demonstrated minimal leakage of contrast media through intervertebral foramina in young patients. Thus, soft tissue (fat) in the extradural space seems most important in the spread of solutions.

The pedicles that join the laminae to the vertebral bodies complete the bony spinal canal that protects the dural sac. Each pedicle is notched, so that pedicles of adjacent vertebral bodies form the intervertebral foramen. The inferior pedicle of each foramen is notched more deeply. The intervertebral foramina are completed posteriorly by the capsule surrounding the articular processes of adjoining vertebrae and anteriorly by an intervertebral disk and the lower part of the body above it. Because the extradural space is continuous with the paravertebral space, it is possible to produce an extradural block by injection close to an intervertebral foramen or to penetrate the dura at the dural cuff region if a needle is inserted into an intervertebral foramen.

The extradural fat extends throughout the spinal and caudal space. It is most abundant posteriorly, diminishes adjacent to the articular processes, and increases laterally around the spinal nerve roots, where it is continuous with the fat surrounding the spinal nerves in the intervertebral foramina and in the paravertebral space. Anteriorly, it is sparse, and thus the dura may lie close to the posterior longitudinal ligament. Overall, the amount of fat in the extradural space tends to vary in direct relation to that present elsewhere in the body, so that obese patients may have extradural spaces that are occupied by generous amounts of fat. Mostly, the fat lies free in the extradural space except near the nerve roots, where connective tissue tends to tether it in the intervertebral foramina. Extradural fat is surprisingly vascular, with small capillaries that form a rich network in its substance. The fat itself has a great affinity for drugs with high lipid-solubility, such as bupivacaine and etidocaine, which may be retained for long periods; uptake of local anaesthetic into extradural fat competes with vascular and neural uptake. The compliance of the extradural fat varies considerably between persons and with increasing age. In children and young adults, it offers little resistance to injection, but in some adults, a low compliance may result in considerable 'drip-back' of injected local anaesthetic.

The dural cuff region is supplied with a rich lymphatic network that conveys debris rapidly from arachnoid villi out through intervertebral foramina to reach lymph channels in front of the vertebral bodies. 9 An extradural catheter may be threaded down the 16 or 18 gauge Tuohy needle or direct injection may be made. The spread of injection through needle or catheter should be controlled. A rapid rate of injection may produce neurological signs (Wildsmith, 1986). Slow injection helps also to identify inadvertent intravascular injection before the onset of toxicity. One test to detect this complication using a single test dose is to administer an adrenaline-containing solution to monitor heart rate (Moore & Batra, 1981).

Incorrect procedure

Incorrect procedure or sometimes inadvertent aberrant needle placement because of anatomical difficulties may result in a different sequence of events than that described above. Failure to define clearly the midline results in needle entry at the side of the supraspinous ligament. If the anaesthetist persists with this unsatisfactory start, it is likely that the needle may enter the interspinous ligament obliquely, resulting in only a transient resistance, followed by loss of resistance, or it may miss the ligament completely, resulting immediately in a feeling of no resistance, in the paravertebral muscles. Both of these situations may be interpreted as rapid entry into the extradural space. However, injection of local anaesthetic is followed by marked 'drip-back', and subsequent attempts to thread an extradural catheter are met with considerable resistance. If the needle is inserted too close to the spinous process (or during any attempt at midline puncture in the midthoracic region), it is not uncommon for the needle to contact the spinous process.

Perhaps the most common obstruction to the needle is the lamina of the vertebral body. Because the posterior surface of the lamina slopes gently down and back from its anterior end to its posterior end (Fig. 58.4), an extradural needle inserted too far laterally may encounter lamina either at a superficial depth or deeper, close to its junction with the ligamentum flavum. Even more extreme lateral insertion or lateral angulation of the needle may result in the needle point contacting the superior or inferior articular processes or the joint space, where their articular facets meet. Since the articular facets have a rich nerve supply, needle trauma may result in sudden severe localized pain on one side of the back with accompanying paravertebral muscle spasm on that side. This pain is not dissimilar to that caused by direct contact with a nerve root: 'radicular pain'. Both may result in pain that radiates into the leg. Radicular pain is usually more discrete with only one area involved (e.g. the inside of the knee for L3 or inside of the leg for L4). Facet pain may radiate but is somewhat more diffuse.

Additional anatomical and technical aspects of spinal subarachnoid anaesthesia

If spinal subarachnoid anaesthesia is planned, the needle is advanced through the extradural space to puncture the dura and enter the subarachnoid space. Formal identification of the extradural space is undertaken rarely; however, it is a useful exercise for the beginner using a 22 gauge needle.

The test of dural puncture is flow of CSF through the needle. In spinal anaesthesia, CSF must be obtained but dural puncture is suspected also sometimes during an extradural block, as indicated in Table 58.2.

Alternative approaches to the extradural space

The technique of spinal injection in the midline has been described. An alternative approach is to use a paraspinous (paramedian or lateral) insertion. The needle should be inserted close to the spinous process because in both lumbar and thoracic regions, the spinous process narrows superiorly and thus guides the needle to a midline entry through the ligamentum flavum.

Extreme lateral angulation of the needle should be avoided, as it may result in oblique penetration of the ligamentum flavum and vascular or neural damage. In most instances, the needle need not be angulated and merely follows the spinous process; thus, 'paraspinous' describes the essence of the technique.

Techniques with extreme angulation of the needle should be discarded in favour of the safer paraspinous approach.

In the lumbar region, infiltration is made 1–1.5 cm lateral to the caudad tip of the inferior spinous process of the chosen interspace. At 9–10 cm, a 22 gauge, spinal needle is used to infiltrate perpendicular to the skin beside the spinous process; this enables the depth of the lamina to be determined before inserting the extradural needle. It is worth noting that for single-shot techniques the extradural space can be identified if an air-filled syringe is attached to the 22 gauge needle and constant pressure is applied to the plunger. However, in most patients an 18 gauge extradural needle is inserted next beside the spinous process and

Table 58.2 Suspected dural puncture. (From Cousins & Bridenbaugh, 1987)

Sign	Cause	Management
Second loss of resistance and fluid flows from needle	Dural puncture	Convert to spinal anaesthetic or move to higher interspace for extradural
Second loss of resistance after identifying ligamentum flavum; no fluid flows from needle, but injected solution; some 'drip-back'	? Entry into subdural space ? Dural puncture	Test 'drip-back' on arm: cold = LA, warm = CSF Drip into container with etidocaine in it: CSF precipitate If drip-back only LA, withdraw needle and re-identify extradural space If drip-back = CSF + LA, move to a rostrad interspace or convert to spinal anaesthetic
One loss of resistance only—'drip-back' at: a shallow level; a deeper level	Interspinous ligament pierced and needle in paravertebral muscle Low compliance of extradural fat Needle only partially through ligamentum flavum	Re-insert needle in midline Test as above, if drip-back only LA: Attempt to pass catheter—easy passage Attempt to pass catheter—does not pass: Superiorly needle can be advanced and then catheter threaded. Inferiorly needle will not advance
	Needle in CSF	Test for CSF; if positive, move to rostrad interspace or convert to spinal

LA = local anaesthetic.
CSF = cerebrospinal fluid.
Do not attempt to withdraw needle into extradural space at the same level, as this may result in subdural cannulation.

angled upwards at 45° to the skin (Fig. 58.4); often the spinous process carries the needle slightly inward 10–15° to the sagittal plane. This may not always be so, and the needle may pass directly to the ligamentum flavum without any necessity for inward angulation. With this technique, resistance to the advancing needle and syringe plunger is encountered only when the needle tip enters the ligamentum flavum. Thus, careful location of the depth of ligamentum flavum is essential; from this point the technique is identical to that at the midline.

In the thoracic region, skin infiltration is made 1–1.5 cm lateral to the caudad tip of the spinous process, *cephalad* to the intended level of needle insertion. Infiltration down to the level of the lamina is carried out as described above. The extradural needle is inserted beside the spinous process and 55–60° to the skin (sagittal plane); a steep angle is required to reach ligamentum flavum caudad to the chosen spinous process. For both thoracic and lumbar paraspinous approaches, the Crawford 18 gauge, thin-wall needle is suitable for single-shot and catheter techniques. The angulation of the needle may permit easier threading of a catheter if a straight-tip Crawford needle is used rather than the Huber tip of the Tuohy needle.

The dural sac ends caudally at the lower border of S2, where it is pierced by the filum terminale. The filum terminale is the terminal thread of the pia mater, which extends from the tip of the spinal cord to blend with the periosteum on the back of the coccyx. The filum terminale anchors the cord and spinal dura, the latter being steadied further in the lower end of the vertebral column by a few fibrous strips from the posterior longitudinal ligament. The spinal dura provides also a thin cover for the spinal nerve roots, becoming progressively thinner near the intervertebral foramina, where it continues as epineural and perineural connective tissue of the peripheral nerves. The dura is the outer of three coverings of the spinal cord (and brain). The middle covering is the delicate non-vascular arachnoid mater. It is attached closely to the dura and ends with it at S2. Between the dura and the arachnoid lies the (potential) subdural space. A technique for entry into this space with X-ray control has been described; after the needle enters the subarachnoid space with flow of CSF, one withdraws the needle until the flow stops, and at this point the bevel of the needle should rest in the subdural space.

This space may be entered unintentionally during spinal administration of local anaesthetics. It may explain some failed spinals despite aspiration of 'some' spinal fluid. The case-reports of subdural injection indicate unilateral, patchy and inordinately high levels of anaesthesia, but usually after volumes of local anaesthetic intended for extradural anaesthesia.

The dura can be considered as a protective tube that is pierced by and gives a short 'cuff' to each pair of spinal nerves; at this point, the dura becomes markedly thinner and is adherent closely to the dorsal surfaces of the dorsal root ganglia as far as the point where anterior and posterior roots fuse to form the spinal nerve. Within these dural cuffs, there is a small blind pocket of CSF, which is separated from the extradural space only by the greatly thinned dura (Fig. 58.7). Here, the dura is pierced by veins, arteries and lymphatics, running to and from the underlying subarachnoid space. Also, the arachnoid membrane pushes small 'granulations' through the dura; these may either indent extradural veins or come into contact with extradural lymphatics, to facilitate drainage of CSF and elimination of foreign material. This region provides also a ready route for passage of local anaesthetics into the spinal fluid. Although the dura and arachnoid are usually in close apposition, they are separated easily and it is possible to insert unintentionally a catheter into the subdural space.

The innermost covering of the cord is the delicate though highly vascular pia mater. It invests the spinal cord closely along its length. The space between pia and arachnoid is the subarachnoid space and contains the CSF, spinal nerves and a large number of trabeculae which run between the two membranes. The denticulate ligaments which are attached to the dura and help to support the spinal cord are lateral projections of the pia mater.

The dorsal and ventral nerve roots are covered only by pia as they traverse the subarachnoid space. They receive a covering of the other two meningeal layers as they pierce the spinal dura and pass through the extradural space. As the dura extends further out to the intervertebral foramina it becomes thinner. The pia and arachnoid extend beyond the dorsal root ganglia as the perineurium of the peripheral nerves.

Spinal cord and nerves

The spinal cord begins at the level of the foramen magnum and ends as the conus medullaris. At birth, the cord ends at the level of L3 but rises with age to end in adults at the lower border of L1 (Fig. 58.8).

There are 31 pairs of spinal nerves. Each is composed of anterior and posterior roots which are formed by coalescence of several rootlets arising from

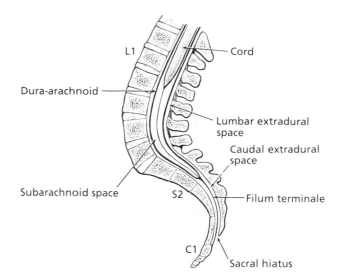

Fig. 58.8 Lumbosacral portion of vertebral column, showing terminal spinal cord and its coverings. (Reproduced from Cousins & Bridenbaugh, 1987.)

the cord. Beyond the end of the cord, lumbar and sacral nerve roots extend as the cauda equina. The nerves in the cauda equina are covered only by a thin layer of pia and have a large surface area from their cord origin to their exits through the dura. They are therefore especially sensitive to local anaesthetics within the CSF.

Cerebrospinal fluid

The CSF is an ultrafiltrate of blood and is contained within the subarachnoid space of spine and cranium. It is clear and colourless in health, has a specific gravity of 1.003–1.009 (mean 1.006) at 37 °C. The total volume of CSF is 120–150 ml but only 25–35 ml is within the spinal subarachnoid space and most of this volume is below the end of the cord.

The baricity of various local anaesthetic spinal solutions is summarized in Table 58.3.

Cerebrospinal fluid is usually homogenous but if conditions change rapidly (e.g. respiratory acidosis) only cisternal values mirror systemic values and the composition of lumbar CSF changes slowly. Cerebrospinal fluid is produced at a constant rate of approximately 0.35 ml/min or 500 ml/day and rate of absorption equals rate of formation. Formation of CSF is increased when serum is hypotonic, and reduced when serum osmolality increases. There is an approximately linear relationship with a 1% change in serum osmolality causing a 6.7% change in production of CSF. In conditions where CSF is lost e.g. postdural-puncture

Table 58.3 Local anaesthetic solutions used in spinal anaesthesia.

Amethocaine (tetracaine)	Solutions can be hyperbaric (0.5% in glucose 8%, SG 1.0203), isobaric (0.5% in N/2 saline, SG 1.066) or hyperbaric (1% in water, SG 1.0007) Maximal intrathecal dose of 20 mg
Bupivacaine (marcain)	Solutions can be (slightly) hypobaric (0.5% in water, SG 1.059) or hyperbaric (0.5% in glucose 8%, SG 1.0278)
Cinchocaine (nupercaine, dibucaine)	Usually a hyperbaric solution (0.5% in glucose 6%, SG 1.024)
Lignocaine (xylocaine)	Solutions may be isobaric (2% in water, SG 1.0066) or hyperbaric (5% in glucose 7.5%, SG 1.0333)

SG measured at 37°C.
SG CSF 1.0069.

headache, it is therefore important at least to prevent dehydration but better to infuse intravenous fluids. Cerebrospinal fluid is produced in the choroid plexuses of the lateral, third and fourth ventricles. There is a concentration gradient of protein from a low level (6–15 mg/dl) in the ventricles to 20–50 mg/dl in the lumbar sac. Anaesthetic drugs have little effect on production of CSF.

The cord is supplied with arterial blood through one anterior and paired posterior arteries (Fig. 58.9). The anterior spinal artery arises above from branches of the vertebral arteries and descends in front of the anterior longitudinal sulcus of the spinal cord. It receives contributions from the spinal arteries which reach the spinal cord by way of the intervertebral foramina and enter the extradural space to reach spinal nerve roots in the region of the dural cuffs. It is thus possible to cause spinal cord ischaemia if a spinal artery is traumatized by a needle inserted towards a spinal nerve root. The spinal cord territory supplied by the anterior spinal artery is most vulnerable, as there is only one anterior artery and the major feeder to this artery usually enters unilaterally (on the left in 78%) by way of a single intervertebral foramen, between T8 and L3. It is termed the artery of Adamkiewicz (radicularis magna). Damage to this vessel may result in ischaemia of the lumbar enlargement of the cord. In a small number of patients, the artery of Adamkiewicz originates at a high level (T5). Iliac tributaries are then larger but these can be damaged during pelvic surgery or lumbar extradural anaesthesia resulting in a lesion of the conus medullaris.

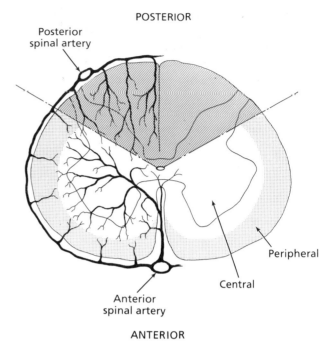

Fig. 58.9 Blood supply of spinal cord, horizontal distribution. The 'central' area, supplied only by anterior spinal artery, is predominantly a motor area (see text). (Redrawn from Cousins & Bridenbaugh, 1988.)

This supports further the practice of ensuring that the needle enters the extradural space in the midline and suggests that the L3–4 interspace is the best choice for beginners.

Anterior spinal artery ischaemia causes a predominantly motor lesion as the anterior two-thirds of the cord including the anterior horn cells are supplied exclusively by this artery. The posterior spinal arteries arise from the posterior inferior cerebellar arteries and they descend on the posterolateral surface of the cord lying medial to the posterior nerve roots. They supply the posterior white columns and some of the posterior grey (Fig. 58.9). In contrast to the six or seven vessels feeding the anterior spinal artery, the posterior longitudinal vessels are fed by 25–40 radicular arteries.

Pharmacology of spinal and extradural anaesthesia

Spinal anaesthesia

Baricity

The inter-relationship between baricity of the local anaesthetic solution and the posture of patient (first described by Barker) is paramount. A local anaesthetic solution with specific gravity less than that of CSF (hypobaric) tends to rise and if the specific gravity is greater than CSF (hyperbaric) it moves downwards whatever position the patient assumes. Spread is therefore determined by the posture the patient is placed in *after* injection, and a knowledge of the spinal curves is important.

Posture

A patient who is placed supine as soon as the subarachnoid injection has been made develops a block to the mid-thoracic level when a hyperbaric solution is used but only to the low thoracic segments with hypobaric or isobaric solutions because of the effect of spinal curves. Isobaric solutions (e.g. plain bupivacaine) give a longer duration of block, regardless of posture. In the sitting patient, hyperbaric solutions may be used to create a 'saddle' block. This is a useful block for operations on the perineum, but if a large volume is used or the patient is placed supine too soon (i.e. less than 5 min) the block spreads as if the patient had been supine from the beginning.

Unilateral blocks can be produced by keeping the patient in a lateral position for at least 5 min. This so-called 'hemi-anaesthesia' reduces the physiological consequences of the block. Unfortunately, the block spreads when the patient turns supine and a unilateral block usually becomes bilateral, although the side which was lower is blocked more profoundly (Wildsmith & Rocco, 1985).

DOSE OF DRUG

Dose of the drug injected is a third major factor affecting spread of subarachnoid injections. Unfortunately, this factor is not constant but varies within the range of volumes used for spinal anaesthesia. Indeed dose, volume and concentration are all inter-related and each plays a part. Thus, injection of isobaric amethocaine 0.5% in a dose of 5, 10 or 15 mg produces blocks of similar spread (usually legs and perineum) (Wildsmith *et al.*, 1981). The same phenomenon occurs with bupivacaine 0.5% but not with a 0.75% solution where increasing the dose increases the spread. If the volume of solution is increased but a constant dose is employed, there is only a small increase in spread, at the cost of increased unpredictability of spread.

Duration

The choice of drug is the main determinant of duration of the block (e.g. lignocaine produces a block lasting approximately 1 hr and bupivacaine and amethocaine at least 2 hr). Drug dose, however, affects duration also, as does the level of block. If a given dose produces a block to the mid-lumbar level it lasts longer than if the same dose spread to block up to the mid-thoracic level.

The addition of vasoconstrictors to subarachnoid injections of local anaesthetic, although safe, results in very little increase in duration. A similar increase can be obtained by increasing the dose of drug by 50% (Wildsmith & Rocco, 1985).

Barbotage

This is the technique of aspirating CSF repeatedly and injecting small volumes of the local anaesthetic (from the French verb *barboter* to mix, dabble or paddle). Greater spread of block is obtained from a given dose, but the result of barbotage is not entirely predictable. Fast injection increases also dispersion of local anaesthetic but this is also unpredictable. Needle size and direction of bevel have little clinical relevance to spread of anaesthesia.

Clinical subarachnoid anaesthesia

The agents available for use are described in Table 58.4. Most studies quote mean level of block. Anaesthetists need to know minimum level (guaranteed efficacy for surgery) and maximum level (risk of hypotension from sympathetic blockade). In practice, only three techniques need be considered to obtain distinctly different levels of block (Wildsmith & Rocco, 1985).

1 For abdominal surgery, block to mid-thoracic segments is necessary. This is achieved best by injecting a hyperbaric solution at the L2–3 or L3–4 interspace and lying the patient supine immediately. The solution runs down the dorsal curve of the spine and excess solution pools opposite the T5 vertebra; it does not spread higher without a steep head-down tilt. The effect of this block on arterial pressure may be profound. Barbotage may increase the height of the block and keeping the patient sitting for a short time after the block may keep the block a few segments lower (e.g. for herniorrhaphy) which may reduce the cardiovascular consequences.

2 For procedures on the perineum, a saddle block is suitable. This is produced by injecting a small volume (0.5–0.75 ml) of hyperbaric local anaesthetic at the L4–5 interspace and keeping the patient in a sitting position for at least 5 min. Arterial pressure is affected rarely by this block. If the patient is to be placed in the

Table 58.4 Spinal anaesthesia—a guide to dosage and effects

Drug	Dose (mg)			Duration (min)
	To L4	To T10	To T4	
Lignocaine 5%	25–50	50–75	75–100	60–70
Bupivacaine 0.5% (Isobaric)	10–15	15–20	—	150–200
Bupivacaine 0.5% (Hyperbaric)	4–8	8–12	14–20	90–110
Cinchocaine 0.5%	4–6	6–8	10–15	150–180

See text for appropriate posture, etc. Approximately 10% increase in duration of effect when vasoconstrictors are added to the solution used.

lithotomy position abduction and flexion of the hip may become uncomfortable and the block described in (3) may be more appropriate.

3 For procedures on the lower limb (or perineum) a block to the level of the inguinal ligament is required. This can be achieved by injecting an isobaric solution at the L2–3 interspace. The risk of hypotension is not high, the hip joint is anaesthetized and unlike the saddle block there is no special positioning required. Dosages for the various local anaesthetics for different levels of block are given in Table 58.4.

Patient factors influencing local anaesthetic distribution in cerebrospinal fluid

When the technique and agent are held constant several patient factors may influence spread of local anaesthetic in CSF:

1 Age. Spread is greater in older patients than in younger ones.

2 Height. The taller the patient the fewer spinal segments are blocked for a given amount of local anaesthetic.

3 Anatomical configuration. A kyphosis or lordosis may affect spread of local anaesthetic and may require extra careful positioning of the patient.

4 Pregnancy, intra-abdominal tumours and ascites. Increased spread of local anaesthetic results from a decrease in CSF volume in these conditions. This is a result of increased intra-abdominal pressure reducing inferior vena caval blood flow and subsequent development of collateral vessels in the extradural space (Fig. 58.6). As the spinal canal has a fixed volume, venous engorgement in the extradural space is accommodated by reduction in the volume of the subarachnoid space.

Segmental levels

In assessing the level of blockade, it is important for the anaesthetist to have a method of using simple surface landmarks to indicate level of dermatomal blockade and hence segmental spinal nerve (and sympathetic) blockade. Table 58.5 lists the key levels. There is no point in testing for blockade of T1–2 by testing above the nipple line, since this area has double innervation from T1 to T2 and C3 to C4, so that normal sensation remains even when T1–2 are blocked. Thus, residual activity in the cardiac sympathetics T1 and T2 is checked by testing skin sensation on the inside of the arm above the elbow (T2) and below the elbow (T1). Residual motor activity in T1 can be checked also by testing the ability of the patient to hold a sheet of paper between the outstretched fingers (interossei C8, T1). In a lightly anaesthetized patient, spinal reflexes may be useful for testing level of blockade: epigastric (T7–8), abdominal (T9, T12), cremasteric (L1, L2), plantar (S1, S2), knee-jerk (L2-4), ankle-jerk (S1, S2).

The fate of local anaesthetic in the CSF

Local anaesthetic disappears from the CSF because of uptake by neuronal tissue or vascular absorption. Four factors govern neuronal uptake:

1 Concentration of local anaesthetic in CSF. Uptake is greatest where the concentration of local anaesthetic in CSF is greatest.

2 Surface area of nerve tissue exposed to local anaesthetic. Both nerve roots and the cord take up CSF. The surface of the cord, lying deep to the pia mater is exposed to local anaesthetic, and deeper structures are exposed also through the spaces of Virchow–Robin which accompany blood vessels penetrating the cord.

Table 58.5 Key levels of dermatomal blockade. (From Cousins & Bridenbaugh, 1988)

Cutaneous landmark	Segmental level	Significance
Little finger	C8	All cardioaccelerator fibres (T1–4) blocked
Inner aspect of arm and forearm	T1 and T2	Some degree of cardioaccelerator blockade
Apex of axilla	T3	Easily remembered landmark
Nipple line (midway sternal notch and xiphistemum)	T4–5	Possibility of cardioacceleratory blockade
Tip of xiphoid	T7	Splanchnics (T5–L1) may become blocked
Umbilicus	T10	Sympathetic blockade limited to lower limbs
Inguinal ligament	T12	
Outer side of foot	S1	No lumbar sympathetic blockade Most difficult nerve root to block

3 Lipid content of nerve tissue. The local anaesthetic agents are lipophilic and are taken up by myelinated tissue within the subarachnoid space.

4 Blood flow to exposed neural tissue. The local anaesthetics are removed from subarachnoid nerve tissue through the blood; blood flow is therefore the most important determinant of concentration of local anaesthetic in cord or nerve whatever the effects of the other factors. The rate at which the local anaesthetic is removed from the subarachnoid space dictates the duration of block; there is no elimination of local anaesthetic in the CSF. The vessel-rich pia mater carries much local anaesthetic, and the greater the spread of a given dose the shorter the duration of action (because of a larger absorptive area exposed). Vasoconstrictors appear to have little effect on this vasculature. Vessels within the cord help also in the removal of local anaesthetic, but decreases in cord blood flow have little effect on the concentration of local anaesthetic in the systemic circulation.

A significant proportion of a dose injected into the subarachnoid space passes across the dura, down a concentration gradient, and is removed by the mechanisms described below for extradural injections. Other substances injected into the subarachnoid space are removed also by vascular absorption including the dextrose used to manufacture hyperbaric solutions. At some time after injection (30–35 min for hyperbaric lignocaine), so much dextrose has been eliminated from the CSF that the remaining solution becomes isobaric. At this time a change in position of patient does not affect the spread of anaesthesia; the level of anaesthesia is then said to be 'fixed'.

Sites of action of local anaesthetic after spinal subarachnoid injection

Subarachnoid neural blockade results from an action of the local anaesthetic on the nerve roots and the dorsal root ganglia; the presence of local anaesthetic in the cord contributes little to the block. The concentration threshold for block (sensitivity) differs between nerve fibre types; the concentration of local anaesthetic in the CSF is reduced with distance from the point of injection. These factors produce *zones of differential blockade*.

Somatic motor nerves are more resistant to blockade than sensory nerves; the level of motor block is correspondingly higher than sensory block (approximately two spinal segments). Motor and sensory block from different agents is compared in Fig. 58.10. In addition, different types of sensory nerves have different sensitivity to local anaesthetic and there is an approximately two-segment discrepancy between the levels of analgesia and anaesthesia.

Traditionally, it is taught that the level of sympathetic blockade is a further two segments higher than the sensory block, thought to result from the preganglion sympathetic nerves being most sensitive to local anaesthetics. Recently, it has become apparent that sensory block may outlast sympathetic block,

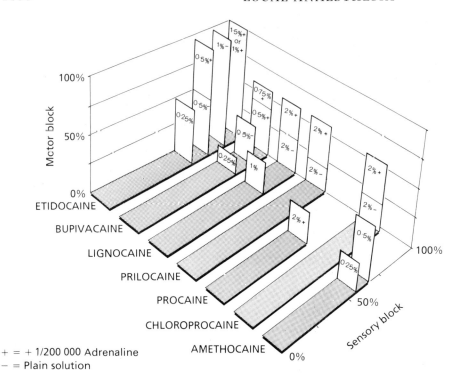

Fig. 58.10 Motor and sensory block percentage success rate. Comparison of agents, concentrations and addition of adrenaline are based on subjective data, so that only approximate comparisons are made. (Reproduced from Cousins & Bridenbaugh, 1988.)

possibly because of sympathetic pathways within spinal cord or resistance to local anaesthetic block of preganglionic sympathetic β-fibres (Bengtsson *et al.*, 1985).

Extradural anaesthesia

The most important factors influencing spread of local anaesthetic in the extradural space are the volume, concentration, dose of injectate and the site of injection.

Injection site

Onset of neural block is most rapid nearest the site of injection and is most intense here. After lumbar extradural injection, there is greater cephalad than caudad spread of analgesia (2:1 segments) and there may also be a delay in onset at the L5 and S1 segments probably because of the large size of these roots (Galindo *et al.*, 1975). After mid-thoracic extradural injection there is even spread of analgesia; repeated doses may cause extensive spread but in addition to L5 and S1, the upper thoracic and lower cervical segments are resistant to block because of their size.

Volume, concentration and dose of injectate

The spread of solutions injected into the extradural space is summarized in Table 58.5. When local anaesthetic solutions are administered, the spread of analgesia for a particular agent is influenced by volume, concentration and dose.

Increasing dosage produces a linear increase in the duration of sensory blockade; increasing the concentration reduces the onset time and increases the intensity of block. Increasing the volume injected increases the longitudinal spread of solution (and also the duration of block); length of the spinal column (i.e. height) is, therefore, an important influence but not a major factor when lumbar injections are made. For lignocaine 2% and bupivacaine 0.5%, a guide for lumbar administration is to use 1 ml per segment to be blocked for 150 cm (5 feet) of height *plus* 0.1 ml per segment for each 5 cm (2 inch) over 150 cm. Having calculated the required dose it must be ascertained that this is a safe dose to administer. For extradural anaesthesia in the mid-thoracic region the dose is reduced by one-third.

Age

There is greater spread of local anaesthetic in the extradural space in the elderly. The consequent declining dose requirements with age can be summarized as:

20–40 yr: 1–1.5 ml/segment adjusted for height.
40–60 yr: 0.5–1 ml/segment adjusted for height.
60–80 yr: 0.3–0.6 ml/segment adjusted for height.

It has been proposed that this phenomenon results from reduced lateral leakage of solution and greater longitudinal spread, but there is conflicting evidence on this subject.

Posture

Whether the patient is sitting or lying has no clinically significant effect generally on cephalad spread although in the obese patient the level of block is lower when the patient is seated. The lateral position does, however, favour spread of analgesia to the dependent side. This is seen in faster onset and longer duration of sensory and motor block (Seow *et al.*, 1983) and greater spread (Husmeyer & White, 1980).

Pregnancy, intra-abdominal tumour or ascites

The potential volume of the extradural space is reduced in these conditions by engorged veins. This makes intravascular injection more likely and increases spread of a given volume. A 30% reduction in volume is recommended.

Speed of injection

Rapid extradural injection must be avoided; it is dangerous and has little effect on spread of analgesia. Rapid injection of a large volume can increase CSF pressure and intracranial pressure (ICP) and compromise spinal cord blood flow. The change in ICP is manifested as headache but cerebral haemorrhage and intraocular haemorrhage have been reported. In addition, slow injection offers the best opportunity to avoid lethal sequelae of intravascular injection of local anaesthetic (see below).

Addition of vasoconstrictors

Great flexibility of sensory and motor blockade and duration are afforded by careful choice of agent. The addition of adrenaline to solutions of lignocaine both prolongs the block and decreases the rate of absorption (see below); addition of adrenaline to solutions of bupivacaine similarly reduces the peak plasma concen-

tration (Burm *et al.*, 1986). Vasoconstrictors have little effect on the duration of block from the long-acting agents bupivacaine and etidocaine. The acidity of commercial local anaesthetic solutions containing adrenaline is increased from approximately pH 6 to pH 3 to maintain stability. It has been recommended that because of this, adrenaline should be added freshly, but this, however, increases the risk of inadvertent overdose of adrenaline (0.2–0.25 ml of 1/1000 adrenaline in 50 ml local anaesthetic is suggested). The effect of adrenaline on motor and sensory block is shown in Fig. 58.10.

pH-ADJUSTED LOCAL ANAESTHETIC SOLUTIONS

Local anaesthetic agents used in extradural anaesthesia

Lignocaine and bupivacaine are used most frequently in the UK. In addition, anaesthetists in the USA may use etidocaine and chloroprocaine. Although an excellent agent, prilocaine is not used frequently for extradural blocks.

Lignocaine (Xylocaine, Lidocaine) is used in 1–2% formulations. It has a short latency of effect of approximately 10 min and a duration of 1–2 hr depending on strength and the presence or absence of adrenaline. Solutions below 1% produce little motor block and 2% may be required for intense muscle relaxation. With repeated doses, *tachyphylaxis* may develop (see below).

Bupivacaine (Marcain) is a long-acting agent available widely in 0.25% and 0.5% formulations (and 0.75% in some countries). Whilst some degree of analgesia may persist for several hours, surgical anaesthesia is provided for 1.5–3 hr by bupivacaine 0.5%. Onset is slower than lignocaine, 20–30 min may be required. Analgesia with little muscle relaxation is provided by 0.25%. The drug can be used with or without adrenaline. Bupivacaine 0.75% has a reputation for severe systemic reactions and the manufacturers do not recommend its use in obstetrics. Use of this formulation requires more care but only because it is more concentrated.

Prilocaine in 1.5, 2 and 3% formulations with adrenaline has been used for extradural anaesthesia. Speed of onset is similar to that with lignocaine but duration is slightly longer.

Etidocaine in 1.0% or 1.5% solution provides rapid onset of analgesia of long duration. There is good motor block but this may exceed the duration of analgesia.

The addition of adrenaline to prolong blockade has been described above; other substances have been added also. Carbonation of local anaesthetic solutions release base readily and have a superior penetrating ability resulting in more rapid onset. The addition of potassium reduces onset time also but the concentration required causes depolarization of nerves which gives rise to muscle spasms. Adjustment of pH with bicarbonate may speed onset of action.

SITE OF ACTION OF EXTRADURAL ANAESTHESIA

The key data were provided by injecting (^{14}C)-labelled lignocaine into the extradural space of dogs and then carrying out autoradiography and tissue assays (Bromage *et al.*, 1963). The data suggested that rapid diffusion of local anaesthetic into the CSF at the dural cuff region is the most important determinant of onset of extradural block: peak local anaesthetic concentrations in the CSF are reached within 10–20 min of extradural injection, and concentrations are high enough to produce blockade in the spinal nerve roots and 'rootlets'. This coincides with the clinical onset of extradural block. The same data showed also that by 30 min after injection, the C_{min} for lignocaine (0.28 μg/mg) had been exceeded in the peripheral spinal cord (1.38 μg/mg) and also in spinal nerves in the paravertebral space (1 μg/mg). Data from other studies in which local anaesthetic was injected directly into the CSF indicate that C_{min} is not exceeded in the dorsal root ganglion or in the more central parts of the spinal cord.

The most likely mechanisms for rapid appearance of local anaesthetic in the CSF relate to the unique anatomy of the dural cuff region. This was reviewed extensively by Shantha and Evans (1972), who observed that arachnoid proliferations and villi are plentiful along both dorsal and ventral roots. Although these 'granulations' are found frequently in quadrupeds, their importance in humans is not certain. They are most plentiful in the region of the dural root sleeves ('cuffs'), immediately proximal to the dorsal root ganglion, where the dura becomes thin and is continuous with the epineurium of spinal nerves (see Fig. 58.7). They provide a mechanism by which arachnoid protrudes either partially or completely through the dura into adjacent subdural and extradural spaces. This implies that local anaesthetics may have to diffuse only across a layer of arachnoid epithelial cells to reach CSF. Even if the granulations are sparse in humans, the dura is thin in the root sleeve area and it is clear from local anaesthetic and opioid studies that these drugs gain access to CSF rapidly. These anatomical and pharmacological data provide strong evidence that the major sites of action of local anaesthetics after extradural block are the spinal nerve roots and spinal cord.

It is most likely that diffusion into intradural spinal nerve roots plays a major role during the early stages of extradural block. This is in keeping with the rapid onset of a segmental pattern of blockade. Subsequently, local anaesthetic seepage through intervertebral foramina may contribute by producing 'multiple paravertebral block'. After lumbar extradural block, diffusion through the CSF to the spinal cord (Fig. 58.7) is probably a secondary phenomenon, although it may occur more rapidly when local anaesthetic is injected closer to the spinal cord in thoracic blockade.

Urban (1973) has reported that regression of analgesia after extradural block follows a circumferential pattern in the sagittal plane, rather than the classic segmental pattern seen during onset of block. This is consistent with a persisting action of local anaesthetic on the peripheral spinal cord after the initial effects on spinal nerve roots have abated. Also, Bromage (1974) has observed reflex changes in lower limbs during thoracic extradural blockade that spares the lumbar segments. Changes typical of an upper motor neurone (long tract) lesion were seen: increased deep tendon reflexes and an upgoing toe on Babinski's reflex. The peripheral part of the spinal cord in the dorsolateral funiculus contains descending excitatory sympathetic fibres, the descending pyramidal tracts, and medullary reticulospinal fibres. The pyramidal tract synapses in Rexed's Laminae IV, V and VI which are involved in the modulation of sensory input. It has been hypothesized that local anaesthetics with a high propensity to penetrate the spinal cord may produce a rapid and long-lasting sympathetic blockade, followed closely by motor blockade because of the superficial placement of the appropriate tracts. At the same time, the modulating influences on Lamina V and VI may be blocked, with a resultant expansion of segmental receptive fields and a relative 'antianalgesic' state. This anatomical basis may be an explanation for the 'sensory motor dissociation' exhibited by drugs such as bupivacaine and etidocaine (see below). Currently, no data support differential penetration of the spinal cord for the various local anaesthetics. Recent support for rapid transport of drugs from extradural space to spinal fluid and spinal cord is provided by studies of extradural opioids.

Some advances in neuroanatomy have helped to explain the segmental onset of extradural blockade. Studies of the size of dorsal roots indicate a considerable variation in size, with large roots at C8 and S1 and a 'valley' between these two peak sizes in the thoracic region. Studies of the number of myelinated and non-myelinated fibres in ventral roots reveal also a peak at S1 and in the lower cervical region at C5–8. This is in keeping with the relative resistance of the lower cervical region and S1 to neural blockade. An alternative explanation of the segmental pattern of onset of extradural block was proposed as an initial action on dorsal root ganglia (Frumin *et al.*, 1953, 1954). Although these data are at variance with some subsequent studies, a definitive *in vivo* study of dorsal root ganglion as a major site of action of extradural local anaesthetics remains to be performed. It has been suggested recently that the pia of the spinal cord and spinal nerve roots is continuous with the perineurium of the spinal nerves. Because the epineurium of spinal nerves is continuous with the dura, this raises the possibility of continuity between the subarachnoid space and a subepineurial space. This would explain reports of transverse myelitis after injection of neurolytic agents directly beneath spinal nerve epineurium. All that is required for rapid spread of injected solution from spinal nerve to CSF is accurate needle placement beneath the spinal nerve epineurium.

CLINICAL EXTRADURAL ANAESTHESIA

In addition to choosing the agent and dose, once the extradural space is located the injection can be made through the needle, or a catheter can be inserted for repeated or continuous administration of local anaesthetic. Actual spread of analgesia cannot be predicted; thus, a catheter technique is recommended generally, as adequate spread with a single shot requires injection of a generous dose. It may not be easy to thread a catheter into the extradural space, and there is an incidence of outright failure with extradural catheter techniques and a higher incidence of complications. For example, Cousins and Mazze found a failure rate of 10%, using catheters without stylets in 80 patients. This compares with a rate of failure of 1.2% in 84 cases when injection was made by needle. The major causes of 'catheter failures' were complete inability to thread the catheter (5%), inability to clear the catheter of

blood (2.5%) and threading the catheter through an intervertebral foramen (1.3%). The use of stylets to introduce catheters may reduce the incidence of failure to thread the catheter but may increase the incidence of vascular cannulation. Even if a catheter does not clear of blood completely, a small test dose of adrenaline-containing solution can be injected to test if the catheter is placed inside a vessel or outside a vessel that has been traumatized. Threading through a foramen can be reduced by inserting only a minimal amount of catheter. Overall the irretrievable failure rate of catheters should be close to one in 100. Catheters inserted via upward-directed needles in the thoracic region tend to travel straight up the extradural space without deviating through paravertebral foramen. Thus, no catheter failures were encountered in a series of 160 blocks performed between T8 and L1 (P.R. Bromage, unpublished data). Only 3–4 cm of catheter should be threaded into the extradural space; this reduces but does not eliminate catheter problems.

Test doses

An effective test dose must be able to demonstrate safely:
1 That the injection is being made into the extradural space and *not* the subarachnoid space.
2 That the injection is not made into a blood vessel in the extradural space.

A 16 or 18 gauge Tuohy needle through the dura usually allows rapid flow of CSF, but not invariably. A tissue plug may prevent it as may the dura itself if the needle tip is only just piercing it. The test dose must therefore be equivalent to a subarachnoid dose e.g. 3–5 ml of isobaric bupivacaine 0.5%. Questioning the patient on warmth and numbness in the legs reveals misplaced administration rapidly; a subarachnoid injection results in almost immediate blockade of β-fibres, difficulty with injection or 'drip-back' of local anaesthetic after disconnecting the syringe is usually a result of superficial injection (e.g. into interspinous ligament). A recent review of fatalities related to extradural anaesthesia revealed that the essential safety checks had been omitted—there is no excuse for this deviation from accepted practice (Prince & McGregor, 1986).

When the injection is made through a catheter, intravascular administration may occur. Usually, blood flows freely through the catheter when an extradural vein is cannulated; a further check is to aspirate gently with a syringe but this is not always effective. One way of demonstrating vascular cannulation is to inject slowly (approximately 10 ml/min) an adrenaline-containing test dose (3–5 ml of 1/200 000 solution) whilst monitoring pulse rate, ECG and arterial pressure (Moore & Batra, 1981). An increase in heart rate gives a prompt warning and should prevent the problems associated with intravenous injection of toxic quantities of local anaesthetic.

If a vessel is cannulated, withdrawing the catheter a little (*not through the extradural needle lest it is sheared*) and flushing the catheter gently with saline may allow the tip to be withdrawn from the vessel but remain within the extradural space.

Multiple dosing, infusions and tachyphylaxis

In its simplest application, the catheter is used to consolidate a block for surgery. A single repeat dose of 20% of the total dose, given 20 min after the main dose, consolidates blockade within the level of blockade established. Thus, a patchy block with missed segments may be overcome without extending the block. Later, during surgery, a dose of approximately 50% of the main dose given after the upper level has regressed by one or two segments restores the block to the initial upper segmental level. This same dose given earlier extends the block.

Mean duration times for a particular anaesthetic dose are shown in Table 58.6. Careful clinical monitoring is necessary to detect signs of regression of block and the requirement for another dose. The intensity of sensory and motor block increases with each successive injection. The analogy of 'repainting the fence' has been suggested by Hingson to describe the deepening of blockade with repeated doses. With dilute solutions (e.g. lignocaine 1% or bupivacaine 0.25%) motor block is limited but as the number of doses increases so does the degree of block.

In some circumstances, the duration and degree of block obtained after repeat doses decreases; this is termed tachyphylaxis. It is manifest clinically as increased dose requirements to maintain a given level of block. Tachyphylaxis has been demonstrated clearly during 'continuous' extradural block produced by administration of the short-acting amide anaesthetics (mostly with lignocaine). It has been suggested that repeat injections induce changes in the pH of spinal fluid resulting in diminished efficacy of the local anaesthetic from alterations in the ratio of the ionized: un-ionized fraction but this is an inadequate explanation. If analgesia from extradural lignocaine is allowed to wear off before there is a repeat dose given, tachyphylaxis is more likely. Bromage *et al.* (1969) have reported that if the 'interanalgesic interval' (time from regression of analgesia from one dose to onset of analgesia from the next) is greater than 10 min, tachyphylaxis is likely. Tachyphylaxis increases with lengthening of the interanalgesic interval up to approximately 60 min and then the effect remains constant; at 60 min there is a 30–40% reduction in effect of repeat doses (Fig. 58.11). Another possible factor in increasing dose requirements is tissue reaction and 'walling off' of the extradural catheter, with a resultant decrease in the amount of local anaesthetic reaching the site of action (Durant & Yaksh, 1986).

Traditionally, extradural analgesia maintained for labour pain or postoperative pain control is *discontinuous*; the patient must complain of pain or discomfort before a repeat dose is given. This would be expected to promote tachyphylaxis but it seems to be uncommon with the long-acting agents bupivacaine or etidocaine.

Table 58.6 Clinical effects of local anaesthetic solutions commonly used for extradural blockade.

Drug	Time spread to + four segments + 1 SD (min)	Approximate time to two-segment regression + 2 SD (min)	Recommended 'top-up' time from initial dose (min)
Lignocaine 2%	15+5	100+40	60
Prilocaine 2–3%	15+4	100+40	60
Chloroprocaine 2–3%	12+5	60+15	45
Mepivacaine 2%	15+5	120+150	60
Bupivacaine 0.5–0.75%	18+10	200+80	120
Etidocaine 1–1.5%	10+5	200+80	120

Note top-up time is based on duration − 2 SD which encompasses the likely duration in 95% of the population. In a conscious, co-operative patient, an alternative is to use frequent checks of segmental level to indicate need to top up. All solutions contain 1/200 000 adrenaline.

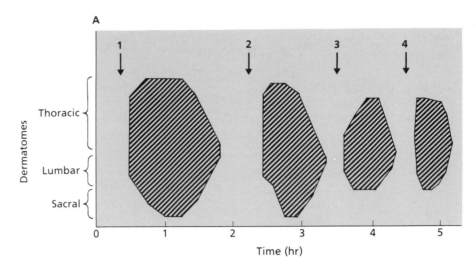

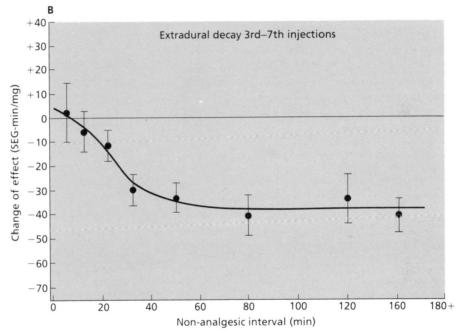

Fig. 58.11 Tachyphylaxis.
A Diminished segmental spread and duration of action of repeated extradural injections of the same dose of local anaesthetic, injected at each arrow. Note re-injection has been made at least 30 min after analgesia has regressed two segments.
B 'Non-analgesic interval'. As the time lag from loss of analgesia to re-injection exceeds 10–15 min, there is a progressive reduction in analgesic effect that reaches a maximum reduction of about 35–40% at 60 min. (Redrawn from Bromage *et al.*, 1969.)

Nevertheless, there is still the humanitarian aspect of only taking 'action on distress' and infusions of local anaesthetic have been introduced in an attempt to provide *continuous* extradural analgesia.

The rate of extradural infusion of local anaesthetic must be a compromise: on one hand the dose must not exceed the maximum recommended dose; on the other, the volume infused must be sufficient to spread within the extradural space and the concentration must be high enough to block the sensory nerves (C_{min}). Several studies using extradural infusions have claimed good results for both labour (Gaylard *et al.*, 1987) and postoperative pain (Scott *et al.*, 1982). There are several advantages for this method: fewer painful intervals, less motor blockade, lower risk of infection with a closed system, greater cardiovascular stability and a lower likelihood of a serious complication following accidental subarachnoid or intravenous injection. Despite some encouraging results, this technique has not gained widespread acceptance, possibly because occasional top-up injections are still required and a higher total dose of local anaesthetic is administered. Thus, the discontinuous technique of intermittent extradural injection on demand still predominates in obstetric practice and after surgery. An alternative approach is to administer extradural top-up doses regularly 'by the clock' before pain returns. Favourable results have been obtained with regular top-up injections for the relief of postoperative pain. Automatic devices to administer regularly timed extradural injections have been described (Scott *et al.*, 1982).

In a study during labour (Purdy *et al.*, 1987), patients receiving regular extradural injections of local anaesthetic complained of much less pain than those receiving injections on demand but received only little more bupivacaine.

Fate of local anaesthetic solutions in the extradural space

The spread of local anaesthetic within the extradural space is summarized in Table 58.7. The local anaesthetic which diffuses across the dura into the CSF is eliminated in the same way as drugs injected directly into it. The majority of the local anaesthetic injected is eliminated from the extradural space. Extradural blockade often requires large doses of local anaesthetic with consequent blood concentrations that are many times higher than those seen after spinal anaesthesia and often nearly toxic (Tucker & Mather, 1975). A thorough knowledge of the pharmacokinetics and toxicity of local anaesthetics is a prerequisite to the safe utilization of extradural anaesthesia.

Extradural injection deposits local anaesthetic some distance from the neural target, so that diffusion across tissue barriers is important. Thus, local anaesthetics with excellent qualities of penetration of lipid are desirable for rapid and effective extradural analgesia. Because a major site of action is within the dural sac, water solubility is of equal importance (see Chapter 36). Thus, agents with a pKa close to physiological pH (e.g. lignocaine, pKa 7.87) are most effective, in that they exhibit readily both lipid- and water-solubility. Procaine and amethocaine, with a high pKa (9.05 and 8.46 respectively), suffer in this respect and perform poorly in extradural blockade.

Extradural fat provides a potential 'reservoir' for deposition of fat-soluble local anaesthetics. Thus, accumulation of long-acting, fat-soluble agents such as bupivacaine, occurs. This is not so for less fat-soluble agents, such as lignocaine. Thus, with repeated injections of bupivacaine, extradural fat concentrations increase but blood concentrations tend to remain the

Table 58.7 Spread of injected solutions in extradural space

Superior and inferior spread is mainly in posterior portion of extradural space between dura and ligamentum flavum
Superiorly to foramen magnum. Note the possibility of diffusion of drugs of low molecular weight across dura at base of brain to cerebral CSF, with possibility of access to cranial nerves, vasomotor and respiratory centres and other vital centres
Inferiorly to sacral hiatus, caudal canal, and through anterior sacral foramina
Laterally through intervertebral foramina to paravertebral space, to produce paravertebral neural blockade. Note rapid access to CSF at 'dural cuff' region to produce spinal nerve root blockade, and subsequent access to spinal cord (see below)
Anteriorly in thin extradural space between dura and anterior longitudinal ligament
Note also: Access to CSF by slow diffusion across spinal dura, subdural space, and subarachnoid membrane into subarachnoid space
Vascular absorption by way of extradural veins may convey drug to heart and brain (see below)
Profuse extradural fat may take up drug

same, provided that dosage is appropriate. Repeated injections of lignocaine result in little accumulation in extradural fat, but progressive accumulation in blood, with a potential for gradually increasing blood concentration.

The extradural venous system provides a rich network of rapid absorption of local anaesthetic. Rapid injection into an extradural vein may despatch local anaesthetic directly to the brain by way of the basivertebral venous system, if flow is reversed by the rapidity of injection. Another risk of rapid intravascular injection is high peak concentrations of local anaesthetic in the myocardium. With bupivacaine, this may lead to serious and prolonged 'cardiac toxicity'. The inclusion of adrenaline in local anaesthetic solutions may reduce vascular absorption greatly and thus enhance neural blocking properties and reduce the likelihood of systemic toxicity.

The time profile of local anaesthetic absorption indicates a peak blood concentration at 10–20 min after injection, so that surveillance is necessary for at least 30 min.

Acid solutions, containing antioxidants to stabilize adrenaline, may release local anaesthetic base with difficulty, and thus spread poorly across lipid barriers. Carbonated solutions release base readily and have superior penetrating ability. pH adjustment with small amounts of bicarbonate may improve neural penetration also.

Plasma protein binding may influence the amount of free local anaesthetic available for placental transfer or for action on the CNS after systemic absorption from the extradural space.

Caudal extradural blockade

In the past, this approach has been used to produce anaesthesia of lumbar and even low thoracic segments by injecting large volumes of solution (often close to or above a recommended maximum dose). This may be dangerous in adults, but can sometimes be useful in children. In adults, caudal anaesthesia is used almost entirely as an extradural technique to provide analgesia anaesthesia of the sacral and low lumbar roots; for high blocks, lumbar or thoracic extradural techniques are used.

Anatomy

The five sacral vertebrae are fused, forming the sacrum. The posterior surface of this triangular-shaped bone is

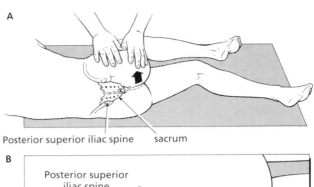

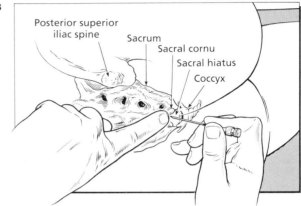

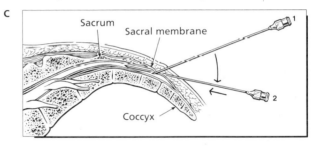

Fig. 58.12 Caudal extradural blockade.
A In the lateral Sim's position, an assistant may be required to reposition the gluteal cleft in the midline.
B Palpation of the sacral hiatus and sacral cornua must not be confused with the sacral foramina. The hiatus should form an equilateral triangle with the posterior superior iliac spines.
C Initial angle of needle insertion should be about 120° to the skin. After penetration of the sacral (sacrococcygeal) membrane the needle is aligned with the long axis of the canal and inserted 1 cm further. (Reproduced from Cousins & Bridenbaugh, 1988.)

convex. Down the middle of the posterior surface runs the sacral crest, composed of three or four remnants of the spinous processes. The laminae of the lowermost vertebra (and sometimes its neighbour) fail to fuse; the resultant gap is the sacral hiatus (Fig. 58.12). The hiatus is bounded laterally by the sacral cornu (these are the remnants of the inferior articular processes of the fifth sacral vertebra) and covered by the sacrococcygeal membrane. This membrane is pierced by the coccygeal and fifth sacral nerves; the first four sacral nerves leave the sacrum through the paired lateral sacral foraminae along the length of the sacrum. The dural sac terminates at the level of the lower border of S2 and below this the canal contains a venous plexus (continuation of the internal vertebral plexus), the filum terminale (continuation of the pia mater), the sacral nerves and fatty tissue. The total mean volume of the canal is 32 ml in females and 34 ml in males.

The anatomy of the sacrum and the sacral canal is *extremely variable*. Most of the abnormalities are readily observable or palpable but they contribute to the less than 100% success rate seen with this block.

Technique

The patient and anaesthetist should be prepared as for extradural or spinal anaesthesia. The usual position for the patient is lateral with hips and knees flexed (Fig. 58.12A), but alternatives are prone (with a pillow under the hips and toes turned in) and the knee–elbow position. The sacral hiatus must be readily palpable. It lies 3.5–5 cm above the tip of the coccyx and at the apex of the triangle formed by it and the posterior superior iliac crest. Lying between the cornu, it often feels triangular in shape. A small weal of local anaesthetic is raised over this point (too much local anaesthetic and the landmarks are obscured). A 23 or 21 gauge needle is inserted at an angle of about 20° to the skin at that point (Fig. 58.12B). The sacrococcygeal membrane is very superficial and a definite 'give' is often felt as it is pierced. The needle is aligned with the anticipated long axis of the canal and advanced no more than 2.5 cm (Fig. 58.12C). In adults, the mean distance from sacrococcygeal membrane to dura is 4.5 cm but it may be much less and aspiration for CSF must precede injection. It is not unusual for the aspiration to reveal blood (there is a rich venous plexus) and the needle should be repositioned. The local anaesthetic should be injected at the rate appropriate for extradural administration (no more than 10 ml/min), and injection of a test dose is recommended. Caudal extradural injection requires very little force: if it does, the needle tip may be deep to the periosteal dura or even within a vertebra. Injection may be easy but superficial to the sacrococcygeal membrane or within a sacral foramina ('decoy hiatus'). During injection, the free hand can be used to palpate for swelling on the back of the sacrum associated with misplaced injections. A test dose of 5 ml of air may be used, after careful aspiration, and palpation performed to check for superficial crepitus.

A Tuohy needle can be used to place a catheter for continuous techniques. They are often difficult to thread because of the variations in diameter and direction of the sacral canal; an alternative is to insert an intravenous cannula.

Indications

Operations on the perineum are the main indication although the technique is useful for providing postoperative pain control. The use of caudal block in obstetrics and paediatrics is discussed in Chapters 38 and 34 respectively.

Drugs

The choice is dependent on the duration of analgesia required. The absorption, disposition, etc. are similar to that of extradural blocks performed higher up the spine. Typically, 15–20 ml may be expected to block to L1. Lignocaine 1 or 2% with adrenaline or bupivacaine 0.5% provide anaesthesia, whereas bupivacaine 0.25% is adequate for postoperative pain control. Injection of large volumes to increase spread is not recommended. A large and variable amount of the injectate leaks out through the sacral foramina (occasionally visible) and this limits the height of block attained. During injection there should be repeated attempts to aspirate the syringe as the needle tip may have been moved. Direct intravascular injection or rapid absorption of local anaesthetic promoted by rapid forceful injection may result in convulsions or cardiac arrest.

Physiology of spinal subarachnoid and extradural blockade

Physiological changes may result from:
1 Consequences of neural blockade—produced mostly by sympathetic blockade but sensory and motor blockade are not wholly benign.
2 Consequences of vascular absorption of drugs used—produced usually by the local anaesthetic agent but the vasoconstrictor may have deleterious effects.

These consequences are summarized in Table 58.8.

Cardiovascular effects

The sympathetic outflow of the cord is from T1–L2 (Fig. 58.13); thus, a block below L2 has little effect on

Table 58.8 Physiological effects of extradural block. (From Cousins and Bridenbaugh, 1988)

Vascular absorption of local anaesthetic (LA) or adrenaline (Ad)	Direct neural blocking effects or indirect results of blockade

Receptor
β-stimulation by Ad
α-stimulation by Ad or phenylephrine
 	
Smooth muscle
Blood vessels, LA or Ad
Heart, LA or Ad
Other organs, LA or Ad
 	
Cardiac muscle
By LA or Ad
 	
Neural tissue
CNS, by LA
Conducting system of heart by LA
 	
Miscellaneous
Neuromuscular junction by LA
	Spinal nerves (roots and trunks) by axonal blockade
	Sympathetic
	   Efferent blockade
	   Peripheral (T1–L2) vasoconstrictor
	   'Adrenal' (T6–L1)
	   'Central' (T1–4) cardiac sympathetic
	Sensory
	   Afferent blockade
	   Reduced peripheral sensation
	   Blockade of visceral pain fibres
	   Reduced efferent neurohumoral responses
	   to surgical or other stimulus within
	   the blocked area
	Motor
	   Efferent blockade
	      Varying degrees of motor paralysis
	      Reflex muscle relaxation without
	      paralysis (deafferentation)
	
	Spinal cord
	Axons
	   Superficial, sensory tracts blocked (e.g. bupivacaine, lignocaine and etidocaine)
	   Deep motor paths blocked (e.g. etidocaine)
	      Dorsal horn modulation of pain transmission (? axons, ? cells)
	      Possibility of 'antianalgesic' effect owing to block of inhibitory paths
	Cells bodies: 'selective' blockade
	
	Secondary changes in parasympathetic activity
	Sympathetic block to T5 + venous return may – vagus
	Sympathetic block to T1 – unopposed vagus

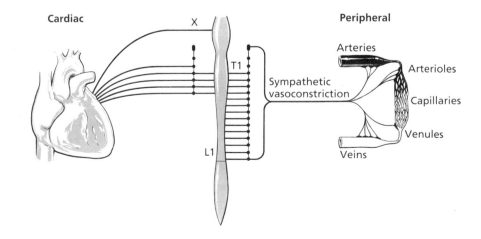

Fig. 58.13 Sympathetic blockade: 'central' (cardiac) and 'peripheral' components. These consist of T1–4 cardiac sympathetic fibres and T1–L2 'peripheral' sympathetic fibres. Note important innervation of veins and venules. Vagal cardiac fibres are also shown. (Reproduced from Cousins & Bridenbaugh, 1988.)

arterial pressure. Blockade above T4 affects not only sympathetic vasoconstrictor fibres but also the sympathetic innervation of the heart (T1–4). There may still be sympathetic tone below the block as tracts within the cord are still functioning (note that spinal and extradural anaesthesia does not produce chemical transection of the cord). The majority of spinal and extradural anaesthetics produce effects that lie between these two extremes and have variable effects on the cardiovascular system (CVS). A block to T10 produces only 'peripheral' sympathetic block and has little effect on the CVS. At this level, only inguinal, perineal and lower limb surgery may be undertaken. Lower abdominal surgery (e.g. appendicectomy, Caesarian section and gynaecological surgery) necessitate block to T4.

A small decrease in arterial pressure usually occurs but the reported incidence of significant hypotension [defined variously as an arterial pressure decrease of greater than 4 kPa (30 mmHg), 20% or 30% of initial pressure] ranges from approximately 3 to 30%. Obviously the height of block is important but the 'category of risk' is also a major factor. There are no data to suggest that hypotension occurs less frequently with extradural or spinal anaesthesia. The level of sympathetic block is the same as (or lower than) sensory with extradural blockade. In comparison, sympathetic block may be two to three segments higher than sensory level with subarachnoid block.

Vascular absorption of local anaesthetic and vasoconstrictor agent may result in significant haemodynamic changes after extradural but not subarachnoid blockade. The reason for this lies predominantly in the much larger doses of drugs used and the proximity of the large extradural veins. The more gradual onset of sympathetic blockade after extradural analgesia compared with subarachnoid block may provide a mechanism for initial responses that are less severe for extradural block. When used extradurally, lignocaine, chloroprocaine, and etidocaine have a rapid onset of sympathetic block (especially etidocaine). This is more evident if adrenaline-containing solutions are used. In comparison, onset of sympathetic block is slower with bupivacaine and there is less tendency for rapid development of hypotension; indeed, sympathetic block may take 25–30 min to develop and even then may be only a 'partial' block. Animal studies have shown that autoregulation at the level of the precapillary sphincters develops within 30 min of complete ablation of neural activity.

Although controlled studies are not available, experience with large series of thoracic extradural blocks administered in intensive therapy units by continuous catheter techniques supports further the allowance of adequate time for autoregulation. A common management protocol for 'topping up' thoracic extradural blockade for chest trauma involves keeping the patient supine during and for 20–30 min after top up. Using this procedure, serious hypotension is uncommon, whereas topping up in the semi-recumbent position or allowing inadequate time in the supine position after blockade may result in large reductions in arterial pressure. With continuous extradural infusions, it is only necessary to lie the patient flat while the loading dose is given.

Blockade below T4

Blockade that is restricted to the level of the low thoracic and lumbar region (T5–L4) results in a 'peripheral' sympathetic blockade with vascular dilatation in the pelvis and lower limbs; if all splanchnic fibres are blocked (T6–L1), pooling of blood in the gut and abdominal viscera may occur also. The peripheral blockade is manifest as an increase in lower limb blood flow by arteriolar vasodilatation and 'pooling' of blood in the venous capacitance vessels. Because the latter contain 80% of blood volume, venodilatation has a potential for dramatic changes in venous return, reduction in right atrial pressure, and reduced cardiac output. The decrease in venous return has been shown to result in increased cardiac vagal tone in young patients. This explains why heart rate remains unchanged or decreased despite hypotension and activation of cardiac sympathetic accelerator fibres.

The patient may compensate for a decrease in mean arterial pressure with a reflex increase in efferent sympathetic vasoconstriction above the level of the block. Thus, blood flow and venous capacitance are reduced in the head, neck and upper limbs. This increased efferent sympathetic activity is mediated predominantly (by means of the baroreceptors) by those sympathetic vasoconstrictor nerves (T1–5) that remain unblocked and by circulating catecholamines released from the adrenal medulla owing to increased activity in any unblocked fibres in the splanchnic nerves (T6–L1). Although blood vessels in some viscera, such as the kidney, appear to be more responsive to direct neural stimuli, in other vascular beds both neural and hormonal influences have major effects, although at different levels of the vasculature. Major arterioles respond mostly to neural stimuli, while small arterioles and venules near the capillary bed respond predominantly to circulating catecholamines. Thus, while any splanchnic fibres remain unblocked, there is a potential for vasoconstrictor activity below (and above) the level of blockade, by release of catecholamines from the adrenal medulla. Finally, the ability of precapillary sphincters to achieve autoregulation within a short time of cessation of neural activity provides a further mechanism for regaining vascular tone and minimizing vascular pooling below the level of blockade.

Increased activity in unblocked cardiac sympathetic fibres (T1–4) may result in increased cardiac contractility and increased heart rate; similar effects are produced by increased levels of circulating catecholamines. Evidence that the latter are important in maintaining homeostasis in some clinical situations is provided by the surprisingly small changes in heart rate and cardiac output (-16%) with blockade of C5–T4, but with splanchnic fibres to the adrenal medulla (T6–L1) intact. Although quite large compensatory cardiac effects may be observed in unmedicated volunteers (e.g. a 20% increase in heart rate and cardiac output), these changes are not seen in premedicated patients (Table 58.8). In premedicated patients, despite decreased peripheral resistance, unchanged heart rate and cardiac output, mean arterial pressure was reduced by only 10%, because total vascular resistances decreased by only 25% as a result of increased sympathetic activity in unblocked areas. The studies by Germann et al. (1979) and others reported changes that are close to those that the anaesthetist may anticipate in clinical practice, although patients in the latter study were not rehydrated. The practice of 'preloading' with intravenous balanced salt solution is capable of maintaining mean arterial pressure close to preblock levels in healthy patients, including parturients, provided the level of blockade is below T4 and inferior vena caval obstruction is avoided. Provided bradycardia is avoided, the healthy supine patient may have little change in arterial pressure. Change in position and ill health may have significant CVS sequelae.

Blockade below T10

With a lower block, fewer vasoconstrictor fibres are included and neither the splanchnic nerves nor the nerve supply to the adrenal medulla are affected. Thus, the potential for hypotension is reduced greatly.

Blockade below L2

There is no sympathetic block and all CVS effects are mediated through absorbed local anaesthetic, etc.

Blockade above T4

In healthy, supine patients there is often surprisingly little effect with a high thoracic block. However, there are no compensatory mechanisms remaining and the anaesthetist must be able to make physiological adjustments rapidly i.e. control of blood volume, heart rate, vascular tone and cardiac contractile state.

EFFECTS OF LOCAL ANAESTHETIC SOLUTIONS ON THE CARDIOVASCULAR SYSTEM

Plain solutions

Whereas the autonomic effects of extradural and spinal block are similar, because of the much larger doses of local anaesthetic used with the former, the CVS consequences of absorbed local anaesthetic are greater. The slow absorption of local anaesthetic from the extradural space has very different effects to rapid inadvertent intravenous injection.

Extradural blockade with lignocaine results in plasma concentrations of approximately 3–5 μg/ml and little effect on the CVS; bupivacaine and etidocaine are similarly benign with slow injection. When an extradural dose is injected rapidly intravenously there may be depression of cardiac contractility and intracardiac conduction which may lead sometimes to cardiac arrest. With lignocaine, the heart responds rapidly to inotropic support, but if bupivacaine has been injected, prolonged vigorous resuscitation including large doses of adrenaline and possibly bretylium may be required to reverse any arrythmias.

Adrenaline-containing solutions

The cardiovascular effects of low-dose adrenaline are different from those of high doses which produce tachycardia, hypertension and peripheral ischaemia. Systemic effects of doses of adrenaline in the range of 80–130 μg, as used in extradural block, are a moderate increase in heart rate, increased cardiac output, decreased peripheral resistance and decreased mean arterial pressure. These changes are, however, greater than if adrenaline without local anaesthetic was administered. This may arise because the degree of sympathetic block is more intense (as with analgesia); the spinal adrenaline itself may cause sympathetic blockade, and the vasodilator β-adrenergic effects of systemically absorbed adrenaline may counteract compensatory vasoconstriction.

FACTORS WHICH MAY MODIFY THE CARDIOVASCULAR EFFECTS OF EXTRADURAL AND SPINAL BLOCKADE

Hypovolaemia

Major conduction blockade should be avoided in patients with uncorrected hypovolaemia; in contrast to the mild changes in normovolaemia, large changes in heart rate, cardiac output and arterial pressures occur. These deleterious changes are reduced by light anaesthesia, suggesting that the sudden CVS collapse seen (precipitated by bradycardia) is a fainting response to decreased venous return mediated by increased vagal activity and by adrenaline-containing solutions (the absorbed adrenaline maintaining an adequate heart rate and cardiac output).

In hypovolaemia, the myocardium receives a greater proportion of cardiac output and may be exposed to a higher concentration of absorbed local anaesthetic. Effects of local anaesthetic on the myocardium are accentuated further by acidosis, which co-exists frequently with hypovolaemia and hypotension, although acidosis does not affect the distribution of local anaesthetic to the heart (Nancarrow et al., 1987).

Cardiovascular disease

Patients with cardiovascular disease have poor compensatory capacity and are more prone to risks of hypotension (Hartung et al., 1986).

General anaesthesia

The effect of general anaesthesia on the CVS changes of extradural and spinal anaesthesia is variable and has been studied little. With an extradural block to mid-thoracic level, a reduction in arterial pressure, heart rate and cardiac output may occur. Whilst arterial pressure is increased by elevating the legs or introducing a head-down tilt, the administration of ephedrine improves all variables. A relative bradycardia responds to atropine. The sequence of induction of regional and general anaesthesia does not affect these changes (Germann et al., 1979).

Intestinal obstruction, ascites, large intra-abdominal tumours and surgery

All these conditions cause inferior vena caval obstruction and limit venous return from below the level of obstruction. When sympathetic block is superimposed, there is an increase in venous pooling and an exaggerated CVS response. Small carefully titrated doses of ephedrine (5–10 mg) restore venous capacitance to a more normal value. Often these conditions cause some arterial obstruction also and when relieved during surgery may result in precipitous hypotension unless adequate amounts of intravenous fluids have been infused, even though ephedrine may be required. Caval obstruction may be caused by poor posturing of the patient and enthusiastic retraction or packing during abdominal surgery.

Advanced pregnancy and labour

The result of this is caval and aortic obstruction; the effects similar to those of intra-abdominal tumours and are discussed in Chapter 38 (see also Fig. 58.6).

Respiratory effects

Extradural or spinal blockade per se have little effect on respiration provided that brain perfusion is maintained. The potential for phrenic nerve (C3–5) block is extremely low. With a high block, the diminished input to the reticular activating system may lead to a drowsy patient with quiet regular respiration, and the sedative effect of blood concentrations of local anaesthetic associated with extradural block may contribute to this.

Continuous extradural blockade for pain relief after surgery improves ability to cough and functional residual capacity in addition to Pao_2 (Spence & Smith, 1971). However, there is no difference in respiratory function tests between this technique of analgesia and opioid analgesia administered optimally.

Visceral effects

Blockade of sacral segments S2–4 results in bladder atonia; it is temporary and causes no, or minimal, increase in postblock bladder dysfunction. Segmental thoracic block may increase bladder–sphincter tone by abolishing reflex sympathetic activity (via T12–L1 segments) and may predispose to acute retention. With continuous extradural block, urinary catheterization is often necessary.

Extradural and spinal block from T5–L1 abolishes splanchnic sympathetic supply and because of parasympathetic tone, results in a contracted small bowel with relaxed sphincters; as there is also relaxation of abdominal muscles, operating conditions are good. There is no evidence that anastomoses are threatened by this technique of anaesthesia.

Major regional blockade obtunds the hormonal and metabolic responses to surgery. This effect is shortlived and once the spinal anaesthesia has worn off the changes are similar to those in patients receiving general anaesthesia. A block to T5 (which includes sympathetic block to this level) abolishes the 'neuro-endocrine' response to surgery temporarily. It is not known what the long-term consequences of this are, although in the short term there have been some advantages reported e.g. reduced catecholamine secretion may reduce the incidence of intraoperative myocardial ischaemia. Continuation of extradural blockade postoperatively modifies some of the components of the stress response, for example urinary nitrogen loss is decreased.

Distribution of blood flow

1 Total peripheral vascular resistance decreases with extradural and spinal block (typically 15–18%); this is a result of differential flow through vascular beds.
2 Pooling in denervated venous capacitance vessels occurs below the level of the right atrium.
3 Blood flow to brain is maintained whilst arterial pressure is within the range of the cerebrovascular autoregulatory mechanisms.
4 Myocardial oxygenation decreases, but in parallel with oxygen requirements which are reduced by decreased ventricular work; studies in animals indicate improved myocardial oxygen supply versus demand and a reduction in the size of an experimentally produced infarction (Reiz et al., 1982; Davis et al., 1986).
5 Hepatic blood flow is reduced; hepatic oxygen extraction increases but in the absence of hypotension hepatic hypoxia does not occur.
6 Renal blood flow is maintained by autoregulation, but, even during severe hypotension, blood flow is usually adequate to oxygenate renal tissues so that renal function returns to normal when arterial pressure is brought back to normal.

Temperature control

The vasodilatation of extensive extradural block may predispose to hypothermia in a cold environment. However, this reduction in body temperature occurs slowly and does not explain the rapid onset of shivering that sometimes immediately follows the injection of local anaesthetic solutions into the extradural space. Various causes of shivering have been proposed in association with extradural blockade:
1 A decrease in core temperature as a result of peripheral vasodilatation caused by sympathetic blockade.
2 An effect of absorbed local anaesthetic on temperature regulatory centres.
3 A differential inhibition of spinal cord afferent thermoreceptor fibres (loss of warm sensation before cold sensation), causing an erroneous indication of a reduction in peripheral temperature.
5 A direct effect of cold local anaesthetic solutions on thermosensitive structures within the spinal cord. (Such structures have been demonstrated in animals, but not in humans.)

The latter explanation (5) is the most likely explanation of the phenomenon although it is not the whole story, and (1), (2) and (3) may contribute. Injection of opioids extradurally usually abolishes shivering in most patients. It has been reported that shivering is more common after bupivacaine, and the slow onset of blockade would certainly permit a longer period of differential loss of warm sensation with associated shivering.

Neurological deficit

A recent extensive review has confirmed that the spinal route of administration of local anaesthetic is extremely safe (Kane, 1981). The spinal cord may be injured by ischaemia, direct trauma and by chemicals. Hypotension is the major cause of ischaemia; consequences range from absent knee or ankle jerks to complete flaccid paraplegia. There are often contributing factors such as surgery affecting the cord (e.g. aortic cross-clamping) or vascular lesions so that all hypotensive episodes must be treated seriously. Trauma and chemicals are infrequent causes of cord damage. In the past, chemicals have been contaminants of local anaesthetic solutions, but they are now administered usually as the result of carelessness. The mechanisms of neurological damage are summarized in Fig. 58.14.

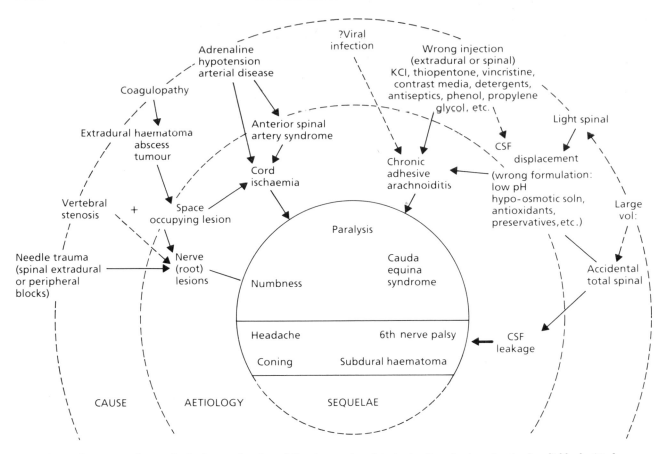

Fig. 58.14 Causation of neurological complications following regional (principally spinal and extradural) block. (Redrawn from Reynolds, 1987.)

Monitoring for major regional blockade

Monitoring heart rate and arterial pressure are mandatory. Heart rate should be monitored by ECG starting before injection of local anaesthetic. Arterial pressure may decrease rapidly and the frequency of measurement should be appropriate for the block. Verbal contact with the patient is a useful monitor of impending problems and complaints e.g. a metallic taste or nausea must receive prompt attention. There may be significant changes in the CVS after repositioning the patient. Oxygenation may be monitored by pulse oximetry. In general, supplemental oxygen should be administered although it may not be necessary for healthy patients with a low level of block.

Sedation

Sedation should be administered carefully. Opioids and benzodiazepines may be used, but these potent drugs are not an alternative to psychological preparation of the patient; 50% oxygen in nitrous oxide (Entonox) by mask is also particularly useful.

Management of hypotension

Peripheral venous pooling from sympathetic blockade reduces preload and hence cardiac output. Myocardial contractility is unchanged by spinal anaesthesia although it may be reduced by systemic absorption of local anaesthetic after extradural administration. There is controversy over the level to which arterial pressure may fall before therapy is required; 33% below resting central values or an absolute level of 10.6 kPa (80 mmHg) systolic in young, normotensive patients may be safe. In conscious patients, a systolic pressure below 10.6 kPa (80 mmHg) frequently precipitates a vasovagal attack and profound hypotension accompanies the bradycardia, nausea and vomiting. The arterial pressure at which regional cerebral perfusion is reduced is not known but symptoms such as restlessness, breathlessness or nausea may indicate the critical value has been reached.

Treatment of hypotension comprises restoration of venous return; the Trendelenberg position or elevation of the legs may achieve this, although greater than $20°$ head-down is counterproductive (and may increase the height of a spinal anaesthetic when hyperbaric solutions are used). Rapid infusion of electrolyte solutions may restore arterial pressure but also increases myocardial oxygen demand in the face of haemodilution.

Large infusions of crystalloids may precipitate heart failure or retention of urine when the block regresses. Bradycardia causing hypotension is treated with small doses (0.2 mg) of atropine. When vasopressors are required, drugs with both α- and β-adrenergic effects (e.g. ephedrine) are used to induce venoconstriction and increase cardiac output (in contrast to the reflex bradycardia which occurs with pure α-agonists). Vigilant monitoring is required to avoid sudden changes of arterial pressure occurring with change in position (e.g. lithotomy to supine) both in the operating room and recovery area.

Postdural-puncture headache

All patients undergoing spinal anaesthesia should be warned of this complication. The headache is bifrontal and occipital and may involve the neck and upper shoulders. It is aggravated by sitting, standing, coughing and straining but often subsides completely when the patient lies down. The headache may be totally incapacitating and is accompanied often by nausea, anorexia, photophobia and neck stiffness. It may persist for many days and causes depression in the patient and anxiety for the anaesthetist. The incidence of headache is proportional to the gauge of needle used; rare after dural puncture with a 25 gauge needle, more frequent with a 22 gauge needle and common with an 18 or 16 gauge extradural needle. Bedrest for 24–48 hr postpones the onset of headache but has no effect on incidence. The complication is usually self-limiting and control of symptoms is achieved by bedrest and simple analgesics administered regularly.

Postdural-puncture headache is presumably a result of continuing leak of CSF through the puncture site resulting in traction on meningeal vessels and nerves. In severe cases, diplopia and other cranial nerve palsies can occur. Therapies aimed at increasing extradural pressure (e.g. extradural infusion of saline and tight abdominal binding), increasing CSF production (e.g.

overhydration of the patient by intravenous or oral fluids at a rate of at least 3 litre/day) and decreasing CSF loss (e.g. by lying flat) are helpful.

The definitive treatment for headache that is severe or refractory to a short trial of conservative measures is extradural injection of autologous blood (extradural 'blood-patch') (Di Giovanni & Dunbar, 1970). Five to 10 ml of blood drawn aseptically from the patient is injected into the extradural space. The success rate is approximately 90–95% after the first injection and the procedure has only a few mild complications of its own (e.g. backache 35%, fever 5%) when infection is avoided.

Spinal opioids

The spinal route of administration of opioids produces a more selective effect on nociception than the axonal blockade of several modalities resulting from local anaesthetics. This method of pain control has developed logically, although the concept progressed extremely fast from laboratory experimentation in animals to man (Cousins & Mather, 1984). The 'gate theory of pain' proposed by Melzack and Wall suggested that nociception could be modulated at spinal cord level. Yaksh and Rudy (1976) reported profound analgesia in rats following spinal administration of opioids. Only 3 yr later, reports of spinal subarachnoid and extradural opioid administration to control cancer pain appeared; prolonged analgesia was achieved with doses a fraction of those used systemically. The first rigorous study of spinal extradural opioid administration for postoperative pain control (Cousins et al., 1979) confirmed that the spinal cord was the site of action and that systemic blood drug concentration was insufficient to produce analgesia. The differences in blood concentrations between CSF and blood are high after extradural administration ranging from $50:1$ to $200:1$ (depending on the opioid and dose), and even higher after spinal subarachnoid dosing. A 0.5 mg spinal subarachnoid dose is huge when compared with the calculated 10 μg which reaches the CNS after a parenteral 10 mg dose, yet despite this, the analgesia is not total. Two reasons are suggested to explain this phenomenon: firstly, a significant proportion of opioid-induced analgesia is mediated through supraspinal opioid receptors (i.e. periaqueductal grey matter neurones in the mid-brain, nucleus raphe magnus and rostral ventral medulla). Secondly, spinal opioids through their action pre- and postsynaptically on small cell networks in the dorsal horn, control pain of a constant ongoing nature (e.g. deep and dull forms of somatic pain) better than pain of a phasic nature (e.g. sharp pain of acute injury and intermittent visceral pain) where large numbers of afferent neurons are recruited rapidly. In practice, this is manifest as the high success rate seen with spinal opioids for control of cancer pain, some success in postoperative pain and poor results with the pain of surgery, acute labour and primary neurological disease.

Pharmacology

The distribution of opioids injected spinally is very similar to local anaesthetics. *In vitro* studies suggest that permeability of the dura to opioids varies inversely with the square of the molecular weight of the drug and that molecular weight is more important than lipid-solubility. *In vivo* transfer of opioid to CNS may occur also by spinal cord blood supply and by diffusion through the dural cuff region of neurones and so there is an interplay of many physico-chemical properties of the agent.

Opioid in the CSF (injected into subarachnoid or diffused from the extradural space) penetrates the spinal meninges and is taken up by the outer layers of the spinal cord at a rate proportional to the agent's lipid-solubility. For analgesia at a spinal level, both superficial and deeper opioid receptors (i.e. Lamina I and II of the dorsal horn) need to be reached by opioid. Thus, even with spinal subarachnoid injection of morphine there is a delay of 30 min before the full effect is achieved. As with local anaesthetics, vascular uptake is the route of elimination from the CSF and this is proportional also to lipid-solubility. Thus, the lipophilic opioids have the most rapid onset of spinal effect but are the most rapidly eliminated.

Opioids can spread in the spinal subarachnoid space both as a result of diffusion and of bulk transport by the circulation of CSF. Because lipophilicity promotes uptake agent, this property is inversely proportional to cephalad spread of drug within the CSF. It is cephalad transport which allows lumbar administration of morphine to be used in upper abdominal and thoracic surgery. However, migration of drug to brain is responsible for the most serious side-effects.

In opioid-naïve subjects, spinal opioids result in a high incidence of non-segmental itching (after about 3 hr following lumbar extradural injection of morphine). Nausea and vomiting is a frequent occurrence several hr after injection. The most serious side-effect is 'delayed' respiratory depression; presumed to be a result of morphine reaching the brain, it can occur from 3 to 12 hr after injection. Early respiratory depression may occur 0–1 hr after extradural or direct spinal subarachnoid injection of lipophilic opioids such as pethidine (see below), alfentanil and even fentanyl. As vascular uptake is competing with CNS uptake, it is not surprising that addition of adrenaline enhances analgesia. Adrenaline has inherent analgesic properties at cord level but it delays drug elimination from CSF also; a consequence of this is more free opioid in the CSF and intensified respiratory depression. Receptor kinetics interplay with lipid-solubility. Thus, sufentanil has a longer duration of action (approximately 6 hr) than fentanyl (2.5–3.5 hr) which, although it is less lipid soluble, has less intense binding.

As cephalad transport of drug is responsible for the most serious yet unpredictable side-effect of spinal opioids, the more lipophilic agents should be safer. The question of relative safety of morphine (hydrophilic opioid) and pethidine (lipophilic opioid) has been considered by Sjöström *et al.* in studies to determine the pharmacokinetics of the two agents after both routes of spinal administration (Sjöström *et al.*, 1987a, b). After extradural or intrathecal administration peak, plasma concentrations of both drugs are attained within 10 min. Pethidine crosses the dura four times more rapidly than morphine, thus the lipophilic drug achieves its peak CSF concentration four times more rapidly than the hydrophilic agent. Similarly, CSF pethidine concentration decreases four times more rapidly than morphine concentration. However, only 4% of the dose of either drug reaches the CSF. The rapid decline in pethidine CSF concentration suggests cephalad transport is unlikely although significant concentrations can be measured at the C7–T1 level 1 hr after lumbar administration (Gourlay *et al.*, 1987). It would therefore appear that respiratory depression following pethidine should occur early (at approximately 1 hr) and be produced both by systemic drug absorption and migration in CSF.

Some other afferent and motor activity may be affected in addition to block of nociception and there can be difficulty with initiating micturition leading to urinary retention; this complication has been reported to occur in up to 90% of males given extradural morphine. Pethidine has a marked local anaesthetic action (Way, 1946) and when administered intrathecally can produce segmental somatic block (Famewo & Naguib, 1985).

Spinal opioids in control of acute pain

POSTOPERATIVE PAIN

Spinal opioids can be extremely effective in postoperative pain therapy. There is a plethora of conflicting reports and opinions on which drug, dose and site of injection is best. If the opioid is injected in the middle of the required dermatomal spread, speed of onset of analgesia is determined by the physico-chemical properties of the drug. If the opioid is injected distant to the required site of action, onset is related to transport of drug in CSF and this may take several hours (Larsen et al., 1985); a larger dose may shorten onset but increases the risk of complications.

There have been few comparisons between drugs and fewer using equipotent doses. Onset of analgesia seems to be slow for morphine (30 min to 1 hr) but is similar for most other opioids. Duration of action varies significantly e.g. morphine (6 mg) 12.3 hr, methadone (6 mg) 8.7 hr, fentanyl (100 μg) 5.7 hr (Torda & Pybus, 1982).

These figures are not as comparable as it may seem, as doses which are equipotent when given intravenously may not have the same ratio of potency by other routes e.g. morphine, 4 mg, extradurally is not as effective as methadone 4 mg. Also, duration of effect is somewhat dose dependent, extradural morphine 5 mg, 7.5 mg and 10 mg are all effective after lower abdominal surgery but the incidence of side-effects is higher with the larger doses. A table suggesting initial doses for extradural morphine for postoperative pain has been prepared by Ready et al. (1988) (Table 58.9). Subsequent doses should be adjusted after observation of degree of analgesia obtained and the severity of any

side-effects (Cousins, 1987). An alternative to morphine is the administration of short-acting opioids with rapid onset by infusion. This technique permits flexibility of rate of drug administration and may avoid 'late' respiratory depression after cessation of therapy. Individualization of dose is stressed; dose–response data suggest that the ratio between analgesic dose and the dose causing life-threatening respiratory depression of spinally administered opioids may be close to two! (Cousins et al., 1987).

There have been no controlled studies comparing spinal subarachnoid with extradural opioids; it appears that the quality of analgesia by the two routes is similar but using a much smaller dose with spinal subarachnoid injection. Unfortunately, ventilatory depression is more common with spinal subarachnoid opioids (Rawal et al., 1987).

The quality of analgesia obtainable with carefully titrated parenteral opioids (e.g. by patient-controlled analgesia) is similar to that from extradural opioids but the profile of side-effects is dissimilar. The extradural route, however, requires less drug for the same effect and patients are therefore less sedated. Respiratory depression is dose dependent with parenteral dosing but less predictable with the spinal route. However, respiratory depression has become less common since smaller doses and 'low-dose infusions' of extradural opioids have been used.

The Swedish Nationwide Follow-up Survey (Rawal et al., 1987) revealed an incidence of ventilatory depression of approximately one in 1100 (0.09%) following extradural morphine and one in 275 (0.36%) following spinal subarachnoid morphine. This survey includes all patients receiving spinal opioids; if only postoperative patients are studied, the incidence is higher. The study identified old age, poor general condition and residual effects of anaesthetic drugs as important risk factors for this complication but more than 50% of patients treated for delayed ventilatory depression had received supplementary local anaesthetic. Naloxone reverses the respiratory depression readily, but obviously patients must be managed in a ward where the condition may be recognized. Measuring respiratory rate alone is a poor monitor; early warning of problems ahead can be obtained from monitoring mental state also. When there has been a sudden deterioration in the conscious level, and/or reduction in respiratory rate, careful titration of naloxone can reverse the adverse effects of the opioid only.

Ventilatory depression can occur 23 hr after spinal subarachnoid opioid administration and may still be

Table 58.9 Suggested starting dose (mg) of spinal extradural morphine for incisional pain.* (From Ready et al., 1988)

Patient age (yr)	Non-thoracic surgery (lumbar or caudal catheter)	Thoracic surgery	
		Thoracic catheter	Lumbar catheter
15–44	5	4	6
45–65	4	3	5
66–75	3	2	4
76+	2	1	2

These doses are guidelines only. Safety and effectiveness of these doses may vary considerably between individual patients.
* Undiluted 0.1% preservative-free morphine is used.

present 16 hr after extradural injection. It has been suggested that when doses of morphine, 4 mg or less, are administered extradurally, surveillance is only necessary for 12 hr (Rawal *et al.*, 1987).

LABOUR PAIN

Although first-stage pain can be controlled with extra-dural opioids alone, active labour cannot. The addition of an opioid to the local anaesthetic allows a lower concentration of local anaesthetic to have the desired effect and can abolish the shivering often seen with local anaesthetic alone: fentanyl, 50–100 μg, or pethidine, 50 mg, in bupivacaine 0.25% are effective (Vella *et al.*, 1985).

Spinal subarachnoid opioids have a high incidence of side-effects (vomiting, urinary retention and itching) when used in labour.

CHRONIC PAIN

Spinal opioids can be effective when satisfactory control is not possible by some other routes.

Their role is controversial and there is only anecdotal evidence that patients who 'fail' with oral opioids obtain better relief when the spinal route is used. Morphine is administered usually, and 5–10 mg is the usual initial dose range extradurally. Ventilatory depression is not a reported feature of chronic dosing. A physiological explanation for this lies in the rapid tolerance of brainstem nuclei to increasing doses of opioids. In *in vitro* preparations of cells from the locus ceruleus (LC), spontaneous discharge of cells can be silenced with morphine; cells in the LC from animals pretreated chronically with morphine require a many-fold increase in applied morphine to have their activity depressed (Andrade *et al.*, 1983). Fortuitously, tolerance in the more caudad nociceptive circuitary develops much more slowly.

Repeat administration of opioid is possible either through conventional transcutaneous extradural catheters (usually tunnelled to reduce the infection risk) or through totally implanted systems requiring repeated percutaneous dosing. Administration through either may be intermittent boluses or continuous infusions. The extradural route is used most frequently because of the absence of headache from dural puncture and the hope that the dura is a barrier to infection. However, spinal subarachnoid administration requires less opioid, migration of the catheter tip does not have dangerous sequelae and there is a lower incidence of pain on injection. There is no evidence for the superiority of one route over the other. Totally implanted pump systems such as the 'Infusaid' have been used with spinal subarachnoid catheters most commonly, but may be used also with extradural catheters.

Dose requirements vary widely, and generally 'tolerance' develops necessitating increased doses. Large doses of morphine may give rise to distressing localized convulsive muscle movement and even hyperaesthesia (Yaksh *et al.*, 1986). In clinical practice, tolerance which has developed at the spinal level can be reversed by 'resting' the receptors by administering spinal local anaesthetic or another spinal analgesic drug such as clonidine for a few days. Once the receptors are 'reset', spinal opioids can be restarted at a much reduced dose.

Many substances are analgesically active when administered spinally e.g. baclofen, calcitonin and clonidine. These are experimental findings and are useful in deducing pain pathways and the associated neurotransmitters (Jordan, 1984) but are not recommended at present for clinical use, until careful studies of neurotoxicity, therapeutic index, etc. are available.

Rather than 'flogging' one pain pathway, co-administration of opioids and non-opioids is being studied. Opioid/local anaesthetic mixtures are extremely effective and in the future non-opioid spinal analgesic agents may be added to spinal opioids or alternated with spinal opioids as tolerance develops to each drug in turn.

References

Andrade R., Vandermaden C.P. & Aghajanian G.K. (1983) Morphine tolerance and dependence in the locus coerdeus: single cell studies in brain slices. *European Journal of Pharmacology* **91**, 161–9.

Barker A.E. (1908) A report on experiences with spinal anaesthesia in 100 cases. *British Medical Journal* **7**, 453–5.

Bengtsson M., Lofstrom J.B. & Malmquist L.A. (1985) Skin conductance responses during spinal anaesthesia. *Acta Anesthesiologica Scandinavica* **29**, 67–71.

Bromage P.R. (1953) The 'hanging-drop' sign. *Anaesthesia* **8**, 237–41.

Bromage P.R. (1974) Lower limb reflex changes in segmental epidural analgesia. *British Journal of Anaesthesia* **46**, 504–8.

Bromage P.R. (1978) *Epidural Analgesia*. W.B. Saunders, Philadelphia.

Bromage P.R., Joyal A.C. & Binney J.C. (1963) Local anaesthetic drugs: penetration from the spinal extradural space into the neuraxis. *Science* **140**, 392–4.

Bromage P.R., Pettigrew R.T. & Crowell D.E. (1969) Tachyphylaxis in epidural analgesia. I. Augmentation and decay of local anaesthesia. *Journal of Clinical Pharmacology* **9**, 30–8.

Bryce-Smith R. (1950) Pressures in the extradural space. *Anaesthesia* **5**, 213–16.

Burm A.G.C., van Kleef J.W., Gladines M.P.R.R., Oltof G. & Spierdijk J. (1986) Epidural anaesthesia with lidocaine and bupivacaine. *Anesthesia and Analgesia* **65**, 1281–4.

Cousins M.J. (1987) Comparative pharmacokinetics of spinal opioids in humans: a step towards determination of relative safety. *Anesthesiology* **67**, 875–6.

Cousins M.J. & Bridenbaugh P.O. (Eds) (1988) *Neural Blockade in Clinical Anaesthesia and Management of Pain* 2nd edn. J.B. Lippincott, Philadelphia.

Cousins M.R., Cherry D.A. & Gourlay G.K. (1987) Acute and chronic pain: use of spinal opioids. In *Neural Blockade in Clinical Anaesthesia and the Management of Pain* 2nd edn. (Eds Cousins M.J. & Bridenbaugh P.O.) pp. 955–1029. J.B. Lippincott, Philadelphia.

Cousins M.J. & Mather L.E. (1984) Intrathecal and epidural administration of opioids. *Anesthesiology* **61**, 276–310.

Cousins M.J., Mather L.E., Glynn C.J., Wilson P.R. & Graham J.R. (1979) Selective spinal analgesia. *Lancet* **1**, 1141–2.

Davis R.F., De Boer W.V. & Maroko P.R. (1986) Thoracic epidural anesthesia reduces myocardial infarct size after coronary artery occlusion in dogs. *Anesthesia and Analgesia* **65**, 711–17.

Di Giovanni A.J. & Dunbar B.S. (1970) Epidural injections of autologous blood for postlumbar puncture headache. *Anesthesia and Analgesia* **49**, 268–71.

Dripps R.D. & Vandam L.D. (1954) Long-term follow-up of patients who received 10,098 spinal anaesthetics: failure to discover major neurological sequelae. *Journal of the American Medical Association* **156**, 1486–91.

Durant P.A. & Yaksh T.L. (1986) Epidural injections of bupivacaine, morphine, fentanyl, lofentanil and DADL in chronically implanted rats: a pharmacologic and pathologic study. *Anesthesiology* **64**, 43–53.

Famewo C.E. & Naguib M. (1985) Spinal anaesthesia with meperidine as the sole agent. *Canadian Anaesthetists' Society Journal* **32**, 533–7.

Frumin M.J., Schwartz H., Burns J.J., Brodie B.B. & Papper E.M. (1953) The appearance of procaine in the spinal fluid during peridural block in man. *Journal of Pharmacology and Experimental Therapeutics* **109**, 102–5.

Frumin M.J., Schwartz H., Burns J.J., Brodie B.B. & Papper E.M. (1954) Dorsal root ganglion blockade during threshold segmental anesthesia in man. *Journal of Pharmacology and Experimental Therapeutics* **112**, 387–92.

Galindo A., Hermandez J., Benavides O., Ortega de Munoz S. & Bonica J.J. (1975) Quality of spinal extradural analgesia: the influence of spinal nerve root diameter. *British Journal of Anaesthesia* **47**, 41.

Gaylard D.G., Wilson I.H. & Balmer H.G.R. (1987) An epidural infusion technique for labour. *Anaesthesia* **42**, 1098–1101.

Germann P.A.S., Roberts J.G. & Prys-Roberts C. (1979) The combination of general anaesthesia and epidural block. I. The effects of sequence of induction on haemodynamic variables and blood gas measurements in healthy patients. *Anaesthesia and Intensive Care* **7**, 229–38.

Gourlay G.K., Cherry D.A., Plummer J.L., Armstrong P.J. & Cousins M.J. (1987) The influence of drug polarity on the absorption of opioid drugs into CSF and subsequent cephalad migration following lumbar administration: application to morphine and pethidine. *Pain* **31**, 297–305.

Hartung H.J., Osswald P.M., Bender H.J. & Lutz H. (1986) Severe hypotension and major conduction anaesthesia. In *Anaesthesiology and Intensive Care Medicine* 176. New Aspects in Regional Anesthesia 4. (Eds Wurst H.J. & Stanton-Hicks M.d'A.) pp. 72–5. Springer-Verlag, Berlin.

Husemeyer R.P. & White D.C. (1980) Lumbar extradural injection pressures in pregnant women. *British Journal of Anaesthesia* **52**, 55–9.

Jordan C.C. (1984) Current views on the mechanism of opiate analgesics and some novel approaches to analgesic drugs. In *Anaesthesia Review*, vol. 2, (Ed. Kaufman L.) pp. 108–36. Churchill Livingstone, Edinburgh.

Kane R.E. (1981) Neurologic deficits following epidural or spinal anesthesia. *Anesthesia and Analgesia* **60**, 150–61.

Larsen V.H., Iverson A.D., Christensen P. & Anderson P.K. (1985) Postoperative pain treatment after upper abdominal surgery with epidural morphine at thoracic or lumbar level. *Acta Anaesthesiologica Scandinavica* **29**, 566–71.

Moore D.C. & Batra M.S. (1981) The components of an effective test dose prior to epidural block. *Anesthesiology* **55**, 693–6.

Nancarrow C., Runciman W.B., Mather L.E., Upton R.N. & Plummer J.L. (1987) The influence of acidosis on the distribution of lidocaine and bupivacaine into the myocardium and brain of sheep. *Anesthesia and Analgesia* **66**, 925–35.

Prince G. & McGregor D. (1986) Obstetric epidural test doses. *Anaesthesia* **41**, 1240–50.

Purdy G., Currie J. & Owen H. (1987) Continuous extradural analgesia in labour. *British Journal of Anaesthesia* **59**, 319–24.

Rawal N., Arner S., Gustafsson L.L. & Allwin R. (1987) Present state of extradural and intrathecal opioid analgesia in Sweden. *British Journal of Anaesthesia* **59**, 791–9.

Ready L.B., Oden R., Chadwick H.S., Benedetti C., Rooke G.A., Caplan R. & Wild L.M. (1988) Development of an anesthesiology-based postoperative pain management service. *Anesthesiology* **68**, 100–6.

Reiz S., Balfors E., Sorenson M.B., Häggmark S. & Nyhman H. (1982) Coronary hemodynamic effects of general anesthesia and surgery: modification by epidural analgesia in patients with ischemic heart disease. *Regional Anaesthesia* **7** (Suppl.), 8–18.

Reynolds F. (1987) Adverse effects of local anaesthetics. *British Journal of Anaesthesia* **59**, 78–95.

Scott D.B., Schweitzer S. & Thorn J. (1982) Epidural block in postoperative pain relief. *Regional Anesthesia* **7**, 135–9.

Seow L.T., Lips F.J. & Cousins M.J. (1983) Effect of lateral posture on epidural blockade for surgery. *Anesthesia and Intensive Care* **11**, 97–102.

Shantha T.R. & Evans J.A. (1972) The relationship of epidural anaesthesia to neural membranes and arachnoid villi. *Anesthesiology* **37**, 543–57.

Sjöström S., Hartvig P., Persson P. & Tamsen A. (1987a) Pharmacokinetics of epidural morphine and meperidine in Humans. *Anesthesiology* **67**, 877–88.

Sjöström S., Tamsen A., Persson P. & Hartvig P. (1987b) Pharmacokinetics of intrathecal morphine and meperidine in humans. *Anesthesiology* **67**, 889–95.

Spence A.A. & Smith G. (1971) Postoperative analgesia and lung function: a comparison of morphine with extradural block. *British Journal of Anaesthesia* **43**, 144–8.

Torda T.A. & Pybus D.A. (1982) Comparison of four narcotic analgesics for extradural analgesia. *British Journal of Anaesthesia* **54**, 291–5.

Tucker G.T. & Mather L.E. (1975) Pharmacokinetics of local anaesthetic agents. *British Journal of Anaesthesia* **47**, 213–24.

Urban B.J. (1973) Clinical observations suggesting a changing site of action during induction and recession of spinal and epidural anesthesia. *Anesthesiology* **39**, 496–503.

Usubiaga J.E., Moya F. & Usubiaga L.E. (1967a) Effect of thoracic and abdominal pressure changes on the epidural space pressure. *British Journal of Anaesthesia* **39**, 612–18.

Usubiaga J.E., Wikinski J.A. & Usubiaga L.E. (1967b) Epidural pressure and its relation to spread of anesthetic solutions in the epidural space. *Anesthesia and Analgesia* **46**, 440–6.

Vella L.M., Willats D.G., Knott C., Lintin D.J., Justins D.M. & Reynolds F. (1985) Epidural fentanyl in labour. *Anaesthesia* **40**, 741–7.

Way E.L. (1946) Studies on the local anaesthetic properties of isonipecaine. *Journal of the American Pharmacological Association* **35**, 44–7.

White D.C. (1982) The epidural space. In *Anaesthesia Review I* (Ed. Kaufman L.) pp. 90–9. Churchill Livingstone, Edinburgh.

Wildsmith J.A.W. (1986) Extradural blockade and intracranial pressure. *British Journal of Anaesthesia* **58**, 579.

Wildsmith J.A.W. (1987) Intrathecal or extradural: which approach for surgery? *British Journal of Anaesthesia* **59**, 397–8.

Wildsmith J.A.W., McClure J.H., Brown D.T. & Scott D.B. (1981) Effects of posture on the spread of isobaric and hyperbaric amethocaine. *British Journal of Anaesthesia* **53**, 273–8.

Wildsmith J.A.W. & Rocco A.G. (1985) Current concepts in spinal anaesthesia. *Regional Anesthesia* **10**, 119–24.

Yaksh T.L., Harty G.J. & Onofrio B.M. (1986) High doses of spinal morphine produce a nonopiate receptor-mediated hyperesthesia: clinical and theoretical implications. *Anesthesiology* **64**, 590–7.

Yaksh T.L. & Rudy T.A. (1976) Analgesia mediated by a direct spinal action of narcotics. *Science* **192**, 1357–8.

59

Upper Limb

W. A. CHAMBERS AND J. A. W. WILDSMITH

Regional anaesthetic techniques, used alone or supplemented by sedation or light general anaesthesia, may benefit patients undergoing surgery to the upper limb in a number of ways. Most obviously, the risk of general anaesthesia may be avoided in certain groups (e.g. emergency operation in patients with a full stomach, rheumatoid patients with cervical spine abnormalities, asthmatic patients, etc.), but regional techniques offer more than the mere avoidance of general anaesthesia e.g. regional anaesthesia can provide very effective postoperative analgesia. If a catheter is inserted, both major (brachial plexus) and minor (e.g. median) nerve blocks may be used to produce analgesia over several days.

Increasing interest in microsurgical reconstruction of the hand and arm after trauma has produced a new indication for brachial plexus anaesthesia, principally because of the sympathetic blockade and consequent vasodilatation that are produced. Also, this is one of the reasons why brachial plexus blockade is useful particularly in patients with renal failure who are having arteriovenous fistulae fashioned for haemodialysis.

Depending on circumstances, it may be possible to choose one of a number of different approaches to produce a regional block. In each case it is necessary to take into account the nerve supply of the operative site, whether or not a tourniquet is to be used, and the likely duration of the procedure. Other important factors are the dose of drug required, the status of the patient and the level of proficiency of the anaesthetist.

Intravenous regional anaesthesia

Injection of a solution of local anaesthetic into an exsanguinated limb was described originally by Bier in 1908, but only became used widely after its re-introduction in the 1960s (Holmes, 1963). Since then, intravenous regional anaesthesia has been used extensively, particularly in accident and emergency departments where its technical simplicity and reliability are suited particularly for many minor procedures to the upper limb. Unfortunately, these features have led to inexperienced clinicians using the technique without understanding its basis and without being able to deal with possible complications. As a result, deaths have been caused by what should be a very safe technique (Heath, 1982).

Intravenous regional anaesthesia (IVRA, Bier's block) provides satisfactory analgesia and muscle relaxation of the hand and forearm in over 95% of patients and it is suitable for many open and closed procedures which are performed distal to the elbow. One of the limiting factors is tourniquet time as some discomfort occurs almost invariably 20–30 min after cuff inflation. This may be alleviated to a limited extent by the inflation of a second cuff immediately distal to the original and deflation of the upper cuff, but even with the use of such a system, it is unwise to embark on a procedure which takes longer than 1 hr.

Although IVRA is used normally for relatively minor procedures, usually in outpatients, it can offer particular advantages in other situations. For example, patients who are tetraplegic may require tendon transfer operations and are at risk of developing postoperative chest infections after general anaesthesia. Thus, local anaesthesia may be preferred. Intravenous regional anaesthesia is tolerated very well by these patients, and tourniquet discomfort from a single cuff is unusual in less than 1 hr.

Another special use of IVRA is in operations where it is desirable for the surgeon to observe movement of the hand before the end of the operation. This may be to ensure correct tension in a tendon graft or to ascertain if adequate tenolysis has been performed. Intravenous regional anaesthesia may be used if continued anaesthesia of the hand is obtained with a wrist block. The operation is carried out under IVRA, and the tourniquet is released after suture of any proximal wounds. Movement of the fingers by action of the long flexors and extensors can be observed, any further dissection or adjustment made and the distal wound sutured without discomfort.

Contra-indications to IVRA include contra-indications to a tourniquet (such as sickle cell disease) and any infective process, the spread of which could be encouraged. It is unwise to use IVRA without other provision for anaesthesia if the intention is to deflate the tourniquet some time before the end of surgery, because the return of sensation may be very rapid. Patients with large lacerations may be unsuitable simply because a large part of the volume injected may escape through the wound.

Technique

The tourniquet should be as simple as possible. The single cuff orthopaedic tourniquet with a 'bicycle-type' pump and high-pressure tubing (Fig. 59.1) has much to recommend it. Double cuffs do not lessen discomfort always and they are dangerous potentially because confusion may lead to accidental deflation of the wrong cuff. Sphygmomanometer cuffs are totally inappropriate and while automatic systems are useful, they can lead to a false sense of security and be confusing to use.

Prilocaine 0.5% (Citanest) is the drug of choice because of its low systemic toxicity. It is available in

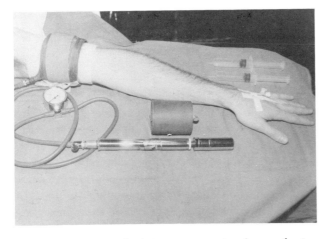

Fig. 59.1 Equipment for intravenous regional anaesthesia.

50 ml single-dose vials, free of any preservative. Forty ml is the standard adult dose, and this may be reduced in frail or elderly patients. Up to 50 ml (or a standard volume of a more concentrated solution) may be used in healthy subjects with muscular, well-built forearms.

Intravenous regional anaesthesia should be undertaken with a care that may appear disproportionate to its technical simplicity. The following guidelines are recommended.

1 The patient should be:
  (a) Fasted for at least 4 hr before elective surgery whenever possible.
  (b) Placed on a tipping trolley or table.
  (c) Supervised closely by an experienced clinician.
2 Venous access should be established in the opposite arm.
3 Full resuscitation equipment must be available immediately.
4 The tourniquet should be checked for leaks before use and observed constantly.

With the patient supine, the arterial pressure is checked. If it is elevated significantly, the need for the procedure to be performed should be reviewed. An intravenous cannula is placed in a vein on the dorsum of the hand or distal forearm of the limb to be blocked. The tourniquet cuff is applied over a layer of orthopaedic felt on the upper arm and inflated after exsanguination of the limb. Rather than apply an Esmarch bandage over a fracture, it may be kinder to ask the patient to elevate the limb for 2 min while the brachial artery is compressed. The cuff should be inflated to 13.3 kPa (100 mmHg) above systolic arterial pressure, and if there is any doubt about occlusion of the circulation, the tourniquet should be released and the procedure restarted. Once it is certain that the limb has been isolated from the circulation, the chosen volume of prilocaine is injected over 1–2 min. Within seconds, the patient may experience paraesthesiae and the skin may appear mottled. Complete sensory block is obtained usually within 10 min, but muscle relaxation may take longer to develop. Throughout the procedure, a careful watch must be kept on the tourniquet which should not be allowed to deflate for at least 20 min after injection of drug. When it is deflated, the patient must be observed closely and kept supine for at least 30 min.

Complications

The major problem is systemic toxicity, and this is associated usually with inadvertent, premature tourniquet deflation because of failure of equipment or technique. There have been reports (Rosenberg *et al.*, 1983) of convulsions (all with drugs other than prilocaine) despite an adequately applied tourniquet. This can be explained only by leakage of local anaesthetic solution past the tourniquet. It has been demonstrated that very high venous pressures, which could cause systemic leakage, may be produced by rapid injection and poor exsanguination (Duggan *et al.*, 1984). The use of antecubital veins contributes to the risk.

The incidence of toxicity when the tourniquet is released after 20 min or more is variable. Minor symptoms (drowsiness, tinnitus, tingling of the lips) are observed even with prilocaine, but neither major systemic toxicity nor met-haemoglobinaemia have been described after IVRA with prilocaine at the recommended dosage.

Nerve damage from tourniquet pressure is extremely rare in association with properly conducted IVRA (Larsen & Hommelgaard, 1987). This complication is more likely when excessive tourniquet times are used and the patient is unlikely to tolerate these with this technique.

Brachial plexus blocks

Although IVRA is useful for minor procedures, brachial plexus blocks have distinct advantages if major surgery is to be carried out using a regional technique. The tissues are not swollen by a large volume of local anaesthetic, and a tourniquet is not necessary. If one is used, the discomfort it causes is minimal. Analgesia may persist well into the postoperative period, and its duration can be varied by using a local anaesthetic agent appropriate to the particular circumstance.

There are disadvantages. A detailed knowledge of anatomy is essential, the procedures take time to perform and the potential for complications is greater.

Anatomy

The nerves of the upper limb derive mainly from the brachial plexus which is formed from the anterior primary rami of the fifth cervical to the first thoracic nerves (Fig. 59.2). Some fibres may be derived also from C4 and T2. The five roots form three trunks, each of which divides into an anterior and a posterior division. These six divisions unite to form three cords, each of which has two terminal divisions which are the nerves that supply most of the upper limb. Branches of the formative parts of the plexus supply the deep structures

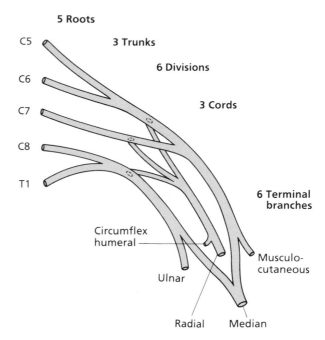

Fig. 59.2 Formative elements of the brachial plexus.

of the shoulder, the skin of this region being supplied by the supraclavicular branches of the cervical plexus. The intercostobrachial nerve (T2) supplies the skin of the inner aspect of the upper arm and, with a branch from the third thoracic nerve, the skin of the axilla. Interbranching within the plexus implies that most of the peripheral nerves carry fibres from several roots. Each nerve supplies a specific area as does each segmental root, but the segmental innervation of deep and cutaneous structures is different.

As they emerge from the intervertebral foramina, the plexus roots lie between the scalene muscles, which join the tubercles of the transverse processes of the cervical vertebrae to the first rib. In the neck (Fig. 59.3), the vertebral artery, the stellate ganglion and the contents of the cervical spinal canal are close relations. The phrenic nerve lies on the anterior surface of scalenus anterior, posterior to the carotid sheath. The recurrent laryngeal nerve lies in the groove between the oesophagus and trachea, and laterally the external jugular vein crosses the interscalene groove at the level of the sixth cervical vertebra and the cricoid cartilage.

As the plexus approaches the first rib the trunks are arranged vertically and are named 'superior', 'middle' and 'inferior'. They are close together, and the subclavian artery lies between the plexus and the scalenus anterior muscle. The dome of the pleura is an important inferomedial relation (Fig. 59.4). At the lateral

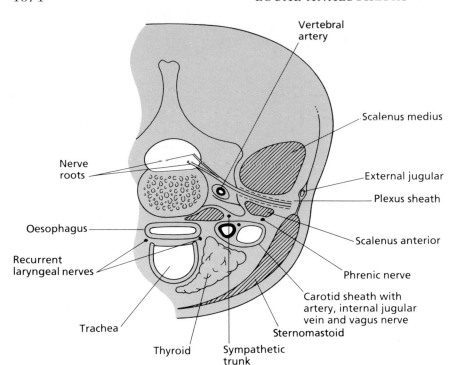

Vertebral artery

Scalenus medius

Nerve roots

External jugular

Plexus sheath

Oesophagus

Scalenus anterior

Recurrent laryngeal nerves

Phrenic nerve

Carotid sheath with artery, internal jugular vein and vagus nerve

Trachea

Sternomastoid

Thyroid

Sympathetic trunk

Fig. 59.3 Transverse section of neck to show relations of brachial plexus.

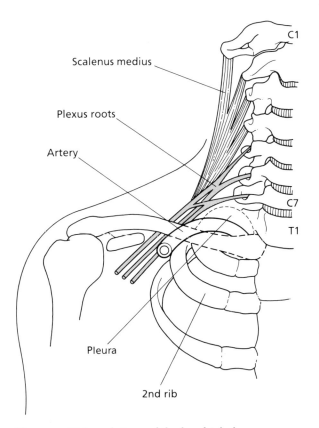

Scalenus medius

Plexus roots

Artery

C1

C7

T1

Pleura

2nd rib

Fig. 59.4 Major relations of the brachial plexus.

border of the first rib, each trunk divides into its divisions and these pass behind and under the clavicle where the cords are formed. In the axilla, the artery is surrounded completely by the components of the plexus, the cords giving rise to terminal branches behind the lateral border of pectoralis minor. The axillary vein lies medial to the artery and the surrounding plexus, overlapping both partially. The musculocutaneous nerve (from the lateral cord) leaves the plexus and enters the substance of the coracobrachialis muscle high in the axilla.

An important feature (Winnie, 1970) is that the plexus lies within a tube of fibrous tissue which extends from the cervical vertebrae, where it is continuous with the prevertebral fascia, to the distal axilla. Any solution injected into the sheath at any point spreads in both directions. Superiorly, the sheath is continuous with that surrounding the cervical plexus, and this explains why block of the cervical nerves is seen occasionally after interscalene block. Radio-opaque dye studies (Thompson & Rorie, 1983) suggest that the sheath is a multi-compartmental structure and this may explain some of the incomplete or delayed blocks which are produced even by experienced clinicians.

Numerous techniques have been described for performing brachial plexus block. From proximal to distal these are:

1 Interscalene (Winnie, 1970).
2 Parascalene (Vongises & Panijayanond, 1978).
3 Subclavian perivascular (Winnie & Collins, 1964).
4 Supraclavicular (Macintosh & Mushin, 1967).
5 Intraclavicular (Raj et al., 1973).
6 Axillary (de Jong, 1961).

Each of these approaches has its advocates (indeed there are variations on each theme), but it is unnecessary for an individual to master all. The supraclavicular is the classical approach and the others have been introduced in an attempt to produce methods which are easier to learn and without the risk of pneumothorax, the major hazard of the classical method. The supraclavicular and subclavian perivascular techniques produce the most complete limb block (Lanz et al., 1983). The axillary approach does not affect the shoulder, and the interscalene often misses the ulnar aspect of the hand and forearm. The axillary method is somewhat easier to learn and perform than the others, and is perhaps the most suitable for the occasional user.

Latency and duration

Onset may be slow with any of these techniques. Most blocks are well established within 20 min, but they may take much longer on occasion. To some extent, this variation is related to the approach and the drug and concentration used. Testing for sensory loss too early may undermine the patient's confidence and at least 10–15 min should elapse before this is done. Motor block becomes apparent often before sensory loss and the earliest sign of a successful axillary block is often inability to extend the elbow. Movement at the shoulder is first affected by interscalene and subclavian perivascular blocks. If there is no evidence of motor weakness within 10 min of injection, success is unlikely.

Duration is variable even if the same drug and dosage are used. For prolonged operations, discomfort at the tourniquet site may become troublesome despite adequate analgesia in the operating field. Lignocaine has a very brief duration unless used with a vasoconstrictor, but a single injection of plain prilocaine provides at least $1\frac{1}{2}$ hr of surgical anaesthesia and bupivacaine 3 hr. Longer durations can be achieved by using a catheter technique and bupivacaine may last occasionally for up to 24 hr.

Toxicity

Brachial plexus block requires the administration of a large dose of local anaesthetic drug regardless of the approach chosen. Thus, even in the absence of direct intravascular injection, significant plasma concentrations of the local anaesthetic may be produced. The addition of adrenaline (1/200 000) produces lower plasma concentrations and is recommended particularly when bupivacaine or lignocaine is used because concentrations near the toxic range may result otherwise (Wildsmith et al., 1977). Similar systemic concentrations are obtained whichever technique is used (McLean et al., 1987) so the risk of toxicity should not be a consideration when deciding which approach to use.

Assessment and preparation

A patient for surgery under brachial plexus block requires the same investigation and preparation as one having a general anaesthetic. Although regional anaesthesia may offer many benefits, this is not a reason to submit patients to surgery in other than optimum condition. In addition, it can never be guaranteed that a patient will not require general anaesthesia because of failure of the block or unexpected operative findings. Premedication is a matter for individual preference, but the patient should not be sedated so heavily that co-operation is lost.

Needles

Short bevel needles are preferable, as penetration of the sheath is appreciated more readily and they decrease the incidence of nerve injury (Selander et al., 1977, 1979). It is helpful also to use the immobile needle technique (Winnie, 1969), in which an extension set connects the needle to the syringe. The set is primed with fluid to avoid air embolism and allows the needle to be held motionless during aspiration, injection and changing of syringes. A strict no-touch technique should be adopted, but gloves are unnecessary for a single injection technique, especially as they may make the palpation of landmarks more difficult. If a cannula is to be inserted, it is probably wiser to 'scrub up' and use gloves and sterile towels. Infection at the site of injection is extremely rare.

Paraesthesiae and nerve stimulators

Before the injection, the patient should be warned about paraesthesiae. It is important to impress on the patient the necessity of reporting paraesthesiae immediately and remaining as motionless as possible at that time. Once paraesthesiae have been elicited, the needle should be held immobile and an aspiration test performed. If blood or air cannot be aspirated then the solution should be injected slowly. Severe pain during injection indicates that an intraneural injection is being performed. This is extremely rare, but if it is the case, the needle must be withdrawn slightly. Some discomfort on initial injection may be caused by over-rapid distension of the plexus sheath and is avoided if the initial part of the injection is made in small increments.

The use of paraesthesiae to determine accurate needle placement depends on having a conscious, co-operative patient who understands clearly the instructions he or she has been given so the use of nerve stimulator allows these techniques to be used on patients who cannot co-operate (Yasuda et al., 1980). This can be useful when a block is performed to provide analgesia after an operation performed under general anaesthesia. However, conscious patients may find the nerve stimulator uncomfortable and in experienced hands its use results only in a marginal increase in the rate of successful blocks.

Management

Once a successful block has been established, patient management varies widely. Healthy, young patients undergoing short procedures may be happy to remain fully conscious during the operation. They should be accompanied at all times so that they can converse and describe any problems they experience. At the other extreme, patients undergoing prolonged procedures require almost certainly some form of sedation or even light general anaesthesia because lying motionless on an operating table for 2 or 3 hr can be very uncomfortable, particularly for patients with other skeletal deformities. If respiratory-depressant drugs have been administered, oxygen should be given by face-mask. It may be appropriate also to monitor the ECG and arterial pressure in patients with systemic disease.

Postoperative care

It is essential that the arm is cared for properly until the block wears off, because the loss of sensory, proprioceptive and motor function can each lead to damage. Hyperextension, especially if it is accompanied by external rotation and traction, can lead rapidly to neural injury.

Interscalene block

The interscalene technique is the most proximal approach to the brachial plexus, local anaesthetic being injected between the scalene muscles at the level of the sixth cervical vertebrae. Pneumothorax should not be a risk, but the method has the disadvantage that the lower roots of the plexus are not blocked consistently. Areas supplied by C5–7, the deep structures of the shoulder, elbow joint and the lateral aspect of the forearm and hand, are blocked reliably. Supplementary blocks may be required for surgery of other parts of the limb, particularly the ulnar aspects of the forearm and hand.

Technique

The patient lies supine with the head resting on one pillow and turned slightly to the opposite side. The arm should be by the patient's side. The lateral border of the sternomastoid is identified. If it is not palpable readily, the patient is asked to lift his or her head just off the pillow as this tenses the muscle. A finger placed in the groove behind the sternomastoid and at the level of the cricoid cartilage lies on the belly of scalenus anterior. The patient is asked to relax completely and the finger rolled laterally over the scalenus anterior until it lies in the groove between the anterior and middle scalene muscles, the interscalene groove. The groove may be made easier to palpate by asking the patient to take a deep breath. The needle is inserted into this groove at the level of the cricoid cartilage. The external jugular vein passes usually near the point of injection and care should be taken to avoid puncturing it.

The needle is inserted at right angles to the skin so that it is directed medially, but also slightly caudally and posteriorly (Fig. 59.5). If it is directed horizontally, it may pass between two cervical vertebrae and could puncture the vertebral artery or enter the intervertebral foramen. The needle is advanced slowly until paraesthesiae are obtained which radiate to the arm or forearm rather than the shoulder tip or scapula. Paraesthesiae in the latter distribution are caused by stimulation of the suprascapular or supraclavicular nerves, which lie outside the sheath. Subsequent injection is thus ineffective. A click may be felt as the needle pierces the plexus sheath and is a useful guide to correct position. If paraesthesiae are not elicited, the

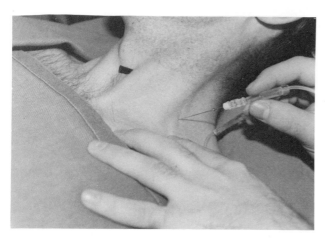

Fig. 59.5 Interscalene block. The tip of the left index finger lies on scalenus anterior.

needle is withdrawn and its angulation checked. It is important to stress that the plexus is rarely more than 2.5 cm from the skin (Yasuda *et al.*, 1980). Once paraesthesiae have been produced, the neck is compressed firmly by a finger placed above the needle to promote caudal spread. After aspiration, the local anaesthetic solution is injected slowly with repeated aspiration.

Volume requirements

Winnie (1984) has determined the spread of different volumes of solution injected into the brachial plexus sheath with the use of local anaesthetic solutions mixed with radio-opaque dye. Injection of 20 ml of solution at the level of C6 results in a block of the lower cervical plexus in addition to the brachial plexus. However, because the injection is made at such a high level, 20 ml is often insufficient to spread far enough inferiorly to reach the lower roots of the plexus, and anaesthesia may be patchy or absent in the distribution of C8 and T1. If the volume is increased to 40 ml, the entire interscalene space is filled from the transverse processes of the upper cervical vertebrae to the cupola of the lung. Usually, this provides anaesthesia of the entire cervical and brachial plexuses.

Digital pressure applied just above the needle during the performance of an interscalene block inhibits cephalad spread and promotes distal flow of the injected solution. Thus, this manoeuvre reduces the volume necessary to produce a complete block of the brachial plexus.

Complications

Phrenic nerve block has been demonstrated radiographically in 36% of patients with interscalene and subclavian perivascular blocks (Farrar *et al.*, 1981), but this causes symptoms rarely unless the patient has severe respiratory disease. Both techniques are associated also with a low incidence of recurrent laryngeal nerve block. This causes hoarseness which is of no clinical significance, but bilateral blocks would cause laryngeal incompetence. Up to 50% of patients who receive these blocks develop Horner's syndrome, and some patients complain of flushing of the face. Unequal pupils may give rise to concern in a patient who has sustained a recent head injury.

Avoidance of vertebral artery injection by careful aspiration and accurate needle placement is essential, as even a small dose of local anaesthetic given by this route causes severe cerebral toxicity. Extradural and subarachnoid injections are possible also and have been reported. These are avoided by correct needle direction and appreciation of the superficial position of the plexus. Finally, all nerve block techniques can be associated with direct nerve trauma. Constant care is needed so that the wrong solution is not injected and paraesthesiae should be elicited gently (Selander *et al.*, 1979). Short bevel needles are to be preferred (Selander *et al.*, 1977).

Subclavian perivascular block

With this technique, the injection is made into the subclavian perivascular space i.e. between the lower ends of the scalene muscles and above the first rib. It differs from the classical supraclavicular approach in that the needle is inserted higher in the neck and also further posteriorly and medially. The needle is directed more caudally and should reach the plexus where the trunks lie on top of each other behind the subclavian artery. The lower trunk of the plexus may be missed occasionally as it lies below the subclavian artery, but this can be overcome to some extent by using a generous volume of solution. The risk of pneumothorax is less than with the classical supraclavicular approach, but is still present, so the method is contraindicated in day-patients.

Technique

The interscalene groove is located (see above) and followed downwards until the pulsation of the subclavian artery can be felt. A finger is placed over the

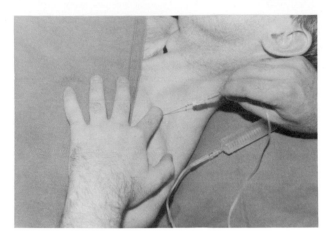

Fig. 59.6 Subclavian perivascular block. The tip of the left index finger is palpating the artery.

artery to mark the site of injection. A needle is inserted in the groove immediately above the artery (Fig. 59.6) and advanced slowly in a caudad direction between the scalene muscles until paraesthesiae are elicited. A click is sometimes felt as the needle penetrates the sheath. If the first rib is contacted before paraesthesiae have been elicited, the needle is withdrawn and redirected more anteriorly or posteriorly. It is important that the needle is not directed medially as this increases the risk of pneumothorax. If the subclavian artery in punctured, the needle should be withdrawn and directed slightly more posteriorly.

Paraesthesiae in the arm or hand indicate that the needle is positioned correctly. Paraesthesiae in any other distribution indicate that the suprascapular, supraclavicular or long thoracic nerves have been stimulated and it is likely that the needle lies outside the sheath.

Volume requirements

Winnie (1984) has again documented the spread of radio-opaque solutions by this approach. Twenty ml provide a block of the entire brachial plexus. However, if the injection is made fairly high in the subclavian, perivascular space, the onset of anaesthesia may be delayed or even absent in the distribution of the inferior trunk, and therefore a slightly larger volume is preferable. If 40 ml of solution are injected, anaesthesia of the lower cervical plexus results.

Complications

Pneumothorax is the principal complication and may become apparent either immediately or up to 24 hr

later. Any coughing during attempts to obtain paraesthesiae should alert the anaesthetist that the needle tip may be near the pleura. Phrenic, recurrent laryngeal and stellate ganglion block (see above) can all occur although they are seldom significant clinically.

Axillary block

This offers the safest and simplest method of blocking the brachial plexus. It produces consistently good anaesthesia of the medial aspects of the arm, forearm and those parts of the hand supplied by the ulnar and median nerves. The lateral aspects of the forearm and hand, supplied by the radial and musculocutaneous nerves, are blocked in some 75% of cases.

Technique

With the patient lying supine, the arm is abducted almost to 90° and rotated slightly externally. It may be helpful to flex the elbow and support the arm on a pillow. If the arm is abducted further, the artery may become more difficult to feel and it is unwise to ask the patient to place his or her palm behind his or her head. The axillary artery is identified as high in the axilla as possible and a needle inserted at an angle of approximately 30° to the skin and directed parallel to the artery (Fig. 59.7). The needle is advanced slowly until it pierces the sheath which lies quite superficially. Evidence that the sheath has been penetrated may take several forms. A 'click' or 'give' may be felt as the needle passes through the sheath and thereafter it can be observed pulsating usually if it is supported gently. Although paraesthesiae are not sought deliberately with this technique, they give additional confirmation

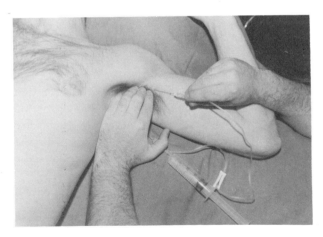

Fig. 59.7 Axillary plexus block. The fingers of the left hand lie over the artery and the needle is inserted just above and parallel to it.

that the tip of the needle is placed correctly if they are elicited. Similarly, if the artery or vein is punctured, this indicates also that the needle tip is within the sheath. In this case, particular care needs to be taken to avoid intravascular injection, and the needle should be withdrawn slowly until blood can be aspirated no longer.

With the needle in the correct position, and connected to a syringe with an extension set, an aspiration test is performed. The injection is made slowly with repeated aspiration. Pressure on the sheath immediately distal to the injection site aids proximal spread of the solution. Digital pressure is more effective in this regard than the use of a rubber tourniquet around the arm. If aspiration reveals that the needle is intravenous before any solution has been injected, then it may be possible to reposition the needle satisfactorily. If the injection has commenced, considerable damage may be caused to the plexus by traumatizing partially blocked nerves, and it may be wise to abandon the method in favour of another. If a vessel has been punctured, it should be compressed for 5 min after the injection to minimize haematoma formation. A finger placed firmly over the artery distal to the injection site during the injection aids proximal spread of the solution and makes block of those nerves which leave the sheath high in the axilla more likely.

An alternative method is to use a 25 gauge needle and puncture the artery deliberately. Once this has been achieved, the needle is advanced slowly while aspiration is continued. As soon as blood can be aspirated no longer (indicating that the needle tip has passed through the artery and is situated posteriorly within the sheath) the needle is fixed and the injection made. Advocates of this method claim that it is more likely to produce block of the radial nerve distribution. In inexperienced hands this may be so, but the deliberate transfixion of a major limb artery seems a high price to pay for this advantage.

Although a needle can be used for axillary block, it is relatively simple to use a cannula technique. The approach is very similar, and once the sheath has been penetrated, the cannula is advanced from the needle. If it is within the sheath, the cannula advances easily and any resistance suggests that it should be withdrawn and re-inserted.

Volume requirements

Twenty ml of solution injected into an adult patient without digital pressure do not spread consistently to reach the level of the cords of the plexus. Sensory loss following such a small volume may provide adequate anaesthesia for hand surgery but the block may not be adequate to prevent discomfort from a tourniquet or to prevent the patient from flexing his or her forearm. If the volume is increased to 40 ml, the solution normally reaches the first rib and thus provides a complete sensory and motor block of the arm. The very large volumes (up to 60 ml) which would be required to produce spread to the cervical portion of the interscalene space are not recommended clinically. Digital pressure applied immediately distal to the injection site prevents distal spread of the solution and encourages proximal flow. This is more effective than the use of a rubber tourniquet because the sheath is situated deeply between coracobrachialis and the long head of triceps. Obstruction to proximal flow can be caused also by the humeral head if the arm remains abducted. Thus, adduction of the arm while maintaining firm digital pressure allows any given volume to reach a higher level within the sheath.

Peripheral nerve blocks

The role of individual nerve blocks in the arm is limited. Because of variations in anatomical course and wide cutaneous sensory overlap, multiple injections with supplementary infiltrations are required for major surgical procedures. Patients obviously object to such techniques. The main value of these blocks is in supplementing the major blocks, providing analgesia for short procedures on the hand (particularly if a tourniquet is not required) and providing also analgesia for physiotherapy and manipulation if this is painful.

For all these blocks, it is important to avoid intraneural injection which can be extremely painful and may produce a neuritis. The longer duration of bupivacaine makes it the most suitable drug in many situations, although lignocaine and prilocaine may be used. The abundance of blood vessels in close proximity to nerves at the elbow and the wrist implies that intravascular injection and haematoma formation are potential complications. Even when blocking small nerves, the action of a local anaesthetic drug is seldom instantaneous and up to 15 min should be allowed for its onset.

Clinically, there is little difference between the effect of nerve block at the elbow or the wrist; and thus, only the simpler methods (at the wrist) are described. Block of the ulnar nerve at the elbow is particularly likely to produce neuritis if injections are made where the nerve lies in the groove behind the medial epicondyle and this approach should be avoided if at all possible.

Ulnar nerve block

The palmar branch of the ulnar is blocked at the level of the styloid process. A fine needle is inserted at right angles to the skin, on the radial side of the tendon of flexor carpi ulnaris and the ulnar side of the ulnar artery (Fig. 59.8). The latter can be palpated usually. If paraesthesiae are produced, the needle is held in place and 2–4 ml of local anaesthetic injected. Even if paraesthesiae are not produced, it is usually possible to obtain adequate anaesthesia by injecting 5–10 ml of solution while the point of the needle is moved from contact with deep fascia and bone until it lies subcutaneously. To block the dorsal branch of the ulnar nerve, a ring of local anaesthetic solution is placed subcutaneously around the ulnar aspect of the wrist from the tendon of flexor carpi ulnaris—approximately 5 ml of solution are required.

Median nerve block

At the level of the proximal skin crease at the wrist, the needle is inserted at right angles to the skin immediately radial to palmaris longus, or if it is absent, 1 cm medial to flexor carpi radialis (Fig. 59.9). The nerve is approximately 1 cm deep at this point, but fanwise movements of the needle in a plane at right angles to the long axis of the forearm may be required to obtain paraesthesiae. When these are elicited, 2–5 ml of

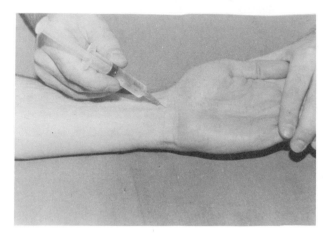

Fig. 59.9 Median nerve block at the wrist.

solution are injected slowly. A further 1 ml may be injected subcutaneously to include the cutaneous branch to the palm of the hand.

Radial nerve block

The terminal part of this nerve can be blocked by infiltrating under the tendon of brachioradialis some 6–8 cm proximal to the wrist, but a simpler and less unpleasant method for the patient is to raise a subcutaneous ring around the radial and dorsal aspects of the wrist joint (Fig. 59.10). Approximately 5 ml of solution are used. The ring of infiltration should not extend around the whole circumference of the wrist and care should be taken to avoid damage to the subcutaneous veins.

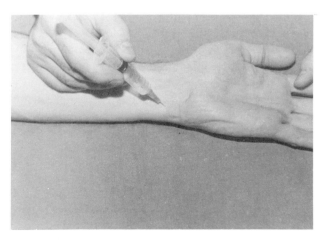

Fig. 59.8 Ulnar nerve block at the wrist.

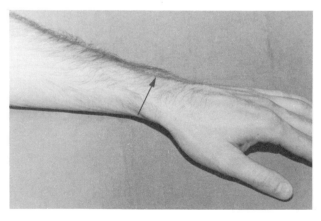

Fig. 59.10 The arrow shows the position and direction of infiltration for radial nerve block at the wrist.

Digital nerve block

This is very effective for procedures on the finger which are carried out on outpatients. Under no circumstances should solutions containing a vasoconstrictor be used. The needle should be inserted from the dorsal aspect and advanced during the injection until pressure is felt on the anaesthetist's finger which should be placed beneath that of the patient's. One to 2 ml of solution are injected subcutaneously on each side of the base of the finger.

Local infiltration

Many minor surgical procedures such as the excision of small tumours and the suturing of wounds can be performed under infiltration anaesthesia. The use of this method in the hand is limited because of the simplicity with which digital nerve or wrist block can be performed. The technique may be useful for suturing wound edges if it is necessary to release the tourniquet before the end of a procedure carried out under intravenous regional anaesthesia.

References

de Jong R. (1961) Axillary block of the brachial plexus. *Anesthesiology* **22**, 215–55.

Duggan J., McKeown D.W. & Scott D.B. (1984) Venous pressure in intravenous regional anesthesia. *Regional Anesthesia* **9**, 20–2.

Farrar M.D., Schebani M. & Nolte H. (1981) Upper extremity block: effectiveness and complications. *Regional Anesthesia* **6**, 133–4.

Heath M. (1982) Deaths after intravenous regional anaesthesia. (Editorial). *British Medical Journal* **285**, 913–4.

Holmes C.M. (1963) Intravenous regional analgesia. *Lancet* **i**, 245–6.

Lanz E., Theiss D. & Jankovic D. (1983) The extent of blockade following various techniques of brachial plexus block. *Anesthesia and Analgesia* **62**, 55–8.

Larsen U.T. & Hommelgaard P. (1987) Pneumatic tourniquet paralysis following intravenous regional anaesthesia. *Anaesthesia* **42**, 526–8.

Macintosh R. & Mushin W. (1967) *Local Anaesthesia: Brachial Plexus* 4th edn. Blackwell Scientific Publications, Oxford.

MacLean D., Chambers W.A., Tucker G.T. & Wildsmith J.A.W. (1987) Plasma prilocaine concentrations after three techniques of brachial plexus blockade. *British Journal of Anaesthesia* **60**, 136–40.

Raj R., Montgomery S., Nettles D. & Jenkins M. (1973) Infraclavicular brachial plexus block; a new approach. *Anesthesia and Analgesia* **52**, 897–904.

Rosenberg P.H., Kalso E.A., Tuominen M.K. & Linden H.B. (1983) Acute bupivacaine toxicity as a result of venous leakage under the tourniquet cuff during Bier's block. *Anesthesiology* **58**, 95–8.

Selander D., Dhuner K. & Lundborg G. (1977) Peripheral nerve injury due to injection needles used for regional analgesia. *Acta Anaesthesiologica Scandinavica* **21**, 182–8.

Selander D., Edshage S. & Wolff T. (1979) Paraesthesia or no paraesthesia. *Acta Anaesthesiologica Scandinavica* **23**, 27–33.

Thompson G. & Rorie D. (1983) Functional anatomy of the brachial plexus sheath. *Anesthesiology* **59**, 117–22.

Vongises P. & Panijayanond T. (1978) A parascalene technique of brachial plexus anesthesia. *Anesthesia and Analgesia* **58**, 267–73.

Wildsmith J.A.W., Tucker G.T., Cooper S., Scott D.B. & Covino B.G. (1977) Plasma concentrations of local anaesthetics after interscalene brachial plexus block. *British Journal of Anaesthesia* **49**, 461–6.

Winnie A.P. (1969) An 'immobile needle' for nerve block. *Anesthesiology* **31**, 577–8.

Winnie A.P. (1970) Interscalene brachial plexus block. *Anesthesia and Analgesia* **49**, 455–66.

Winnie A.P. (1984) *Plexus Anaesthesia*, vol. 1. Schultz/Churchill Livingstone, Edinburgh.

Winnie A. & Collins V. (1964) The subclavian perivascular technique of brachial plexus anesthesia. *Anesthesiology* **25**, 353–63.

Yasuda I., Hirano T., Ojima T., Ohhira N., Kaneko T. & Yamamuro M. (1980) Supraclavicular brachial plexus block using a nerve stimulator and an insulated needle. *British Journal of Anaesthesia* **52**, 409–11.

Further reading

Eriksson E. (Ed) (1969) *Illustrated Handbook in Local Anaesthesia*. Munksgaard, Copenhagen.

Wildsmith J.A.W. & Armitage E.N. (Eds) (1987) *Principles and Practice of Regional Anaesthesia*. Churchill Livingstone, Edinburgh.

Winnie A.P. (1984) *Plexus Anesthesia*, vol. 1. Schultz/Churchill Livingstone, Edinburgh.

60

Plexus and Peripheral Blocks of the Lower Limb

F. P. BUCKLEY

The nerve supply to the leg differs from that to the arm in a number of respects. The arm derives its nerve supply from five root levels (C5–T1) which merge to form a single brachial plexus which is contained for a considerable distance of its course within the brachial plexus sheath, where it may be blocked conveniently with a needle inserted at one location. The leg derives its nerve supply from seven nerve roots (L2–S3) which form the lumbosacral plexus, the two elements of which are separated widely anatomically, and which then branches into several major peripheral nerves. Thus, to block either the plexi or the peripheral nerves to the leg, two or more needles must be inserted. The dermatomal and myotomal distributions of the nerve roots, and the distributions of the peripheral nerves supplying the leg are shown in Figs 60.1, 60.2 and 60.3 respectively. The anatomy of the lumbar plexus is shown in Figs 60.4 and 60.5 and that of the sacral plexus in Fig. 60.9.

As nerve blocks of the lower extremity are performed relatively infrequently and rely on deep landmarks, they often have a high failure rate in the hands of the novice. To reduce the failure rate, a number of measures may be used:

1 Do not attempt them in patients with indistinct anatomical landmarks.
2 Provide the patient with sufficient analgesia and sedation to ensure a static and co-operative target.
3 Position the patient carefully and accurately.
4 Identify and mark all anatomical landmarks accurately.
5 If the nerve is to be identified by eliciting paraesthesiae ensure that the distribution of paraesthesiae is consistent with the peripheral distribution of the nerve.
6 Consider the routine use of a peripheral nerve stimulator (PNS) and an insulated needle to assist in accurate nerve location. Stimulation frequencies of 1.0–2.0 Hz should be used. The general position of the nerve should be identified with a stimulation intensity of 2.0 mA, and more accurate and final needle tip placement, closely adjacent to the nerve, accomplished using lower stimulation intensities of 0.5–0.7 mA. This should produce a readily perceptible twitch in the distant muscles supplied by the nerve. The anaesthetist should not be misled by muscle twitches at or around the site of needle insertion as these may be caused by direct muscle stimulation. While a PNS is a valuable tool it does not correct errors made by incorrect positioning and inaccurate identification of landmarks.

The solutions which should be used for leg blocks are lignocaine 1%, mepivacaine 1%, bupivacaine 0.25–0.5% or etidocaine 0.75–1.0%, all with adrenaline 1/200 000. The choice between these agents should be determined by the desired duration of anaesthesia. Because relatively large masses of drug may be used for leg blocks, care should be taken to stay within the safe maximal dose of any drug for each individual patient.

The lumbar plexus (Figs 60.4 and 60.5)

The lumbar plexus is formed by the roots of L2, 3 and 4. It supplies the skin of the medial, anterior and lateral portions of the thigh, and the psoas, quadratus lumborum, quadriceps and adductor muscles. The plexus divides into anterior and posterior divisions within the psoas muscle, the anterior division forming the obturator nerve, and the posterior forming the femoral and lateral femoral cutaneous nerves. As the nerves leave the psoas, they are encased within a fascial sheath

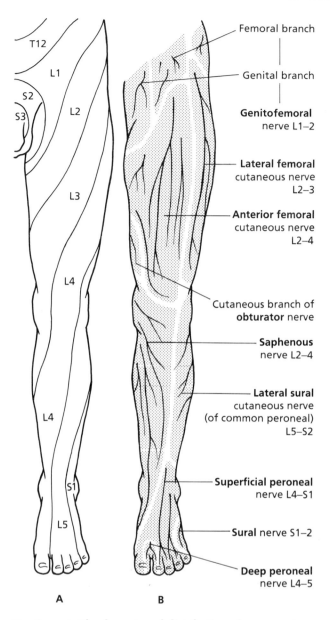

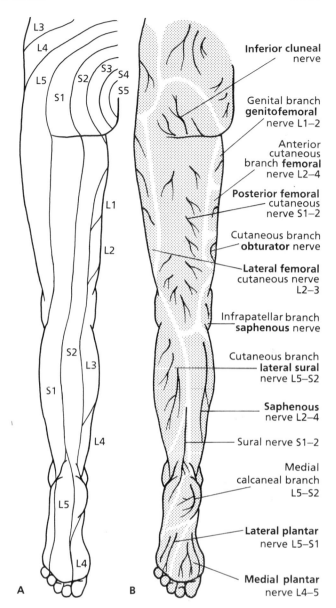

Fig. 60.1 A The dermatomal distribution of nerve roots on the anterior surface of the leg.
B The distribution of cutaneous nerves to the anterior aspect of the leg. The area of distribution of the obturator, lateral femoral cutaneous and saphenous nerves is very variable in extent.

Fig. 60.2 A The dermatomal distribution of nerve roots on the posterior aspect of the leg.
B The distribution of cutaneous nerves to the posterior aspect of the leg.

which continues with the nerves when they emerge into the leg.

Lumbar plexus block (psoas compartment block)
(Chayen *et al.*, 1976)

As the lumbar plexus is formed, it lies within its fascia between the quadratus lumborum posteriorly and the psoas anteriorly. The plexus may be blocked by a posterior approach. The landmarks and practical details of this technique are shown in Fig. 60.6. This block produces anaesthesia in the femoral, obturator and lateral femoral cutaneous nerve distributions, but rarely beyond these. The block may be used in concert with a sciatic nerve block to produce anaesthesia of the whole leg. A catheter may be inserted into the sheath to

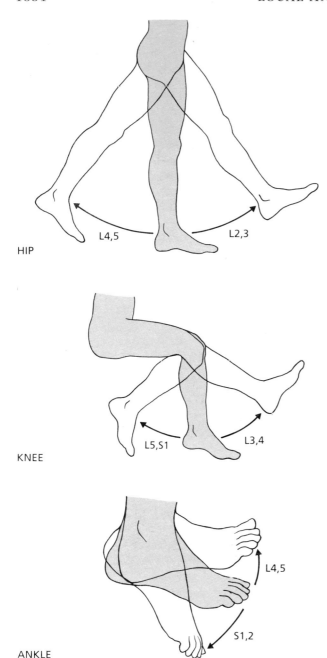

Fig. 60.3 The segmental innervation of the muscles of the leg.

permit repeated injections of local anaesthetic solution (Brands & Callanan, 1978).

FEMORAL NERVE

The femoral nerve emerges from the lateral border of the psoas muscle in the iliac fossa and runs deep to the iliac fascia in a groove between the psoas and iliacus muscles (Fig. 60.5). It emerges into the thigh lateral to

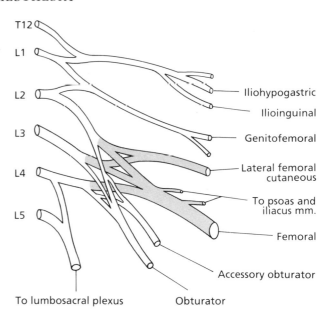

Fig. 60.4 The anatomy of the lumbar plexus. The anterior divisions of the anterior primary rami form the obturator nerve while the posterior divisions (shaded) form the femoral and lateral femoral cutaneous nerves.

the femoral artery, from beneath the inguinal ligament, enclosed within its fascial sheath. The femoral nerve supplies the muscles of the anterior compartment of the thigh and the skin of the anterior surface of the thigh (Figs 60.1 and 60.3). Its terminal branch, the saphenous nerve, follows the long saphenous vein, emerging from beneath the sartorius muscle at the medial side of the knee. It usually supplies an area of skin on the medial side of the leg to at least the level of the medial malleolus, and frequently beyond, up to the base of the great toe (Fig. 60.1).

Femoral nerve block

The landmarks and technical details of this block are shown in Fig. 60.7. This block produces anaesthesia of most of the anterior surface of the thigh. It may be used alone for anaesthesia of its area of distribution or in concert with other blocks to produce anaesthesia of the whole leg. A catheter may be introduced in a similar fashion to that described in Fig. 60.7 to permit repeated injections of local anaesthetic solution (Rosenblatt, 1980).

LATERAL FEMORAL CUTANEOUS NERVE

This nerve is formed by contributions from L2–3 within the psoas muscle. It emerges from beneath the muscle

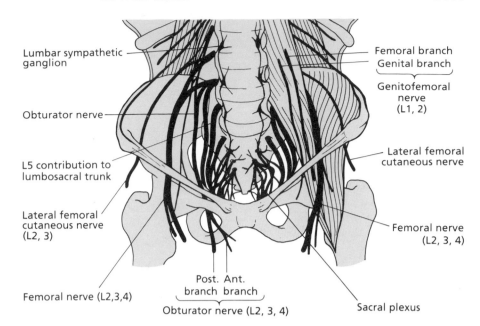

Fig. 60.5 The lumbar plexus anatomy on the posterior abdominal wall. On the left the psoas major and minor muscles have been removed to reveal the plexus more completely.

at the level of the iliac crest, and crosses the iliac fossa. It emerges into the thigh by piercing the inguinal ligament approximately 1–2 cm medial to the anterior superior iliac spine. Approximately 2–4 cm distal to the inguinal ligament, the nerve divides into anterior and posterior branches and pierces deep fascia to supply the skin on the lateral side of the leg as far as the knee. The area of distribution is very variable, and may encompass almost the whole of the anterior surface of the thigh (Figs 60.1 and 60.2).

Lateral femoral cutaneous nerve block

The landmarks and the technical details of this block are given in Fig. 60.7. A recently described alternative approach (Brown & Dickens, 1986) is to perform this block at the anterior superior iliac spine. A 22 gauge needle is inserted vertically immediately medial to the anterior superior iliac spine. As the needle passes through the external and internal oblique muscles, resistance to injection is felt, which is lost as the tip of the needle enters the canal which contains the nerve. Two to 4 ml of solution are injected. Irrespective of the technique used, blocks of this nerve may be used alone to provide anaesthesia on the lateral side of the thigh (e.g. for harvesting small skin grafts) or in concert with other blocks for anaesthesia of the whole leg.

OBTURATOR NERVE

The obturator nerve emerges from the medial border of the psoas muscle at the level of the brim of the true

pelvis, crosses the ala of the sacrum and passes along the wall of the pelvis (Fig. 60.5). It emerges into the thigh through the obturator canal at the antero-medial point of the obturator foramen. In the leg, it divides into anterior and posterior divisions, the former supplying the adductors and an area of skin of variable size on the medial side of the thigh, the latter providing motor innervation to the adductors in addition to a small terminal sensory branch to the knee joint.

Obturator nerve block

The landmarks and technical details for performing this block are shown in Fig. 60.8. This is a technically difficult block to perform and lacks aesthetic appeal for both operator and patients. It has a high failure rate and thus the use of a PNS is invaluable. If a block of only the obturator nerve is desired for diagnostic purposes, only an obturator block suffices. However, as the block is performed usually in concert with femoral and lateral femoral cutaneous nerve blocks to provide surgical anaesthesia, it is worthwhile considering using the 'three-in-one' block which anaesthetizes these three nerves with a high degree of reliability (see below) and is easier technically and quicker than having to perform three separate blocks.

'Three-in-one' block (Winnie et al., 1973)

As the femoral, lateral femoral cutaneous and obturator nerves are formed within the psoas, they are enclosed within a fascial sheath which continues to

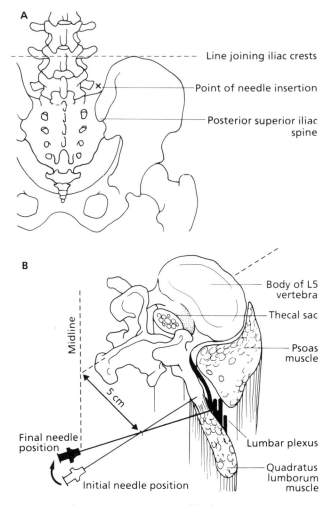

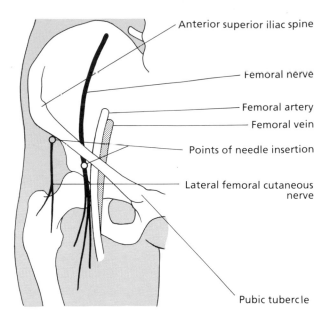

Fig. 60.7 Femoral and lateral femoral cutaneous nerve blocks.

Fig. 60.6 The psoas compartment block.

A The landmarks. The most superior points of the iliac crests should be identified and a line drawn to join them. Three cm caudad from this line, a second line 5 cm in length should be drawn laterally to the point of needle insertion. This point should overlie the transverse process of L5.

B The technique. The patient should lie in the lateral position, curled up as if for a spinal or extradural block. A 15 cm, 22 gauge needle should be inserted perpendicular to the skin at the point shown in (**A**) until it strikes the transverse process of L5. An air-filled syringe should be attached to the needle, pressure applied to the plunger of the syringe and the needle stepped off the transverse process cephalad and 5° laterally. As the tip of the needle enters the dense fascia on the posterior surface of the quadratus lumborum, tight resistance to injection should be felt. As the needle emerges into the plane which contains the plexus, a distinct loss of resistance should be felt. The plane can then be distended with 20–30 ml of air and 25–30 ml of solution injected (Chayen *et al.*, 1976) or, if a PNS is used, the needle tip adjusted to give optimal twitches in the adductor or quadriceps muscles, and 20–30 ml of solution injected. It is possible to place a needle or catheter close to the plexus at levels above L5 (Brands & Callanan, 1978).

The patient should lie in the supine position with the hip slightly abducted and externally rotated. The anterior superior iliac spine and the pubic tubercle are identified. A line joining these two structures overlies the inguinal ligament. The femoral artery is identified at the point where it emerges from beneath the inguinal ligament, and this point is marked. Femoral nerve block is accomplished by placing the index finger at the lateral side of the femoral artery to 'guard' it. The point of needle insertion is 2 cm lateral to the point where the artery emerges from beneath the inguinal ligament. A 5 cm, 22 gauge needle is inserted perpendicular to the horizontal to pierce first the fascia lata which is usually 1.5–3 cm deep in a normal-sized adult, and then the fascia iliaca approximately 0.5 cm deeper. Passing through each fascial layer is usually perceived as a 'pop'. Once the needle tip has passed through the fascia iliaca, the solution may then be injected as a bolus (Khoo & Brown, 1983), or infiltrated as a fan across the path of the nerve. Alternatively, paraesthesiae or, if a PNS is used, a twitch in the quadriceps muscles, sought and solution injected as a bolus. It may be difficult to obtain paraesthesiae or a twitch as at this point in its course the femoral nerve may have divided into a number of branches which slide away from any advancing needle rather easily. An alternative to a discrete femoral nerve block is to use the 'three-in-one' block (see text). The volume of injectate for femoral nerve block is 10–15 ml.

For lateral femoral cutaneous nerve block the point of needle insertion is 2 cm medial and 3 cm distal to the anterior superior iliac spine. A 5 cm, 22 gauge needle is inserted perpendicular to the horizontal. Five to 8 ml of solution are injected deep to the fascia which is usually encountered 1.5–2.5 cm deep to the skin. An alternative method of this block is given in the text.

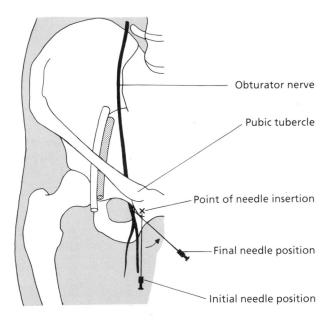

Fig. 60.8 Obturator nerve block.

The patient should lie in the supine position with the hip abducted 10–15° and in full external rotation. The pubic tubercle should be identified and marked. A line 3 cm in length drawn caudal to the pubic tubercle and at its termination a further line 2.5 cm in length drawn laterally, to the point of needle insertion. An 8 cm, 22 gauge needle should be inserted at 90° to the ischiopubic ramus (usually approximately 45° to the horizontal) parallel to the midline. At approximately 3–4 cm depth, the tip strikes the ischiopubic ramus. The needle is then withdrawn approximately 2 cm and 'walked' laterally and anterior until it slides off the lateral surface of the ischiopubic ramus and/or the inferior surface of the iliopubic ramus. The needle tip should then enter the obturator canal and drug may be injected blind, a paraesthesia sought, or a twitch of the adductor muscles obtained if a PNS is being used. See text for recommendations concerning this block. The volume of injectate should be 10–15 ml.

encase the nerves on their journey to the periphery. Placing a sufficient volume of injectate within this sheath and encouraging its proximal spread to the lumbar plexus or nerve roots results in a high incidence of block of all three nerves. Practically, this is achieved by using the landmarks shown in Fig. 60.7 and is performed best with the assistance of a PNS. A 6–8 cm, 22 gauge needle is inserted as for a femoral nerve block but at an angle at 45° to the horizontal, aiming the tip of the needle for the manubrium sterni. The nerve is sought, usually being found lateral to this position at a depth of 3–4 cm, and the position of the tip of the needle adjusted to obtain an appreciable twitch of the rectus femoris and vastus intermedius. At this point, the tip of the needle lies under the inguinal ligament and in the

centre of the nerve (by moving the needle from medial to lateral twitches of the vastus medialis and lateralis, respectively, may be obtained as the needle sweeps across the nerve). The position of the tip of the needle should be adjusted so that a twitch of vastus medialis and rectus femoris is obtained at a stimulation intensity of 0.4–0.6 mA. To prevent distal spread of the injectate, the sheath distal to the point of injection should be occluded digitally, and 30 ml of solution injected. Digital pressure should be maintained for approximately 5 min. This technique results in proximal spread of injectate to the plexus, and even root level, with a high incidence of block of all three major branches of the lumbar plexus (J.E. Charlton, personal communication; Patel *et al.*, 1986). If a prolonged block is required, an 18 gauge or 20 gauge catheter may be introduced into the sheath using this technique, and analgesia maintained with injections of 20–25 ml of bupivacaine 0.25% every 6 hr (Rosenblatt, 1980).

The sacral plexus

This plexus is formed by the anterior and posterior divisions of the primary rami of L5 and S1–3, with a small contribution from L4 (Fig 60.9). These contributions pass over the lateral portion of the sacrum to merge as the sciatic nerve and its branches at the sciatic notch.

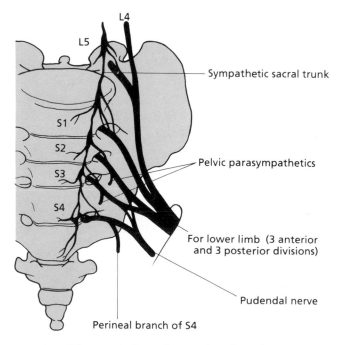

Fig. 60.9 The sacral plexus from within the pelvis.

THE SCIATIC NERVE

The sciatic nerve emerges into the buttock via the sciatic notch, often splitting the pyriformis muscle in the process (Fig. 60.10). It runs caudad on the posterior surface of the gemelli and the quadratus femoris muscles, and is covered posteriorly by the gluteal muscles. The sciatic nerve supplies the sensory and motor innervation to the posterior compartment of the

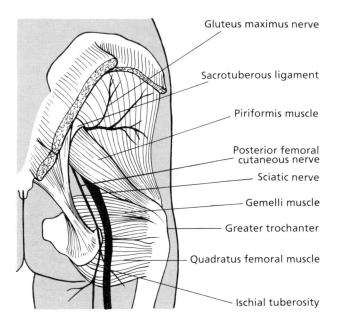

Fig. 60.10 The sciatic nerve in the buttock area. The sciatic nerve emerges into the buttock via the greater sciatic notch, often splitting the pyriformis muscle in the process. It curves over the lateral portion of the sacral spinous process and then runs caudad on the posterior surface of the gemelli and quadratus femoris muscles. It is covered superficially by the glutei.

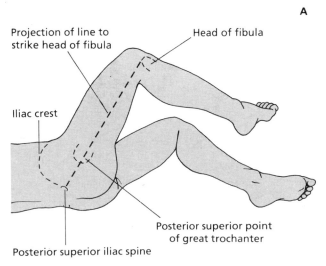

Fig. 60.11A

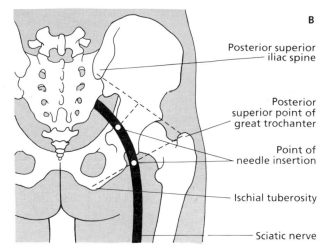

Fig. 60.11 The sciatic nerve block by the posterior approach.

A The position of the patient. The patient should be placed in the lateral position with the lower leg straight and the upper leg flexed at 45° and adducted so that the knee rests on the bed anterior to the lower leg (Sims' position). The posterior superior iliac spine and the posterior superior end of the greater trochanter should be identified, marked and a line joining those two points drawn. A further refinement of positioning is to place the upper leg so that, when viewed from above, a projection of the line between the anterior superior iliac spine and the greater trochanter strikes the very tip of the head of the fibula.

B Landmarks and technique of sciatic nerve block by the posterior approach.

The patient should be positioned as in (**A**). For the classical approach (Labat) the posterior superior iliac spine and the posterior superior point of the greater trochanter are identified, marked and a line joining those two points drawn. The mid-point of this line should be marked and a second line drawn at 90° to the first line in a caudad direction. The point of needle insertion is 2.5–3 cm along this line. (An alternative is to identify the caudal hiatus and draw a line from it to the greater trochanter. Where this line intersects with the perpendicular is the point of needle insertion.) A 10 cm, 22 gauge needle is inserted at 90° to the skin in all planes. It should encounter the sciatic nerve as it crosses the lateral portion of the ischial spine. If the nerve is not encountered, a series of needle insertions along the plane of the second line should be performed. A PNS is a helpful tool for this nerve block but care should be taken only to inject solution when twitches of the distal musculature supplied by the sciatic nerve i.e. muscles to the foot and ankle, are produced. For the alternative approach, the ischial tuberosity and the posterior superior end of the greater trochanter should be identified and a line drawn joining those two points. The midline of this line overlies the sciatic nerve as it crosses the quadratus lumborum muscle. A 10 cm, 22 gauge needle should be inserted at this point at 90° to the skin in all planes. If the nerve is not encountered, a series of passes along the line, at 90° to the course of the nerve, should be made. Again, a PNS is a useful tool. The volume of injectate should be 20–25 ml.

lower extremity. The dermatomal and myotomal distributions and the areas supplied by the sciatic nerve and its branches are shown in Figs 60.1 and 60.2.

Sciatic nerve block

The nerve is blocked classically in the buttock by a posterior approach. The landmarks and techniques are detailed in Fig. 60.11. Both of these techniques may be performed with the patient in Sims' position. The more distal block, between the ischial tuberosity and the greater trochanter, may be performed also with the patient in the lithotomy position (Raj *et al.*, 1975).

In the patient who cannot adopt the Sims' or lithotomy position e.g. a patient with a fractured femur, the nerve may be blocked also by an anterior approach (Fig. 60.12). The anterior technique is difficult to perform and has a high failure rate. Whichever technique is employed to block the sciatic nerve, meticulous attention to positioning, identification of landmarks and correct needle placement is essential.

Sciatic nerve blocks may be used in combination with femoral, lateral femoral cutaneous and obturator blocks (or the three-in-one block) to produce anaesthesia of the whole leg, with saphenous nerve blocks for anaesthesia of the leg below the knee, or alone for anaesthesia of the foot. A technique for introducing a catheter close to the sciatic nerve for repeated injections of local anaesthetic has been described (Smith *et al.*, 1984).

Nerve blocks around the knee

Saphenous nerve block

The saphenous nerve is the only component of the femoral nerve which has a distribution below the knee. It emerges from beneath the sartorius muscle on the medial side of the knee and accompanies the long saphenous vein, usually lying just posterior to the vein, over the medial side of the tibia. It is distributed to the medial side of the leg and the dorsum of the foot (Fig. 60.1).

The saphenous nerve should be blocked at a point 4–6 cm distal to the joint line of the knee on the medial side of the tibia. If the long saphenous vein can be identified at this level, a 2–4 ml infiltration on both sides of the vein blocks the nerve. If the vein cannot be identified, a band of infiltration of 8–10 ml of solution running from the posterior border of the tibia to the

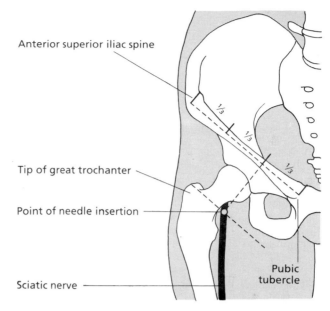

Fig. 60.12 Sciatic nerve block by the anterior approach.

The patient should lie supine with the hip abducted at 10° and in full external rotation. The anterior superior iliac spine and the pubic tubercle should be identified, marked and a line joining those two points drawn and divided into three equal lengths. At the junction of the medial and middle thirds, a perpendicular should be drawn caudally and laterally. The superior part of the greater trochanter should be identified, marked and a line drawn parallel to the line between the iliac spine and pubic tubercle, passing through the superior part of the greater trochanter. The point of needle insertion is where this last line and the perpendicular meet. A 15 cm, 22 gauge needle should be inserted perpendicular to the horizontal, with an air-filled syringe attached and with pressure applied to the plunger of the syringe. The needle usually strikes the medial surface of the femur at a depth of 7–8 cm. The needle should be angled medially to slide off the medial surface of the femur. At this point the tip of the needle passes through the origins of the adductors and there is resistance to injection. As the needle tip enters the posterior compartment, this resistance to injection is lost and drug may be injected. This block has a fairly high failure rate and the use of a PNS is valuable. The volume of injectate should be 20–25 ml.

tibial tubercule anteriorly blocks the nerve. Saphenous nerve blocks may be used in conjunction with sciatic or common peroneal and tibial nerve blocks for anaesthesia of the lower leg and foot.

The common peroneal and tibial nerve blocks

At a variable point in its course through the posterior compartment of the thigh, the sciatic nerve divides into its two major terminal branches, the common peroneal and tibial nerves. These nerves become accessible at the apex of the popliteal fossa where they may be blocked. The landmarks and technique are given in Fig. 60.13. This block may be used alone, or with saphenous nerve blocks, for lower leg and foot anaesthesia.

The common peroneal nerve block

This nerve leaves the popliteal fossa, coursing superficial to the lateral head of the gastrocnemius and, having curled around the lateral surface of the fibula

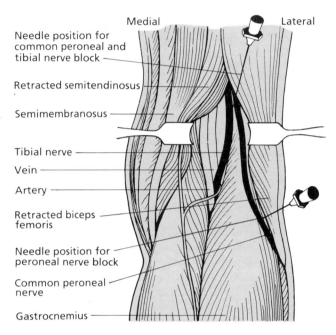

Fig. 60.13 Nerve blocks around the knee. The contents of the popiteal fossa with the medial and lateral hamstrings retracted to show the contents.

Common tibial nerve blocks. With the patient prone and the knee flexed, the superior end of the diamond-shaped popliteal fossa should be identified and marked. The knee should then be extended and the popliteal artery palpated at the marked apex of the popliteal fossa. If identification of the artery is difficult, a Doppler probe may be helpful. A 10 cm, 22 gauge needle is inserted immediately lateral to the artery and advanced until paraesthesiae are obtained or a twitch produced, if a PNS is used. This is usually at a depth of 3–5 cm, and 3–5 cm superficial to the posterior surface of the femur. The volume of injectate should be 8–10 ml. Prior to and during injection of solution careful aspiration of the needle is essential to ensure that injection of solution into the closely adjacent artery and vein does not occur.

Common peroneal blocks. This nerve should be blocked just before it curls around the head of the fibula. It can usually be palpated at this point and a 5 cm, 22 gauge needle inserted by a posterior or lateral approach. The volume of injectate should be 4–6 ml.

some 3 cm distal to the head of the fibula, enters the anterior compartment of the leg.

The nerve should be blocked by a posterior approach approximately 1.5–3 cm proximal to the point where it begins to curl around the head of the fibula. Three to 5 ml of solution should be used. This block has minimal usefulness on its own, but being performed easily may be useful as a 'back up' where other blocks are not possible, or have failed.

Nerve blocks at the ankle

The nerve supply to the foot is derived mainly from the branches of the common peroneal and tibial nerves, with a variable contribution from the saphenous nerve. The areas of cutaneous distribution are shown in Figs

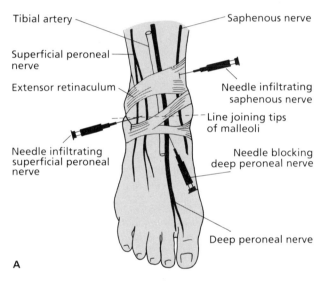

A

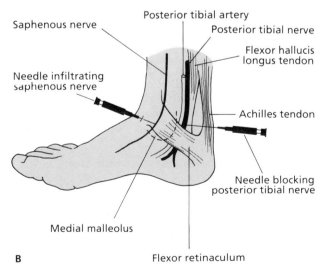

B

Fig. 60.14A and B

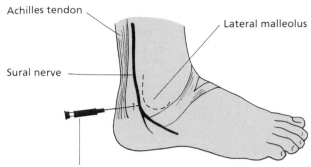

Achilles tendon

Lateral malleolus

Sural nerve

Needle infiltrating sural nerve

C

Fig. 60.14 Nerve blocks at the ankle.
A Anterior view of the ankle.

A line should be drawn joining the tips of the two malleoli. The saphenous nerve is blocked 2–3 cm above this line, either by infiltrating on both sides of the long saphenous vein, or by infiltrating a cuff of solution from the anterior to the posterior border of the medial malleolus. Four to 6 ml of solution should be used. The superficial peroneal nerve should be blocked by a band of infiltration along the line joining the two malleoli, superficial to the extensor retinaculum, from the anterior border of the lateral malleolus to the midpoint of the ankle. Four to 6 ml of solution should be used. The deep peroneal nerve should be blocked by infiltrating on the lateral side of the tibialis anterior tendon, medial to the anterior tibial artery, either at the level of the line between the two malleoli, or 2.5–3 cm distal to that point. Two to 3 ml of solution should be used.

B Medial view of the ankle.

The posterior tibial nerve should be blocked at the upper border of the flexor retinaculum, 2.5 cm proximal to the tip of the medial malleolus. The nerve lies immediately posterior to the tibial artery and anterior to the tendon of flexor hallucis longus. These structures should be identified and, with an index finger 'guarding' the posterior tibial artery, a 2 cm, 25 gauge needle inserted from a posterolateral direction. Paraesthesiae may be obtained, or 3–5 ml of solution infiltrated immediately posterior to the artery. The nerve is usually 1–1.5 cm deep to the skin.

C Lateral view of the ankle.

The sural nerve should be blocked by infiltrating a band of solution 2 cm proximal to the tip of the lateral malleolus from the lateral border of the tendo achilles to the posterior border of the lateral malleolus. Four to 6 ml of solution should be used.

60.1 and 60.2. The various nerves and the techniques used to block them are shown in Fig 60.14. The techniques described in Fig. 60.14 are aimed at the nerves at or above the extensor and flexor retinacula.

The various nerves may be blocked also below the retinacula (Sharrock et al., 1986).

Intravenous regional anaesthesia of the leg

Intravenous regional anaesthesia (IVRA) is an appealing, simple technique, but is not applied as readily to the leg as to the arm. If the tourniquet is placed around the thigh, large volumes of injectate, and therefore masses of drug, are necessary to produce satisfactory anaesthesia. With these large masses of drug, toxicity is likely to occur when the drug is released into the systemic circulation at the time of tourniquet release. If the tourniquet is placed above the malleoli, adequate tourniquet occlusion pressures (13.3 kPa, 100 mmHg, above systolic pressure), slow injection (over 2–3 min) and modest volumes of drug (20–30 ml lignocaine 0.5%) are used, satisfactory and safe anaesthesia may be produced (Davies & Walford, 1986). Similar precautions to those taken when IVRA is used in the arm should be observed at the time of tourniquet deflation.

References

Brands E. & Callanan V.L. (1978) Continuous lumbar plexus block. Analgesia for femoral neck fractures. *Anaesthesia and Intensive Care* **6**, 265–9.

Brown T.C.K. & Dickens D.R.V. (1986) A new approach to lateral femoral cutaneous nerve of thigh block. *Anaesthesia and Intensive Care* **14**, 126–7.

Chayen D., Nathan H. & Chayen M. (1976) The psoas compartment block. *Anesthesiology* **45**, 95–9.

Davies J.A.H. & Walford A.J. (1986) Intravenous regional anaesthesia for foot surgery. *Acta Anaesthesiologica Scandinavica* **30**, 145–7.

Khoo S.T. & Brown T.C.K. (1983) Femoral nerve block—the anatomic basis for a single injection technique. *Anaesthesia and Intensive Care* **11**, 40–2.

Patel N.J., Flashburg M.H., Paskin S. & Grossman R. (1986) A regional anesthetic technique compared to general anesthesia for outpatient arthroscopy. *Anesthesia and Analgesia* **65**, 185–7.

Raj P.P., Parks R.I., Watson T.D. & Jenkins M.T. (1975) A single position supine approach to sciatic–femoral nerve block. *Anesthesia and Analgesia* **54**, 489–93.

Rosenblatt R.M. (1980) Continuous femoral anesthesia for lower extremity surgery. *Anesthesia and Analgesia* **59**, 631–2.

Sharrock N.E., Waller J.F. & Fierro L.E. (1986) Midtarsal block for surgery of the forefoot. *British Journal of Anaesthesia* **58**, 37–40.

Smith B.E., Fischer H.B.J. & Scott P.V. (1984) Continuous sciatic nerve block. *Anaesthesia* **39**, 155–7.

Winnie A.P., Rammamurthy S. & Durrani Z. (1973) The inguinal paravascular technique of lumbar plexus block—the '3-in-1' block. *Anesthesia and Analgesia* **52**, 989–96.

61

Surface and Infiltration Anaesthesia

K. HOUGHTON AND J. B. BOWES

Surface or topical application of local anaesthetic agents may be employed to relieve or alleviate pain or to allow pain-free surgery to take place. It comprises the blockade of touch sensation in skin or mucous membrane. Whilst penetration through intact skin is difficult to achieve, absorption through mucous membrane may be rapid. Although methods such as the application of sprays, cold temperature, counter-irritation, acupuncture and massage may be used also for the transient relief of pain, this section deals only with the use of local anaesthetic techniques.

Drugs suitable for use as surface local anaesthetics

Local anaesthetics are, by definition, drugs which block nerve conduction when applied locally to nerve tissue. In clinical use, their action must be followed by complete recovery of conduction. An agent is suitable for surface anaesthesia only if it is able to penetrate the surface to which it is applied. Penetration through intact skin is generally poor unless high concentrations of certain agents are used and the contact time is long (Covino & Vassallo, 1976; Ritchie & Greene, 1985). In contrast, absorption through mucous membranes may be very rapid and therefore a detailed knowledge of the properties and toxicity of the drugs employed is essential and those with low systemic toxicity are preferred. Agents should not be irritating to the tissues to which they are applied. The pharmacological preparation in which the drug is supplied is relevant in relation to the site where it is applied. The (acidic) salt of the local anaesthetic base is supplied usually in aqueous solution and may be applied by direct instillation, on swabs, as a spray or aerosol, paste, ointment, cream, lotion, suppository or gel (Atkinson *et al.*, 1982).

Objective assessment of the relative efficacy of different agents for surface anaesthesia is difficult because of the variability in the site of application and the diversity of the forms in which an agent may be applied (Covino & Vassallo, 1976). Similarly, the speed of onset of anaesthesia and its duration depends on the agent used, its vehicle and the site to which it is applied. In general, higher doses and concentrations shorten onset time and prolong duration of anaesthesia. Cocaine is the only agent which causes vasoconstriction and this reduces bleeding and improves operating conditions. The addition of phenylephrine 0.005% gives similar conditions but adrenaline is unable to penetrate mucous membranes and is ineffective.

Agents suitable for surface use are shown in Table 61.1. Preparations available in the UK are described below (British National Formulary, 1987).

Lignocaine

Lignocaine is absorbed effectively through mucous membranes, and is the most commonly used agent.

Uses

Mucous membranes, skin and cornea.

Preparations

1 Gel. Lignocaine hydrochloride 1–2% with chlorhexidine gluconate solution 0.25% in a sterile lubricant water-miscible base.
2 Ointment. Lignocaine 5% in a water-miscible base.
3 Aerosol spray. Lignocaine 10% with cetylpyridinium chloride 0.01% in a metered spray container supplying 10 mg lignocaine/dose.

Table 61.1 Local anaesthetic agents for surface use

Agent	Typical conc. used	Max. safe dose mg/kg (max. dose)	Onset (min)	Duration (min)
Lignocaine	2–4%	3 (200 mg)	<5	20–30
Prilocaine	4%	6 (400 mg)	<5	20–30
Cocaine	4%	3 (200 mg)	<5	30–60
Amethocaine	0.2–1.0%	– (40 mg)	3–8	30–60
Benzocaine	1–2%		Slow	Prolonged
Cinchocaine	0.1%	Used rarely	No data	
Eye preparations				
Oxybuprocaine	0.4%			
Proxymetacaine	0.5%			
Colorectal				
Pramoxine	1%			

4 Topical solution. Anhydrous lignocaine hydrochloride 4%.

5 Oral solution. Anhydrous lignocaine hydrochloride 2%.

6 Cream. Lignocaine 50 mg + hyaluronidase 150 μg for application to mucous membranes of the mouth.

7 Eye drops. Lignocaine 4% with fluoroscein.

8 EMLA cream. Lignocaine 2.5% + prilocaine 2.5% as a 5% oil-in-water emulsion cream.

Particular attention should be given to the dose of lignocaine used in sites where absorption is rapid such as the trachea. Its use is contra-indicated in patients with myasthenia gravis, complete heart block and in hypovolaemia. It should be used with caution in those with epilepsy, hepatic impairment or abnormal cardiac conduction.

Toxicity

Hypotension, bradycardia, cardiac arrest, sleepiness, agitation, euphoria, respiratory depression and convulsions.

Prilocaine

Prilocaine is similar to lignocaine but less toxic.

Uses

Mucous membranes and skin.

Preparations

1 Prilocaine 3% with felypressin 0.03 unit/ml for injection.

2 EMLA cream (see under lignocaine).

3 Although not available commercially in the UK, a topical formulation may be prepared from imported prilocaine powder.

Toxicity

As for lignocaine but in addition, oxidation of haemoglobin by a breakdown product of prilocaine, *o*-toluidine, can occur if high doses are used, causing met-haemoglobinaemia.

Cocaine

Cocaine, now used solely for surface anaesthesia, penetrates mucous membranes easily and is extremely effective. It potentiates the action of adrenaline by blocking the re-uptake of transmitter at sympathetic nerve endings and thus cocaine and adrenaline should not be used in combination. It is soluble in water and alcohol. Solutions should be protected from light.

Uses

Nasopharynx, cornea.

Preparations

1 Solution 4–10%.

2 Paste 25%.

3 Eye drops 2–4%.

Toxicity

Excitation of the central and sympathetic nervous systems, depression of the cardiovascular system, respiratory stimulation followed by arrest, pyrexia, clouding of the corneal epithelium; and long-term ischaemia of tissues. Contra-indicated in closed-angle glaucoma. Hypersensitivity reactions may occur.

Amethocaine

Amethocaine is an effective surface anaesthetic which is absorbed rapidly through mucous membrane and should not be applied to inflamed, traumatized or highly vascular surfaces such as the respiratory tract where lignocaine is safer. Solutions should be protected from light.

Uses

Ophthalmology, skin, oropharynx.

Preparations

1 Eye drops, 0.5% and 1%.
2 Cream. Amethocaine hydrochloride 1% in water-miscible base or in combination with other local anaesthetics.

There are no commercial preparations available for surface or infiltration anaesthesia in the UK.

Toxicity

Cardiac asystole or ventricular fibrillation. Hypersensitivity has been reported. Amethocaine causes stinging in the eye and may produce sensitization of the skin with prolonged use.

Benzocaine

Benzocaine is an agent with low potency and low toxicity. Onset of anaesthesia is slow and of prolonged duration. It is used only for surface anaesthesia where it is absorbed too slowly to be toxic.

Uses

Relief of pain and irritation of the oropharynx and perianal area. It is safe to leave in contact with wounds and ulcerated surfaces.

Preparations

1 Lozenges. Benzocaine 10 mg, 100 mg.
2 Gel. Benzocaine 1% + cetylpyridinium chloride 0.01%.

3 Ointment (for rectal use). Benzocaine 2% in various compound preparations.
4 Lotion.
5 Spray 5% with triclosan 0.1%.

Toxicity

Prolonged use causes sensitization of skin.

Cinchocaine

Cinchocaine is highly potent, toxic and has a prolonged duration of action.

Uses

Minor skin and anorectal conditions.

Preparations

It is available only for surface use as a 1.1% ointment, or as an ingredient in various compound local anaesthetic creams and suppositories. The 0.1% solution has been reported for use for corneal analgesia. No topical solution is available commercially.

Toxicity

It is more toxic than cocaine or lignocaine.

Miscellaneous

PRAMOXINE

This agent is too irritating for application to the eye or nose, and its use is limited to preparations for dermatoses and painful perineal and anorectal conditions. It is included in various creams and suppositories in concentrations of approximately 1%.

OXYBUPROCAINE AND PROXYMETACAINE

These are used exclusively for surface analgesia of the eye.

ETHYL CHLORIDE

This was used extensively in the past as a local spray for dental extraction where, as a result of its extreme potency, general anaesthesia was known to supervene on occasions! It is now used only occasionally as a spray for incision of small abscesses, before injections, etc. It renders skin anaesthetic by freezing.

ANTIHISTAMINES

These have some local anaesthetic effect when used topically but are not recommended as they cause sensitization of the skin.

Infiltration anaesthesia

This is the production of regional analgesia by direct infiltration of the incision, wound or lesion. Local anaesthetic solution is injected around and into the site which is to be rendered pain-free in order to prevent the appreciation of pain, although the sensation of touch may persist. No attempt is made to identify individual nerves. Results are most likely to be successful if systematic injection is carried out commencing with dermis, followed by subcutaneous tissue, fascia and then muscle, as appropriate to the plane through which the nerves to be anaesthetized pass (Moore, 1978). Aspiration tests should be performed whenever any quantity of solution is injected in one place to avoid intravascular injection. Various adjuvants may alter the duration of action or rate of spread of the agent used. As only the distal portions of the nerves and nerve endings are blocked, a greater volume of local anaesthetic solution is required when compared with specific nerve blocks and therefore care is needed to avoid toxic doses of both local anaesthetic and vasoconstrictor (if used).

Infiltration anaesthesia in infected areas is likely to be ineffective because of the lower pH of infected tissue which reduces penetration of the local anaesthetic agent. It is considered by some to be contra-indicated. A small weal raised over a pointing abscess, however, may prove simple and useful for drainage without serious risk of disseminating infection (Eriksson, 1979).

Complications include neuritis, sloughing of tissue and necrosis of wound edges, particularly if large volumes and vasoconstrictors are used.

A *field block* is produced when a wall of anaesthesia surrounds the operative field (Moore, 1978), thus interrupting the passage of nerve impulses from the operative site to the CNS. Individual nerves are not sought specifically but are anaesthetized in the tissue plane or planes in which they lie. Infiltration should be performed in the area and direction from which the nerves supplying the operative site arise, ensuring that all layers are anaesthetized. Where the nerve supply comes from more than one direction, the site may be outlined geometrically and several points of infiltration used (Fig. 61.1). The latter technique is suitable for skin graft donor areas, biopsies, removal of small lumps, etc.

Drugs suitable for use in infiltration anaesthesia

Lignocaine, prilocaine and bupivacaine are the drugs used most commonly for infiltration anaesthesia. Procaine is used rarely, as, although it has equivalent potency to lignocaine, it has a shorter duration of action and produces less intense analgesia. It is usually used therefore with adrenaline 1/200 000. It is metabolized to para-aminobenzoic acid which inhibits the action of sulphonamides. Cinchocaine is not used as it produces a high incidence of tissue slough. Amethocaine is more toxic than lignocaine and is now used rarely.

Effective infiltration anaesthesia can be obtained with 0.5–1.0% solutions (Table 61.2) (Scott & Cousins, 1980), although higher concentrations are used frequently in dental practice. Onset of analgesia is virtually instantaneous with all agents. Duration of analgesia varies with the agent and increases with higher concentrations and with the addition of other substances (Concepcion & Covino, 1984).

Maximum safe doses depend on the patient's age, weight, physique and clinical condition. The vascu-

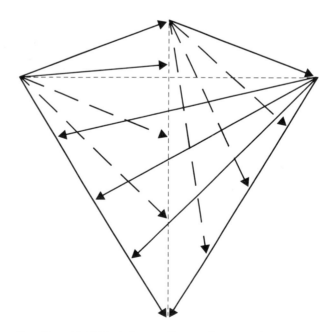

Fig. 61.1 Field block for small operative procedures.

Table 61.2 Local anaesthetic agents for infiltration

Agent	Typical conc. used	Equivalent conc.	Approx. duration of action (min)	
			− Adren.	+ Adren. 1/200 000
Short-acting				
Procaine	0.5–2%	2%	15–30	30–90
Chloroprocaine*				
Intermediate				
Lignocaine	0.5%	1%	30–60	120–360
	1%		120	400
Prilocaine	0.5–1%	1%	120	360
Mepivacaine*	0.5–1%	1%	120	360
Long-acting				
Bupivacaine	0.25–0.5%	0.25%	180	420
Etidocaine*	0.5–1%		180	420

* Not available in UK.

Table 61.3 Guide to doses of drugs for infiltration

Agent	Maximum safe doses (mg/70 kg adult)	
	− Adren.	+ Adren.
Procaine	800	1000
Chloroprocaine	800	1000
Lignocaine	200	500
Prilocaine	400	600
Mepivacaine	300	500
Bupivacaine	150	225
Etidocaine	300	400
Amethocaine	—	200

larity of the area to which the drug is applied must be considered also. A guide to dosage is given in Table 61.3.

Substances affecting action of local anaesthetics

VASOCONSTRICTORS

Vasoconstrictors may decrease bleeding, decrease plasma levels of local anaesthetic drug and increase operating time. They are more effective when added freshly to local anaesthetic solutions. They should never be used for infiltration of appendages or digits.

Adrenaline

The addition of adrenaline increases the duration of infiltration anaesthesia of all agents but particularly lignocaine (Covino & Vassallo, 1976) and prilocaine (Hassan *et al.*, 1985). Concentrations of 2–5 µg/ml (1/200 000–1/500 000) are usual although higher concentrations (12.5 µg/ml or 1/80 000) are used frequently in dentistry where the total dose is small. The total dose should not exceed 0.5 mg, but, as plasma catecholamine concentrations vary markedly with the site of application, the safe dose varies also (Cotton *et al.*, 1986). Its use is contra-indicated in patients taking tricyclic or related antidepressants (as arrhythmias may result) and in thyrotoxicosis (Boakes *et al.*, 1973).

During halothane anaesthesia the 'safe' dose of adrenaline is said to be 1.0 µg/kg. This is said to be reached with doses of approximately 10 ml of 1/100 000 concentration injected every 10 min. The maximum used should be 30 ml/hr and carbon dioxide retention should be avoided. Signs of toxicity are pallor, tachycardia and syncope. However, the recommendation should be qualified, as it is known that adrenaline is absorbed much more rapidly from nasal or aural infiltration than from an axillary brachial plexus block (Cotton *et al.*, 1986).

Noradrenaline

Concentrations of 20–40 µg/ml (1/50 000–1/25 000) may be required for vasoconstriction, but these may cause severe hypertension. It is contra-indicated in hypertensive patients and those in whom adrenaline is inadvisable (Boakes *et al.*, 1972, 1973). It is not indicated for routine use.

Phenylephrine

Also an α-receptor stimulant, this may be used in place of adrenaline. It does not cause cerebral stimulation or tachycardia. The usual dose is 0.25–0.5 ml of 1% solution per 100 ml of local anaesthetic solution.

Felypressin

The synthetic polypeptide is related to vasopressin, although it lacks antidiuretic and oxytocic effects and is a less toxic alternative to adrenaline. It is used commonly in combination with prilocaine as it has a more prolonged action than adrenaline, particularly in dentistry. It is safe for use with antidepressants. Typical concentration is 0.03 unit/ml.

DEXTRANS

Dextrans have been used in the past to prolong the duration of local anaesthetics but there is some controversy regarding their efficacy. This is discussed on p. 1019 in Chapter 57.

HYALURONIDASE

This is an enzyme which inactivates the hyaluronic acid which inhibits diffusion of invasive substances. It appears to be particularly active in subcutaneous tissues and should therefore enhance the rate and distance of spread of local anaesthetic. It is not toxic and may be used concurrently with adrenaline, the addition of which prevents any reduction in duration of anaesthesia caused by enhanced diffusion.

Hypersensitivity has been reported. A dose of 1500 units is a suitable dose to use in any volume of local solution. Its use limits the dosage which can be used because of enhanced absorption, unless adrenaline is used also. It is available as a powder for reconstitution in 1500 unit ampoules.

Individual blocks

Before performing these blocks, the patient should have the procedure explained fully and a suitable premedication such as temazepam 20 mg orally may be prescribed. Resuscitation equipment and oxygen should always be available. If relevant, the skin is prepared.

The techniques employed may not be suitable in children and nervous adults.

Scalp

Uses

Suture or debridement of wounds and removal of small lesions.

Ventriculography, intracranial biopsy, and burr hole exploration especially in cases of acute head injury.

As an adjunct to general anaesthesia to reduce blood loss and allow a lighter plane of anaesthesia to be employed.

Anatomy (Williams & Warwick, 1980)

The sensory supply is shown in Fig. 61.2.

The layers of the scalp are shown in Fig. 61.3 and comprise:
1 Skin.
2 Subcutaneous tissue.
3 Epicranial aponeurosis (galea aponeurotica) which is adherent firmly to subcutaneous tissue above and is

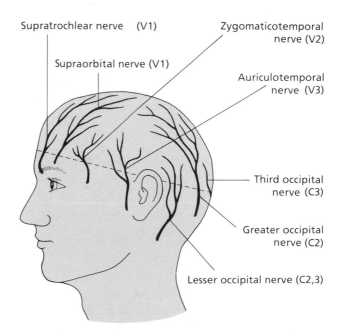

Fig. 61.2 Nerve supply to the scalp with level of circumferential injection for field block of the scalp.

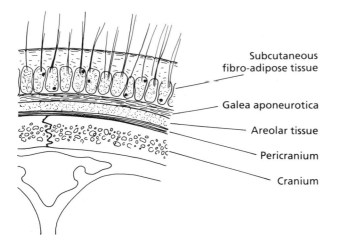

Fig. 61.3 Coronal section through the scalp.

continuous anteriorly and posteriorly with occipitofrontalis and laterally with temporoparietalis muscle. In combination they form a fibromuscular layer over the upper part of the cranium.

The upper three layers are adherent firmly and remain connected when torn.

4 Subaponeurotic areolar tissue.
5 Pericranium.

Technique

For a limited area of analgesia, solution should be injected in skin and subcutaneous tissue above the aponeurosis, as nerves (and vessels) lie here, followed by infiltration below it in the area required. For a wider area of blockade, a skull cap distribution of analgesia may be produced by circumferential infiltration along a line passing above the ear from glabella to occiput (Fig. 61.2). It is along this line that the sensory branches of nerves supplying the scalp become subfascial. The landmarks are found by palpation and a circle of anaesthesia produced by systematic infiltration of all layers, accompanied by careful aspiration. In the temporal region, the muscle layer is thicker and the nerves may lie more deeply so more local anaesthetic may be required. Periosteal injection is necessary only if bone is to be removed. Lignocaine or prilocaine 0.5% are suitable and the addition of adrenaline is advisable, as the soft tissues are highly vascular (Macintosh & Ostlere, 1967; Eriksson, 1979; Atkinson *et al.*, 1982).

Ear, nose and throat surgery

Advantages of local anaesthesia include avoidance of emergence problems from general anaesthesia, inhala-

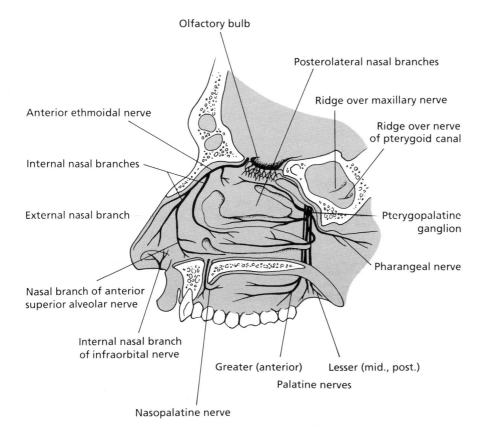

Fig. 61.4 Nerve supply to the lateral wall of the nasal cavity.

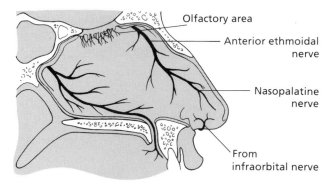

Fig. 61.5 Nerves of the nasal septum.

tion of blood and sore throat from the use of a throat pack.

NASAL CAVITIES

Uses

Surgery on the nasal septum, submucous resection, cautery or diathermy, polypectomy, turbinectomy.

Anatomy (Williams & Warwick, 1980)

The sensory nerve supply to the nasal cavity and septum originates from the trigeminal nerve (V) via its ophthalmic (V1) and maxillary (V2) divisions (Figs 61.4 and 61.5). The main supply is from:

1 The *anterior ethmoidal nerve* supplying the anterior third of the septum, roof and lateral walls of the nasal cavity. This is a branch of the nasociliary nerve which arises from V1.

2 The pterygopalatine ganglion which arises from V2 gives off the greater and lesser palatine nerves. The nasal branches of the lesser palatine nerves are the *lateral* and *medial posterior superior nasal nerves*. These, together with the *posterior inferior nasal branches* of the greater palatine nerve supply the posterior two-thirds of the lateral wall, roof, floor and septum.

A small supply is received also from:

3 The *infraorbital nerve* (V2) and its branch, the *anterior superior alveolar (dental) nerve*, supply the vestibule and a part of the septum and floor near the anterior nasal spine and the anterior part of the lateral wall as high as the opening of the maxillary sinus.

4 Branches from the *nerve of the pterygoid canal* (from V2) supply the upper and back part of roof and septum.

Vasomotor sympathetic nerves accompany the sensory fibres and supply the vessels.

Techniques

Packing. The nasal cavities are sprayed with cocaine 4–10% solution and then packed with gauze soaked in cocaine 4–5% solution. Use of a 10% solution with 1/1000 adrenaline has been described, although the powerful vasoconstrictor property of cocaine makes the use of adrenaline superfluous. Adrenaline has the additional disadvantages of potentiating the cardiac sympathomimetic properties of cocaine and of causing reactive vasodilatation when it wears off. The gauze must contact all areas, but in particular the area behind the middle meatus (where it anaesthetizes the greater and lesser palatine nerves) and the cribriform plate (close to the anterior ethmoidal nerve branches). It should remain in place for 10 min. The base of the columella must be injected separately for septal operations.

Direct application. After spraying the cavities with cocaine 4% solution, cocaine paste (e.g. 2 g of a paste containing 25% cocaine and soft paraffin) may be pasted to the areas described above using a wool-covered probe. In particular, the cribriform plate (anterior ethmoidal nerve) and the area behind the middle meatus (where the sphenopalatine ganglion lies) should be pasted. The dose of cocaine is higher than that recommended normally, as absorption is slow in this formulation.

Sluder (1913) described the use of wool mounted on four narrow applicators and then dipped into adrenaline solution and cocaine crystals or cocaine paste. After initial spraying with cocaine, two applicators were placed for 5 min on each side between middle turbinate and septum, one anteriorly and one posteriorly.

For *antral puncture*, applicators with wool soaked in cocaine 4% solution or lignocaine 4% with 2–3 drops (0.15 ml) of adrenaline 0.1% per 5 ml of solution may be placed under the middle and inferior turbinates for 10 min and the mucosa sprayed with lignocaine 10% aerosol spray (Atkinson *et al.*, 1982).

These methods require considerable skill, are time-consuming, unpleasant for the patient and may cause mild trauma.

Instillation of solution

1 Moffett (1947) described a method in which Moffett's solution comprising 2 ml cocaine hydrochloride 8%, 2 ml sodium bicarbonate 1% and 1 ml adrenaline 1/1000 is instilled into the nose with the

patient adopting three different positions, each of which must be maintained for 10 min.

Firstly, the patient lies on the left side with a pillow under the left shoulder. Using this as a fulcrum, the head is allowed to extend until it is at 45° to the vertical. One-third of the above solution is drawn up and half is instilled into each nostril. The needle used is 5 cm long and angled at 45° with three lateral holes near the blunt end.

Secondly, a third of the solution is divided between the nares and the patient asked to pinch his or her nose and turn immediately prone.

Thirdly, the patient is positioned as for the first stage but lying on the right side and the final third of the solution instilled. This provides a very satisfactory block with good operating conditions but is time-consuming and uncomfortable for the patient. It was modified by Curtiss in 1952.

2 Curtiss (1952) showed radiographically that in each of Moffett's positions, the solution came to lie in the region of the sphenopalatine recess. He showed that the same effect could be obtained by positioning the patient with the head fully extended over the end of the trolley and instilling 2 ml of Moffett's solution into each of the nares. The same type of needle is inserted with the tip directed along the floor of the nose and when the angled part has entered the nose, the direction of the tip is altered to point towards the roof of the nose. When the tip impinges on the bony roof, 2 ml of solution are administered. The same procedure is followed on the other side. The patient remains in position for 10 min.

As with Moffett's method, the pool of solution deposited affects the sphenopalatine ganglion, its branches and the anterior ethmoidal nerve. The main trunk of the maxillary division of the Vth nerve appears to be affected as the area under the inferior turbinate is anaesthetized (this is supplied by the anterior and posterior alveolar nerves). The floor and lateral walls of the antrum are therefore rendered anaesthetic also, allowing antral operations to be performed e.g. Caldwell–Luc (see below).

3 Macintosh and Ostlere (1967) described a method employing the same position and instilling 2.5 ml of cocaine 5% solution after spraying the mucosa.

4 Bodman and Boyes-Korkis (1960) used 40 ml lignocaine 1.25% with 0.5 ml adrenaline added, with 20 ml being poured into each nostril with the head in hyperextension. The patient breathes through the mouth for 3 min and then sits up and blows excess solution out.

These methods are nerve blocks, albeit adminis-

tered via the topical route. They are time-consuming and uncomfortable for the patient, and toxicity is a risk, particularly if the mucous membrane is inflamed.

MAXILLARY ANTRUM

Uses

Caldwell–Luc and other antral operations.

Anatomy

The sensory supply is from branches of the infraorbital nerve.

Technique

The gingiva should be sprayed first with lignocaine 4%. Infiltration of the alveolar–buccal mucosa above the premolars with lignocaine 0.5–1% with vasoconstrictor blocks branches of the infraorbital nerve. Further injections may be made into and under the mucous membrane. The nose can be packed with gauze soaked in lignocaine 4% or one of the methods of direct instillation of solution described above may be used. Further solution may be sprayed into the antrum if anaesthesia is incomplete (Oldham, 1968; Bryce-Smith, 1976; Eriksson, 1979; Morrison et al., 1985).

OUTER NOSE AND SEPTUM

Uses

Operations on the outer nose and septum.

Anatomy

The skin of the nose is supplied by branches of the trigeminal nerve (V).

The skin over the upper part of the nose is supplied by the *nasociliary nerve* (a branch of the ophthalmic nerve, V1). The skin between the palpebral fissure and nostril is supplied by the *infraorbital nerve*, the continuation of the maxillary nerve (V2).

Technique

Subcutaneous infiltration at the tip of the nose and then from the glabella down over the lateral aspects of the nose are made while withdrawing the needle to avoid undue tissue distension. Infiltration can be commenced from either glabella or tip. Four tracks of infiltration are made on each side with lignocaine 1%. The nasal cavities are dealt with separately as are the membranous septum and columella. This technique should not be used in a fractured nose (Eriksson, 1979).

EAR

Uses

Paracentesis of the eardrum, tympanotomy, myringotomy and radical mastoidectomy.

Anatomy (Williams & Warwick, 1980)

The sensory supply to the ear is described below (Fig. 61.6A, B).

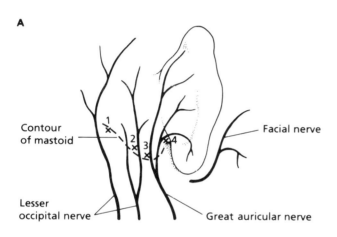

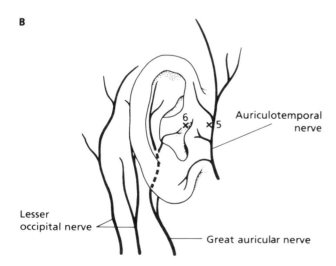

Fig. 61.6 Sensory supply to the auricle showing injection sites for radical mastoidectomy.
A Cranial aspect.
B External aspect.

Auricle

1 The *great auricular nerve* (a branch of the cervical plexus, C2 and 3) supplying the helix, antihelix, lobule and most of the cranial surface of the auricle.
2 The *lesser occipital nerve* supplying the upper part of the cranial surface.
3 The *auricular branch of the vagus* supplying the concavity and posterior part of the concha.
4 The *auriculotemporal nerve* (a branch of the mandibular nerve) supplying the tragus and adjacent part of the helix.
5 The *facial nerve* which together with the auricular branch of the vagus supplies small areas of skin on both aspects of the auricle, in the conchal depression and over its eminence.

External auditory meatus

1 The *auriculotemporal nerve* supplying the skin of the anterior and upper wall of the meatus.
2 The *auricular branch of the vagus* supplying the posterior wall and floor.

Tympanic membrane

1 The tympanic nerve (a branch of the glossopharyngeal nerve). The auriculotemporal nerve (a branch of the mandibular nerve).
2 The *auricular branch of the vagus*.

Techniques

Paracentesis of the eardrum. Two or three spray doses (20–30 mg) of lignocaine 10% aerosol spray are directed towards the upper wall of the auditory canal and allowed to run down over the eardrum. This can be repeated after 2 min and is then left for 3–5 min.

Radical mastoidectomy. Several injections of 1–2 ml of solution made over the mastoid process behind the ear anaesthetizes the great auricular nerve (Fig. 61.6A, injection sites 1,2,3). Two to 3 ml injected into the skin of the floor of the auditory canal and periosteal injection on the anterior part of the mastoid process (4) blocks the auricular branch of the vagus. Infiltration of the skin and periosteum over the auditory canal in front of the ear blocks the auriculotemporal nerve (Fig. 61.6B, site 5). To include its tympanic branch another injection must be made in the anterior wall of the auditory canal between bony and cartilaginous parts (6).

A few drops of more concentrated topical solution may be instilled into the meatus for surface anaesthesia of the mucous membrane, and tympanic membrane.

Lignocaine 4% may be used for topical application and lignocaine 0.5–1.0% with adrenaline for infiltration.

Tympanotomy. Blockade of the auriculotemporal nerve and its tympanic branch should be performed as above (Fig. 61.6B, injections 5 and 6). If a wide incision is contemplated, the full block should be performed as for radical mastoidectomy.

Mouth and pharynx

DENTAL PROCEDURES

Uses

Extraction of all teeth except lower molars, some conservation work, periodontal surgery e.g. gingivectomy.

Anatomy (Williams & Warwick, 1980)

The sensory supply to the teeth is from branches of the trigeminal nerve (V). Maxillary branches supply the upper jaw and mandibular branches supply the lower jaw as follows (Fig. 61.7).

Upper jaw

1 The *superior alveolar nerves* (branches of the infraorbital nerve, V2) supply the upper teeth, buccal gingiva and periosteum.
2 The *nasopalatine nerve* (one of the posterior nasal branches of the maxillary nerve, V2) supplies the mucosa, gingiva and periosteum of the anterior part of the hard palate.
3 The *greater palatine nerve* supplies the mucous membrane of the hard palate and palatal aspect of gum.

Lower jaw

4 The *buccal nerve* supplies the gum between the second molar and second premolar teeth on the buccal aspect.
5 The *inferior alveolar nerve* supplies the teeth and gums of the lower jaw on the lingual aspect.
6 The *lingual nerve* supplies the lingual gingiva and the floor of the mouth.

Technique

A surface anaesthetic can be applied to the gingiva in the area to be infiltrated.

Because of the tautness of the tissues, it is only possible to use a small volume of local anaesthetic solution, and this must diffuse through periosteum and compact bone to reach the nerve supply to the pulp, periodontum and jaw bone. Using a 26 gauge needle, solution is injected at the junction of adherent muco-periosteum of buccal gingiva and mucous membrane of cheek, parallel with the long axis of the tooth. One-half to 1 ml of solution is deposited close to the apex in the buccal fold. Two to 3 ml injected in one site anaesthetizes two to three teeth. It is usually necessary also to anaesthetize the palatal or lingual aspect of the tooth. The mucosa is applied so closely to the periosteum of the hard palate that 0.1 ml of solution is sufficient and should be injected very slowly. One-tenth to 1 ml may be used on the lingual aspect of the lower teeth. For all injections, it is important that the tip of the needle lies just above the periosteum. In the lower jaw, injection must be close to bone to avoid depositing solution in the chin or muscles of the lower lip. All injections should be preceded by aspiration in this vascular area and should be made very slowly to avoid pain and damage to tissues induced by counter-pressure. Infiltration blocks do not last as long as nerve

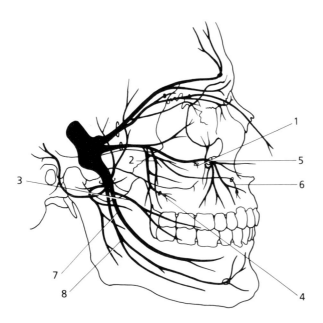

Fig. 61.7 Nerve supply to the upper and lower jaw.
1 and 2 Anterior and posterior superior alveolar nerves.
3 Buccal nerve.
4 Greater palatine nerve.
5 Infraorbital nerve.
6 Nasopalatine nerve.
7 Lingual nerve.
8 Inferior alveolar nerve.

blocks as the vascularity of the buccal fold aids rapid transport of solution away from the site of injection.

Anaesthesia may be inadequate for operations on pulp which is more richly innervated than the periodontal gingival and bone tissues. Infiltration blocks are unsuitable for procedures on the lower molars and premolars because of the large mass of mandibular bone. Haematoma and prolonged anaesthesia may result from damage to nerves and blood vessels, which is particularly likely to occur if the needle tip enters a foramen.

Solutions used commonly include lignocaine 2% with 1/80 000 adrenaline and prilocaine 3% with felypressin 0.03 IU/ml (Haglund & Evers, 1984).

TONSILLAR BLOCK

Uses

Tonsillectomy. Although not used often as the sole anaesthetic, local anaesthesia may be useful with general anaesthesia in adults or children (Boliston & Upton, 1980).

Anatomy

The *tonsillar branch of the glossopharyngeal nerve* forms a plexus around the tonsil with branches of the *middle* and *posterior (lesser) palatine nerves*, which are branches of the maxillary nerve. Filaments are sent to adjacent soft palate and fauces.

Technique

The patient may be given a benzocaine lozenge 30 min before spraying mouth and pharynx with approximately 1 ml of cocaine 4–10% solution or lignocaine 4% or prilocaine 4% (repeated after 5 min).

Infiltration injections are then made (Fig. 61.8):
1 Under the mucous membrane of the posterior palatal arch.
2 Under the mucous membrane of the anterior palatal arch, sufficient to make both oedematous.
3 Into remaining peritonsillar tissue, below and above the tonsil. Infiltration into the supratonsillar fossa above is facilitated by drawing the tonsil medially.

Ten to 15 ml of either lignocaine 0.5–1.5% or prilocaine with adrenaline (e.g. 1/200 000) are used for infiltration on each side.

Some operators do not like the loss of cough reflex and the risk of aspiration which may occur with good pharyngeal spraying.

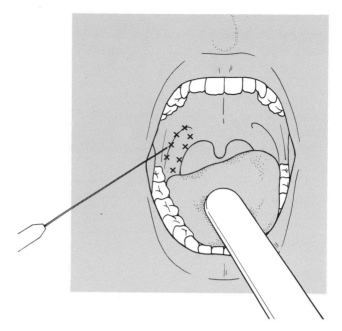

Fig. 61.8 Injection sites for tonsillectomy.

GASTROSCOPY, OESOPHAGOSCOPY

Technique

Premedication is helpful, and the patient is asked to suck a benzocaine lozenge 30 min before the procedure. Intravenous sedation with a benzodiazepine e.g. diazemuls or midazolam in 2 mg increments is often necessary.

Surface anaesthesia of the mouth and pharynx is accomplished by:
1 Spraying with a suitable topical agent e.g. cocaine 4%, lignocaine 4%, amethocaine 1%.
2 Swallowing a viscous lignocaine preparation (2%) (Williams *et al.*, 1968; Atkinson *et al.*, 1982).

LARYNX, TRACHEA AND BRONCHI

Uses

Laryngoscopy, tracheoscopy, bronchoscopy, bronchography and blind nasal intubation.

Anatomy

Larynx, trachea and bronchi. The sensory nerve supply is from the vagus via its superior and recurrent laryngeal branches.

The *superior laryngeal nerve* passes deep to the external and internal carotid arteries and there divides into a small motor external branch and a larger *internal branch* which pierces the posteroinferior part of the thyrohyoid membrane above the superior laryngeal artery and provides sensory supply to the laryngeal surface of the epiglottis, aryepiglottic folds and the interior of the larynx as far down as the vocal cords.

The terminal (inferior) branch of the *recurrent laryngeal nerve* ascends to the larynx in the groove between oesophagus and trachea together with the laryngeal branch of the inferior thyroid artery. It is sensory to the mucosa of the larynx below the cords, and to the trachea and bronchi.

Technique

Sedative premedication may be given 1 hr preoperatively and intravenous sedation at the time of the procedure is helpful although not essential (Pearce, 1980).

The mouth and pharynx are prepared as for oesophagoscopy (see above). For passage of a nasal endotracheal tube or flexible bronchoscope, one nostril may be sprayed or packed with local anaesthetic (e.g. with cocaine 5%, lignocaine 4%). The nostril and tube may be lubricated also with lignocaine gel. This may be sufficient for laryngoscopy if inspection of the cords only is intended.

If the cords are to be touched or biopsied, the larynx itself must be anaesthetized. The internal branches of the superior laryngeal nerve may be anaesthetized as they pass beneath the mucosa of the pyriform fossae (Macintosh & Ostlere, 1967) by applying swabs soaked in local anaesthetic solution and held in Krause's forceps (or other curved forceps such as Jackson's or Moynihan's). These are then passed over the back of the tongue until the fossae are reached and held in position there for a short time. The swab should then be palpable through the skin near the tip of the hyoid bone. This procedure is easier if the tongue is held in a gauze swab and brought forward gently. The epiglottis and vocal cords are sprayed, or local anaesthetic solution may be dropped directly onto them under direct vision using a mirror and laryngeal syringe, or injected via the side arm of a flexible bronchoscope. The glottis is rendered anaesthetic by holding a swab soaked in local anaesthetic solution in it for a short time. If solution has been dripped directly onto the larynx this should not be necessary.

Surface anaesthesia of the upper airway may be combined with block of the superior laryngeal nerve performed percutaneously (Gotta & Sullivan, 1981).

The trachea is anaesthetized either by allowing solution dropped onto the glottis to run down the trachea or by injecting 2–4 ml of solution through the cricothyroid membrane into the trachea. Cricothyroid puncture is performed using a 22 gauge needle with syringe attached. The patient lies supine with neck extended and the anaesthetist stands as if for intubation. The cricothyroid membrane is palpated and the needle advanced perpendicularly in the midline until air is aspirated, confirming the presence of the needle tip in the trachea. The solution is then injected at the end of a maximal expiration. Inspiration and coughing then normally ensure spread throughout trachea and bronchial tree (Moore, 1978).

It is possible to produce anaesthesia throughout the respiratory tract using nebulized lignocaine. Methods have been described which utilize either a small disposable type of nebulizer (Vuckovic *et al.*, 1980) or an ultrasonic nebulizer (Christoforidis *et al.*, 1971). The patient mouth-breathes through a mask until 6–10 ml of lignocaine 4% solution is nebulized fully. If a few minutes of positive-pressure breathing via a face-mask can be tolerated, solution can be dispensed via a nebulizer and ventilator (e.g. Bird MK 7).

Patients should have no oral intake for 3 hr after the procedure to ensure return of laryngeal reflexes.

Absorption from the respiratory tract is rapid, and levels equivalent to intravenous injection may be achieved. Toxic levels of anaesthetic agent may be reached more readily if the mucosa is inflamed or traumatized. Chronic bronchitics may require higher doses for adequate analgesia, and particular care must be taken to avoid toxicity. When any type of spray is used, the accuracy of the dispensing apparatus must be considered. A local technique is contra-indicated in patients with a full stomach.

Cricothyroid puncture should not be performed in patients who have a bleeding disorder, local sepsis or tumour. Complications include breakage of the needle during transtracheal injection, subcutaneous emphysema and haematoma, penetration of the posterior wall of the trachea leading to mediastinitis or mediastinal emphysema and vocal cord damage. Inadvertent submucosal injection could produce airway obstruction (Gold & Buechel, 1939; Newton & Edwards, 1979; Prithvi-Raj, 1983; Morrison *et al.*, 1985).

Lignocaine 4% (max. 5 ml) or prilocaine 4% (max. 10 ml) are suitable. Lignocaine 10% aerosol spray may be used with caution.

TRACHEOSTOMY

Technique

Infiltration of skin and subcutaneous tissues at the site of the proposed incision followed by infiltration of deeper layers as necessary provides adequate anaesthesia. Transtracheal injection of 2–3 ml of lignocaine 4% is advisable to prevent excessive coughing on entering the trachea (Morrison *et al.*, 1985).

Eyes

General anaesthesia is now used more commonly than local anaesthesia, as it is safer for the less healthy patient and its effects on the eye are more clearly understood. However, as the eye is such a well-defined organ, it is easily amenable to blockade, and local techniques are still very suitable in many instances if full co-operation and immobility on the part of the patient can be attained. For intraocular surgery, there is less reduction in intraocular pressure than with a well-managed general anaesthetic. Premedication helps to produce a calm patient, and an antiemetic is a useful component.

CONJUNCTIVA AND CORNEA

Uses

Tonometry, removal of foreign bodies, syringing and probing of tearduct and as part of the technique for any eye surgery.

Anatomy

The sensory supply to the ocular conjunctiva and the conjunctiva of the upper eyelid arises from branches of the ophthalmic division of the trigeminal nerve. The conjunctiva of the lower eyelid is supplied by branches from its maxillary division.

The cornea is supplied with numerous nerves from branches of the ophthalmic nerve, particularly the long ciliary nerves.

Technique

One to two drops of solution are instilled into the open eye. Discomfort is allowed to settle (30–60 sec) and then a further instillation is made. This may be repeated until adequate anaesthesia is obtained.

If solution is syringed into the tearduct, probing can be performed.

A number of local anaesthetic agents are suitable including lignocaine 4%, prilocaine 4%, oxybuprocaine 0.2–0.4%, proxymetacaine 0.5% and amethocaine 0.5–1.0%. The latter stings less if used in solutions containing methyl cellulose, but such solutions increase the viscosity of the preparation and may penetrate the eyeball and should be avoided. Adrenaline may be added to any of these solutions to produce ischaemia although corneal damage can result from vasoconstriction.

Cocaine 2–4% is still used occasionally if prolonged and intense analgesia is required. It causes vasoconstriction which is useful, but the resultant corneal clouding limits its use. It should not be used in closed-angle glaucoma as it causes mydriasis (Allen & Elkington, 1980; Morrison *et al.*, 1985).

EYELIDS

Uses

For removal of superficial lesions e.g. retention cysts, papillomata, basal cell carcinomata, correction of ectropion or entropion and to enable retraction of the eyelids during intraocular surgery.

Anatomy

The upper eyelid is supplied medially by the *supratrochlear nerve* (a branch of the frontal nerve from V1), the infratrochlear, lacrimal and supraorbital nerves.

The lower eyelid is supplied by the *palpebral branches of the infraorbital nerve* (V2) and the *facial and zygomaticofacial nerves* (the latter being a branch of the facial nerve).

Technique

Both skin and conjunctival aspects of the eyelid must be injected if surgery involves the whole thickness of the lid because the tarsal plate in the eyelid limits spread of infiltrated solution. This can be accomplished in one manoeuvre. The needle is inserted at the lateral margin of the tarsal plate and subcutaneous infiltration is first performed with 2–3 ml of solution. The eyelid can then be everted over the needle which is then advanced and when its tip is seen under the conjunctiva, further infiltration can be made subconjunctivally.

Lignocaine or prilocaine 1–2% with adrenaline are suitable. Hyaluronidase aids spread and hastens the onset of anaesthesia (Eriksson, 1979; Allen & Elkington, 1980).

EYEBALL

Uses

Intraocular surgery requires anaesthesia of the eyeball in addition to that of the eyelids, cornea and conjunctiva. It is necessary also for enucleation and photoelectric coagulation of the retina.

Anatomy

The nerve supply is from the oculomotor nerve (III) via the *long and short posterior ciliary nerves* and the *ciliary ganglion* which lie within the muscle cone. Some of the short ciliary nerves pass into the ciliary ganglion which lies between the optic nerve (II) and the lateral rectus muscle. Others pass into the long ciliary nerves which lie close to the ganglion and in turn join the nasociliary nerve.

Technique

Blockade of these nerves abolishes pain and also paralyses the extraocular muscles, an absolute requirement for intraocular surgery as these muscles may cause movement or distortion of the globe and a consequent increase in intraocular pressure. These may all be blocked together by a single infiltration (retrobulbar block), following surface anaesthesia of cornea and conjunctiva.

Retrobulbar block is performed in one of two ways.
1 The patient looks upwards and inwards while a 4–5 cm needle is inserted through a skin weal at the outer inferior angle of the orbit (Fig. 61.9). Alternatively, the needle may be inserted directly through the conjunctiva with the lower eyelid retracted. The needle is advanced for about 3 cm upwards, backwards and medially towards the apex of the orbit. The needle tip should then lie within the cone formed by the extraocular muscles. After aspiration, 2 ml of solution are injected. This is the commonest method employed.
2 The patient looks downwards and the needle is passed through a weal in the centre of the tarsal plate of the upper eyelid and advanced 3 cm backwards and slightly inwards and downwards. Two ml solution are injected.

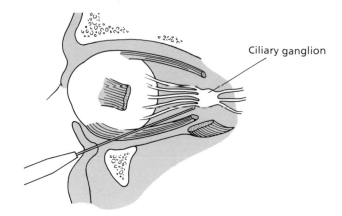

Fig. 61.9 Retrobulbar block. Site and direction of injection.

The block is effective after approximately 5 min. It causes also pupillary dilatation, exophthalmos and a modest decrease in intraocular pressure.

Two ml lignocaine 2% or prilocaine are used usually. Four ml may be used for enucleation. The addition of hyaluronidase 6–10 TRU per ml aids diffusion of solution.

The *orbicularis oculi muscle* must be paralysed for all intraocular surgery to prevent movement of the eyelids (blepharospasm). It is innervated by the terminal branches of the facial nerve and these must be blocked near the lateral canthus. A weal is raised at the inferolateral angle of the orbit and the needle inserted at right angles to the skin. Tissues are infiltrated down to bone. The needle is advanced subcutaneously along the lateral and inferior margins of the orbit and further infiltration made (van Lint's method). Alternatively, the facial nerve may be blocked over the condyle of the mandible (O'Brien's method) (Macintosh & Ostlere, 1967; Allen & Elkington, 1980; Morrison *et al.*, 1985).

Retrobulbar block may result in retrobulbar haematoma with resulting marked proptosis. Operation must be deferred until it resolves and this block should not be performed for emergency surgery. Other complications include perforation of the globe (Ramsay & Knobloch, 1978) and convulsions (Duncalf & Rhodes, 1963; Meyers *et al.*, 1978).

Abdomen

Uses

Infiltration of the abdominal wall and rectus sheath block may be used for procedures where profound muscle relaxation is not required and in which there is no great degree of visceral pain. It may be used for Caesarean section in exceptional circumstances (Ranney & Stanage, 1975), herniorrhaphy (inguinal and femoral), pyloric stenosis in babies and suprapubic cystotomy.

Anatomy (Williams & Warwick, 1980)

The superficial layers of the anterior abdominal wall (from exterior to interior) are:

1 Skin.
2 Superficial fascia from xiphisternum to a point midway between umbilicus and pubis.
3 Superficial (Scarpa's) fascia and deep (Camper's) fascia.
4 Four large flat sheets of muscle (external oblique, internal oblique, transversus abdominis and rectus abdominis) and pyramidalis (Fig. 61.10).

The *external oblique* is the most superficial, with fibres passing downwards and medially from their origins on the lower eight ribs to insert into the anterior superior iliac spine of the iliac crest and into its aponeurosis which ends medially in the linea alba from the xiphoid process to the pubic symphysis. It inserts inferiorly into the pubic symphysis and crest as far as the pubic tubercle. Between this point and the iliac crest insertion on the anterior superior iliac spine, it folds in on itself and forms the *inguinal ligament*.

The *internal oblique muscle* lies beneath the external oblique and arises from the lateral two-thirds of the inguinal ligament, from the iliac crest and from the thoracolumbar fascia between the 12th rib and the iliac crest. Its fibres pass upwards and medially. Superiorly, some fibres attach to the lower three to four ribs but most fibres end in an aponeurosis, the upper two-thirds of which splits at the lateral border of the rectus abdominis and encloses this muscle, reuniting in the midline to help form the linea alba. The anterior layer blends with the aponeurosis of the external oblique and the posterior layer with that of transversus abdominis. The whole lower one-third of the aponeurosis passes anterior to the recti to end in the linea alba. Fibres arising from the inguinal ligament join the aponeurosis of transversus abdominis and form the *conjoint tendon*.

The *transversus abdominis* lies beneath the internal oblique and arises from the lateral one-third of the inguinal ligament, the iliac crest, the thoracolumbar fascia and the lower six costal cartilages. The fibres pass transversely and medially to end in an aponeurosis whose upper two-thirds lie behind rectus abdominis,

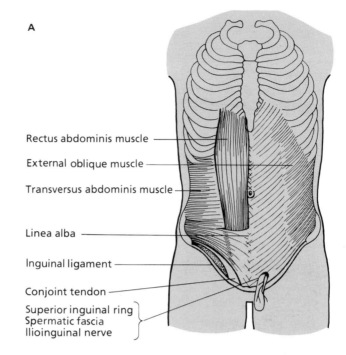

A

- Rectus abdominis muscle
- External oblique muscle
- Transversus abdominis muscle
- Linea alba
- Inguinal ligament
- Conjoint tendon
- Superior inguinal ring
  Spermatic fascia
  Ilioinguinal nerve

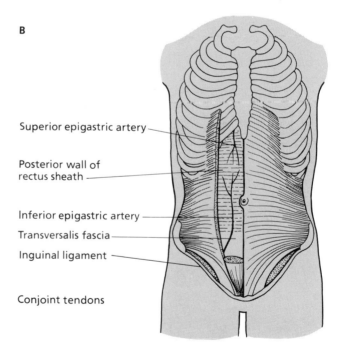

B

- Superior epigastric artery
- Posterior wall of rectus sheath
- Inferior epigastric artery
- Transversalis fascia
- Inguinal ligament
- Conjoint tendons

Fig. 61.10 Muscles of the anterior abdominal wall.
A The external oblique and transversus abdominis muscles.
B The internal oblique muscles.

whilst the lower third passes in front of it. It inserts medially into the linea alba with the lower fibres curving downwards and medially to form the *conjoint tendon* with the aponeurosis of the internal oblique. This tendon is inserted into the pubic crest.

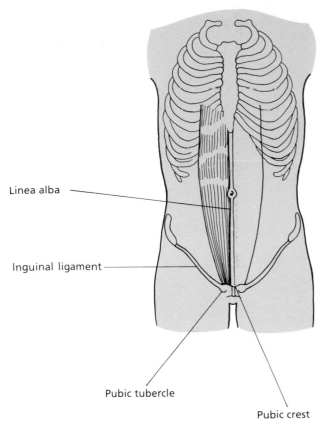

Linea alba

Inguinal ligament

Pubic tubercle

Pubic crest

Fig. 61.11 Rectus abdominis muscle showing tendinous intersections.

The two *recti abdomini* are separated by the linea alba and extend from their origins on the fifth, sixth and seventh costal cartilages to the pubis (Fig. 61.11). The muscle is enclosed in the rectus sheath which is formed by the split in the internal oblique aponeurosis which fuses anteriorly with the aponeurosis of the external oblique and posteriorly with that of transversus abdominis as far down as a point midway between umbilicus and symphysis pubis. Below this point, the three aponeuroses all pass anterior to the muscle which is separated from peritoneum by a thin connective tissue layer (transversalis fascia) and fat. Each rectus muscle is intersected within the rectus sheath by three tendinous intersections at the level of the xiphisternum, umbilicus and a point half-way between. They are attached usually to the anterior layer of the rectus sheath but do not pass normally right through the muscle to the posterior layer, and therefore when local anaesthetic is infiltrated, these intersections may limit spread anteriorly but not posteriorly.

The two small *pyramidalis muscles* lie in front of the lower part of the rectus muscles and within the sheath.

They arise from the pubis and insert into the linea alba at a point midway between pubis and umbilicus.

The nerve supply to the muscles of the abdominal wall is from T7–12 and L1. The terminal portions of the intercostal nerves 7–12 enter the abdominal wall between the diaphragm and transversus abdominis, and come to lie between the internal oblique and transversus abdominis. They enter the rectus sheath laterally and run within it posteriorly before piercing the recti to supply the overlying skin. L1 makes its contribution inferiorly through the iliohypogastric and ilioinguinal nerves.

Posteriorly, the rectus sheath is pierced by the superior and inferior epigastric vessels.

Techniques

Abdominal field block provides anaesthesia from skin down to peritoneum. The intercostal nerves (T7–12) are blocked as they enter the anterior abdominal wall just below the costal margin. Three weals are raised (Fig. 61.12).

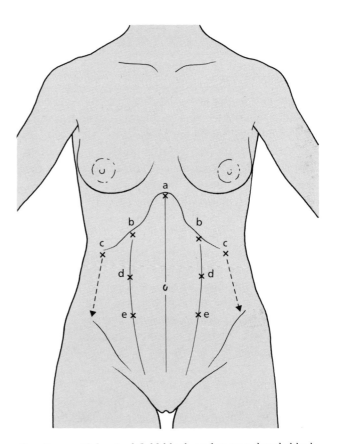

Fig. 61.12 Abdominal field block and rectus sheath block.

1 Below the xiphisternum.

2 Below the ninth costal cartilage on each side where the rectus muscle crosses it.

3 At the lower borders of the costal margins laterally.

Infiltration is made between these points through subcutaneous tissues and muscle layers to form a continuous line of infiltration along the lower costal margin, bearing in mind that the nerves lie in a plane between the internal oblique and transversus abdominis muscles. Further infiltration is made down the lateral side of the abdominal wall as far as the iliac crest.

Rectus sheath block. If this is also performed, a higher success rate is likely. Rectus sheath block performed alone does not produce relaxation of the other abdominal muscles (external and internal oblique and transversus abdominis). This is performed by raising three weals as for (1) and (2) above (Fig. 61.12), followed by:

4 At the lateral borders of the rectus muscles just above the umbilicus.

5 In the same lateral lines just below the umbilicus.

The needle is advanced at right angles to the skin, and when it is felt that the rectus sheath has been pierced anteriorly, it is advanced a further 0.5 cm, and 5 ml of solution are injected. The needle is then directed upwards and downwards and further solution deposited at each of the three sites. The aim is to deposit solution in the posterior part of the rectus sheath where the tendinous intersections are incomplete. If the costal margin has not been infiltrated, the skin weals are joined by subcutaneous infiltration.

One hundred to 200 ml of dilute solution e.g. lignocaine 0.25–0.5% or bupivacaine 0.25% can be used with care without reaching toxic levels because of the relative avascularity of the abdominal wall. Adrenaline 1/200 000 is a helpful addition.

Success depends largely on injections being made in the correct plane which may prove difficult, particularly in the obese patient. Relaxation of abdominal musculature may not be complete. Near toxic doses of agent may be used and the size of the patient should be considered. Pain from viscera is not obtunded unless a coeliac plexus block is performed also.

For Caesarean section, injections should be made parallel with the skin, as the abdominal wall is thin and there is danger of perforating the uterus. The deeper layers may be infiltrated by the surgeon as surgery advances. Traction on the uterus may still be painful and this technique is used best only to supplement light general anaesthesia e.g. where tracheal intubation has failed and spontaneous respiration is proceeding (Macintosh & Bryce-Smith, 1962; Bryce-Smith, 1976; Atkinson *et al.*, 1982; Scott, 1983).

PYLORIC STENOSIS IN BABIES (RAMMSTEDT'S OPERATION)

Technique

Correction of fluid and electrolyte imbalance must precede surgery and premedication is desirable e.g. morphine, 0.1–0.2 mg/kg i.m., or chloral hydrate, 30 mg/kg orally. Intravenous access is secured and the baby is bandaged to a cross-splint and maintained in a warm environment. Local infiltration of the abdominal wall is made subcutaneously between umbilicus and costal margin on the right followed by a right or bilateral rectus sheath block, depending on the incision to be used. A rectus sheath block alone may be adequate. The peritoneum may be infiltrated under direct vision by the surgeon.

Lignocaine 0.25–0.5% is suitable, and adrenaline 1/400 000 should be used to retard absorption. A volume of 13 ml of 0.25% solution may be used in a 3.5 kg baby (Black & Love, 1957; Leatherdale, 1958).

SUPRAPUBIC CYSTOTOMY

Technique

A bilateral rectus sheath block performed through weals raised at the lateral margin of the rectus from umbilicus to pubis may be adequate. In addition, the weals may be joined by subcutaneous and intradermal infiltration. A weal is raised also in the midline, 3 cm above the symphysis pubis, and a needle inserted through it in a backwards and downwards direction to enter the retropubic space, where 30 ml of solution are injected (Leatherdale & Ellis, 1958).

INGUINAL HERNIA

Anatomy (Williams & Warwick, 1980)

The sensory supply to the inguinal area is from three nerves, all derived from the lumbar plexus (Fig. 61.13):

1 The iliohypogastric nerve (L1).

2 The ilioinguinal nerve (L1).

3 The genitofemoral nerve (L1 and L2).

The first two arise from the lumbar plexus within psoas muscle, cross quadratus lumborum, pierce transversus abdominis and come to lie between it and the

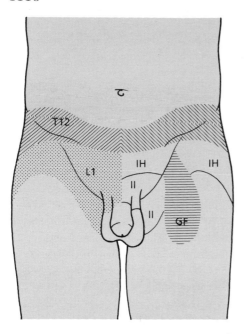

Fig. 61.13 Sensory supply to the inguinal region.

internal oblique near the iliac crest (Fig. 61.14). The iliohypogastric nerve pierces the internal oblique and supplies skin over the lowest part of the abdominal wall and pubis. The ilioinguinal nerve runs parallel to and 1 cm below the iliohypogastric (both now lying between the external and internal oblique muscles). It enters the inguinal canal posteriorly to accompany the spermatic cord or round ligament and becomes superficial after passing through the external ring to supply the skin of the scrotum or labia majora and adjacent thigh.

The genitofemoral nerve divides into a *genital branch* which follows the spermatic cord through the inguinal canal and supplies cremaster muscle plus the skin of the scrotum or labia majora and a *femoral branch* which supplies skin over the upper part of the femoral triangle.

Skin and muscles of the lower abdomen are supplied also by T11 and T12 which run medially from near the iliac crest between transversus abdominis and the internal oblique.

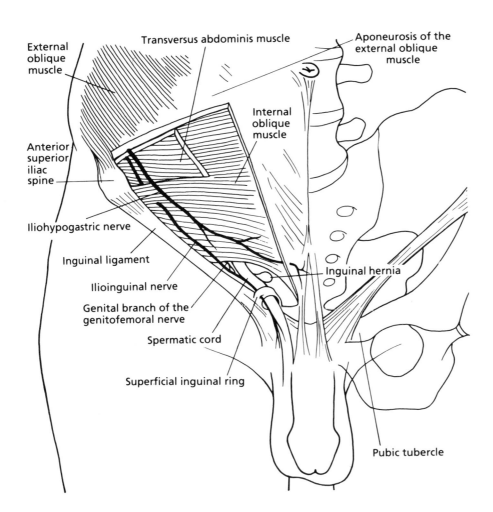

Fig. 61.14 Anatomy of the inguinal region.

The spermatic cord and testis receive also an autonomic supply.

Technique

Both skin and the hernial sac must be anaesthetized. The iliohypogastric and ilioinguinal nerves, T11 and T12 may all be blocked by infiltration in the region of the iliac crest. A weal (X, Fig. 61.15) is raised two fingers breadth medial to the anterior superior iliac spine and a needle inserted perpendicular to the skin until it strikes the medial wall of the iliac bone. Fifteen to 20 ml of solution are infiltrated into the muscle layers as the needle is withdrawn slowly. At the same site, a further 15–20 ml of solution should be injected in a caudal and mediocaudal direction under the aponeurosis of the external oblique (Fig. 61.15, injections a and b). This may be detected more easily if a short-bevelled needle is used, when a click may be felt.

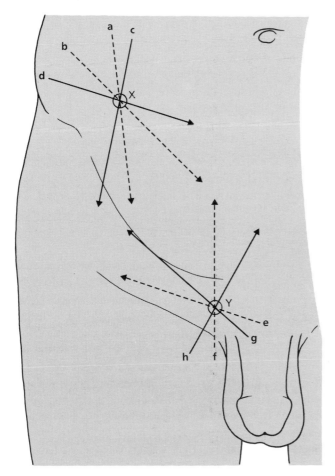

Fig. 61.15 Injections for inguinal herniorrhaphy. (See text for discussion.)

Subcutaneous injections can be made also from the same site in a lateral direction towards the inguinal fold and mediocaudally (c and d) towards the midline using a further 10–30 ml of solution.

Another weal (Y) is raised just proximal to the pubic tubercle, and infiltrations made extraperitoneally along the upper border of the pubic bone (e), then within the external oblique aponeurosis and in a more cranial direction (f). Subcutaneous injections are made at the same site in a fan from the inguinal ligament (g) to midline (h). The injections towards the midline should anaesthetize any overlapping nerve supply from the opposite side. Five ml of solution should be used for each injection.

To anaesthetize the contents of the sac, a percutaneous injection of 20 ml of solution may be made above the mid-point of the inguinal ligament after penetration of the aponeurosis of the external oblique in order to anaesthetize the contents of the inguinal canal. However, this is undertaken best by the surgeon, under direct vision, along the spermatic cord at the superficial inguinal ring or when the inguinal canal has been opened. In the latter case, the sac is opened, the hernia reduced and the neck of the hernia is injected medially and laterally from inside the sac in an outward direction. This renders further manipulation painless. If the hernia is irreducible, the sac may be injected from the outside. Infiltration along the line of incision may also be necessary. Success rate is low in the very obese with irreducible herniae.

Sixty to 90 ml of lignocaine or prilocaine 0.5% may be used. The addition of adrenaline helps to reduce plasma concentrations of local anaesthetic (Bryce-Smith, 1976; Eriksson, 1979)

FEMORAL HERNIORRHAPHY

Technique

As for inguinal herniorrhaphy with the addition of intradermal and subcutaneous infiltration around the lump. Alternatively, a femoral nerve block anaesthetizes the skin over the thigh.

URETHRA

Uses

Bouginage, catheterization, urethrocystography and possibly cystoscopy.

Anatomy

The nerve plexus supplying the urethral mucosa lies directly beneath it. Local anaesthetic placed in contact with the mucosa diffuses easily across it to render the urethra anaesthetic.

Technique

Male. Glans and foreskin are cleaned and the penis held in a dry swab. Either an aqueous solution of local anaesthetic or a gel may be used, although the latter is more favoured, as it lubricates the mucose and remains in contact with it for longer. The plastic nozzle of a tube of gel is inserted into the urethra and the contents of the tube squeezed gently into the urethra. After the first few ml, the patient should be asked to strain as if passing urine and the rest of the gel is inserted. This manoeuvre should allow gel to enter the prostatic urethra. A penile clamp should be applied just below the glans and left for 10–15 min. Ten to 15 ml of gel are used.

Female. An applicator (e.g. a throat swab) covered with cotton wool along 4 cm of its length is dipped in gel and inserted into the urethra and left *in situ* for 10 min with the patient lying on her back.

Rupture of the mucosa may occur, making it possible for injection to be made into the circulation if the patient has bulbocavernous reflux. Gels containing methylcellulose have caused serious systemic reactions. Instillations should therefore be made slowly under low pressure and agents of low toxicity used. Bleeding may occur.

Ten to 15 ml of lignocaine gel 1–2% or prilocaine gel 2% are used, or 30 ml of a solution containing cocaine 0.5% and sodium bicarbonate 0.5%.

Pyribenzamine 2% (an antihistamine) may give reasonable analgesia in patients in whom local anaesthetics are contra-indicated (Bryce-Smith, 1955; Dix & Tresidder, 1963).

PERINEUM

Uses

Episiotomy, repair of lacerations, outlet forceps (in combination with pudendal nerve block).

Anatomy

The sensory supply to the vulva is from the *genito-femoral and ilioinguinal nerves* anteriorly and from the *perineal branch of the posterior femoral cutaneous nerve* posteriorly. The perineum is supplied by branches of the *pudendal nerve* (S2, 3, 4).

Technique

For performing an episiotomy, infiltration is made between perineal skin and vaginal mucosa where the incision is to be made. For repair of an episiotomy or lacerations, infiltration should be performed parallel to both perineal skin and vaginal mucosa.

A spray may be applied to vulva and perineum as an adjunct to pudendal nerve block for normal or forceps delivery but this is not employed normally.

Lignocaine 0.5–1.0% for infiltration or a 10% spray should be used. Particular care is needed in calculating dosage in this highly vascular area.

ANUS

Uses

Field block of the anal region may be used for lateral sphincterotomy, excision of skin tags, thrombosed haemorrhoids and diagnostic procedures such as proctoscopy, sigmoidoscopy and colonoscopy in patients with painful anal lesions.

Anatomy

The perianal region is supplied by the inferior haemorrhoidal branches of the pudendal nerve (S2, 3 4).

Technique

To attain satisfactory analgesia, deep injections should be made at 3, 6, 9 and 12 o'clock around the anal margin and approximately 5 ml injected at each site. Subcutaneous circumferential injection is made prior to this through two initial weals on each side of the anus and 2.5 cm from it, using 20 ml of solution. A finger in the rectum should prevent inadvertent perforation of its mucous membrane. Compliance is understandably low even following premedication and intravenous sedation. Techniques have been devised to allow simultaneous injection at all four sites using a four-needle adaptor fitted to a syringe (Dodi, 1986).

Bupivacaine 0.5% with adrenaline 1/200 000 provides a longer period of analgesia than lignocaine or prilocaine.

Miscellaneous

FRACTURE HAEMATOMA BLOCK

Uses

Recent fractures, such as Colles', Pott's, metatarsal, metacarpal and femoral fractures. Although analgesia is usually imperfect, this technique may be useful in mass casualty situations.

Technique

A weal is raised over the fracture site and a needle introduced towards the fracture site until aspirated blood confirms that the tip lies in the associated haematoma. Slow injection of solution without vasoconstrictor is made. Volume depends on the fracture site e.g. 15–20 ml for a Colles' fracture, 20–30 ml for a femoral fracture. Hyaluronidase appears to be a useful addition. Ten min is allowed to elapse before reduction is attempted.

The block should not be performed in the presence of overlying sepsis. Toxicity may occur from rapid absorption of solution.

Lignocaine or prilocaine 1–2% with or without hyaluronidase (1000 unit/20 ml solution) are suitable.

INTACT SKIN

Penetration of intact skin by a local anaesthetic depends on the available concentration of its uncharged base form and a high water content. Pharmacologically, this has always proven difficult to achieve as the uncharged base is poorly soluble in water and combination of the active base with water is only possible in an oil-in-water emulsion. In such an emulsion, the maximum achievable concentration of local anaesthetic in a droplet is 20% and this is too low for effective analgesia. This problem has been overcome partly by the formulation of eutectic mixtures of local anaesthetics (EMLA). Lignocaine and prilocaine crystals, when mixed in equal amounts, melt to form an oil (eutectic mixture) at room temperature. When this oil is used in an emulsion, the droplet concentration of local anaesthetic base is raised to 80%, although the total anaesthetic concentration is only 5%. If such a mixture is allowed contact time with skin of 30–60 min, good analgesia can be obtained.

Uses

Painless venepuncture particularly in children and skin graft donor sites. EMLA cream may in future prove useful for other purposes.

Technique

EMLA cream (lignocaine 2.5% plus prilocaine 2.5% as a 5% oil-in-water emulsion cream) is applied 30–60 min prior to venepuncture over a suitable site and covered with an occlusive dressing. Transient skin blanching, erythema and oedema may occur and methaemoglobinaemia has been reported in an infant when a large area was covered, although toxic plasma levels were not reached (Hallen *et al.*, 1985; Scott, 1986).

References

Allen E.D. & Elkington A.R. (1980) Local anaesthesia and the eye. *British Journal of Anaesthesia* 53, 689–94.

Atkinson R.S., Rushman G.B. & Lee J.A (1982) Regional analgesia. In *A Synopsis of Anaesthesia* 9th edn. John Wright & Sons Ltd, Bristol.

Black G.W. & Love S.H.S. (1957) Anaesthesia for Rammstedt's operation. *Anaesthesia* 12, 430–4.

Boakes A.J., Laurence D.R., Lovel K.W., O'Neil R. & Verrill P.J. (1972) Adverse reactions to local anaesthetic/vasoconstrictor preparations. A study of the cardiovascular responses to Xylestesin and Hostacain-with-noradrenaline. *British Dental Journal* 133, 137–40.

Boakes A.J., Laurence D.R., Teoh P.C., Barar F.S.K., Benedikter L.T. & Prichard B.N.C. (1973) Interactions between sympathomimetic amines and antidepressant agents in man. *British Medical Journal* 1, 311–15.

Bodman R.I. & Boyes-Korkis F. (1960) Anaesthetizing the nose. *British Medical Journal* 2, 1956.

Boliston T.A. & Upton J.J.M. (1980) Infiltration with lignocaine and adrenaline in adult tonsillectomy. *Journal of Laryngology and Otology* 94, 1257–9.

British National Formulary (1987) No. 13. British Medical Association and The Pharmaceutical Society of Great Britain.

Bryce-Smith R. (1955) Topical analgesia for the urethra. *British Medical Journal* 1, 462.

Bryce-Smith R. (1976) In *Monographs in Anaesthesiology*, vol. 5. Practical Regional Analgesia (Eds Lee J.A. & Bryce-Smith R.). Excerpta Medica, Amsterdam.

Christoforidis A.J., Tomashefski J.F. & Mitchell R.I. (1971) Use of an ultrasonic nebulizer for the application of oropharyngeal, laryngeal and tracheobronchial anesthesia. *Chest* 59, 629–33.

Concepcion M. & Covino B.G. (1984) Rational use of local anaesthetics. *Drugs* 27, 256–70.

Cotton B.R., Henderson H.P., Achola K.J. & Smith G. (1986) Changes in plasma catecholamine concentration following infiltration with large volumes of local anaesthetic solution containing adrenaline. *British Journal of Anaesthesia* 58, 593–7.

Covino B.G. & Vassallo H.B. (1976) Clinical aspects of local anesthesia. In *Local Anesthetics. Mechanisms of Action and Clinical Use*. pp. 89–92. Grune and Stratton, New York.

Curtiss E.S. (1952) Postural nerve block for intranasal operations. *Lancet* 1, 989–91.

Dix V.W. & Tresidder G.C. (1963) Collapse after use of lignocaine jelly for urethral anaesthesia. *Lancet* 1, 890.

Dodi G. (1986) An improved technique of local anal anaesthesia. *Diseases of the Colon and Rectum* 29, 71.

Duncalf D. & Rhodes D.H. (1963) In *Anesthesia in Clinical Ophthalmology*. Wilkins & Wilkins, Baltimore.

Eriksson E. (1979) In *Illustrated Handbook in Local Anaesthesia* 2nd edn. Lloyd-Luke, London.

Gold M.I. & Buechel D.R. (1939) Translaryngeal anaesthesia: a review. *Anaesthesia* 20, 181.

Gotta A.W. & Sullivan C.A. (1981) Anaesthesia of the upper airway using topical anaesthetic and superior laryngeal nerve block. *British Journal of Anaesthesia* 53, 1055–7.

Haglund J. & Evers H. (1984) In *Local Anaesthesia in Dentistry*. Zohlbergs Tryckeri, Malmo.

Hallen B., Carlsson P. & Uppfeldt A. (1985) Clinical study of a lignocaine–prilocaine cream to relieve the pain of venepuncture. *British Journal of Anaesthesia* 57, 326–8.

Hassan H.G., Renck H., Lindberg B., Akerman B. & Hellquist R. (1985) Effects of adjuvants to local anaesthetics on their duration I. *Acta Anaesthesiologica Scandinavica* 29, 375–9.

Leatherdale R.A.L. (1958) Anaesthesia for Rammstedt's operation. *Lancet* 1, 932–5.

Leatherdale R.A.L. & Ellis H. (1958) Prostatectomy: anaesthetic technique and other factors affecting prognosis. *Lancet* ii, 1189–92.

Macintosh R.R. & Bryce-Smith R. (1962) *Local Analgesia: Abdominal Surgery* 2nd edn. Churchill Livingstone, Edinburgh.

Macintosh R.R. & Ostlere M. (1967) *Local Analgesia, Head and Neck* 2nd edn. Churchill Livingstone, Edinburgh.

Meyers E.F., Ramirez R.C. & Boniuk I. (1978) Grand mal seizures after retrobulbar block. *Archives of Ophthalmology* 96, 847.

Moffett A.J. (1947) Nasal analgesia by postural instillation. *Anaesthesia* 2, 31–4.

Moore D.C. (1978) In *Regional Block* 4th edn. Charles C. Thomas, Springfield, Illinois.

Morrison J.D., Mirakhur R.K. & Craig H.J.L. (1985) In *Anaesthesia for Eye, Ear, Nose and Throat Surgery* 2nd edn. Churchill Livingstone, Edinburgh.

Newton D.A.G. & Edwards G.F. (1979) Route of introduction and method of anesthesia for fiberoptic bronchoscopy. *Chest* 75, 650.

Oldham K.W. (1968) A simple technique for anaesthesia of the nose for intranasal surgery. *British Journal of Anaesthesia* 40, 979–83.

Pearce S.J. (1980) Fibreoptic bronchoscopy: is sedation necessary? *British Medical Journal* 281, 779–80.

Prithvi-Raj P. (1983) In *Practical Regional Anaesthesia* (Eds Henderson J.J. & Nimmo W.S.). Blackwell Scientific Publications, Oxford.

Ramsay R.C. & Knobloch W.H. (1978) Ocular perforation following retrobulbar anesthesia for retinal detachment surgery. *American Journal of Opthalmology*. 86, 61–4.

Ranney B. & Stanage W.F. (1975) Advantages of local anesthesia for Cesarean section. *Obstetrics and Gynecology* 45, 163–7.

Ritchie J.M. & Greene N.M. (1985) In *The Pharmacological Basis of Therapeutics* 7th edn. (Eds Goodman-Gilman A., Goodman L.S., Rall T.W. & Murad F.). Macmillan Publishing Co. Inc., New York.

Scott D.B. (1983) In *Practical Regional Anaesthesia* (Eds Henderson J.J. & Nimmo W.S.). Blackwell Scientific Publications, Oxford.

Scott D.B. (1986) Topical anaesthesia of intact skin. *British Journal of Parenteral Therapy* , 134–5.

Scott D.B. & Cousins M.J. (1980) In *Neural Blockade in Clinical Anesthesia and Management of Pain* (Eds Cousins M.J. & Bridenbaugh P.O.) pp. 91–2. J.B. Lippincott Co., Philadelphia.

Sluder G. (1913) Nerve trunk anesthesia and carbolisation in nasal surgery. *Laryngoscope* 23, 1078.

Vuckovic D.D., Rooney S.M., Goldiner P.L. & O'Sullivan D. (1980) Aerosol anesthesia of the airway using a small disposable nebulizer. *Anesthesia and Analgesia* 59, 803–4.

Williams D.G., Truelove S.C., Gear M.W.L., Massarella G.R. & Fitzgerald N.W. (1968) Gastroscopy with biopsy and cytological sampling under direct vision. *British Medical Journal* 1, 535–9.

Williams P.L. & Warwick R. (Eds) (1980) *Grays Anatomy* 36th edn. Churchill Livingstone, Edinburgh.

62

Thorax, Abdomen and Perineum

E. N. ARMITAGE

In clinical practice, local anaesthesia of the thorax, abdomen and perineum is obtained usually with a central block, such as a spinal, extradural or caudal, and the effects of almost all the blocks described in this chapter can in fact be obtained with these regimens. However, central blocks may be contra-indicated occasionally or difficult to perform, whereas a peripheral block may be appropriate and feasible technically. In such circumstances, the benefits of local anaesthesia to the patient need not be lost if the anaesthetist is capable of performing a suitable peripheral block.

Disadvantages of central blocks

A central block involves the introduction of a needle between two vertebral spines or laminae, through the ligaments connecting them, into the extradural or subarachnoid space. Anatomical abnormality of the bony spine and calcification or ossification of the intervertebral ligaments can make it difficult or impossible to insert the needle. Similar difficulty may be encountered in the grossly obese patient in whom bony landmarks may be impalpable and in whom spinal flexion, which opens up access to the extradural space, is limited. In such cases, a peripheral block may be easier.

Although it is possible to confine the effects of a central block to a limited area by careful attention to factors such as the site of needle insertion, the position of the patient and the dose of drug injected, such blocks usually act bilaterally and extend over a greater area than that required for the surgical procedure. Not only is this lack of specificity inelegant, but it is not appreciated by the patient if it causes widespread impairment of sensory and motor function, and particularly if it results in urinary retention.

Some degree of autonomic denervation usually accompanies spinal and extradural anaesthesia, and hypotension, produced by sympathetic block, is common. Although this is no longer considered an undesirable side-effect and may actually be an advantage in some cases, it is contra-indicated in patients in whom maintenance of cardiovascular stability is paramount. Severe hypotension is not tolerated well by the conscious patient in whom it causes faintness and nausea. In both these groups, therefore, a peripheral block may be preferable because extensive sympathetic denervation is avoided.

Skin sepsis at the site of needle insertion is considered rightly to be a contra-indication to a nerve block. The skin over the back of the elderly, bed-ridden patient is often unhealthy and if this is the case, central blocks should not be performed. However, it is in patients such as these that regional anaesthesia has so much to offer and a peripheral block may be an acceptable alternative.

Because all central blocks involve the insertion of a needle (and perhaps a catheter) into deep tissues which are surrounded largely by bone, any bleeding in these tissues cannot be controlled directly. This is of little clinical consequence in the presence of normal clotting mechanisms, but patients may already be receiving anticoagulant therapy when they undergo surgery, and some may require anticoagulants during the operation. Also, it is now common surgical practice to give low-dose subcutaneous heparin before the start of all but the smallest surgical procedures. Although there is evidence from two large series (Rao & El-Etr, 1981; Odoom & Sih, 1983) that central blocks may be performed safely in these three groups, the risk of an extradural haematoma, with its potentially serious neurological consequences, deters many anaesthetists.

Advantages of specific blocks

Peripheral blocks may be feasible when anatomical abnormalities or skin sepsis preclude a central block, but they have advantages in their own right also. They produce generally a comparatively localized area of anaesthesia which may match the surgical field more exactly. A haematoma produced during the performance of a peripheral block can be controlled almost always by direct pressure. Unwanted side-effects e.g. hypotension, motor blockade and disturbance of bladder function, are rare. Thus, patients can stand and walk immediately after surgery. This is an important consideration at a time when day-case surgery is increasing in popularity.

Disadvantages of specific blocks

Whereas central blocks achieve their effects with a single injection, most peripheral blocks require several, and their disadvantages stem mainly from this. Multiple injections may be unacceptable to the patient and, where they are required, the performance of the block and the development of complete anaesthesia may take some time. There is always the possibility that one of the injections may be ineffective, therefore peripheral blocks requiring multiple injections tend to be somewhat less reliable than central ones. In such cases, the anaesthetist may assess the overall anaesthesia as, say, 80% effective, but the patient is more likely to mark it down as a complete failure. Absorption of a local anaesthetic drug from more than one site e.g. after multiple intercostal blocks, results in comparatively high plasma concentrations, and systemic toxicity can be a problem.

Large peripheral nerves run with arteries and veins frequently, and attempts to block such a nerve may cause damage to one of the accompanying vessels and may result in a haematoma. Injection of local anaesthetic into one of these vessels is a possible hazard.

For a peripheral block to be successful, local anaesthetic must be deposited close to the nerve. The nerve may be located by probing with a needle until paraesthesiae are elicited, but this method requires a conscious, co-operative patient, and it can be very uncomfortable. It may also damage the nerve. A nerve stimulator can be used to avoid these disadvantages.

Paravertebral block

Although this block is used rarely in present-day anaesthesia, it is of some historical interest. In 1927,

Cleland set out to determine the nerve supply to the uterus. Six years later, after preliminary studies on animals, he was able to conclude that, in the human, the pain of labour from uterine contraction 'is transmitted by afferent fibers through the eleventh and twelfth thoracic roots' and that 'paravertebral block of the eleventh and twelfth thoracic roots will abolish the pain of uterine contraction. . .' (Cleland, 1933).

Anatomy

The paravertebral space is the space which a spinal nerve enters immediately after it has left the intervertebral foramen, and theoretically, therefore, there is a space corresponding to each foramen. However, in practice, only the thoracic and lumbar paravertebral spaces are sufficiently well defined and accessible to be of use to the anaesthetist. Spaces in the sacral region are of no clinical importance because it is impossible to gain access to them by the posterior approach, and those in the cervical region are more apparent than real because there are no ribs or costotransverse ligaments to bound the space posteriorly and no pleura anterolaterally. Nevertheless, deep cervical plexus block may be thought of as a cervical paravertebral block. The space, seen in transverse section (Fig. 62.1) is triangular with its apex pointing laterally. The base of the triangle is formed by the posterolateral surface of the vertebral body and the intervertebral foramen. The posterior side is made up of the superior costotransverse ligament which runs from the lower border of a transverse process to the upper border of the rib below. The anterolateral side of the triangle is formed by the pleura.

There is no direct communication between paravertebral spaces because, anterolaterally, the pleura is applied closely to the anterior surfaces of the ribs and, posteriorly, the inferior costotransverse ligament runs forward from the transverse process to its own rib and thus seals off the space above and below (Fig. 62.2). Medially, however, it is possible for injected solution to spread up and down in the loose areolar tissue lining the base of the triangle. A single injection of local anaesthetic can therefore produce anaesthesia of more than one segment.

Purcell-Jones et al. (1987) studied the behaviour of radio-opaque solution after paravertebral injection. Using image intensification and computerized tomography (CT) scanning, they found that the spread was unpredictable and in only 10% of cases did the solution remain confined to the paravertebral space. In most

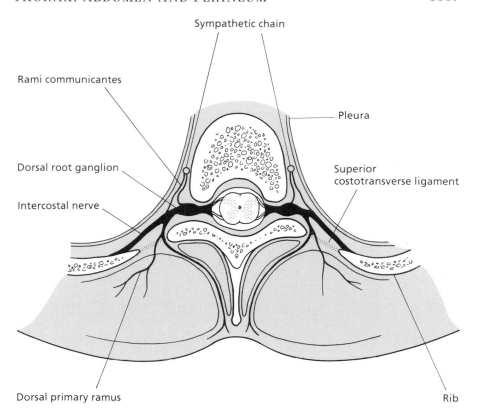

Fig. 62.1 Relations of paravertebral space. (Redrawn from Eason & Wyatt, 1979.)

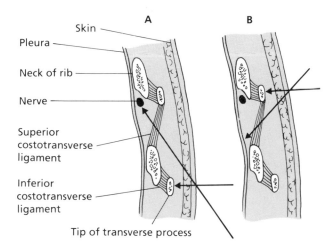

Fig. 62.2 Longitudinal section of paravertebral space.
A Direction of needle above transverse process or rib.
B Direction of needle below transverse process or rib.
(Redrawn from Eason & Wyatt, 1979.)

cases, the solution could be seen in the extradural space, sometimes extending bilaterally and spreading over as many as 12 segments. Pleural spread was also demonstrated occasionally.

The spinal nerve enters the paravertebral space through the intervertebral foramen and divides imme-diately into anterior and posterior primary rami. The posterior ramus runs posteriorly, winds round the medial edge of the superior costotransverse ligament and leaves the paravertebral space. The anterior ramus runs laterally and becomes one of the intercostal nerves. Both rami contain sensory and motor fibres. Rami communicantes are given off and run anteriorly to connect with the sympathetic chain which occupies the anterior angle of the space. Injection of local anaesthetic into the paravertebral space therefore affects sensory, motor and sympathetic fibres (Fig. 62.3).

Indications

Paravertebral block should be considered when unilat-eral anaesthesia of limited extent is required. Because of the medial communication between paravertebral spaces described above, it is possible to produce anaes-thesia of at least four segments with a single injection (Eason & Wyatt, 1979). Thus, the technique can provide analgesia for unilateral fractured ribs and for Kocher's subcostal incision for cholecystectomy. It can be used also in cases where access to the extradural space is impossible because of kyphoscoliosis or ossific-ation of the supraspinous and interspinous ligaments;

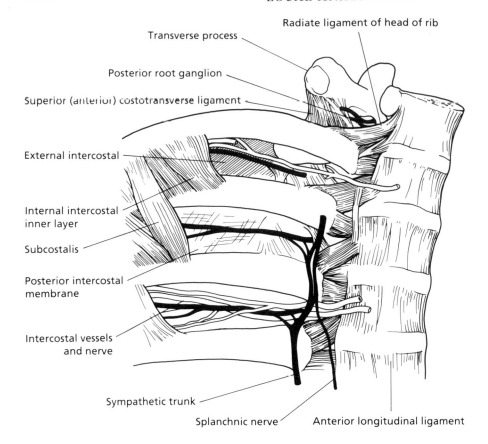

Radiate ligament of head of rib

Transverse process

Posterior root ganglion

Superior (anterior) costotransverse ligament

External intercostal

Internal intercostal inner layer

Subcostalis

Posterior intercostal membrane

Intercostal vessels and nerve

Sympathetic trunk

Splanchnic nerve   Anterior longitudinal ligament

Fig. 62.3 Vertebral end of an intercostal space and the costo-vertebral ligaments. (Redrawn from Williams & Warwick, 1980.)

and it has a limited application in certain chronic pain conditions where it is important to know the effect of a comparatively localized segmental block before a more radical neurolytic or surgical procedure is undertaken. However, in view of the unpredictable spread of injected solutions, a diagnostic block in such cases cannot be regarded as reliable and may actually be dangerously misleading (Purcell-Jones *et al.*, 1987).

Paravertebral block may be regarded as midway between extradural and intercostal block not only anatomically, but clinically, in that it usually produces localized, unilateral, segmental anaesthesia without the need for multiple injections.

Technique

The patient may be placed in either the sitting or lateral position. The author finds it easier to visualize the underlying anatomy when the patient is sitting, and patients themselves often find this position more comfortable. The transverse process must be located. It cannot be palpated, but in the upper and mid-thoracic regions, it lies level with the spine of the vertebra above. A skin weal of local anaesthetic is raised 3 cm lateral to

the appropriate vertebral spine. A 3.8 cm, 21 gauge needle is inserted through the weal at right angles to the skin and the deeper tissues are infiltrated until bone is encountered, usually at a depth of about 3 cm. It may occasionally be necessary to use a 5 cm needle in obese subjects.

The choice of needle for the block itself depends on whether or not a single shot or continuous block is required. For the former, a 9 or 10 cm, 18 or 20 gauge needle, with a stilette, is suitable. However, it may be preferable to insert a catheter at the outset, and for this a Tuohy extradural needle is suitable. The needle is introduced through the skin weal and advanced through the infiltrated tissues until the bone of the transverse process is felt. The depth at which it strikes bone is noted. It is then withdrawn slightly, re-angled cephalad and inserted again. This process is repeated until the needle clears the superior edge of the transverse process and lies in the costotransverse ligament. The stilette is then removed, a syringe of air or saline is attached to the needle, and the whole assembly is advanced until loss of resistance is felt to pressure on the plunger. This indicates that the needle tip has penetrated the costotransverse ligament and now lies in the paravertebral space. An aspiration test should be performed to exclude air in addition to blood and cerebrospinal fluid (CSF). If a catheter is to be passed, the depth of the space from the skin is noted with reference to the graduations on the Tuohy needle. Eason and Wyatt (1979) recommend that less than 1 cm of catheter should project into the space and an end-hole-only type is therefore required. These authors found that 15 ml of 0.375% bupivacaine anaesthetizes at least four segments.

Complications

Pleural tap and intravenous cannulation can occur, but dural tap has not been described when the above approach has been used, and hypotension is not a problem even in the presence of high blocks. This is presumably because sympathetic activity on the contralateral side remains unimpaired. However, it should be remembered that diffusion centrally into the extra-dural space is a theoretical possibility and if this were to occur, bilateral sympathetic block, and bilateral anaesthesia, would result.

Intercostal nerve block

Anatomy

An intercostal nerve is the lateral continuation of a thoracic anterior primary ramus. It is described classically as running inferior to its corresponding rib, in the subcostal groove, accompanied by the intercostal ar-

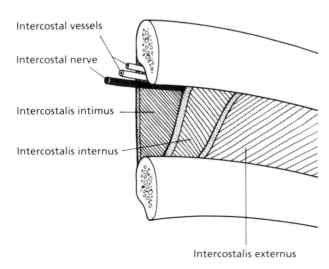

Fig. 62.4 Dissection of part of the thoracic wall showing the position of the intercostal vessels and nerve. (Redrawn from Williams & Warwick, 1980.)

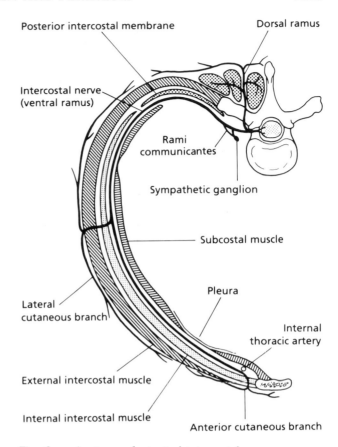

Fig. 62.5 Anatomy of a typical intercostal nerve. (Redrawn from Wildsmith & Armitage, 1987.)

tery and vein (Fig. 62.4). In the posterior part of its course, it is bounded laterally by the inferior notched aspect of the rib and the posterior intercostal membrane which lines the medial surface of the external intercostal muscle (Fig. 62.5). Anteriorly, the posterior intercostal membrane is replaced by the internal intercostal muscle. Medially, the intercostal nerve is bounded by the subcostal muscle in the posterior part of its course and by the intercostalis intima anteriorly. The pleura lies medial to both these muscles. Detailed examination of postmortem specimens has shown that there is considerable variation within this basic arrangement (Nunn & Slavin, 1980). For example, in some cases, the nerve was not a single structure, but consisted of three or four separate bundles, and although the posterior intercostal membrane was always defined clearly and impermeable to India ink injected in the cadaver, the intercostalis intima was found to consist of separate fasciculi between which India ink could pass medially to the subpleural space. It could then track up and down and re-enter adjacent intercostal spaces (Fig. 62.6).

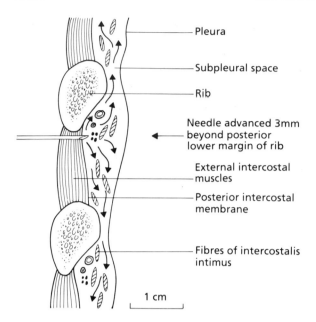

Fig. 62.6 The spread of India ink between pleura and internal surfaces of the ribs. (Redrawn from Nunn & Slavin, 1980.)

These anatomical studies showed also that at a point 7 cm from the posterior midline, the rib was relatively thick and the pleura lay, on average, 8 mm deep to its lower edge.

Each intercostal nerve has two main branches. The lateral cutaneous branch arises approximately at the mid-axillary line and divides into anterior and posterior branches which supply the skin over the scapula and back and the anterolateral part of the abdominal wall. The anterior cutaneous branch supplies the skin of the anterior abdominal wall. If all the components of an intercostal nerve are to be blocked, it is clear that local anaesthetic must be injected at a point posterior to the origin of the lateral cutaneous branch i.e. posterior to the mid-axillary line (Fig. 62.5).

Indications

Intercostal blocks can provide unilateral, segmental anaesthesia of the thorax and abdomen without sympathetic block. They are valuable in cases of fractured ribs for initial analgesia and before subsequent chest physiotherapy sessions. They are also suitable for a subcostal (Kocher's) surgical incision, and Nunn and Slavin (1980) found that blocks from T5 to T11 inclusive produced satisfactory analgesia for at least 5 hr after cholecystectomy. However, unilateral blocks

are inadequate for a paramedian incision because the area adjacent to the anterior midline receives its innervation from both sides.

Techniques

BOLUS INJECTIONS

The block may be performed with the patient in the prone, sitting or lateral position. The shoulders should be abducted and the arms moved forward to lift the scapula clear of the angles of the ribs. The posterior angles of the ribs are easily palpable in most subjects, but in the very obese it may be necessary to locate the rib near the posterior axillary line forward of the anterior border of latissimus dorsi.

A short-bevelled, 25 gauge needle is introduced at right angles to the skin and level with the lower half of the rib. When contact with the rib is made, a small amount of local anaesthetic may be injected to render the periosteum insensitive. The depth at which the needle meets bone is noted. The needle is then withdrawn into the subcutaneous tissues and the skin is moved downwards until the needle is judged to be level with the inferior border of the rib. The needle is advanced again and if bone is still encountered, this manoeuvre is repeated until the needle clears the lower border of the rib. The needle is then advanced, in a slightly cephalad direction, 3 mm deeper than its point of contact with the rib. This takes it through the external intercostal muscle and the posterior intercostal membrane, but should leave it well clear of the pleura. An aspiration test is carried out for air and blood before 3–5 ml of local anaesthetic are injected. During aspiration and injection, the patient should be asked to hold his or her breath. This minimizes damage to the pleura and lung if the needle has punctured them accidentally.

Choice of drug

For bolus dose intercostal blockade, a long-acting agent such as bupivacaine has advantages, but multiple injections can result in very high plasma bupivacaine concentrations, second only to those obtained after intravenous or tracheal administration (Braid & Scott, 1965). Furthermore, these concentrations are achieved very rapidly. Systemic toxicity is therefore a real possibility, and prilocaine is safer for poor risk cases and those in whom bilateral block is required.

Murphy (1983) introduced an extradural catheter through a Tuohy needle into the intercostal space of patients who had undergone cholecystectomy through a subcostal incision. He chose the T7–8 or T8–9 interspace, inserted the needle 3 mm under the rib, directed the bevel medially and passed the catheter 3–4 cm into the intercostal space. Twenty ml of bupivacaine 0.5% were injected. The mean duration of the initial dose was approximately 7 hr, but top-up injections did not last so long, and in one (and possibly two) cases in his series of 25, the catheter migrated from the intercostal space into the subcutaneous tissues.

CRYOANALGESIA

This is performed by the surgeon before the closure of a thoracotomy wound (Glynn *et al.*, 1980). It has the advantage that the intercostal nerves can be identified and exposed, and the cryoprobe can be applied directly to them. The technique is very effective, but it may be 3 months before sensation is restored fully (Palmer, personal communication).

Complications

There is a risk of *pneumothorax* each time an intercostal block is performed, and several blocks are required usually for surgical analgesia. It is a life-threatening complication and specific measures must be taken to avoid it and to minimize the effects if it occurs. Injections should be made at the posterior angle of the ribs where the intercostal space is at its widest, and the needle should not be advanced more than 3 mm deep to the inferior border of a rib. Stimulation of the pleura with a needle is said to provoke coughing, and the needle should be withdrawn if this occurs. The patient should be encouraged to breathe quietly while the needle is being inserted and, if possible, should hold his or her breath during the injection. Bilateral blocks should be avoided. It is unwise to perform intercostal blocks on outpatients even if a chest X-ray taken after the procedure is normal. Symptoms appear often several hours after the block and may be severe before any radiographic abnormality is apparent.

There are several reasons why *systemic toxicity* may occur after intercostal block. Local anaesthetic deposited in the intercostal space is in close contact with the neurovascular bundle and is therefore absorbed readily. However, any solution which tracks medially into the subpleural space is absorbed also very rapidly by the pleura itself. Therefore, a single intercostal injection results in both vascular and pleural absorption. Because multiple blocks are almost always required, high plasma concentrations of local anaesthetic are achieved rapidly. This is a situation which may predispose to the appearance of toxic symptoms, as the latter are determined not only by the absolute plasma concentration, but by the rate at which it has been reached (Scott, 1975).

Moore *et al.* (1976) measured plasma concentrations in patients having bilateral intercostal blocks from T6 to T12 inclusive. They injected 5 ml of bupivacaine 0.5% with adrenaline 1/320 000 into each of the 14 intercostal spaces so the patients received a total of 70 ml. Bupivacaine 350 mg was therefore used for the blocks, but a further 10 ml of solution were infiltrated into the skin and subcutaneous tissues, bringing the total to 400 mg. The mean peak arterial and venous plasma concentrations achieved were 3.29 μg/ml (range 1.72–4.0 μg/ml) and 2.52 μg/ml (range 1.4–3.45 μg/ml) respectively. These peaks occurred 10–20 min after injection. No systemic toxic reactions were observed. However, all the patients had received opioid premedication and they were given methohexitone 100–150 mg intravenously before and during performance of the blocks.

The systemic effects of adrenaline have to be considered also. Eighty ml of bupivacaine with adrenaline 1/320 000, the total amount used in Moore's cases, contains 0.25 mg of adrenaline, but the commercially prepared solution contains adrenaline 1/200 000. Therefore, 70 ml of bupivacaine with adrenaline (the amount actually needed for the intercostal blocks) contains 0.35 mg adrenaline.

Haemorrhage is a possible hazard when a needle is placed close to a neurovascular bundle. Intercostal vessels which lie snugly in the subcostal groove are protected to some extent, but dissections of the intercostal space show that there is considerable anatomical variation in the individual relationships and sizes of the vessels (Nunn & Slavin, 1980).

Dorsal nerve of penis (penile) block

Anatomy

The penis consists of the corpus spongiosum, which contains the urethra, and the right and left corpora cavernosa which lie dorsally. Each of the three corpora are enclosed by a tough, inelastic fibrous membrane,

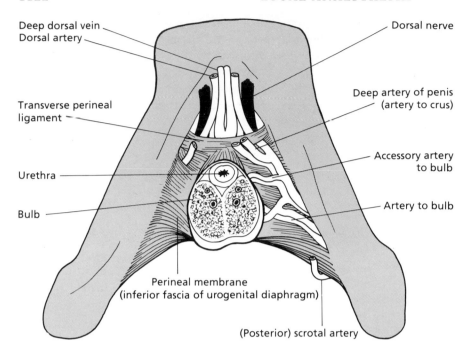

Deep dorsal vein
Dorsal artery

Transverse perineal
ligament

Urethra

Bulb

Dorsal nerve

Deep artery of penis
(artery to crus)

Accessory artery
to bulb

Artery to bulb

Perineal membrane
(inferior fascia of urogenital diaphragm)

(Posterior) scrotal artery

Fig. 62.7 To show the inverted V formed by the right and left pubic arches and the symphysis pubis, the perineal membrane and the emergence of the dorsal nerves inferior to the symphysis. (Redrawn from Boileau, 1951.)

the tunica albuginea, and all the corpora are surrounded by a looser layer of fibrous tissue—the fascia penis or Buck's fascia—which is penetrated easily by a needle.

The nerve supply to almost all the penis is derived from the second, third and fourth sacral roots (S2,3,4).

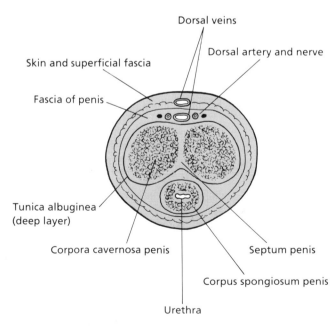

Dorsal veins

Dorsal artery and nerve

Skin and superficial fascia

Fascia of penis

Tunica albuginea
(deep layer)

Corpora cavernosa penis

Septum penis

Corpus spongiosum penis

Urethra

Fig. 62.8 Cross-section of the penis to show the position of the dorsal nerves. (Redrawn from Wildsmith & Armitage, 1987.)

Fibres travel first in the pudendal nerve and then in one of its terminal branches, the dorsal nerve of the penis. This nerve emerges from the pelvis by penetrating the perineal membrane just inferior to the symphysis pubis (Fig. 62.7). It then runs deep to the fascia penis, with the dorsal artery of the penis, along the dorsal surface of the corpus cavernosum which it supplies (Fig. 62.8). Its terminal branches pierce the fascia and supply the skin of the penis and the glans. The autonomic supply to the penis comes from the inferior hypogastric plexus. Fibres may reach the penis by travelling either with the somatic nerves or with the arteries.

Two important practical points must be considered when penile block is being planned. The penile urethra is supplied throughout its length by the perineal branch of the pudendal nerve. Block of the dorsal nerve does not therefore provide anaesthesia for catheterization. The block is also inappropriate for operations on the base of the penis and the scrotum since these areas are supplied by the genital branch of the genitofemoral nerve.

Indications

Penile block is suitable for operations on the shaft of the penis, the glans and the foreskin. It provides very localized anaesthesia for circumcision, dorsal slit and chordae correction in cases where more extensive blocks, such as a caudal or lumbar extradural are inappropriate.

Technique

The nerve may be blocked at the root of the penis where it emerges through the perineal membrane. The symphysis pubis is palpated, a skin weal of local anaesthetic is raised over it and a 4 or 5 cm, 23 gauge needle is introduced until the symphysis is felt by the needle tip. A small amount of local anaesthetic solution may be injected at this point. The needle is then withdrawn into the subcutaneous tissues and the palpating finger moves the skin and needle inferiorly so that when the needle is advanced again, it clears the lower border of the symphysis. After careful aspiration, bupivacaine 0.5% is injected. This process of aspiration and injection is repeated as the needle is advanced down to the dorsal surface of the corpora cavernosa. A total of 10 ml of *plain* solution should be injected. It is essential that adrenaline is *not* used.

Although this approach almost certainly results in a satisfactory block, additional local anaesthetic can be deposited more distally, deep to the fascia penis. The needle is again withdrawn to the subcutaneous tissues, angled distally and advanced until it is felt to have pierced the fascia. Up to 5 ml of solution are injected if no blood appears on aspiration. Finally, the needle is once more withdrawn through the fascia—this sensation is often easier to appreciate than the initial insertion—and a ring of local anaesthetic is infiltrated circumferentially in the subcutaneous layer. This ensures that fibres running superficial to the fascia penis are anaesthetized also.

Therefore, it is possible to block the dorsal nerves at three sites—below the symphysis, and deep and superficial to the fascia penis—with a needle inserted through a single skin weal. A total of 20 ml of solution are required.

Essentially, the same technique may be used in children. Yeoman *et al.* (1983) located the symphysis pubis and then redirected the needle 2 mm inferior to it. They injected bupivacaine 0.5% in a dose of 1 ml for boys up to the age of 3 yr and 0.3 ml/yr of age thereafter. They had one failure in 19 cases. White *et al.* (1983) used the more distal approach and gave bupivacaine 0.5% in a dose of 0.2 ml/kg body weight. They injected two-thirds of this deep to the fascia penis and the remaining one-third circumferentially in the subcutaneous layers.

Complications

The penis is a highly vascular organ and the most common complication of penile block is *haematoma*.

This may result from damage to the corpora cavernosa; White *et al.* (1983) reported two small haematomas in their series of 27 paediatric cases. It may result also from puncture of the dorsal vein of the penis when a needle is introduced in the midline. Although bleeding from this vein is not serious and can be controlled easily with pressure, it is superficial and therefore the bruising is obvious to the patient. Identification and avoidance of the dorsal vein before insertion of the needle eliminates the problem.

Arterial blood enters the penis through vessels which lie close to the dorsal nerves and run distally with them. These vessels are in effect end-arteries and any vasoconstrictor in the local anaesthetic solution may cause ischaemia and necrosis of tissue distal to the site of injection, with disastrous results. It cannot be emphasized too strongly that only plain solutions of local anaesthetic must be used for penile block.

Coeliac plexus block

Anatomy

The coeliac plexus lies at the level of the junction of the 12th thoracic and the first lumbar vertebrae. It is composed, in part, of two main ganglia which are interconnected and which lie anterior to the crura of the diaphragm and to the aorta at the origin of the coeliac artery, and anterolateral to the vertebral bodies (Fig. 62.9). Preganglionic sympathetic fibres carried in the greater (T5–10), lesser (T10–11) and least (T12) splanchnic nerves relay in the coeliac ganglia, which receive also parasympathetic fibres from the coeliac branch of the right vagus nerve. Postganglionic fibres form a network anterior to the aorta and the whole complex of nerve tissue at this site forms the coeliac plexus (Fig. 62.10). The plexus lies posterior to the stomach, the pancreas and the left renal vein.

Indications

It is occasionally necessary to perform upper abdominal surgery on a patient in whom general anaesthesia is contra-indicated. In such a case, extradural anaesthesia provides somatic, motor and sympathetic block, but it leaves the parasympathetic supply to the abdomen unaffected. Coeliac plexus block is therefore required if all sensation is to be abolished. Under these circumstances, the block is performed usually by the surgeon as soon as the abdomen is opened.

It is used more commonly in the treatment of painful conditions, such as malignant disease of the

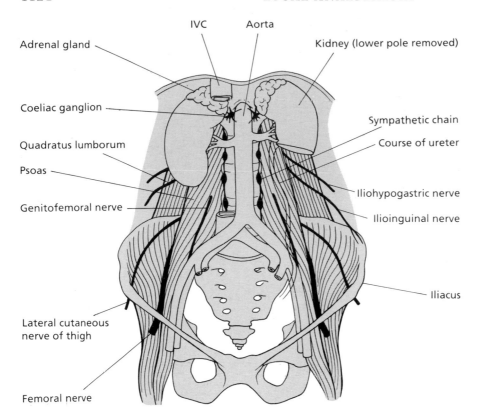

Fig. 62.9 Posterior abdominal wall to show the position and relations of the coeliac plexus. IVC = inferior vena cava. (Redrawn from Wildsmith & Armitage, 1987.)

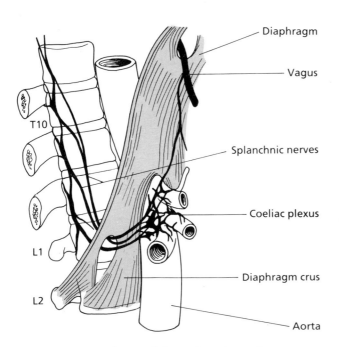

Fig. 62.10 Lateral view of the coeliac plexus showing its relations to the vertebral bodies, diaphragm and vagus. (Redrawn from Wildsmith & Armitage, 1987.)

upper abdomen and chronic pancreatitis. Local anaesthetic can be injected initially to see if the benefits are sufficient to justify the later ablation of the plexus with alcohol.

Technique

The coeliac plexus is related to important blood vessels and viscera, so needles and solutions (particularly neurolytic ones) must be placed accurately. Because the plexus is also deeply situated, accuracy can be guaranteed only if the block is performed under X-ray control. A C-arm image intensifier enables the position of the needles to be checked in both posteroanterior and lateral planes.

The patient is placed prone on the X-ray table with a pillow under the chest. The iliac crests are marked. A line joining them crosses the spine of the fourth lumbar vertebra or the interspace below it. From this landmark, the 12th thoracic spine and the 12th ribs are identified and marked (Fig. 62.11).

Skin weals of local anaesthetic are raised approximately 7–12 cm from the midline just inferior to the

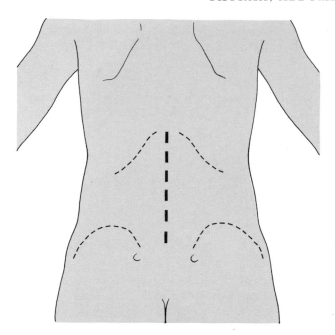

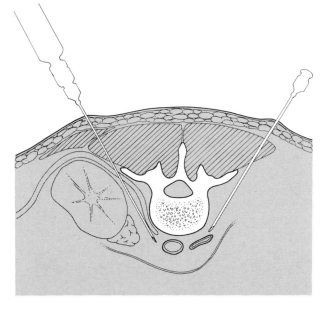

Fig. 62.11 Landmarks and needle alignment for coeliac plexus block. (Redrawn from Wildsmith & Armitage, 1987.)

Fig. 62.12 Correct position of needles for coeliac plexus block. (Redrawn from Cousins & Bridenbaugh, 1987.)

12th rib on each side, the greater distance being chosen for the larger patients. A 15 cm, 20 gauge needle with stilette is introduced through each skin weal and advanced under the 12th rib, anteriorly, medially and cephalad, until it strikes the body of the 12th thoracic vertebra. Where the needle strikes bone and at any point where it causes localized discomfort, local anaesthetic solution should be infiltrated. If paraesthesiae are elicited, indicating that a somatic nerve is being stimulated, the needle should be withdrawn and re-inserted at a slightly different angle. When the needle tip contacts the vertebral body, the hub of the needle is held between the thumbs and middle fingers, and the index fingers mark a point along the needle shaft 2–3 cm from the skin. The needle is then withdrawn partially and inserted in the same medial and cephalad directions, but more anteriorly. If bone is encountered again, the position of the index fingers is adjusted so that they are once more 2–3 cm from the skin, and the needle is inserted still more anteriorly. This manoeuvre is repeated until the needle clears the anterolateral border of the vertebral body. The position of the needle must now be checked radiographically and adjusted so that, in the lateral view, it lies approximately 2 cm anterior to the body and, in the anteroposterior view, approximately one-third of the way across it (Fig. 62.12). When the position of both needles is satis-

factory radiographically, aspiration tests should be performed and the position adjusted if blood is obtained.

Correct placement of the needles is confirmed if injected radio-opaque dye spreads up and down in a narrow strip in front of the vertebral body. Any resistance to injection indicates that the needle tips lies in the wall of a major blood vessel, a viscus or a muscle, from which it must be withdrawn before the injection is continued.

Injection in the region of the coeliac plexus causes severe burning abdominal pain. This is usually transient when local anaesthetic is used, but it may be necessary to induce general anaesthesia before injection of a neurolytic agent. For a diagnostic block, 25 ml of lignocaine 1% or bupivacaine 0.25% are injected on each side. For neurolysis, 25 ml of 50% alcohol are required on each side and the needles should be cleared of alcohol by the injection of 1 ml of air before they are withdrawn. This prevents necrosis of tissues lying in the track of the needle.

Complications

These may be classified as *technical* and *physiological*.

Technical complications include damage to somatic nerves and dural tap produced by penetration of the intervertebral foramen if initial insertion of the needle is too posterior; haematoma from trauma to the closely related great vessels, and, as a late complication, aortoduodenal fistula resulting from necrosis of the intervening tissue.

The commonest physiological complication is hypotension. This is often first noticed a few min after injection, but it can occur also when the patient stands up for the first time after the block, and he or she must be forbidden to attempt this unless supervised. Ablation of the coeliac plexus results in impotence, and the patient must be informed of this when neurolysis is being considered.

Lumbar sympathetic block

Anatomy

The sympathetic supply to the lower limb comes from the second, third and fourth lumbar sympathetic ganglia. These ganglia receive preganglionic sympathetic fibres from the lower thoracic sympathetic chain, and preganglionic somatic fibres from the first and second lumbar nerves. Postganglionic sympathetic fibres emerge from the ganglia, run initially with the spinal nerves, continue with the femoral, saphenous and obturator nerves and supply the closely related arteries and their branches. They are vasoconstrictor to the arterioles and pilomotor and sudomotor to the skin within the distribution of the nerves. It is obvious therefore that block of the lumbar sympathetic ganglia causes absence of sweating, warm dry skin, and vasodilatation in the lower limb. Other postganglionic sympathetic fibres leave the ganglia, but they have no relation with any somatic nerves and run as the hypogastric nerves to enter the hypogastric plexus.

The above anatomical arrangement varies considerably. Accessory ganglia occur sometimes at the level of the first and second lumbar vertebrae, embedded in the body of the psoas muscle, and their presence may result in a block being incomplete in the L1–2 distribution.

The ganglia lie anterolateral to their vertebral bodies and on the medial border of psoas muscle. They are placed less anteriorly than the coeliac plexus. The genitofemoral nerve runs down the surface of psoas and is therefore a lateral relation, with the kidney and ureter more lateral still. On the left side, the aorta lies anteriorly and on the right side, the inferior vena cava (IVC) (Fig. 62.13).

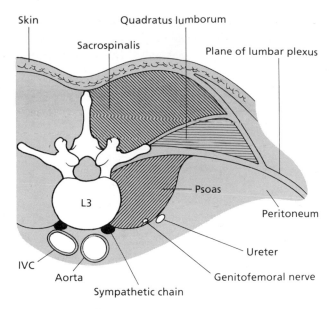

Fig. 62.13 Transverse section through L3 to show the position and relations of the lumbar sympathetic chain. (Redrawn from Wildsmith & Armitage, 1987.)

Indications

Chemical lumbar sympathectomy has been advocated for the diagnosis and treatment of a very wide range of symptoms and pathologies, and it has been used empirically often. Its popularity has declined as the measurement of arterial blood flow, the diagnosis of arterial occlusion and the surgical management of arteriopathy have improved. It is now used mainly to alleviate the rest pain of chronic, peripheral, obliterative vascular disease, such as atherosclerosis and thromboangiitis obliterans in patients who are unsuitable for surgery (Reid et al., 1970) and it may improve vasospastic conditions, such as Raynaud's disease, post-traumatic vasospasm, embolism and cold injury.

It is useful also for delineating potentially viable, proximal tissue, capable of responding to the effects of sympathetic denervation, from unsalvageable distal tissue. Therefore, it can help to determine the most suitable site for amputation. Lumbar sympathetic block is performed sometimes to increase the blood supply to the skin flaps after amputation, and to assist the healing of gangrenous areas of skin, 65% of which show some improvement (Lofstrom & Zetterquist, 1969).

The benefits obtained after lumbar sympathetic block depend not only on the increase in total arterial flow to the lower limb, but also on the effects of any redistribution of flow. In the resting limb, most of the increase is to the skin, and this accounts for the finding that over 70% of patients treated for rest pain obtain benefit for at least 6 months (Lofstrom & Zetterquist, 1969), although the muscle blood flow under these conditions may actually decrease (Cousins & Wright, 1971). However, because claudication is improved in up to 20% of patients, some increase in muscle blood flow may apparently occur.

LOCAL ANAESTHETIC BLOCK

Local anaesthetic should be used when some indication is sought on whether or not a more permanent sympathectomy, neurolytic or surgical, is likely to be effective. It can be used also for the treatment of conditions such as phantom limb pain for which a permanent block would be too radical. The block may have to be repeated several times in such cases.

NEUROLYTIC BLOCK

Destruction of the sympathetic ganglia with phenol should result theoretically in permanent sympathectomy and relief of symptoms. In practice, some return of sympathetic activity occurs commonly and, because the course of the underlying condition is likely to be one of steady deterioration, symptoms may reappear after a few months. However, neurolytic blocks may be repeated with success and arteriopathic patients can be given long-term relief often before amputation becomes inevitable.

Technique

The procedure is carried out with X-ray monitoring and the patient may be placed prone or in the lateral position. The former facilitates the palpation and drawing of landmarks; the latter is more comfortable for the anaesthetist. The iliac crests are marked. The line joining them crosses the fourth lumbar spine or the interspace below it and from this landmark, the spines of the second, third and fourth vertebrae are identified and marked. A line is drawn, parallel to the vertebral column, 7–11 cm from the midline on the side to be blocked (Fig. 62.14). Three skin weals of local anaesthetic are raised along this line opposite the second, third and fourth vertebral spines and, at each level, the deeper tissues are infiltrated through a longer needle directed medially towards the vertebral body. A 15 cm, 20 gauge needle with stilette is inserted through each skin weal and advanced medially and slightly cephalad

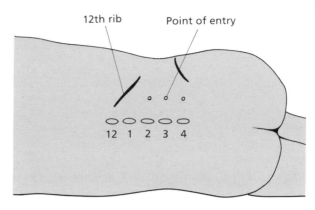

Fig. 62.14 Landmarks and angle of needle insertion for lumbar sympathectomy.

until bony contact is felt. This should be the vertebral body, but may be the transverse process if contact is made within the first few cm. Withdrawal of the needle and insertion with a greater cephalad angle should take the needle clear of the transverse process. When the vertebral body has been located, a small amount of local anaesthetic may be injected as the contact is often painful and more than one probing may be necessary. The hub of the needle is held between the thumbs and middle fingers while the index fingers mark the shaft approximately 2 cm from the skin. The needle is withdrawn into the superficial tissues and is re-inserted more anteriorly. If it strikes the vertebral body again, the position of the index fingers is adjusted so that they are once more 2 cm from the skin, and the manoeuvre is repeated until the needle tip clears the anterolateral border of the body. The needle is advanced a further 2 cm until the index fingers are flush with the skin. The position of the needle must now be checked radiographically and adjusted until, in the anteroposterior plane, the tip lies one-quarter of the way across the transverse diameter of the vertebral body and, in the lateral plane, level with its anterior border (Fig. 62.15). An aspiration test should be negative and there should be minimal resistance to injection of a small quantity of saline.

Although the author prefers to insert needles at the second, third and fourth vertebral level, some anaesthetists take advantage of the fact that solution injected in the correct plane spreads up and down freely, and they therefore insert only one needle, at L3.

If local anaesthetic is to be used, bupivacaine 0.5% or lignocaine 1% is injected in a total volume of 15–20 ml. Before a neurolytic block, there must be radiographic evidence that the solution is confined to

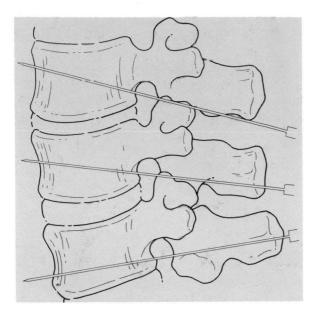

Fig. 62.15 Correct needle position for lumbar sympathectomy. (Redrawn from Wildsmith & Armitage, 1987.)

the correct plane, so the radio-opaque dye Conray 280 is injected slowly while the patient is screened in the lateral plane. The dye should spread as a thin line up and down from the injection site. Posterior spread may result in damage to somatic nerve roots. Anterior spread indicates that the needle tip has entered the peritoneum and if a full neurolytic dose is deposited there, an aortoduodenal fistula may develop eventually. Spread down the surface of psoas is also unsatisfactory as the genitofemoral nerve may be affected, causing numbness or paraesthesiae over the front of the upper thigh. In such cases, the dye tracks downwards, but in the lateral view, it tends to run somewhat anteriorly as it does so, whilst in the anteroposterior view, lateral spread may be seen. Phenol 7.5% in Conray 280 is injected slowly in a total volume of 10–15 ml and its spread is monitored radiographically. The injection must be stopped if the patient complains of pain, and the position of the needle should then be adjusted. At the end of the procedure, the lumen should be cleared by the injection of a small amount of air, so that when the needle is withdrawn, phenol is not deposited along its track.

Complications

If the initial angle of insertion of the needle is too medial, the tip may enter an intervertebral foramen and puncture the dura. This is not an indication for abandoning the block, but it does show that the needle needs to be directed much more anteriorly. Damage to blood vessels and aspiration of blood is common. The aorta on the left side, the inferior vena cava on the right and the lumbar vessels on both sides may be punctured. Some bleeding presumably occurs after such damage, so it is essential that the block is not performed on patients with abnormal clotting mechanisms. Significant intravascular injection should be avoided if a careful aspiration test is negative, but it is seen occasionally on screening.

Spinal nerves may be traumatized during insertion of the needle. If paraesthesiae are elicited, the needle should be withdrawn and re-angled. The patient should be asked to describe, but not to touch, the area affected, as this gives some indication of the spinal level involved. Phenol may also cause damage to somatic nerves (such as the genitofemoral nerve mentioned above), to the ureter if the needle has been placed too laterally, and to the psoas muscle, although pain on injection gives warning of this.

Caudal (sacral extradural) block

Anatomy

Viewed in the anteroposterior plane, the sacrum is an equilateral triangle with its apex pointing inferiorly. Most of its posterior aspect is bony and is formed by the fusion of the spines, laminae and articular processes of the upper four sacral vertebrae. No posterior fusion takes place at the fifth vertebra at which level the articular processes are represented by rounded horns, the sacral cornua. The bony defect, or sacral hiatus, between the cornua and laminae on each side and the vestigial fourth vertebral spine above, is covered by the sacrococcygeal ligament. The lower part of the sacrococcygeal ligament runs from the base of the sacrum to the coccyx. The upper part can be thought of as an isosceles triangle with its apex pointing superiorly, the basal angles being formed by the sacral cornua, and the apex by midline bony fusion at the fourth sacral level (Fig. 62.16).

The extradural space runs from the foramen magnum to the base of the sacrum where it is sealed off by the sacrococcygeal ligament. In most adults, the dural sac ends at the inferior border of the second sacral vertebra, and the spinal cord at the inferior border of the first lumbar vertebra (Fig. 62.17), but in the newborn, the cord and dura extend lower. At all ages, there is much variation and both the cord and dura

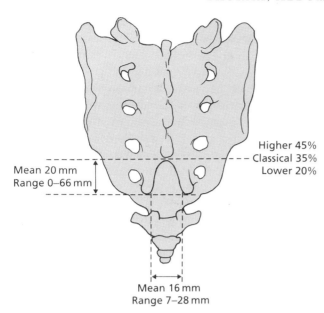

Higher 45%
Classical 35%
Lower 20%

Mean 20 mm
Range 0–66 mm

Mean 16 mm
Range 7–28 mm

Fig. 62.16 Posterior aspect of sacrum showing cornua and triangular shape of sacral hiatus. (Redrawn from Wildsmith & Armitage, 1987.)

may be found higher or lower than these points (Lanier *et al.*, 1944). Indeed, all aspects of sacral anatomy may vary, including the level and degree of bony fusion and the prominence and symmetry of the cornua (Trotter & Lanier, 1945; Trotter, 1947).

Because the cord is shorter than the bony spine, the lower lumbar and sacral spinal roots have to run inferiorly in the extradural space, forming the cauda equina, before emerging from their intervertebral foramina at the appropriate level.

Indications

Caudal block is suitable for surgery of the perineum, either as the sole regimen in patients in whom general anaesthesia is contra-indicated or, more usually, in combination with light general anaesthesia. Operations such as haemorrhoidectomy, anal dilatation and circumcision are notoriously stimulating, and, when performed under general anaesthesia alone, can induce laryngospasm and marked cardiovascular responses. Caudal block performed before surgery eliminates these problems and allows general anaesthesia to be maintained at a relatively light plane. Extension of analgesia into the postoperative period is an additional benefit.

Some relaxation of the anal sphincter is usual after a caudal. This may not always be desirable surgically and the surgeon should be consulted in doubtful cases.

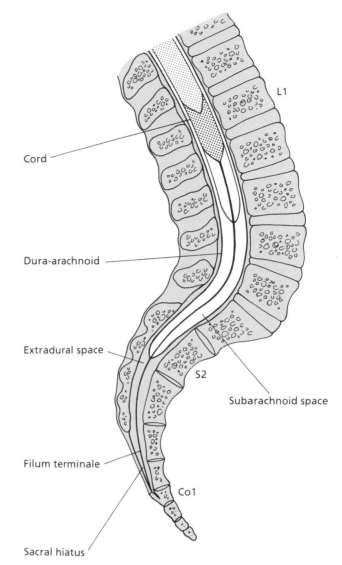

Cord

Dura-arachnoid

Extradural space

Filum terminale

L1

S2

Subarachnoid space

Co1

Sacral hiatus

Fig. 62.17 Sagittal section of lumbar and sacral regions of the spine. (Redrawn from Wildsmith & Armitage, 1987.)

The caudal has a special place in paediatric anaesthesia. This is principally because a child's extradural fat is less dense than an adult's. Injected solution can therefore spread more easily and blocks extending to the umbilicus and higher can be obtained. As a result, inguinal herniotomy, orchidopexy and surgery of the lower limb come within the scope of a paediatric caudal.

Although caudal block has a historical place in obstetric analgesia (Edwards & Hingson, 1942), it has been superseded largely by the lumbar extradural approach, but it is still useful occasionally as a single injection technique in the second stage of labour.

Technique

The key to successful caudal block is the accurate identification of the sacral cornua. The patient may be placed prone or in the lateral position. Landmarks are easier to feel when the patient is prone because the buttocks tend to fall away from the midline, but the lateral position is more suitable for maintenance of general anaesthesia and the author prefers it. When the triangular outline of the sacrum is visible, the approximate position of the sacral cornua can be estimated. The cornua are not midline structures, and palpation should therefore be from side to side. In the obese, considerable pressure may be required for which the thumb is better than the index finger. The sacral cornua were described classically as lying under the proximal interphalangeal joint of the anaesthetist's index finger when its tip was palpating the end of the coccyx, but the anatomy in this region is so variable that this method is unreliable and frequently gives too low a position for the sacral hiatus.

When the cornua have been located, the thumb is drawn cephalad until bone is felt in the midline. This is the apex of the triangle formed by the superior part of the sacrococcygeal ligament. A 19 gauge disposable needle is inserted, immediately caudad to the thumb, at a cephalad angle of approximately 45°. Resistance is felt after a few millimeters as the needle engages in the ligament, followed by sudden loss of resistance as it penetrates it and enters the sacral extradural space. The angle of insertion is now changed so that it is parallel with the long axis of the sacrum, and the needle is advanced to the hub. An aspiration test should be performed. If the bevel of the needle lies against the intima of a blood vessel, blood does not necessarily appear. One ml of saline should therefore be injected before aspiration. A caudal need not be abandoned if blood is seen on aspiration, but the needle must be withdrawn or repositioned until the test is negative. Very rarely, the aspiration test may yield CSF. The exact incidence of this complication is unknown, but is probably of the order of one in 1000.

Injection should be easy. If resistance is met, the needle should be rotated through 90° initially. It should be removed and re-inserted if there is persistent difficulty. Lignocaine, prilocaine and bupivacaine are used in their standard concentrations and a volume of 20 ml is adequate for perineal procedures.

If repeated caudal injections are likely to be needed, an 'intravenous' cannula can be inserted, the injection site sealed with an occlusive dressing, and the cannula connected to the syringe by a length of extension tubing and a bacterial filter.

In children, the technique requires some modification. A 21 gauge needle is used for all but the smallest infants in whom a 23 gauge is more suitable. When the needle has penetrated the sacrococcygeal ligament, it should not be re-angled and advanced to the hub as this is more likely to result in a vascular or dural tap, and the needle does not have to be advanced cephalad for high blocks to be obtained. Advance of 2–3 mm is all that is required.

PAEDIATRIC DOSAGE

The spread of a caudal dose of local anaesthetic solution correlates best with the age of a child, but also very satisfactorily with the weight and height (Schulte-Steinberg & Rahlfs, 1970). The equation worked out by these workers (Schulte-Steinberg & Rahlfs, 1977) has been simplified by Hain (1978): volume of drug = [Age (yr) + 2 ml] divided by 10, per segment to be blocked, using lignocaine 1% or bupivacaine 0.25%. Although this formula is used widely, it is not entirely satisfactory for infants, some of whom may have been born very prematurely and whose 'age' was obstetrically determined. Another disadvantage is that, because anaesthesia of several segments is invariably required, the arithmetic is not always simple.

The author prefers to use weight as the index and to calculate the volume of drug required to provide anaesthesia in three anatomical areas—lumbosacral, thoracolumbar and lower thoracic. With lignocaine 1% or bupivacaine 0.25%, 0.5 ml/kg body weight is required to block the lumbosacral distribution, 1 ml per kg for the thoracolumbar, and 1.25 ml per kg for the lower thoracic. When this calculation gives a volume greater than 20 ml, one part of saline is added to three parts of drug and the calculated volume of the diluted drug is injected.

Complications and disadvantages

The commonest complication of a caudal is inability to locate the sacral cornua and, thus, failure to deposit local anaesthetic in the sacral extradural space. The success rate in adults is rarely higher than 95% and often considerably lower. In children, on the other hand, landmarks are much easier to feel, and blocks are almost always successful.

The sacral extradural space is capacious, and comparatively large volumes of solution are needed to anaesthetize relatively few segments. In adults, this is of no clinical significance if the block is confined to the sacral distribution, but if it is used for anaesthesia of the lumbar segments, systemic toxicity is a potential hazard and the lumbar extradural route is to be preferred.

Accidental intravascular injection can produce a plasma concentration of local anaesthetic high enough to cause a toxic reaction. The author has data which show that intravascular injection can occur even after a negative aspiration test, and plasma concentrations obtained when the injection follows an initial bloody tap tend to be higher than normal.

Some workers use continuous caudal anaesthesia and give top-up injections or infusions during and after surgery. However, many anaesthetists feel that the skin puncture site, being close to the anus, is difficult to keep sterile and is therefore unsuitable for the insertion of a caudal catheter, although there is no good evidence that a caudal carries a higher risk of infection than any other form of extradural.

Paracervical block

Anatomy

Paracervical block anaesthetizes three types of nerve running to and from the uterus in the broad ligament.

The motor supply to the upper uterine segment is derived from sympathetic fibres which travel in the splanchnic nerves and the coeliac, aortic, renal and hypogastric plexuses and then enter the broad ligament, accompanying the uterine vessels, to reach the uterus.

The sensory supply is conveyed by visceral afferents which run with the sympathetic fibres in the broad ligament. They enter the cord at the 11th and 12th thoracic and first lumbar level. Some sensory fibres, supplying the fundus of the uterus, travel occasionally with the ovarian vessels and are therefore unaffected by paracervical block.

The pelvic splanchnic nerves run in the broad ligament also and contain visceral afferent and efferent fibres. The former are sensory to the cervix and upper vagina, and they enter the cord at the second, third and fourth sacral level.

Paracervical block therefore prevents the pain of uterine contraction, unless a significant proportion of this is transmitted by fibres accompanying the ovarian vessels. It prevents also the pain of cervical dilatation, but sensation to the lower vagina, vulva and perineum is unimpaired.

Indications

Bilateral block provides analgesia for the first stage of labour and may be sufficient also for the second stage, if bilateral pudendal block is added. Because it can be performed easily by the obstetrician, the technique was very popular in the days before extradural services, provided by anaesthetists, were available.

It has no regular place in modern obstetric practice because it has been found to cause fetal bradycardia and depression of the neonate. This was thought initially to result from high concentrations of local anaesthetic reaching the fetal myocardium, but more recently it has been shown that the uterine artery constricts when local anaesthetic is applied directly to it (Cibils, 1976; Greiss et al., 1976) and impairment of uterine blood supply is the more likely cause.

Pudendal nerve block

Anatomy

The pudendal nerve is derived from the second, third and fourth sacral roots. It leaves the pelvis through the greater sciatic notch and, lying medial to the pudendal artery, winds round the lateral side of the ischial spine where it can be blocked. It then runs anteriorly in the pudendal canal, medial to the ramus of the ischium and lateral to the ischiorectal fossa, and emerges at the ischial tuberosity. It supplies the perineum and pelvic floor through its inferior haemorrhoidal and perineal branches, and the penis and clitoris through the dorsal nerve to those organs.

The pudendal nerve is not the only sensory nerve to the perineum. The labia majora are supplied by the terminal branches of the ilioinguinal and genito-femoral nerves, and part of the perineal body is supplied by the perineal branch of the posterior cutaneous nerve of the thigh. These areas are anaesthetized usually by local infiltration, although if the transperineal approach is used for pudendal nerve block, the perineal branch of the posterior cutaneous nerve of the thigh can be blocked where it runs under the ischial tuberosity.

Indications

These are almost entirely confined to obstetrics. Pudendal nerve block provides adequate analgesia for low forceps delivery. It is performed usually by the obstetrician and, in an emergency, is quicker and safer than general anaesthesia. It can be used also for episiotomy and for the repair of perineal lacerations, but supplementary local infiltration may be needed. It has no effect on the pain of uterine contraction or cervical dilatation.

Technique

TRANSVAGINAL APPROACH

The patient is placed in the lithotomy position and the ischial spine is palpated through the lateral vaginal wall. The sacrospinous ligament can be felt running posteriorly from the spine. A deep injection is required and the operator has very little space in which to work, so accurate insertion of a long needle is difficult. An introducer, approximately 140 mm long with a blunt, bulbous end, is therefore passed along the palpating fingers until it lies medial and slightly posterior to the ischial spine. A needle long enough to project 10 mm beyond the end of the introducer is then passed through it. With the needle and introducer directed a little laterally, the needle is advanced beyond the end of the introducer so that it penetrates the anterior part of the sacrospinous ligament. After careful aspiration, 10 ml of lignocaine, prilocaine or bupivacaine are injected and the procedure is repeated on the other side.

TRANSPERINEAL APPROACH

This allows the pudendal nerve to be blocked at the ischial tuberosity in addition to the ischial spine. A skin weal of local anaesthetic is raised midway between the posterior limit of the vagina and the ischial tuberosity, and a 150 mm needle is inserted through it. Palpation of the ischial tuberosity through the vagina assists in directing the needle towards it. Five ml of local anaesthetic injected on the medial side of the tuberosity block the pudendal nerve as it emerges from the pudendal canal on the medial aspect of the ischial ramus, and the same amount deposited inferiorly blocks the perineal branch of the posterior cutaneous nerve of the thigh as it runs under the tuberosity. With the palpating fingers now marking the ischial spine, the needle is advanced along the ischiorectal fossa (medial to the tuberosity and ramus) and through the sacrospinous ligament where a further 10 ml of local anaesthetic are injected.

Complications and disadvantages

The pudendal nerve is related closely to the pudendal vessels. Haematoma may result if the latter are damaged and systemic toxicity may occur if an accidental intravascular injection is made. Bilateral blocks are always required, so the risks of complications are compounded.

Pudendal nerve block has no effect on the pain of uterine contractions and although it provides the sensory supply to the greater part of the perineum, it does not give complete perineal analgesia. Supplementary local infiltration is therefore usually required and Scudamore and Yates (1966) believe that this makes a major contribution to the efficacy of the block.

References

Boileau G. (1951) *Grants Atlas of Anatomy* 3rd edn, p. 180. Bailliere Tindall, London.

Braid D.P. & Scott D.B. (1965) The systemic absorption of local anaesthetic drugs. *British Journal of Anaesthesia* 37, 394–404.

Cibils L.A. (1976) Response of human uterine arteries to local anesthetics. *American Journal of Obstetrics and Gynecology* 126, 202–10.

Cleland J.G.P. (1933) Paravertebral anesthesia in obstetrics. Experimental and clinical basis. *Surgery, Gynecology and Obstetrics* 57, 51–62.

Cousins M.J. & Bridenbaugh P.O. (Eds) (1988) *Neural Blockade in Clinical Anaesthesia and Management of Pain* 2nd edn. J.B. Lippincott, Philadelphia.

Cousins M.J. & Wright C.J. (1971) Graft, muscle, skin blood flow after epidural block in vascular surgical procedures. *Surgery, Gynecology and Obstetrics* 133, 59.

Eason M.J. & Wyatt R. (1979) Paravertebral thoracic block—a reappraisal. *Anaesthesia* 34, 638–42.

Edwards W.B. & Hingson R.A. (1942) Continuous caudal anesthesia in obstetrics. *American Journal of Surgery* 57, 459–64.

Glynn C.J., Lloyd J.W. & Barnard J.D.W. (1980) Cryoanalgesia in the management of pain after thoracotomy. *Thorax* 35, 325–7.

Greiss F.C., Still J.G. & Anderson S.G. (1976) Effects of local anesthetic agents on the uterine vasculature and myometrium. *American Journal of Obstetrics and Gynecology* 124, 889–98.

Hain W.R. (1978) Anaesthetic doses for extradural anaesthesia in children. *British Journal of Anaesthesia* 50, 303.

Lanier V.A., McKnight H.E. & Trotter M. (1944) Caudal analgesia: an experimental and anatomical study. *American Journal of Obstetrics and Gynecology* 47, 633–41.

Lofstrom B. & Zetterquist S. (1969) Lumbar sympathetic blocks in the treatment of patients with obliterative disease of the lower limb. *International Anesthesia Clinics* 7, 423–38.

Moore D.C., Mather L.A., Bridenbaugh P.O., Bridenbaugh L.D., Balfour R.I., Lysons D.F. & Horton W.G. (1976) Arterial and venous plasma levels of bupivacaine following epidural and intercostal nerve blocks. *Anesthesiology* 45, 39–45.

Murphy D.F. (1983) Continuous intercostal nerve blockade for pain relief following cholecystectomy. *British Journal of Anaesthesia* 55, 521–4.

Nunn J.F. & Slavin G. (1980) Posterior intercostal nerve block for pain relief after cholecystectomy. Anatomical basis and efficacy. *British Journal of Anaesthesia* **52**, 253–60.

Odoom J.A. & Sih I.L. (1983) Epidural analgesia and anti-coagulation therapy. Experience with 1000 cases of continuous epidurals. *British Journal of Anaesthesia* **38**, 254–9.

Purcell-Jones G., Pither C.E. & Justins D.M. (1987) Paravertebral block—a misnomer? In *Abstracts of Scientific Papers, 6th Annual Meeting of the European Society of Regional Anaesthesia* p. 182.

Rao T.L.K. & El-Etr A.A. (1981) Anticoagulation following placement of epidural and subarachnoid catheters: an evaluation of neurologic sequelae. *Anesthesiology* **55**, 618–20.

Reid W., Kennedy-Watt J. & Gray T.G. (1970) Phenol injection of the sympathetic chain. *British Journal of Surgery* **57**, 45–50.

Schulte-Steinberg O. & Rahlfs V.W. (1970) Caudal anaesthesia in children and spread of 1 per cent lignocaine. A statistical study. *British Journal of Anaesthesia* **42**, 1093–9.

Schulte-Steinberg O. & Rahlfs V.W. (1977) Spread of extradural analgesia following caudal injection in children. A statistical study. *British Journal of Anaesthesia* **49**, 1027–34.

Scott D.B. (1975) Evaluation of the clinical tolerance of local anaesthetic agents. *British Journal of Anaesthesia* **47**, 328.

Scudamore J.H. & Yates M.J. (1966) Pudendal block—a misnomer? *Lancet* i, 23–4.

Trotter M. (1947) Variations of the sacral canal: their significance in the administration of caudal analgesia. *Anesthesia and Analgesia* **26**, 192–202.

Trotter M. & Lanier P.F. (1945) Hiatus canalis sacralis in American whites and negroes. *Human Biology* **17**, 368–81.

White J., Harrison B., Richmond P., Procter A. & Curran J. (1983) Postoperative analgesia for circumcision. *British Medical Journal* **286**, 1934.

Wildsmith J.A.W. & Armitage E.N. (Eds) (1987) *Principles and Practice of Regional Anaesthesia.* Churchill Livingstone, Edinburgh.

Williams P.L. & Warwick R. (Eds) (1980) *Grays Anatomy* 36th edn. Churchill Livingstone, Edinburgh.

Yeoman P.M., Cooke R. & Hain W.R. (1983) Penile block for circumcision? A comparison with caudal blockade. *Anaesthesia* **38**, 862–6.

63

Head and Neck

R. S. NEILL

The classic text, *Regional Anaesthesia* by Labat, written in 1928 includes several chapters on the techniques and indications for regional nerve blocks in the head and neck, ranging from removal of sebaceous cysts to total laryngectomy. With the development of safe and routine tracheal intubation, modern anaesthetic practice has relegated regional nerve block to a minor role in head and neck surgery (Murphy, 1986).

Ophthalmic, ear, nose and throat (ENT), and maxillofacial surgeons continue to use regional anaesthesia for very large numbers of relatively minor surgical procedures, not involving specialist anaesthetists, and where general anaesthesia would be inappropriate (Allen & Elkington, 1980; Jahrsdoerfer, 1981; Martof, 1981; Stromberg, 1985). The specialist anaesthetist has therefore tended to concentrate on improvements in general anaesthetic techniques for major surgery, and few have explored the possibilities of regional anaesthesia, although most have experienced its benefits in the dental chair.

Innervation of the head and neck

The structures of the head and neck are supplied by 12 cranial and four cervical nerves. The majority of this supply is of a specialized sensory or secretomotor nature, and has no relevance to nerve block for surgery. A distinctive feature of the nerves to the head and neck is the almost complete separation of sensory and motor function, allowing sensory block to be achieved without motor paralysis. Intraoral blocks may be performed without endangering control of the airway muscles. At other sites it may be important to block both motor and sensory nerves. Anaesthesia for cataract extraction requires block of the orbital branches of the facial nerve to minimize the risk of iris or vitreous prolapse (Boberg-Ans & Barnes, 1980).

For the purposes of nerve block for surgery, a detailed knowledge of the sensory supply to the skin of the head and neck and mucous membranes of the airway is required. The anatomical relations of the major motor supply should be known also. Close study of the bony skeleton and dissection specimens help to develop a three-dimensional picture of the anatomy, essential for accurate deposition of the local anaesthetic agent.

Trigeminal nerve

The trigeminal (fifth), the largest cranial nerve, supplies sensation to the face, greater part of the scalp, the teeth, mouth and nasal cavity and through its small motor branch controls the muscles of mastication (Figs 63.1 and 63.2). The trigeminal (Gasserian) ganglion lies in a recess near the apex of the petrous temporal bone.

On leaving the ganglion, the sensory root divides into three divisions: ophthalmic, maxillary and mandibular. The motor root lies inferior to the ganglion and joins the mandibular division.

The ophthalmic nerve enters the orbit through the superior orbital fissure and divides into frontal, lacrimal and nasociliary nerves. The terminal cutaneous branches of the frontal are the supraorbital and supratrochlear; of the nasociliary the infratrochlear and external nasal; the lacrimal is inconstant and is replaced sometimes by a branch of the maxillary nerve.

The maxillary nerve leaves the cranial cavity through the foramen rotundum, crosses the pterygopalatine

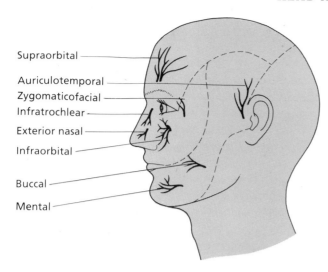

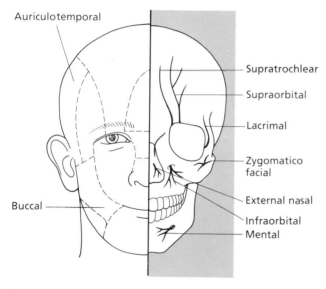

Fig. 63.1 Sensory distribution of the divisions of the V cranial nerve: trigeminal.

Fig. 63.2 Sensory distribution of the distal branches of the V cranial nerve: trigeminal.

posterior trunk. At this point the nerve lies in the pterygopalatine fossa, anterior to the neck of the mandible and posterior to the lateral pterygoid plate. The anterior trunk supplies the muscles of mastication and sensation to the skin branch—the buccal nerve.

The posterior trunk is sensory (apart from one branch to the mylohyoid muscle) with three main branches—the auriculotemporal, inferior dental and lingual nerves.

The auriculotemporal emerges from behind the temporomandibular joint to supply sensation to the external auditory meatus and temple. The inferior dental nerve enters the foramen on the medial side of the ramus of the mandible to run through the bone and emerge at the mental foramen, as the mental nerve.

The lingual nerve runs between the ramus of the mandible and the medial pterygoid muscle to lie on the deep surface of the mandible at the third molar, at which point it is covered only by mucous membrane. The lingual nerve supplies sensation to the anterior two-thirds of the tongue and adjacent mucous membrane.

Facial nerve

The facial (seventh) is the motor nerve of the face—supplying the muscles of expression and most importantly the muscles controlling eyelid closure and oral competence.

The nerve runs between the deep and superficial lobes of the parotid gland. As it does so, it divides into five main branches which fan out to supply their respective areas of the face—temporal, zygomatic,

fossa to enter the orbit through the inferior orbital fissure, enters the infraorbital canal, and emerges from the infraorbital foramen as the infraorbital nerve.

An inconstant branch may arise in the infraorbital fissure which emerges as the zygomaticotemporal nerve; a connection between this and the lacrimal nerve may replace one or other of these nerves.

The mandibular nerve is the largest division of the trigeminal. The sensory and motor roots leave the skull through the foramen ovale before uniting and redividing to form the small anterior trunk and larger

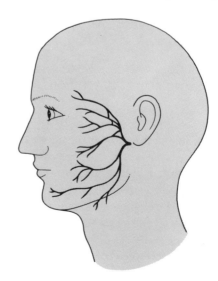

Fig. 63.3 Facial nerve.

buccal, mandibular and cervical. The mandibular branch runs forward below the angle of the mandible before turning upwards to supply the angle of the mouth (Fig. 63.3).

Glossopharyngeal nerve

The glossopharyngeal (ninth) nerve supplies sensation to the posterior part of the tongue, pharynx and tonsil, secretomotor fibres to the parotid and motor fibres to the stylopharyngeus. It emerges from the jugular foramen in close relationship to the internal jugular vein and internal carotid artery, then runs forward on the stylopharyngeus muscle to pierce the superior constrictor muscle of the pharynx.

Vagus nerve

The branches of the vagus (10th) of importance in the head and neck supply sensory and motor innervation to the larynx.

The superior laryngeal nerve arises from the inferior ganglion of the vagus to run downwards, forwards and medially to the greater cornu of the hyoid where it divides into two branches. The internal branch pierces the thyrohyoid membrane to supply sensation to the larynx above the level of the vocal cords. The external branch is motor to the cricothyroid muscle.

The recurrent laryngeal nerve loops around the aorta on the right and the subclavian on the left before ascending in the groove between the oesophagus and trachea to enter the larynx between the articulation of the inferior cornu of the thyroid and cricoid cartilages. It provides sensation to the larynx below the vocal cords and motor fibres to all the laryngeal muscles except cricothyroid.

Hypoglossal nerve

The hypoglossal (12th) nerve is the motor nerve to the tongue. It leaves the base of the skull related closely to the glossopharyngeal and vagus nerves, lying between the internal jugular vein and internal carotid arteries. At the angle of the mandible, it crosses both internal and external carotid arteries to run downwards and forwards to the greater cornu of the hyoid where it enters the tongue. It supplies branches to the thyrohyoid, styloglossus, hyoglossus, geniohyoid and genioglossus muscles.

Cervical nerves

The skin over a wide area of the scalp, back of the neck and shoulders, the 'cape' area, is supplied by sensory branches of the upper four cervical nerves (Fig. 63.4). Dorsal rami of C2–4 supply the back of the neck and scalp—the greater occipital nerve. Ventral rami of C1–4 form the cervical plexus which may be considered as two separate entities. The deep branches supply the muscles of the neck and the diaphragm. The superficial branches, which pierce the deep fascia at the middle of the posterior border of sternomastoid, fan out to provide sensation from the lower border of the mandible to the level of the second rib. The branches are the great auricular, lesser occipital, the transverse cervical and the supraclavicular.

Clinical applications

The use of regional anaesthesia in the head and neck may produce significant advantage in certain groups of patients.

Outpatients

The majority of dental surgery is performed on outpatients under local anaesthesia, supplemented frequently by intravenous sedation. When general anaesthesia is employed, nerve block has been advo-

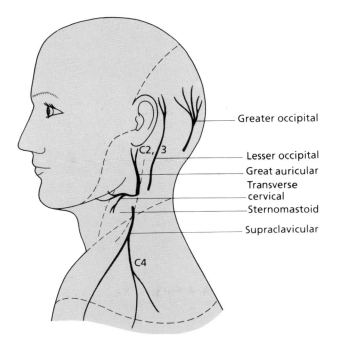

Fig. 63.4 Sensory distribution of the cervical plexus.

cated as a possible method of reducing intraoperative arrhythmias (Plowman *et al.*, 1974).

Postoperatively, the continuing action of the local anaesthetic drug provides a period of analgesia without central depression, reduces general systemic upset and permits early ambulation.

Similar techniques may be employed with advantage to the increasing numbers of patients undergoing day-case surgery. Szmyd *et al.* (1984) have described a technique for stabismus surgery in adults involving the use of retrobulbar nerve block combined with intravenous sedation. Ocular discomfort occurred 1.5–2 hr after the block. Visual acuity and extraocular muscle function were restored fully after 4 hr allowing strabismus to be corrected by adjusting sutures early in the postoperative period.

Attwood and Evans (1985) employed a regional anaesthetic technique for correction of prominent ears in a mixed group of patients in which 20% were under the age of 13 yr. The majority were in favour of local rather than general anaesthesia and 30% 'enjoyed' the experience.

Poor-risk patients

Carefully selected regional anaesthetic techniques can avoid or reduce greatly the need for general anaesthesia. Backer *et al.* (1980) reported no myocardial re-infarction following 288 ophthalmic procedures under local anaesthesia, in 195 patients with a history of a previous myocardial infarction.

Lynch *et al.* (1974) compared general anaesthesia with local anaesthesia for cataract surgery and found a significantly higher risk of nausea and vomiting following general anaesthesia. This was attributed to the earlier requirement for postoperative analgesia.

Donlon (1986) compared the mortality rates of local and general anaesthetic groups and found them almost equal. However, the patient groups were unequal, as physical status influenced choice and local anaesthesia may be safer in older age groups. Memory performance of patients undergoing extraction of senile cataracts under local anaesthesia with sedation or general anaesthesia was similar 1 week after surgery (Karhunen & Jönn, 1982).

The ophthalmic surgeon can perform most of his or her surgery with local anaesthesia; however, co-operation of an anaesthetist familiar with these techniques can contribute greatly to the care of patients with eye problems. The choice of anaesthesia can range from local anaesthesia with varying amounts of sed-ation, to general anaesthesia. If both doctors can perform the regional technique, delays between operations can be minimized (Allen & Elkington, 1980; Jolly, 1980).

Nerve block using small amounts of local anaesthetic with added vasoconstrictor produces effective haemostasis (Keoshian, 1980). The excellent operating conditions can be used as an alternative to induced hypotension in major eyelid surgery in elderly, poor-risk patients (Neill, 1982).

Impaired cerebral circulation

Regional anaesthesia in the awake patient has been advocated as the method of choice for patients requiring carotid endarterectomy following transient ischaemic attacks (Spencer & Eiseman, 1962; Connolly, 1985). The technique permits continuous assessment of neurological status and requirement for shunt (Jopling *et al.*, 1983).

Peitzman *et al.* (1982) found the technique safe and reliable with the same rate of neurological complication but a lower rate of non-neurological complications than general anaesthesia. Prough *et al.* (1984) found a low incidence of intraoperative arrhythmias and no perioperative myocardial infarction.

Awake intubation of the trachea

Certain patients have airway abnormalities of such severity that tracheal intubation or tracheostomy should be performed before induction of general anaesthesia. This may be accomplished by a combination of nerve block and topical application of local anaesthetic, using a short-acting agent to limit the time to return of protective laryngeal reflexes (Brown & Sataloff, 1981; Gotta & Sullivan, 1981; Murrin, 1985; Donlon, 1986).

Postoperative airway problems

Proximal block of the trigeminal nerve with a long-acting agent offers high quality analgesia and reduced dependence on opioid analgesics to patients in whom the airway may be at risk following major maxillofacial surgery (Murphy, 1980).

Intractable pain

Neurolysis with alcohol or phenol is now reserved for patients with intractable pain from inoperable tumours. Good results can be obtained from proximal block of the trigeminal nerve at the foramen ovale, and cervical plexus at the transverse process (Lipton, 1979; Carron, 1981).

Patients following successful block have a lowered dependence on potent opioid analgesics with an improvement in quality of life (Dwyer & Gibb, 1980).

Nerve block or local infiltration

Basal cell carcinoma, the most common skin tumour, occurs frequently on the face and neck. Patients are often frail and elderly, with multiple and extensive lesions, and may be dealt with on an outpatient basis.

Infiltration techniques distend and distort the tissues making accurate definition of the lesion difficult; when multiple lesions are present, the volume of local anaesthetic required may cause anxiety if all lesions are to be removed at one visit. Nerve block supplemented by minimal local infiltration offers a solution (Murphy, 1980).

Volume of local anaesthetic is much reduced, a wide area of anaesthesia is provided with little or no tissue distortion and fear of toxicity removed.

Balanced anaesthesia

Nerve blocks may be used as the analgesic component of a balanced anaesthetic regimen, the residual effects of the local anaesthetic agent extend into the postoperative period ensuring a pain-free recovery with reduced requirement for analgesics. Great auricular nerve block with a long-acting agent is of special benefit to children who have had surgical correction of prominent ears.

Careful identification of the branches of the facial nerve is essential during surgery of the parotid gland. The combination of light general anaesthesia and cervical plexus block in a spontaneously breathing patient provides a clear operating field and the ability to assess facial nerve function continuously.

Techniques ranging from profound hypotension to local infiltration of large volumes of vasoconstrictors have been used to control bleeding during corrective rhinoplasty. Regional nerve block in combination with light general anaesthesia can provide comparable conditions to profound hypotension, with little or no tissue distortion from local infiltration (Neill, 1983).

Reconstructive techniques in major intraoral cancer surgery often involve free tissue transfer (Soutar et al., 1983). The reduction in the sympathetic tone produced by a deep cervical plexus block can help in the establishment of an adequate circulation to the transferred tissue (Neill, 1983).

Possible blocks, problems and hazards

The cranial nerves may be blocked proximally as they leave the base of the skull, but more frequently, block is confined to the distal branches. The anatomical relationship of the nerves to each other and to the major vessels (the carotid artery and internal jugular vein), as they leave the base of the skull creates a significant risk of intravascular injection, haematoma formation and nerve damage.

The major complication following retrobulbar nerve block is haemorrhage from accidental puncture of an orbital vein. This produces proptosis, and an increase in intraoptic pressure which necessitates postponement of the surgery (Allen & Elkington, 1980). Accidental injection into the ophthalmic artery incurs the risk of retrograde spread to the internal carotid and consequent acute cerebral toxicity.

Idiopathic trigeminal anaesthesia has caused trophic ulceration of the ala nasae (McLean & Watson, 1982). This has also followed damage to the infraorbital artery if the needle is introduced deeply into the infraorbital foramen during an infraorbital nerve block (Moore, 1975; Garber, 1980).

Therapy of trigeminal neuralgia by chemical ablation of the affected division of the nerve has been superseded by radiofrequency coagulation (Lipton, 1979; Wise, 1984). Chemical ablation was associated with a 0.9% fatality rate, and a danger of permanent blindness if the injection of the maxillary nerve was misplaced in the infraorbital fissure (Swerdlow, 1980).

Total spinal anaesthesia has followed both trigeminal and anterior ethmoidal nerve block (Nique & Bennett, 1981; Hill et al., 1983). The injections perforated the dura of the foramen ovale and cribiform plate. Both patients recovered following immediate aggressive therapy, and were fortunate that an ablative agent had not been used.

The close association of the glossopharyngeal, vagal and hypoglossal nerves at the styloid process creates a significant risk of impairment of motor and sensory supply to the airway from local spread of small volumes of correctly positioned agents. Respiratory obstruction caused the death of a patient who received a vagal nerve block as therapy for a postcricoid carcinoma (Dwyer & Gibb, 1980).

Less serious but distressing complications can follow correctly placed nerve blocks. They are self-

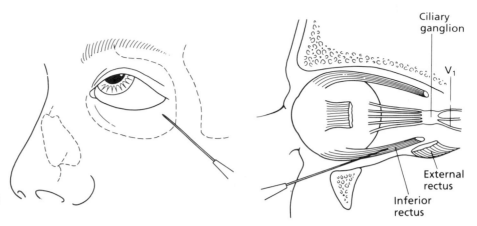

Fig. 63.5 Retrotubular nerve block. (Redrawn from Boberg-Ans & Barnes, 1980.)

limiting and related to the duration of action of the anaesthetic agent e.g. diplopia following maxillary block (Kronman & Kabani, 1984) or Horner's syndrome following a stellate ganglion block. All patients should be given a clear explanation of these complications and reassurance as to the outcome.

Precise anatomical knowledge and meticulous technique can minimize the risk of these mishaps, but few opportunities to acquire these skills exist outside specialist units, and these complex methods offer little advantage over the more distal blocks. These are less demanding technically and may be employed reliably even by the occasional user with benefit to patient and operator, either alone or as a component of balanced anaesthesia (Neill, 1983).

Techniques of nerve block

Trigeminal

All divisions of the nerve may be blocked as they emerge from the foramina on the base of the skull.

BLOCK OF FIRST DIVISION (OPHTHALMIC)

To perform this block, a 4 cm, 25 gauge needle is inserted slightly above the bony orbital margin in the lower lateral quadrant (Fig. 63.5). The patient is instructed to look upwards and inwards to move the internal oblique muscle and the fascia between the lateral and inferior rectus muscles out of the path of the advancing needle. The needle is advanced along the orbital floor beyond the globe, then directed upwards towards the apex of the orbit to a total distance of 2.5–3.5 cm. It is now inside the muscle cone adjacent to the ciliary ganglion. Following careful and repeated aspiration 2–2.5 ml of local anaesthetic are injected slowly.

BLOCK OF SECOND AND THIRD DIVISIONS (MAXILLARY AND MANDIBULAR)

These may be blocked using either a lateral or an anterior approach.

Lateral approach

One or both divisions may be blocked from a single entrance point using the landmarks which define the coronoid notch i.e. the zygomatic arch, the ramus and the coronoid process of the mandible (Fig. 63.6).

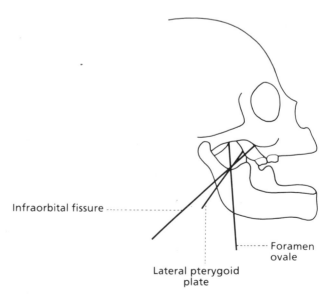

Fig. 63.6 Block of the V second and third divisions: landmarks.

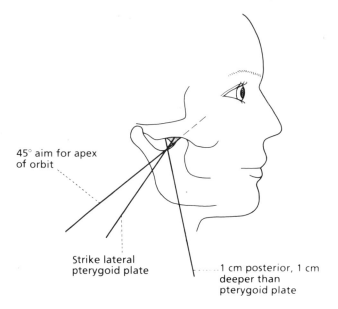

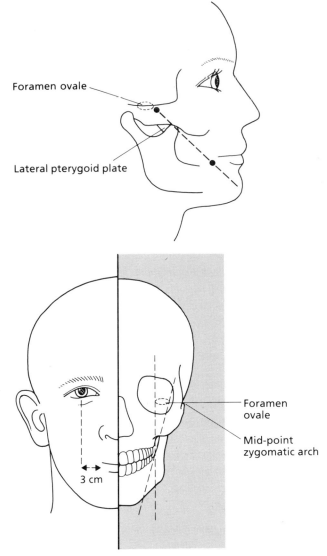

Fig. 63.7 Block of the V second and third divisions: lateral approach.

To block the maxillary division of the nerve, a 23 gauge spinal needle is introduced through the coronoid notch below the midpoint of the zygomatic arch (Fig. 63.7). It is directed at an angle of 45° to the vertical, aiming for the apex of the bony orbital cone, to strike the medial edge of the lateral pterygoid plate or the body of the maxilla. Care must be exercised to prevent damage to the optic nerve if the needle enters the infraorbital fissure. Following careful aspiration, 2–5 ml local anaesthetic solution are injected.

To block the mandibular division, the same landmarks are used. In this instance, the needle is directed at 90° in both planes to strike the posterior edge of the lateral pterygoid plate. It may then be retracted to the skin and re-introduced aiming for a point 1 cm posterior to and 1 cm more deeply than previously, to slide past the edge of the plate. This step may be omitted (Moore, 1975), as sufficient anaesthetic filters around the pterygoid plate if injection is made at the point of bony contact. Paraesthesiae are not essential for either of these blocks.

Anterior approach

The essential landmarks are the midpoint of the zygomatic arch and the pupil. With the patient's head resting on a 'donut' to provide stability, the midpoint of the zygomatic arch, and a point 3 cm lateral to the angle of the mouth are marked (Fig. 63.8).

Fig. 63.8 Block of V second and third divisions: anterior approach.

Through the latter mark the introducer needle for a 25 gauge spinal needle is inserted. The spinal needle is advanced towards the base of the skull aligning it with the pupil in the vertical plane and 1 cm anterior to the mid-point of the zygoma in the horizontal. The needle strikes the sphenoid anterior to the foramen ovale. It should now be redirected in line with the midpoint of the zygoma and at the same depth should enter the foramen ovale (Fig. 63.8).

This approach to the divisions of the trigeminal nerve has a high risk of serious complications. Involvement of the first division causes loss of corneal sensation, and corneal reflex with the possibility of corneal ulceration. Accidental injection into the cranial cavity can lead to paralysis of other cranial nerves (Nique & Bennett, 1981). Meticulous attention to technique, with careful repeated aspiration is mandatory. Paraesthesiae should be sought always, and it is recommended that this route be used only for treatment of intractable cancer pain.

Glossopharyngeal nerve

This nerve may be blocked, as it lies close to the posterior edge of the styloid process. The block is required infrequently and carries an exceedingly high risk of accidental intravascular injection and spread to hypoglossal, vagus and accessory nerves (Dwyer & Gibb, 1980).

Cervical plexus

The classical method of deep cervical plexus block involves injections on to the transverse processes of C2, 3 and 4 vertebrae.

To locate the relevant transverse processes, a line is drawn from the tip of the mastoid process to the

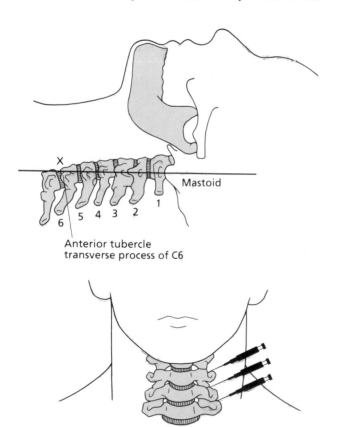

Fig. 63.9 Deep cervical plexus block: injection onto transverse process, needle direction caudad.

transverse process of C6, which is readily palpable, The transverse processes of C2, 3 and 4 lie approximately 0.5 cm posterior to this line with C2 palpable 2 cm caudad to the mastoid process (Fig. 63.9).

C3 and C4 are palpated a further 1 cm apart and slightly anteriorly. As each landmark is identified, a 23 gauge needle is inserted in a caudad direction to rest on the transverse process. This should avoid puncturing the vertebral artery or penetrating the dural space (Winnie *et al.*, 1975). The needle should be maintained in contact with bone during aspiration and injection of anaesthetic agent 5–10 ml at each site.

An alternative technique (Winnie *et al.*, 1975) involves a single injection site. Local anaesthetic 10–20 ml is placed at the C4 transverse process. Successful block depends on spread within the fascial sheath. As C4 is a major component of the phrenic nerve, bilateral deep cervical plexus blocks are inadvisable.

Stellate ganglion

This block is requested sometimes as a diagnostic tool or therapeutic aid in circulatory disturbances of the upper limb e.g. Raynaud's phenomenon. The ganglion lies between the base of the transverse process of C7 and the neck of the first rib behind the carotid sheath. It is related more closely to the pleura on the right than on the left.

The position of C7 transverse process is determined by placing a mark 3 cm lateral to the middle of the clavicular notch and 3 cm vertical to the clavicle—two fingerbreadths in each direction. Palpation of C6 transverse process should confirm this mark, as it lies 1.5 cm cephalad to C7.

The carotid sheath and sternomastoid are retracted laterally as the needle is inserted perpendicularly through the mark. It impinges normally on the transverse process but should be redirected if paraesthesiae occur in the brachial plexus or if bone is not contacted.

Following the normal careful aspiration, a small amount is injected as a test dose, as a precaution against injection into the vertebral artery.

Techniques of nerve block—distal

Trigeminal nerve

The areas of skin supplied by the terminal branches of the trigeminal are illustrated in Fig. 63.2. The three main branches emerge from the supraorbital notch, the infraorbital foramen and the mental foramen. These exit points lie on a line 1.5 cm from the alar margin which is of especial help in determining the site of injection when blocking these branches in the edentulous patient.

SUPRAORBITAL AND SUPRATROCHLEAR NERVES

Block of both these nerves, bilateral if necessary, can be achieved from a single injection site on the nasal bridge. The needle is first directed downwards and laterally towards the medial canthus, and then directly laterally under the orbital rim to a point 1 cm beyond the supraorbital notch. Injection should be continuous as the needle is advanced, essential if non-aspirating dental cartridge syringes are used. One to 2 ml are adequate for both blocks.

INFRAORBITAL NERVE

The infraorbital foramen is located 1 cm below the orbital rim 1.5 cm lateral to the nasal bone. The nerve may be blocked by direct skin puncture at this point or alternatively by entering the buccal sulcus at the upper premolar directing the needle upwards to the orbital rim. A finger should be placed on the orbital rim to prevent damage to the orbit or its contents.

The infraorbital canal should not be entered; it is both unnecessary and potentially hazardous. The floor of the orbit is punctured easily; damage to the infraorbital artery can cause ulceration of the infraorbital skin (Moore, 1975).

Zygomatico facial and lacrimal nerves

The zygomatic foramen can be palpated 1–2 cm below the lower lateral orbital margin. The area immediately around the foramen should be infiltrated with 1–2 ml of anaesthetic as the nerve breaks into radiating branches immediately it emerges from the foramen. From the same injection site, infiltration past the lateral canthus to the outer third of the upper eyelid will anaesthetize the lacrimal nerve.

Mental nerve

The mental foramen is situated below the first premolar halfway between the gum margin and the lower border of the mandible. In the edentulous patient the position may be confirmed using the straight line relationship between the foramina (Fig. 63.10). As with the

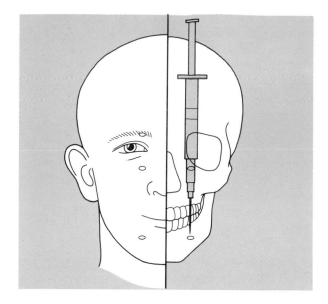

Fig. 63.10 Mental nerve block: approach through buccal sulcus using 'straight-line' relationship between foraminae.

infraorbital nerve block, the injection may be made through the skin, but the buccal sulcus is used more frequently. The application of anaesthetic gel to this site makes the injection pain-free.

Inferior dental and lingual nerves

These may be injected at the foramen which lies in the centre of the medial aspect of the ascending ramus of

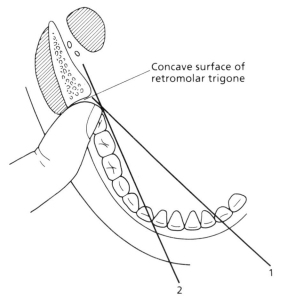

Concave surface of retromolar trigone

Fig. 63.11 Inferior dental nerve block.

the mandible. To locate the foramen, the ramus is palpated with the index finger, the pulp resting on the concavity of the retromolar trigone, the nail identifying the medial ridge. With the barrel of the syringe resting on the contralateral premolars, the needle is directed parallel to the occlusal surface of the mandibular molars to penetrate the mucosa just beyond the midpoint of the palpating finger (Fig. 63.11). As the injection is made, the syringe is swung across to allow the insertion to continue parallel to the mandibular ramus for a distance of 2 cm. Injection of 2 ml will block both nerves.

Buccal nerve

The needle is inserted into the mucous membrane of the cheek at the level of the first mandibular molar and directed backwards. Injection of 2–3 ml is made as the needle is advanced parallel to the lateral aspect of the mandibular ramus.

Akinosi (1977) described a method of mandibular nerve block in which it was not necessary for the patient to open his or her mouth. The injection is made into the tissues between the vertical ramus of the mandible and the maxillary tuberosity (Fig. 63.12). Using this approach, buccal anaesthesia occurs in 80% of cases (Sisk, 1986).

Auriculotemporal nerve

Injection of 2 ml of anaesthetic between the superficial temporal artery and the ear is normally sufficient to produce block of this branch.

Anterior ethmoidal—external nasal nerves sphenopalatine ganglion

The sensory supply of the mucosa lining the nasal passage is derived from these nerves. The external nasal branches supply the skin on the tip of the nose related to the alar cartilages. Block of the nasal mucosa is achieved normally by packing with cocaine-soaked gauze or mounted pledgets (Q-tips) placed strategically above and below the superior and middle turbinates.

The external nasal nerve is blocked readily with a 1 ml injection at the junction of the bony and cartilaginous nose.

Cervical plexus—superficial block

The superficial branches of the plexus emerge at the midpoint of the posterior border of the sternomastoid muscle. The external jugular vein normally crosses the muscles 1–2 cm below this point. This posterior border of the muscle is identified by asking the patient to raise his or her head, and the injection point marked. Solution is directed upwards and downwards from this point and if made within the correct tissue planes will be seen to 'flow' along the border of the muscle. Five to 10 ml are sufficient and bilateral blocks may be used with safety (Fig. 63.13).

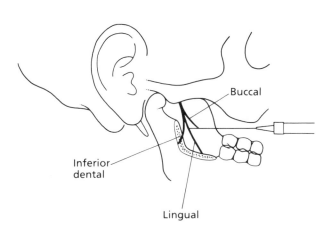

Fig. 63.12 Inferior dental nerve block (Redrawn from Akinosi, 1977).

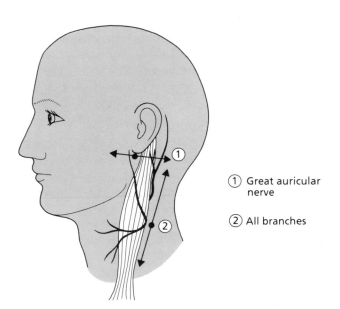

① Great auricular nerve

② All branches

Fig. 63.13 Block of the superficial branches of the cervical plexus.

Great auricular nerve

The great auricular nerve divides into pre- and postauricular branches to supply the greater part of the ear.

Both branches may be blocked with a single injection of 2–3 ml infiltrated 2–3 cm from the tip of the mastoid process in anterior and posterior directions (Fig. 63.13).

Anaesthetic agents

Surface anaesthesia: cocaine 2%–10%, lignocaine 4%.

Infiltration anaesthesia: lignocaine + adrenaline, prilocaine + octapressin, bupivacaine 0.25% or 0.5%.

Nerve block
1 Anaesthesia: lignocaine + adrenaline, prilocaine + octapressin, bupivacaine.
2 Ablation: aqueous phenol, alcohol.

Analgesia and sedation

Regional anaesthesia requires the same detailed attention to assessment and preparation as general anaesthesia (p. 430). Preoperative medication and intraoperative sedation should result in a patient who is calm, drowsy, devoid of anxiety yet capable of arousal and co-operation (Pratt, 1985). This may be achieved using combinations of opioids, short-acting barbiturates, benzodiazepines and butyrophenones given intravenously in very dilute concentration. Individual anaesthetists favour differing combinations of these agents, no one regimen attains universal approval. Sedation must be regarded always as complementary to the regional nerve block and cannot be used as a substitute for inadequate anaesthesia.

References

Akinosi J.O. (1977) A new approach to the mandibular nerve block. *British Journal of Oral Surgery* **15**, 83.

Allen E.D. & Elkington A.R. (1980) Local anaesthesia and the eye. *British Journal of Anaesthesia* **52**, 689.

Attwood A.I. & Evans D.M. (1985) Correction of prominent ears using Mustarde's technique: an outpatient procedure under local anaesthetic in children and adults. *British Journal of Plastic Surgery* **38**, 252.

Backer C.L., Tinker J.H., Robertson D.M. & Vlietstra R.E. (1980) Myocardial reinfarction following local anaesthesia for ophthalmic surgery. *Anesthesia and Analgesia* **59**, 257.

Boberg-Ans J. & Barnes S.S. (1980) Neural blockade for ophthalmic surgery. In *Neural Blockade* (Eds Cousins M.J. & Bridenbaugh P.O.) p. 458. Lippincott, Philadelphia.

Brown A.C.D. & Sataloff R.T. (1981) Special anaesthetic techniques in head and neck surgery. *Otolaryngologic Clinics of North America* **14.3**, 587.

Carron H. (1981) Control of pain in the head and neck. *Otolaryngologic Clinics of North America* **14.3**, 631.

Connolly J.E. (1985) Carotid end arterectomy in the awake patient. *American Journal of Surgery* **150**, 159.

Donlon J.V. jr. (1986) Anesthesia for eye, ear, nose and throat. In *Anesthesia* 2nd edn., vol. 3 (Ed. Miller R.D.) p. 1837. Churchill Livingstone, New York.

Dwyer B. & Gibb D. (1980) Chronic pain and neurolytic neural blockade. In *Neural Blockade* (Eds Cousins M.J. & Bridenbaugh P.O.) p. 642. Lippincott, Philadelphia.

Garber J. (1980) Neural blockade for dental, oral and adjoining areas. In: *Neural Blockade* (Eds Cousins M.J. & Bridenbaugh P.O.) p. 423. Lippincott, Philadelphia.

Gotta A.W. & Sullivan G.A. (1981) Anaesthesia of the upper airway using topical anaesthetic and superior laryngeal nerve block. *British Journal of Anaesthesia* **53**, 1055.

Hill J.N., Gershon N.I. & Gargiulo P.O. (1983) Total spinal blockade during local anaesthesia of the nasal passages. *Anesthesiology* **59**, 144.

Jahrsdoerfer R.A. (1981) Anesthesia in otologic surgery. *Otolaryngologic Clinics of North America* **14.3**, 699.

Jolly C. (1980) Clinical use of nerve blocks in relation to surgery. In *General Anaesthesia* 4th edn., vol 1. (Eds Gray T.C., Nunn J.P. & Utting J.E.) p. 381. Butterworths, London.

Jopling M.W., de Sanctus C.A., McDowell D.E., Savarin R.A., Martinez O.A. & Gray D.F. (1983) Anaesthesia for carotid endarterectomy: a comparison of regional and general techniques. *Anesthesiology* **59**, A217.

Karhunen U. & Jönn G. (1982) A comparison of memory function following local and general anaesthesia for extraction of senile cataract. *Anaesthesiologica Scandinavica* **26**, 291.

Keoshian L.A. (1980) Neural blockade for plastic surgery. In *Neural Blockade* (Eds Cousins M.J. & Bridenbaugh P.O.) p. 642. Lippincott, Philadelphia.

Kronman J.H. & Kabani S. (1984) The neuronal basis for diplopia following local anaesthetic injections. *Oral Surgery, Oral Medicine, Oral Pathology* **58**, 533.

Labat G. (1928) *Regional Anaesthesia its Technic and Clinical Application* 2nd edn. pp. 75–323. W.B. Saunders, Philadelphia.

Lipton S. (1979) *Relief of Pain in Clinical Practice* p. 324. Blackwell Scientific Publications, Oxford.

Lynch S., Wolf G. & Berlin I. (1974) 2200 cases of cataract surgery under general anaesthesia. *Anesthesia and Analgesia* **53**, 909.

Martof A.B. (1981) Anesthesia of the teeth supporting structures and oral mucous membrane. *Otolaryngologic Clinics of North America* **14.3**, 653.

McLean N.R. & Watson A.C.H. (1982) Reconstruction of a defect of the ala nasi following trigeminal anaesthesia with an innervated forehead flap. *British Journal of Plastic Surgery* **35**, 201.

Moore D.C. (1975) *Regional Block.* pp. 77–111. Charles C. Thomas, Illinois.

Murphy T.M. (1980) Somatic blockade. In *Neural Blockade* (Eds Cousins M.J. & Bridenbaugh P.O.) p. 423. Lippincott, Philadelphia.

Murphy T.M. (1986) Nerve blocks in the head and neck. In *Anaesthesia* 2nd edn., vol. 2 (Ed. Miller R.D.) p. 1044. Churchill Livingstone, New York.

Murrin K.R. (1985) Awake intubation. In *Difficulties in Tracheal Intubation* (Ed. Latto I.P. & Rosen M.) p. 90. Bailliere Tindall, W.B. Saunders, Eastbourne.

Neill R.S. (1982) Regional anaesthesia for major eyelid surgery in the elderly—an alternative to induced hypotension. *British Journal of Plastic Surgery* **36**, 29.

Neill R.S. (1983) Head and neck surgery. In *Practical Regional Anaesthesia.* (Eds Henderson J.J. & Nimmo W.S.) p. 165. Blackwell Scientific Publications, Oxford.

Nique T.A. & Bennett G.R. (1981) Inadvertent brainstem anesthesia following extraoral trigeminal V2–V3 blocks. *Oral Surgery, Oral Medicine, Oral Pathology* **51**, 468.

Peitzman A.B., Webster M.W., Loubeau J.M., Bahnson H.T. & Grundy B.L. (1982) Carotid endarterectomy under regional (conductive) anaesthesia. *Annals of Surgery* **196**, 59.

Plowman P.C., Thomas W.J.N. & Thurlow A.C. (1974) Cardiac dysrhythmias during anaesthesia for oral surgery. *Anaesthesia* **52**, 689.

Pratt J.M. (1985) Analgesics and sedation in plastic surgery. *Clinics in Plastic Surgery* **12**, 73.

Prough D.S., Scuderi P.E., Stullken E. & Davis C.H. (1984) Myocardial infarction following regional anesthesia for carotid endarterectomy. *Canadian Anaesthetists' Society Journal* **31**, 192.

Sisk A.L. (1986) Evaluation of the Akinosi mandibular block technique in oral surgery. *Journal of Oral Maxillo-Facial Surgery* **44**, 113.

Soutar D.S., Scheker L.R., Tanner N.S.B. & McGregor I.A. (1983) The radial forearm flap: a versatile method for intra-oral reconstruction. *British Journal of Plastic Surgery* **36**, 1.

Spencer F.C. & Eiseman B. (1962) Technique of carotid endarterectomy. *Surgery, Gynecology and Obstetrics* **115**, 115.

Stromberg B.V. (1985) Regional anesthesia in head and neck surgery. *Clinics in Plastic Surgery* **12**, 123.

Swerdlow M. (1980) Complications of neurolytic neural blockade. In *Neural Blockade* (Eds Cousins M.J. & Bridenbaugh P.O.) p. 547. Lippincott, Philadelphia.

Szmyd S.M., Nelson L.B., Calhoun J.H. & Harley R.D. (1984) Retrobulbar anaesthesia in strabismus surgery. *Archives of Ophthalmology* **102**, 1325.

Winnie A.P., Ramamurthy S., Durrani Z. & Radonjic R. (1975) Interscalene cervical plexus block a single injection technique. *Anesthesia and Analgesia* **54**, 370.

Wise R.P. (1984) Pain clinic and operative nerve blocks. In *Wylie and Churchill Davidson's: A Practice of Anaesthesia* (Ed. Churchill Davidson H.C.) p. 893. Lloyd Luke (Medical Books) Ltd., London.

SECTION IV
ACUTE AND CHRONIC PAIN

64

Assessment of Pain

C. R. CHAPMAN

Basic concepts

Pain

Most anaesthetists think of pain as an aversive sensation arising from tissue damage or stress. For most situations in day-to-day clinical life, this is an adequate working definition, but it falters when applied to the distressed patient with labour pain, the querulous postoperative patient or the burn patient terrified of debridement. The concept fails altogether on a chronic pain service where pain complaint often bears little or no relationship to organic pathology. Experience with awake, suffering patients convinces inevitably even the staunchest purist that human pain is linked intimately with emotion, altered powerfully for better or worse by a patient's expectations and beliefs, and correlated imperfectly with tissue injury. Many chronic pain problems seem to be more under the control of psychological factors than of physical disease processes.

It is hardly surprising, therefore, that a confluence of clinical wisdom from many settings and of theory from basic science areas has occurred in the last decade. It is now held that sensory processes signalling tissue injury (nociception) are necessary but not sufficient for a working definition of pain. Wall emphasized this point recently in introducing his textbook on pain (Wall, 1984): 'A revolution is in progress against classical pain mechanisms although even here a few intellectual dodos honour the moribund and sterile corpse'.

A comprehensive conception of pain is needed when one sets out to design a study or assess patients in pain in a specific clinical setting. There is no single solution for how pain should be defined for there are many types of pain, both acute and chronic, in many

different patient populations and settings. The exact working definition chosen must fit the circumstances whilst taking advantage of the state of knowledge in the field.

At present, theory varies with the writer but, in general, pain is seen as a complex and multi-dimensional human perception which involves sensory, affective and cognitive aspects. For the purposes of scaling pain in the individual patient, these dimensions can be considered features or *attributes*, each of which requires a separate operation for number assignment. This brings us to the concept of measurement.

Measurement

As ordinary daily life and clinical practice involve frequent measurements, it seems superfluous to define what it means. Nonetheless, there is disagreement on what the term should mean when subjective states are quantified (Michell, 1986). Before pursuing definitions, it is useful to consider the different types of operations performed under the rubric of pain measurement.

TWO TYPES OF MEASURES

The term 'pain measurement' encompasses two rather different procedures that need to be considered separately. Pure forms of these procedures are described below as types of measurement but in practice, the two are often intertwined.

Type I measurement is objective and typically observational. It occurs when the investigator or clinician assigns numbers to persons (patients or subjects) in order to scale them on one or more attributes. This allows one to test the effects of therapeutic interventions, describe samples or populations of patients or characterize situations that produce pain. In brief, the scores obtained make it possible to compare patients with one another. For example, a set of procedures for scoring patients with low back pain on pain behaviour was used by Keefe and Block (1982) to measure each patient in a sample on the basis of several pain-related attributes (e.g. groaning, sighing). In Type I measurement the criteria for scoring are well defined and independent of the patient.

Type II measurement takes place when numbers are assigned to scale the subjective experience of pain itself i.e. pain is the 'object' being measured and the numbers scale features of the pain such as its intensity or severity. A cardinal characteristic of Type II measurement is that the patient assigns the numbers him- or herself because the experience is private and inaccessible to others. Thus, the measurement is in the hands of the patient rather than of the investigator or clinician, although the latter can provide guidelines or rules to follow.

The contrast of Type I and II measurements exceeds the familiar distinction between objective and subjective; there is a fundamental difference in what is being scaled. In Type I measurement, numbers are assigned to an attribute of the patient whilst in Type II measurement it is the pain itself that is the object of number assignment.

Naturally, controversy exists on whether or not the latter should qualify as scientific measurement, as the investigator does not perform a measurement. We would not normally accept a patient's best estimate of a physiological variable as a valid measure, and critics see no reason to suppose that self-report of pain is any more valid than, say, guessing one's own pulse rate. Defendants of Type II measurement point out that such numbers, when collected carefully, are typically consistent, behave as they should across conditions in which injury varies or drugs are given, and conform to theoretical predictions.

In practice, Type II measurements are treated often as though they were the results of Type I scaling. That is, they become the basis of comparing each patient with another, evaluating effects of treatment, or characterizing patient populations. Although the numbers are merely scores created by each patient to characterize his or her personal experience, typically they are treated as numbers which scale patients relative to one another on an attribute. There are problems inherent in this practice and, indeed, in any form of casual number assignment.

BASIC PROBLEMS IN NUMBER ASSIGNMENT

It is useful to keep in mind that Type I or Type II number assignment itself can always be achieved, but number assignment does not imply that the results are meaningful. For example, in Chinese medicine there are 12 pulses at the wrist, each with several measurable features (six on each side). It is said that it takes at least a decade to master the skill, but supposedly a master of oriental medicine can diagnose conditions very accurately. If a coding scheme is developed carefully and a group of 20 masters is recruited for a study of, say, migraine headache, Type I number assignment proceeds well. Patients can be measured during headache, and while pain-free by each of the masters, and the results can be compared. But are consistent judgements obtained? Does this constitute measurement?

Similarly, a psychiatrist may theorize that anxiety is a feature of pain in certain types of patients and develop a Type II self-report scale in which patients indicate by numbers the anxiety aspect of certain painful events. But patients are not trained to distinguish between arousal and anxiety. Nor do they know the distinction between fear and anxiety (the former has a definite object, the latter is diffuse). The patients will yield numbers and these are probably consistent; but is the psychiatrist scaling what he or she thinks is being measured? Can we presume that we have scaled what we set out to scale because patients co-operated cheerfully and provided numbers that fitted our expectations?

These examples show that, although assigning numbers is necessary for measurement, it may not be sufficient. Correct measurement requires always:

1 Reliability. Measurements should yield consistent outcomes when performed under similar conditions or when repeated under similar circumstances.
2 Validity. Measurements should scale precisely what they purport to scale.

While the clinical investigator must be careful to use reliable and valid measurements, he or she must also be pragmatic. Measurement is constrained by the health of patients, limited manpower and the nature of the clinical situation. When obtaining data from patients, it is important to impose the smallest possible responder burden and still obtain the highest quality of information possible under the circumstances.

A final consideration (although not a requirement for measurement) is precision: the random error associated with measurement should be small. Ideally, measurement should be reasonably sensitive to differences and should reflect such differences faithfully. As described below, the interpretation of these principles depends in practice upon which measurement tradition is followed.

Three traditions of measurement

Michell (1986) has reviewed three traditional approaches to measurement of subjective and behavioural variables:
1 Classical theory.
2 Operational theory.
3 Representational theory.

Classical theory

This approach clearly dominates contemporary science and the practice of measurement in the field of pain. Classical theory is concerned with scoring objects according to attributes which they possess i.e. quantifying 'how much' of an attribute an object has. In order to qualify for measurement, an attribute must be quantitative. The classical theorist seeks to quantify the patient or research subject as an end in itself; rather, the goal is to discover numerical relations between variables by the process of measurement.

Duncan (1975) asserted that science should begin with a highly refined theoretical basis from which one can derive models or predictions. The models specify relationships among theoretical constructs and measures, and must be defined algebraically by a set of equations. For Duncan, the purpose of science is to test and refine such models; the goal of research is to produce equations or models that are 'true' i.e. mathematically unambiguous and coherent. The most important criterion for identifying an attribute to measure is the theory within which one is working. In this measurement tradition, rating scale data, test scores and other types of subjective reports have meaning so long as they reflect the structure of *theoretical* variables. Although these variables are not in themselves measurable, the scores obtained are considered to provide valid representations of latent (theoretical rather than actual) variables.

While classicists assume that an attribute to be measured must be quantitative, they put no limits on the evidence necessary for support of this assumption. Therefore they accept numbers that have been generated by the objects of measurement themselves (e.g. pain reports—Type II measures) provided that theory allows one to equate self-reports with attributes that objects possess. Measures, however obtained, are considered always to be unconstrained numbers and any form of statistical manipulation may be imposed on such numbers. The issue of what a self-report of pain really means is one that is to be resolved by theory alone.

Operational theory

The operationalist perspective is six decades old and owes its identity to Bridgman (1927) who contended that a theoretical concept was equivalent to and defined by a corresponding set of operations. For the operational theorist, measurement is simply an operation that produces numbers. Measures are consistent numerical assignments produced by precisely defined operations, and quantitative relations among operations are held to be very important. Few, if any, pure operationalists remain, but their fundamental principle can be found: a single measure of a thing, clearly defined by an operation, suffices.

Certain psychological ability tests of performance yield scores that qualify as measurements for most operationalists because they are produced by clearly defined operations. However, self-reports generated by the objects of study themselves (pain reports produced by patients in pain) lack a set of clearly defined operations on the part of the investigator and therefore fail to qualify as valid measures.

The operational approach, which holds that a single score yielded by an operation undertaken by the investigator is a pain measurement, has been resisted by many investigators because it is limiting. Some contend that such an approach oversimplifies scientific processes greatly. The operationalist cannot account for hypothetical constructs derived from theory which are necessary for many complex calculations in the physical, natural and social sciences as these numbers do not qualify as measures. Operational traditions appeal to some clinicians who attempt to assess and treat chronic pain patients. The popularity of this approach has been enhanced by the lack of consistent, effective psychological theory to account for and guide interventions for chronic pain problems.

Representational theory

Stevens (1946, 1975) has influenced strongly the practice of measurement in psychology and related areas through his arguments that numbers represent empirical relations amongst the objects that are measured. For those who follow this persuasion, measurement produces a numerical representation of empirical fact. Variables and relationships between variables exist in nature, and the purpose of measurement is to characterize these relationships through number assignment. If this is true, the subject matter of science can be manipulated statistically. Obviously, it is critical that the numbers be faithful representations of the true relationships among the variables in nature.

The representationalists argue that there are different types of relationships between scales. The simplest form of a relationship is classification. One might classify patients with postoperative pain in three categories: abdominal, orthopaedic, and head and neck. This type of categorization would be called a *nominal* scale.

Another type of scale is characterized by weak order. One type of object may be said to be greater with regard to some attribute than another. Thus, one might argue that a thoracotomy (score = 12) produces more postoperative pain than a gastrectomy (score = 8) which in turn produces more pain than an appendicectomy (score = 4). This statement of rank order is termed an *ordinal* scale. The investigator can talk about greater than or less than but can make no more precise statements than those of order. It is meaningless to ask if the difference in pain between the thoracotomy and gastrectomy patient is of the same magnitude as that between the gastrectomy and appendicectomy patient. The only information in ordinal data lies in the greater than or less than relationship. The scale would convey exactly the same information on the three patients if the scores were 250, 18 and 1 instead 12, 8 and 4.

In the third type of scale, the *interval* scale, the numbers assigned to the objects permit one to interpret the differences between scores. The Fahrenheit scale of temperature provides a good example of an interval scale. In this case 0° does not mean a total absence of heat (it is an arbitrary number), but one can say that $40\,°F - 30\,°F = 80\,°F - 70\,°F$.

Finally, the *ratio* scale is characterized by an absolute zero. The length of a surgical incision provides an example in which zero has an absolute meaning (total absence of surgical insult). The patient with a 20 cm incision has a wound four times as long as the patient whose incision is 5 cm and (although it is pointless) one could calculate the total length of surgical incisions in patients operated upon by surgeon X and compare those with similar scores from a set of matched patients operated upon by surgeon Y. In this case, the numbers are meaningful relative to an absolute 0.

The strong influence of the representationalists in measurement is derived from their conviction that there are different types of measurement scales (nominal, ordinal, interval and ratio) and that one should classify all scores according to scale type. They have contended that statistical manipulation of the numbers obtained by measurement should be appropriate for the type of scale involved. Although conventional statistics are appropriate for ratio and interval scales, means and variances should not be calculated on ordinal or nominal scales. Such manipulation of numbers would distort the relationship between the scores and the actual variables as they exist in nature. On ranked scores the investigator must use non-parametric statistics suitable for ordinal data. Similarly, calculation of medians for scores which are characterized by nominal scaling would be forbidden and only statistical techniques suitable for categorized data (frequency counts) could be employed. It has been argued often by representationalists that subjective report data derived from rating scales must not be subjected to normal statistical manipulation (cannot be characterized by means, standard deviations, etc.) and can only be treated by statistics designed to handle rank order.

Michell (1986) has pointed out that the statistical restriction principles of the representationalists can be applied only to representationalists themselves, and that researchers who operate from a basis of classical theory are not obliged to follow them. The classicist would argue that, in common with the operationalists, the representationalists are guilty of oversimplifying the conduct of science. By and large, scientists do not work with numbers as representations of otherwise inaccessible relationships among variables in nature. Rather, scientists operate on the basis of theory (or models) and hypothesize such relationships. Therefore, the meaning one can derive from a scaling procedure depends on the theory from which one operates and blind commitment to a set of rules on how one handles numbers statistically may impose an unnecessary constraint on scientific endeavour.

Theory and current practices

There are many procedures for measuring pain; most reflect classical theory but the strong influence of the operationalists and representationalists is seen in cur-

Table 64.1 Type I methods used for the evaluation of pain

Physiological
Increased plasma cortisol
Increased plasma catecholamine
Changes in cardiovascular variable (heart rate,
arterial pressure, cardiac output)
Changes in respiratory variables (frequency, VC,
$FEV_{1.0}$, PEFR)

Neuropharmacological
Correlates inversely with plasma β-endorphin
Change in skin temperature

Neurological
Nerve conduction velocity
Evoked potentials
Single positron emission tomography
Microneurography

VC = vital capacity.
$FEV_{1.0}$ = forced expiratory volume in 1 sec.
PEFR = peak expiratory flow rate.

rent practice. It is helpful to recognize the theoretical basis for measurement in research or clinical practice.

Procedures for measuring pain (Table 64.1)

Clinical investigators have attempted to quantify pain using physiological, subjective report and behavioural variables. The scientific and clinical inference permitted by these approaches depends on the theoretical perspective of the investigator, the measurement tradition in which he or she is working and the limitations inherent in the measurements themselves. A review of pain measurement follows, and the advantages and limitations of the various approaches are discussed.

Physiological indicators of pain

PATHOPHYSIOLOGICAL CORRELATES

Both acute and chronic pain states may be associated with pathophysiological changes detected by examination or investigation (Syrjala & Chapman, 1984; Chapman *et al.*, 1985).

Moore and McQuay (1985) have described the response of the adrenal cortex to a surgical insult. Plasma cortisol increases with the start of surgery. The degree of this response is a function of the size of the incision. Increased plasma cortisol concentrations continue into the postoperative period for one or more days, but marked decreases in plasma cortisol occur when the anaesthetic is terminated. Large systemic

doses of opioids such as morphine, fentanyl or sufentanil decrease cortisol responses to surgery and administration of a high dose of naloxone antagonizes this effect. However, this response is independent of consciousness, and plasma cortisol concentrations vary with the anaesthetic alone. Although it may be an indicator of stress, it is an imperfect correlate of pain.

Acute pain states such as postoperative pain are accompanied often by motor reflexes that produce muscle spasm or splinting. For example, surgical trauma to the chest or abdomen may result in impaired ventilation. Gastrointestinal and genito-urinary inhibition, which encompass both ileus and smooth muscle spasm, reflect autonomic reflexes associated with acute pain (Chapman & Bonica, 1983). In addition, increases in arterial pressure and cardiac output and increased respiratory rate are associated with catecholamine release. Thus, variables which are monitored routinely postoperatively may reflect the presence of pain (see Chapter 66, p. 1180).

The presence of pain may be accompanied by trophic changes in certain chronic pain syndromes. In the older patient with clearly defined trigger points and myofascial pain, subtle indicators of autonomic dysfunction such as enhanced pilomotor segmental reflex, vaso- and pseudomotor disturbances of the skin in addition to trophoedematous changes in subcutaneous tissues may be observed (Gunn & Milbrandt, 1978; Gunn, 1988).

Neuropharmacological correlation

Intense interest in the endorphins in recent decades has led to the development of elaborate neurophysiological models for the modulation of pain. Both β-endorphin and β-lipotropin (its precursor) are thought to be released during acute pain. As β-endorphin is an endogenous opioid, pain intensity should be diminished in its presence. Szyfelbin and Osgood (1985) measured endorphin concentration in the plasma of patients in pain and found that it was correlated negatively with acute pain report i.e. the greater the β-endorphin concentrations, the lower the reported pain. Because of its inverse relationship to pain report, endorphin concentration may be a better indicator of endogenous pain modulation than of pain itself. A major limitation of this approach is that endorphins have been linked also to stress. Their presence does not provide unequivocal evidence of the existence of pain because they may be released as part of a global stress reaction.

When pain is chronic, pathophysiological changes may be detected sometimes at the site of the pain. *Thermography*, the measurement of skin temperature patterns, has received considerable attention in recent years. Thermographers contend that skin temperature may be used in the evaluation of certain types of chronic pain (Rubal *et al.*, 1982). It is well known that dysautonomias including reflex sympathetic dystrophy produce temperature changes in the affected extremities (Bonica, 1980). Skin temperature is low in the afflicted area in myofascial pain syndromes, certain cancer pain syndromes, and a few other pain states. This temperature change is probably indicative of altered sympathetic nervous system function. Conversely, arthritis may produce abnormal warmth because of acute inflammation.

Neurological measures

Painful and non-painful peripheral neuropathies, entrapment syndromes and nerve injuries are evaluated sometimes by studies in which *nerve conduction velocities* are assessed in the larger nerves of an extremity. A skin electrode is used to stimulate the nerve and its discharge is recorded distally. Such measures are non-specific as all components of the nerve are activated, and, because nerve endings are not activated, pathology and other factors specific to them cannot be evaluated. Activity in the larger and faster conducting fibres may obscure responses in the smaller and slower conducting fibres which carry nociceptive information. Altered nerve conduction velocities are not synonymous with the presence of pain. Some patients demonstrate abnormal nerve conduction velocities despite being asymptomatic neurologically, whilst others who take medication such as phenytoin may show reduced conduction velocities in the absence of structural changes in peripheral nerves (Thomas, 1984).

Short-latency, *evoked potentials* are used sometimes to study peripheral neuropathology including pain-related neurological dysfunction. They are used also for surgical monitoring. For example, Campbell and Lipton (1985) recorded intraspinal somatosensory-evoked potentials associated with median nerve stimulation during percutaneous cervical cordotomy performed to relieve chronic pain. This type of approach does not lead easily to the independent scaling or even verification of clinical pain as median nerve stimulation is unrelated to clinical pain state. The use of long-latency, evoked-potential procedures in volunteers who undergo painful dental or cutaneous stimulation has been reviewed by Chudler and Dong (1983) and Chapman and Saeger (1985). However, these methods have not been used with pain patients or in clinical research.

A new scanning technology, *single positron emission tomography* (PET), seems promising for evaluation of certain pain states. It allows the study of regional cerebral blood flow and regional glucose metabolic rate. It employs low intensity radioactive isotopes attached to metabolically active molecules to provide markers for the amount of neurological activity in various parts of the brain. It may be used to identify foci in patients with partial epilepsy or to characterize brain activity patterns in schizophrenics. As with other neurological measures, this technology should be used concomitantly with subjective report of pain in order to be valid. If extended studies of thalamus or other brain areas prove promising, PET may help to validate pain complaint in the absence of other organic evidence.

Finally, extensive development of *microneurography* and the related procedure of intraneural stimulation appears promising as a technology for assessing chronic pain related to peripheral neuropathy (Ochoa *et al.*, 1985). In this technically demanding procedure, electrodes must be placed accurately upon fibres within a peripheral nerve. By delivering low levels of electrical currents to target fibres, a neurologist can activate primary sensory units or sets of units in combination, and abnormal firing patterns may be identified. When this has been accomplished successfully, the neurologist is able to identify precisely the peripheral origin of a neuropathical pain problem and he or she may replicate the pain by electrical stimulation of the involved pathways. Work performed so far indicates that fibre type is the important determinant of pain rather than pattern of discharge. The quality of pain varies with fibre type whether Aδ or C.

To be meaningful, microneurography data require concomitant verbal report of pain by the patient. The electrical signals obtained do not yield unequivocal evidence on the activation of nociceptive processes or even Aδ- versus C-fibre pain. This approach represents surely a major advance in pain diagnosis, but it does not offer a definitive or fully objective measure of pain.

Advantages and limitations of physiological approaches

Most physiological indicators of pain are correlates of nociception. In common with alterations in muscle tone, trophoedema and other autonomically mediated indicators occur concomitantly with pain but for the most part do not play a causal role. The value of correlates as measures depends on the theoretical perspective of the investigator or clinician. From the viewpoint of the classical theorist such indicators may prove to be powerful measures given that basic relationships among variables have been established clearly by preliminary work and a well-developed model for these relationships has been defined.

Measures of neurological function appear to offer considerable promise for the evaluation of certain types of pain. However, the major problems seen on a chronic pain service (back pain and headache) cannot be evaluated by these approaches. Moreover, neurological methods cannot stand alone. Abnormal neurological function can be observed in the absence of pain, and it is only the co-existence and correspondence of verbal report with neurological abnormality that allows correct diagnosis or scientific inference. This being the case, it is often most cost effective to depend upon verbal report alone.

Self-report measurement procedures (Table 64.2)

All self-report techniques are Type II measures i.e. the patient performs the act of number assignment. There are many variations on this approach, and they include both single- and multi-dimensional methods. These are evaluated below and examples are provided in Fig. 64.1.

SINGLE-DIMENSION METHODS

The simplest and most frequently used procedures for subjective pain report are:
1 Category scales.

Table 64.2 Type II methods used for the evaluation of pain

Single-dimension methods
Category scales
Numerical rating scales
Visual analogue scales

Multi-dimensional methods
McGill pain questionnaire
Dartmouth pain questionnaire
West Haven–Yale multi-dimensional pain inventory
Brief pain inventory
Pain perception profile
Behavioural observational techniques
Pain diaries
Physician pain rating
Sickness impact profile
Rehabilitation tests

CATEGORY SCALE (CS)
Please check the category that best describes your pain:
____Mild   ____Horrible
____Discomforting ____Excrutiating
____Distressing

NUMERICAL RATING SCALE (NRS)
Please choose a number from 0 to 100 to describe the intensity of your pain. Zero indicates no pain and 100 means that the pain is as bad as it can be.

VISUAL ANALOGUE SCALE (VAS)
Mark the line below to indicate the intensity of your pain.

No pain   Pain as bad as
                                            it can be

Fig. 64.1 Typical scales for subjective pain report (shown with instructions to patient).

2 Numerical rating scales.
3 Visual analogue scales.

Each of these represents a simple paper and pencil instrument which the patient uses to produce a record of his or her pain report.

Category scales (CSs) make minimal demand upon the patient; it is necessary only to choose the best word descriptor for the pain. Test devices of this nature are known sometimes as verbal rating scales. They are employed commonly for both nominal and ordinal scaling, depending on whether or not the category descriptors connote a ranking among the categories. Sometimes category methods are used to produce interval scales, and Borg (1982) has developed a ratio category scale which combines adjectives and adverbs with the numbers 1 to 10.

An example of an ordinal category scale is given by Melzack and Torgerson (1971) who introduced a scale which is still used extensively for describing pain intensity (Fig. 64.1). Any suitable set of categories can be constructed depending on what one wishes to measure. Moreover, CSs are not limited to words. A facial expression picture scale involving eight cartoon faces ranked according to expressed displeasure has been developed for pain assessment (Frank et al., 1982). The obvious advantage of the category scale approach is its simplicity and suitability for all types of patients. Its major disadvantage is statistical. It produces simple category data with a limited range. In practice, patients tend to use the middle rather than the ends of category scales and thus the range of responses is reduced further and to some extent distorted.

Numerical rating scale (NRS) (Fig. 64.1). Patients are asked to indicate how intense their pain feels (any dimension can be measured in this way, such as aversiveness) on a scale of 0–10. In effect, this scale uses 10 categories, but the categories are ranked in a way that implies interval scaling. Most patients can comprehend the scale and it can be administered easily.

Visual analogue scale (VAS) is perhaps the most intensively studied method. This consists typically of a 10 cm line with verbal anchors at both ends (Fig. 64.1). Scoring may be accomplished by the patient marking the line and measuring the length of the line to the mark. There are many variations of this approach. Tick marks may be placed upon the line or numbers may be placed below the line. The scales may be arranged horizontally or vertically. The important consideration is that the patients understand the two end-points and that they are free to indicate a response at any point in the scale.

Such methods are more demanding of patients than CSs. Researchers have found that 7–11% of patients cannot complete the VAS, or find it confusing (Revill *et al.*, 1976; Kremer *et al.*, 1980a) and in one report 26 of 98 patients in a particular sample were unable to complete a VAS (Walsh & Bowman, 1984). Sometimes patients who have difficulty with the VAS, including elderly patients and those with limited education, can be trained to use it through examples with familiar pain problems.

Critical evaluation of the VAS was undertaken by Carlsson (1983) who examined it as an indicator of both pain state and pain relief and chronic pain in patients. She compared different forms of the scale and found that reliability as judged from consistency of response to two different forms was low. This led Carlsson to conclude that the validity of the VAS procedure for chronic pain assessment may be unsatisfactory. There are other studies, however, which support both the reliability and validity of the VAS as a measure of pain and change in pain (Revill *et al.*, 1976; Kremer *et al.*, 1980a).

Advantages and disadvantages of single-dimensional scaling

The broad advantages of single-dimensional scaling methods are their simplicity and efficiency. They provide only a minimal responder burden for patients. The same scale can be used in a wide variety of different settings and most patients can understand the task of measuring pain with these technologies. They produce numbers directly and do not require elaborate scoring. In addition, they make sense intrinsically both to the patient and to the data collector (that is, they have high face validity).

On the negative side, these methods are subject to subtle distortions and may be misused by patients who appear to understand them but do not. More importantly, they oversimplify the complex human experience of pain. A data collector may ask for sensory intensity but obtain a response that reflects emotional arousal or aversiveness. Despite these limitations, unidimensional self-report methods remain the most efficient and popular way of scaling pain in a clinical setting.

Which of the three methods is the best? Jensen *et al.* (1986) evaluated several types of scales for administering pain and concluded that the NRS was the most practical index. They recommended developing an NRS that includes 100 points which scale pain in addition to a 0 which indicates no pain. However, the investigator or clinician should consider all three carefully in light of his or her own unique needs and patient population before arriving at a decision. There is no substitute for careful pilot trials which compare the different methods available.

MULTI-DIMENSIONAL SELF-REPORT:
CLASSICAL TRADITION

The requirements for comprehensive measurement of pain are:
1 The investigator should adopt or develop a model for pain perception that involves multiple dimensions.
2 Instruments for the simultaneous measurement of these dimensions (each being an attribute of pain) be employed.

The most pragmatic approach to this problem is use of several VAS or NRS scales but this causes inherent problems. First, it is impossible to ensure that responses to the different scales are not correlated with one another. Basically, the response to the first scale administered will probably influence the response to following scales. It is important that patients respond to each scale without the opportunity to compare the present response with other, earlier responses (Carlsson, 1983).

Several complex pencil and paper tests have been developed to allow simultaneous multi-dimensional scaling. The best known and most extensively tested multi-dimensional scale is the *McGill pain questionnaire*

(MPQ). The method is designed to scale pain in three dimensions: sensory, affective and evaluative. Patients are presented with 20 sets of words that describe pain and are asked to select those sets which seem relevant to their pain. They are instructed to circle the words within each set that best describes the pain. There are from two to six words within each set, and these vary in intensity for the quality described by that set. Sensory qualities are represented by the first 10 sets. The following five indicate affective quality, the 16th set is evaluative and the last four sets are miscellaneous words. There are methods for scoring each dimension and also to obtain a total score.

A supplement to the MPQ, the *Dartmouth pain questionnaire* (DPQ) has been developed to allow the assessment of three additional factors. These include a general affective dimension, an indication of the time course and intensity of the pain, and a record of behaviour affected by the presence of pain (Corson & Schneider, 1984). An advantage of the DPQ is its consideration of those remaining positive aspects of functioning in chronic pain patients; most methods simply assess impairment.

The MPQ has been studied extensively and has shown to have high reliability and strong concurrent validity in addition to adequate factor structure (Syrjala & Chapman, 1984; Chapman *et al.*, 1985). Its advantage in pain measurement is its comprehensiveness. On the negative side, the MPQ has a much greater responder burden. It takes 5–15 min to complete, and the vocabulary used by the test exceeds the language capability of some patients. Moreover, the scoring procedures, whilst straightforward, are simple compared with those of most mental tests of comparable size. Turk *et al.* (1985) argue that the total score derived from the MPQ is valid as a general measure of pain severity; however, individual scale scores should not be interpreted according to their unique scales because adequate discriminate validity cannot be demonstrated. Walsh and Bowman (1984) reported that patients who complete the MPQ in the presence of their spouses may give responses that reflect spouse interference or opinion.

Despite criticism, the MPQ is a standard in the field of pain measurement and it remains the first choice for assessing the quality or character of a patient's pain, particularly its sensory aspects and affective impact. Although the responder burden is substantial, the scale may be determined by reading out each word set and having patients indicate responses verbally. This allows even very sick patients to complete the test. (If this alternative is chosen, it is necessary to maintain a standard format; Klepac *et al.*, 1981.)

Kerns *et al.* (1985) have offered the *West Haven–Yale multi-dimensional pain inventory* (WHYMPI) as an alternative to the MPQ. This method is briefer and more classic in its psychometrics than the MPQ. There are three parts to this 52-item test. The first provides five general dimensions of the experience of pain, interference with normal family and work function, and social support. The second is concerned with patient perception of how others respond to displays of pain and suffering. The third concerns the frequency with which the patient engages in common daily activities as a function of pain. From the viewpoint of classical measurement theory this method has been derived from cognitive behavioural models of chronic pain and assesses constructs appropriate to such models. In this sense, it is far more focused than the MPQ, but the meaning of the outcome obtained is more model dependent.

The MPQ, DPQ and WHYMPI have all been designed to examine problems of chronic pain. Sometimes the investigator or clinician needs to assess acute or persisting pain problems of a progressive nature such as cancer pain or the pain of an arthritic condition. In these cases, it is not always necessary to conduct extensive evaluation of social contingencies for pain behaviour. A short and efficient measure of worst, average and current pain may be obtained by using the *brief pain inventory* (BPI) developed by Cleeland and colleagues (Daut *et al.*, 1983; Cleeland, 1985). This method scales pain relief also from medication and the extent to which pain interferes with the quality of life.

MULTI-DIMENSIONAL SELF-REPORT:
REPRESENTATIONAL TRADITION

Investigators who embrace representational theory when conducting clinical measurement are dissatisfied with most subjective report techniques as they do not follow the rules for scaling nor do they permit the use of normal parametric statistics by the criteria of the representationalist. These investigators have approached multi-dimensional scaling by using a psychophysical technique known as *cross-modality matching*. With this technique, a sensory experience is quantified by matching it to the experience of a precisely controlled stimulus in another sensory modality. One might, for example, produce a safe experimental pain by pressing with controlled force on a finger at the base of the nail and ask the patient to match the intensity of the pain produced to the loudness of a tone that he or she controls by adjusting decibels. A complex technology is used to relate spontaneous pain of natural origin to control stimuli in other sense modalities (Stevens, 1975).

In pain research, words describing pain are matched typically to line length or hand grip, both of these are matched to an experimental pain, and then scaling standards for the relationship for words describing pain to clinical pain are derived. Once this operation has been performed, the technique can be applied to clinical pain assessment. There is no limit to which or how many dimensions of pain one can scale. Gracely et al. (1979) used this approach to scale both pain intensity and unpleasantness.

Tursky et al. (1982) have used a cross-modality matching approach to develop a procedure for assessing clinical pain, the *pain perception profile*. This method measures sensation threshold, employs magnitude estimation procedures to judge induced pain, scales pain on intensity, reaction and sedation dimensions (employing verbal pain descriptors), and permits the registration of these three dimensions in a diary format for repeated assessment over time. In brief, it assesses pain through the use of psychophysically scaled verbal descriptors. This type of procedure is shorter and less demanding for patients than the MPQ, once the psychophysical scaling has been completed.

Potentially, the data obtained by cross-modality matching should be more reliable and valid than those of these simpler unidimensional self-report scales such as VAS. It is uncertain to what extent independent validation is required for different pain populations. Use of this approach probably necessitates substantial development including experimental pain testing before one could interpret confidently scores obtained from pain patients. Future development of this approach may yield substantial advances in pain measurement technology, but the disparity in philosophy of measurement between classicists and representationalists may limit its adoption.

MULTI-DIMENSIONAL BEHAVIOURAL SCALING:
OPERATIONAL TRADITION

For the behaviourist, who is concerned with what people do, pain as a subjective state is meaningless. It can be defined only as a pattern of behaviour. Measurement consists of identifying behaviours and scoring them according to frequency, speed, rate or accuracy. Because behaviours differ markedly with different pain

syndromes, methods analogous to the MPQ do not exist within this approach. Methods are highly specific, and back pain has been studied more extensively than other pain problems.

Keefe and Block (1982) and Keefe and Hill (1985) have shown that patients with back pain engage in grimacing, guarding their movements, rubbing the affected body area and sighing. Measures of these behaviours proved reliable and valid in relation to pain reports, and they occurred more frequently in pain patients than in either normals or depressed control patients. Pain behaviour patterns can be quantified in terms of frequency or rate of occurrence and scaled by trained observers either directly or with the use of video-taped records of patients in selected settings involving specific task performance. Behaviour patterns that are non-trivial are invariably complex, and most behavioural observational systems are correspondingly multi-dimensional. In general, behaviours are tallied over time and scored by frequency counts.

Behavioural observational techniques may include measures derived by mechanical force transducers or other monitors of behaviour. Keefe and Hill (1985) employed a transducer placed in the patients' shoes in order to assess walking parameters. During video taping, both patients and normal controls were required to walk 5 metres. Guarding, bracing, rubbing the painful area, sighing and grimacing were scored by judges. Investigators found that patients walked more slowly than normals, took smaller steps, did not show a normal symmetrical gait pattern and in general exhibited more pain behaviour. This study serves as an excellent demonstration of how behavioural observation may be employed for study of chronic pain.

Whilst these methods are potentially powerful, they are extremely specific. Patients with headache, for example, would probably appear indistinguishable from normals on the test basis developed by Keefe and Hill (1985). In light of this limitation, Keefe et al. (1985) evaluated pain in patients with head and neck cancer using behavioural techniques. These patients displayed their pain primarily through facial expression rather than through guarded movement or postural changes.

A solution to the problem of specificity in behavioural measures might lie with the identification of broad behavioural indicators of pain that are common to different clinical populations. Linton (1985) investigated the general level of activity in chronic back pain patients, hypothesizing that reported pain intensity is related inversely to general level of activity. This activity was measured by self-monitoring or observed behaviour in a test situation. The reported intensity of chronic pain was unrelated to general activity level; and thus, general activity does not appear to be a suitable global indicator of pain state.

MULTI-DIMENSIONAL SELF-REPORT OF BEHAVIOURS: PAIN IS INFERRED FROM REPORTS ON COMPLEX ACTIVITIES

Type II measures of pain behaviours are gathered sometimes because it is more efficient and cost effective to ask people about behaviour and habits than to video tape and score such activity formally. In some cases it is not the patient who is asked but the spouse or some other daily observer who lives with the patient. Strictly speaking, the use of formal test instruments to yield scores is viable behaviourism; however, the pure behaviourist would be loathe to accept self-report of activities as measures of those activities. It is the business of the behaviourist to score the patient; it is less than legitimate for the patient to score him- or herself. Using the spouse to score the patient is viable behaviourism provided that the spouse qualifies as a trained and objective observer. From the classical viewpoint, what one makes of a self-reported record of behaviour depends on the theoretical perspective of the investigator. Cognitive behavioural psychologists have elaborate models for how thinking and beliefs affect behaviour; for them, this type of approach can be a rich source of information.

Chronic pain clinics sometimes use the *pain diary* for behavioural self-report. These records consist typically of a log of daily activities allocated to small intervals of time. The activities recorded are relevant to pain and would be allocated to sitting, standing and walking, and reclining, for example. The patient notes the specific activity within the appropriate category and indicates the time and duration of the activity. In most instances, clinicians ask the patient also to provide an NRS for pain level for each hour and to indicate the medications taken.

There are strong advantages associated with pain diaries. Because these measures are obtained daily, they are distorted neither by memory nor by the mental attitude of the patient. Moreover, the diary relates pain to patterns of normal activity as opposed to contrived activities such as those used in video-tape observational studies. Extended time patterns involving days or weeks may be derived from examination of pain diaries as may any relationship between pain, activity and medication intake.

A limitation of the pain diary is that its reliability is unknown and may vary greatly from patient to patient. The record produced day by day is disturbing to some patients because their less than ideal habit patterns become apparent over time, and they may refuse to complete it or may distort it. Others complete the diary retrospectively just before appointments, thus defeating the purpose of the measurement.

In using the pain diary or any other similar device, the clinician presumes the patient or the spouse is a reliable historian and capable of accurate record keeping. Ready *et al.* (1982) examined reported medication uses in patients with chronic pain and found that these patients reported drug consumption 50–60% lower than actual drug usage. Kremer *et al.* (1980b) found discrepancies when they compared patient records with staff observations of patient activity or social behaviour. Similarly, Sanders (1983) compared the activity time reported by pain patients with records derived from automatic monitoring of activity in normal controls, psychiatric patients and patients with chronic back pain. All three groups reported less activity than the automated monitoring equipment indicated, but the discrepancy was greatest in chronic back pain. These studies challenge the validity of self-report methods as indicators of behaviours. Until further information is available or these methods are refined further, they are regarded best as doubtful methods with a high liability for patient response bias.

Physicians set up sometimes a standardized system for *health care provider patient pain rating*. The simplest form of this type is classification of patients (nominal scaling). Whether this can be termed measurement is debatable, but representationalists may argue that categorical scaling is the simplest form of measurement. Typically, diagnostic data and medical history are employed to categorize patients with pain. The diagnostic value of physician measures has been investigated by Tearnan and Dar (1986).

In some circumstances it is useful to provide a rating of patients (e.g. none, mild, moderate or severe pain) based on what the patient does when faced with certain tasks such as lifting a standard weight. This is a form of *ability testing* which is scaled rather simply. This may be biased if the rater knows the patient's diagnosis or medical condition, and it is difficult to avoid stereotyping patients on the basis of age, sex or racial categories. When these methods are used, it is critical that raters be trained carefully with well-defined criteria for judgement.

MULTI-DIMENSIONAL SCALING OF PAIN-RELATED FUNCTION: CLASSICAL TRADITION

The measurement of functional status is a good example of classical measurement. It is difficult to interpret any measures of function apart from a well-defined concept of sickness impact or disability. The presence of persisting pain disturbs usually the ability of the patient to function normally, and this can be quantified if representative behaviours sensitive to pain are identified and measured. For example, patients with low back pain spend more time reclining or in bed because of the pain, restrict normal social and recreational activities, and have difficulty maintaining gainful employment. These disturbances can be defined as sickness impact. They can be measured by activity diaries or by any method which scales systematically typical physical, social and psychological limitations imposed by painful illness.

A global indicator of sickness impact which has been well validated is a *sickness impact profile* or SIP (Bergner *et al.*, 1981). This method is not pain specific but provides a general indicator of health status. It is designed to be self-administered but can be given via structured interview if necessary. Three aspects are measured: physical, psychosocial and overall. Follick *et al.* (1985) found that chronic pain patients seen at a multi-disciplinary pain service showed impaired function on the SIP. The psychosocial dimension of the method correlated significantly with scores from the Minnesota multi-phasic personality inventory (MMPI) and the physical dimension score related inversely to independent measures of activity.

Mayer *et al.* (1986) have developed a set of rehabilitation-focused tests which consists of mostly *objective physical function measures* suitable for patients with low back pain. In combination with psychological measures, these tests provide eight categories of scaling:

1 Range of motion.
2 Cardiovascular fitness and muscular endurance.
3 Gait speed.
4 Time on simulated daily activities.
5 Static lifting.
6 Lifting under load.
7 Isometric and isokinetic dynamic trunk strength.
8 Global effort.

These measures provide a comprehensive assessment of functional capacity which can be obtained repeatedly through the course of treatment. The method was used in a therapeutic trial with a group of patients whose initial unemployment rate was 92%. Eighty-two percent of these patients returned to work following treatment with this rehabilitation model combined with psychological intervention. Patients who were rehabilitated successfully maintained high VAS pain reports, indicating that rehabilitation may be achieved without major reduction in reported pain. This outcome stresses the need for comprehensive, multi-dimensional assessment when complex clinical issues are under investigation.

Bias and pain measurement

The quantification of pain may be inaccurate systematically if any or all of three factors influence the measurements:

1 Investigator bias.
2 Patient bias.
3 Consistent technical errors in data collection or scoring.

Both Type I and Type II measures are sensitive to these three sources of bias.

Investigator bias in Type I measures has been noted above. Knowledge of a patient's history, interaction with a patient or beliefs regarding the patient's medical condition may affect scoring. To obviate this, raters must perform their tasks objectively and have had no prior knowledge of, or contact with, the patient being evaluated. Strictly defined criteria help also to protect against bias.

Investigator bias may interact with patient bias in Type II measurement when patient's expectations or beliefs are shaped by statements or actions on the part of physicians. Patients tend to do what is expected of them in most circumstances, and in chronic pain certain patients exaggerate pain complaint in an attempt to enhance the credibility of a pain problem which exists in the absence of organic disease.

Patient bias is always a problem in Type II measurement, as the investigator exercises no control over the patient's report. Although this type of bias may be offset by clear instructions and guidance, patients' responses are shaped inevitably by beliefs on personal health, expectations surrounding their present situation and possibly personal social or financial goals.

The pain report may vary greatly as a function of the presence or absence of family members. The patient who appears tranquil and resigned on the first day following major surgery is sometimes seen to break into tears and display exaggerated pain behaviour when the spouse enters the room. Pain reports collected in the presence of the spouse may differ markedly from those collected when the spouse is absent.

Patient bias may arise also when the patient is asked to recall past pain states or to scale pain that is no longer present or has changed. It has been shown that the ability of patients to remember pain while in a relatively pain-free state is reasonably accurate for approximately a week after surgery (Hunter et al., 1979; Kwilosc et al., 1984). However, when pain continues for a prolonged period and comparisons of pain are made over time, the pain intensity of the present moment can distort systematically the accuracy of memory for prior pain (Eich et al., 1985). This problem presents major obstacles for studies of chronic pain in which investigators may wish to compare present pain with past pain.

When therapeutic trials are undertaken, systematic biases in reporting pain after treatment occur. These are referred to often as the placebo effect (Shapiro, 1971). In general, the placebo refers to the tendency of the patient to report a favourable outcome in order to please the therapist or satisfy the hopes of his or her family or him- or herself. Placebo trials are included often in therapeutic studies in order to gauge the extent to which this source of bias occurs. Ineffectual treatments are given sometimes so that patients may have the opportunity to demonstrate this type of bias.

It has become conventional to use the term placebo effect for any form of bias which represents the patient's beliefs or expectations about the situation and the measurement of pain or its opposite (pain relief). Such bias is affected by any psychological variable impinging upon the patient. There are some patient populations in which the therapeutic opposite of this phenomenon can be observed. Patients who are subjected to surgery which should alleviate a chronically painful condition may insist that the pain is unchanged or even worse following the operation despite correction of the underlying pathology. This is observed most often in patients who have a long history of illness behaviour or a commitment to the illness role. It is sometimes associated with secondary gain such as successful litigation.

Finally, poor method design can produce bias in pain measures. Under ideal conditions, a simple method such as a VAS should yield a normal distribution of scores characterized by a wide range. Many years ago, a colleague of the author designed a VAS which had anchors at both ends of a 10 cm line and small tick marks were placed at 2.5, 5.0 and 7.5 cm. This instrument was used routinely in a clinical setting until several years later when it was observed that the

scores had a trimodal distribution i.e. instead of marking the score along its full 10 cm length, patients tended to mark it at one of the three tick marks, and what should have been a normal distribution of scores was reduced to a set of three categories with frequency counts at each. Systematic measurement error is a major source of bias in pain studies that have not been planned carefully.

Pain assessment in paediatrics

Measurement of pain in children is considerably more difficult than in adults and requires attention to developmental stage. Developmental change with age influences behaviour patterns strongly, verbal proficiency, and the ability of the child to follow instructions. Because individual children vary in their rate of development, it is difficult to assign firm rules about what type of measurement is suitable for what age. Pain measurement in children has been reviewed by Lavigne et al. (1986) and by Thompson and Varni (1986).

The most difficult problem is the assessment of pain in infants. In this case, the investigator must use gross motor indicators such as generalized body reaction, reflex withdrawal or crying as an indicator of pain. This is far from satisfactory as these are not definitive pain measures and the presence of pain cannot be validated by verbal report. Pain in toddlers may be evaluated through more complex behaviour patterns which include pressing the lips together, rocking, rubbing the affected part, kicking, hitting or biting, attempting to escape the situation, or opening the eyes wide (Jeans, 1983).

The situation is better for children older than 3 yr as limited methods for self-report and behavioural observation are available. Children older than 5 yr can complete reliably the VAS and related simple interdimensional scaling instruments (Scott et al., 1977; Abu-Saad & Holzmer, 1981). Paediatric investigators find it useful to practise these methods with children on familiar problems before using them to scale pain.

A number of methods has been designed for use with children. These include a colour-matching procedure in which patients indicate the colour that represents pain best (Elend, 1981), and a picture scale known as 'Oucher' (Beyer, 1984). The MPQ has been validated in children 12 yr and over (Jeans, 1983).

Can pain really be measured in children? There is still not a definitive answer to this question. Certainly, children are unable to differentiate conceptually between sensory and affective dimensions of pain, and any scores obtained on a single dimension of pain reflect probably a composite expression of distress rather than an accurate quantification of pain intensity.

Scales of behavioural distress have been developed for use with children (Katz *et al.*, 1980; Jay *et al.*, 1983; Jay & Elliott, 1984; LeBaron & Zeltzer, 1984). These methods observe typically behaviours such as crying, screaming, requests for emotional support, muscular rigidity and verbal expressions. Distress in children can be complicated by parental anxiety. It can be difficult to quantify either distress or pain in a young child independent of its parent. It is sometimes impossible to assess a child in the absence of parent, or to separate parent–child as suffering unit.

Guidelines for undertaking pain research

There are several steps that can be followed when initiating pain measurement procedures in a clinical setting. These considerations facilitate the development of pain measurement and ensure its quality.

DEFINE THE POPULATION BEING TESTED

Pain measurement requires that patients understand the instructions given and are able to perform the tasks necessary. Age is an important factor. Similarly, educational level and grasp of English as a language are important determinants of whether or not measurement will succeed. Finally, patients in different situations have different levels of energy to contribute. Young adults recovering from elective surgery can perform much more demanding tasks than can elderly patients with advanced cancer. Thus, the methods chosen must fit the patients being tested.

When undertaking research, it is essential to define explicit inclusion and exclusion criteria for participation in a study. When assessing pain for clinical purposes, it may be valuable to define a minimally demanding alternative strategy. For example, patients who cannot complete the MPQ may be able to complete a simple category scale. Pilot data that define the relationship between the complex test scores and the simple test scores will make interpretation of the alternative measures possible.

DEFINE THE GOALS OF MEASUREMENT

In most cases, measurement is undertaken to permit the evaluation of a patient, to permit the comparison of one patient with another or to make possible the comparison of groups or populations of patients. This is Type I scaling. In other cases, pain measurement is undertaken to characterize certain pain syndromes such as pain related to cancer of the pancreas, tic douloureux or thalamic pain. This is Type II scaling. Some methods are better suited to one type of scaling than the other, and the method chosen should fit the goal as well as possible. For example, the MPQ is well suited for characterizing a unique pain problem as it records quality differences in pain states while behavioural observation methods offer no data of value for Type II measurement.

ESTABLISH A WORKING MODEL FOR THE PAIN IN QUESTION

The classical tradition biases of the author cannot be hidden here. It seems inconceivable that either science or clinical evaluation could be undertaken in the absence of some set of assumptions on the nature of pain. Such matters are discussed rarely, but decisions to select or reject a possible method for pain measurement are often (and appropriately) coloured by what the investigator believes pain is and how the concept of pain fits into his or her beliefs about sickness, suffering and disability in general.

One factor that requires attention is whether the pain in question is acute or chronic. Acute pain is unstable and may vary from moment to moment. Measures of acute pain should be administered rapidly and should be sensitive to rapid change. In contrast, chronic pain is often comparatively stable. Minor variations from day to day or moment to moment are of little interest in a study of therapeutic outcome. Changes in acute pain over 2 hr following dental extraction in patients with a non-steroidal, anti-inflammatory drug versus a placebo are of interest, but changes over 2 hr in a chronic pain patient taking the same drug are not. One needs to know if the drug alters daily or weekly trends in activity, job performance, family life and recreational habits. Only then can conclusions be drawn on whether or not the drug is effective for a given type of pain. A clearly thought-out model for what constitutes a meaningful outcome is fundamental to definitive research for clinical decision making.

ASSESS SEVERAL ALTERNATIVES

It is often wise to select several alternatives and assess them simultaneously in the test situation before making a final decision on the best choice of method for pain measurement. Sometimes an apparently good method is distasteful unexpectedly to patients, hard to understand or difficult to score. Time invested in preliminary assessment is rarely, if ever, wasted.

When conducting preliminary studies, assess if the scores obtained are reliable i.e. if similar scores occur in similar situations or with repeated measures of the same person in the same situation (Harms-Ringdahl *et al.*, 1986). Between patients the scores should show a good range. If everyone yields low or high scores when pain varies between patients, it is likely that the scaling is not meaningful. Also, a test method should be sensitive to differences between patients with obviously different pain intensities and the effects of known interventions. Finally, the scores obtained should approximate to a normal distribution unless one is undertaking non-parametric scaling.

ANTICIPATE AND CONTROL SOURCES OF BIAS

One of the goals of any measurement is to minimize error. It is probably impossible to devise a system for data collection in a clinical setting that is free from systematic error (bias). It is a good idea to anticipate from the beginning what the most likely sources of bias may be and to conduct continuous surveillance as data collection proceeds in an attempt to minimize it. Effort expended to control bias is often a seemingly thankless task, but it is usually an important investment of research or clinical resources.

KNOW THE LIMITS OF THE METHODS CHOSEN

The scientific or clinical inference that can be derived legitimately from a pain measurement technique may be less than one would like. However, many of the problems that ensue from pain studies or the use of pain measurement techniques in diagnosis result from overinterpretation of the data. The inference value of a pain score is largely a matter of what it means within the context of an overriding theoretical framework, as discussed above. Much depends on the careful development of a theoretical perspective at the outset of a project. In choosing a pain-measurement technology, swift action is always a poor substitute for careful planning.

Conclusion

There are many approaches to the measurement of pain but all are rooted in three traditions of measure-

ment. Review of these approaches and careful consideration of one's objectives narrow greatly the range of choices. There is no single, maximally advantageous method. The important considerations in choosing a method for pain research are:

1 Is the method meaningful for the theory, model or set of assumptions used by the investigator or clinician?
2 Is the method sensitive to differences and reliable?
3 Is the responder burden imposed by the method appropriate for the patients studied?

Careful planning and preliminary assessment are indispensable in establishing satisfactory procedures for measuring pain.

Acknowledgement

This work was supported in part by grant number CA 38552 from the National Cancer Institute of the National Institutes of Health, United States Public Health Service.

References

Abu-Saad H. & Holzmer W.L. (1981) Measuring childrens' self-assessment of pain. *Issues in Comprehensive Pediatric Nursing* **5**, 337–49.

Bergner M., Bobbitt R.A., Carter W.B. & Gilson B.S. (1981) The Sickness Impact Profile: development and final revision of health status measure. *Medical Care* **19**, 787–805.

Beyer J.E. (1984) Development of a new instrument for measuring intensity of childrens' pain. IV World Congress on Pain, Seattle, Washington. *Pain* (Suppl. 2), S421.

Bonica J.J. (Ed.) (1980) Introduction. In *Pain: Research Publications in Nervous and Mental Disease*, vol. 58, pp. 1–17. Raven Press, New York.

Bonica J.J. (1983) (IASP Presidential Address) Pain research and therapy: achievements of the past and challenges of the future. In *Advances in Pain Research and Therapy*, vol. 5 (Eds Bonica J.J., Lindblom U. & Iggo A.) pp. 1–36. Raven Press, New York.

Borg G. (1982) A category scale with ratio properties for intermodal and interindividual comparisons. In *Psychophysical Judgment and the Process of Perception* (Eds Geisler G-G. & Petzold P.) pp. 25–34. VEB Deutscher Verlag der Wissenschaften, Berlin.

Bridgman P.W. (1927) *The Logic of Modern Physics*. Macmillan, New York.

Campbell J.A. & Lipton S. (1985) Intraspinal somatosensory evoked potentials in man. In *Evoked Potentials: Neurophysiological and Clinical Aspects* (Eds Morocutti C. & Rizzo P.A.) pp. 37–43. Elsevier, New York.

Carlsson A.M. (1983) Assessment of chronic pain. I. Aspects of the reliability and validity of the visual analogue scale. *Pain* **16**, 87–101.

Chapman C.R. & Bonica J.J. (1983) Acute pain. In *Current Concepts* p. 44. Upjohn Company, Kalamazoo, Michigan.

Chapman C.R., Casey K.L., Dubner R., Foley K.M., Gracely R.H. & Reading A.E. (1985) Pain measurement: an overview. *Pain* **22**, 1–31.

Chapman C.R. & Saeger L.C. (1985) The use of evoked potentials in the assessment of analgesic states In *Quantitation, Modelling and Control in Anaesthesia* (Ed. Stoeckel H.) pp. 108–22. Thieme Inc., New York.

Chudler E.H. & Dong W.K. (1983) The assessment of pain by cerebral evoked potentials. *Pain* **16**, 221–4.

Cleeland C.S. (1985) Measurement and prevalence of pain in cancer. *Cancer Pain* **1**, 87–92.

Corson J.A. & Schneider M.J. (1984) The Dartmouth Pain Questionnaire: an adjunct to the McGill Pain Questionnaire. *Pain* **19**, 59–69.

Daut R.L., Cleeland C.S. & Flanery R.C. (1983) Development of the Wisconsin Brief Pain Questionnaire to assess pain in cancer and other diseases. *Pain* **17**, 197–210.

Duncan O.D. (1975) *Introduction to Structural Equation Models.* Academic Press, New York.

Eich E., Reeves J.L., Jaeger B. & Graff-Radford S.B. (1985) Memory for pain: relation between past and present pain intensity. *Pain* **23**, 375–9.

Elend J.M. (1981) Minimizing pain associated with prekindergarten intramuscular injections. *Issues of Comprehensive Pediatric Nursing* **5**, 352–72.

Follick M.J., Smith T.W. & Ahern D.K. (1985) The Sickness Impact Profile: a global measure of disability in chronic low back pain. *Pain* **21**, 67–76.

Frank A.J.M., Moll J.M.H. & Hort J.F. (1982) A comparison of three ways of measuring pain. *Rheumatology and Rehabilitation* **21**, 211–17.

Gracely R.H., Dubner R. & McGrath P. (1979) Narcotic analgesia: fentanyl reduces the intensity but not the unpleasantness of painful tooth pulp sensations. *Science* **203**, 1261–3.

Gunn C.C. (1988) Musculoskeletal pain of neuropathic origin: a model and treatment rationale. *Pain* (In press).

Gunn C.C. & Milbrandt W.E. (1978) Early and subtle signs in low-back sprain. *Spine* **3**, 267–81.

Harms-Ringdahl K., Carlsson A.M., Ekholm J., Raustorp A., Svenson T. & Toresson H-G. (1986) Pain assessment with different intensity scales in response to loading of joint structures. *Pain* **27**, 401–11.

Hunter M., Phillips C. & Rackman S. (1979) Memory for pain. *Pain* **6**, 35–46.

Jay S.M. & Elliott C. (1984) Behavioral observation scales for measuring children's distress: the effects of increased methodological rigor. *Journal of Consulting and Clinical Psychology* **52**, 1106–7.

Jay S.M., Ozolins M., Elliot C.H. & Caldwell S. (1983) Assessment of childrens' distress during painful medical procedures. *Health Psychology* **2**, 133–47.

Jeans M.E. (1983) The measurement of pain in children. In *Pain Measurement and Assessment* (Ed. Melzack R.) pp. 183–9. Raven Press, New York.

Jensen M.P., Karoly P. & Braver S. (1986) The measurement of clinical pain intensity: a comparison of six methods. *Pain* **27**, 117–26.

Katz E.R., Kellerman J. & Figel S.E. (1980) Distress behavior in children with cancer undergoing medical procedures: developmental considerations. *Journal of Consulting and Clinical Psychology* **48**, 356–65.

Keefe F.J. & Block A.R. (1982) Development of an observation method for assessing pain behavior in chronic low back pain patients. *Behaviour Research and Therapeutics* **13**, 363–75.

Keefe F.J., Brantley A., Manuel G. & Crisson J.E. (1985) Behavioral assessment of head and neck cancer pain. *Pain* **23**, 327–36.

Keefe F.J. & Hill R.W. (1985) An objective approach to qualifying pain behavior and gait patterns in low back pain patients. *Pain* **21**, 153–61.

Kerns R.D., Turk D.C. & Rudy T.E. (1985) The West Haven–Yale multidimensional pain inventory (WHYMPI). *Pain* **23**, 345–56.

Klepac R.K., Dowling J., Rokke P., Dodge L. & Schafer L. (1981) Interview vs. paper and pencil administration of the McGill Pain and Questionnaire. *Pain* **11**, 241–6.

Kremer E.F., Atkinson J.H. & Ignelzi R.J. (1980) Measurement of pain: patient preference does not confound pain measurement. *Pain* **10**, 241–8.

Kremer E.F., Block A.J. & Gaylor M.S. (1980) Behavioral approaches to treatment of chronic pain: the inaccuracy of patient self-report measures. *Archives of Physical Medical Rehabilitation* **62**, 188–91.

Kwilosc D.M., Gracely R.H. & Torgerson W.S. (1984) Memory for post-surgical dental pain. IV World Congress on Pain, Seattle, Washington. *Pain* (Suppl. 2), S426.

Lavigne J.V., Schulein M.J. & Hahn Y.S. (1986) Psychological aspects of painful medical conditions in children. I. Developmental aspects and assessment. *Pain* **27**, 133–46.

LeBaron S. & Zeltzer L. (1984) Assessment of acute pain and anxiety in children and in adolescents by self-reports, observer reports, and a behavior check list. *Journal of Consulting and Clinical Psychology* **52**, 729–38.

Linton S.J. (1985) The relationship between activity and chronic back pain. *Pain* **21**, 289–94.

Mayer T.G., Gatchel R.J., Kishino N., Keeley J., Mayer H., Capra P. & Mooney V. (1986) A prospective short term study of chronic low back pain patients utilizing novel objective functional measurement. *Pain* **25**, 53–68.

Melzack R. & Torgerson W.S. (1971) On the language of pain. *Anesthesiology* **34**, 50–9.

Michell J. (1986) Measurement scales and statistics: a clash of paradigms. *Psychological Bulletin* **100**, 398–407.

Moore R.A. & McQuay H.J. (1985) Neuroendocrinology of the postoperative state. In *Acute Pain* (Eds Smith G. & Covino B.G.) pp. 133–54. Butterworths, London.

Ochoa J.L., Torebjörk E., Marchettini P. & Sivak M. (1985) Mechanisms of neuropathic pain: cumulative observations, new experiments, and further speculation. In *Advances in Pain Research and Therapy*, vol. 9 (Eds Fields H.L., Dubner R. & Cevero F.). Raven Press, New York.

Ready L.B., Sarkis E. & Turner J.A. (1982) Self-reported vs. actual use of medications in chronic pain patients. *Pain* **12**, 285–94.

Revill S.I., Robinson J.O., Rosen M. & Hogy M.I.J. (1976) The reliability of a linear analogue for evaluating pain. *Anaesthesia* **31**, 1191–8.

Rubal B.J., Traycoff R.B. & Ewing K.L. (1982) Liquid crystal thermography. A new tool for evaluating low back pain. *Physical Therapy* **62**, 1593–6.

Sanders S.H. (1983) Automated vs. self-help monitoring of 'up-time' in chronic low back pain patients: a comparative study. *Pain* **15**, 399–405.

Scott P.J., Ansell B.M. & Huskinsson E.C. (1977) Measurement of pain in juvenile chronic polyarthritis. *Annals of Rheumatic Diseases* **36**, 186–7.

Szyfelbin S.K. & Osgood P.F. (1985) The assessment of pain and plasma α-endorphin immunoactivity in burn children. *Pain* **22**, 173–82.

Shapiro A.K. (1971) Placebo effects in medicine, psychotherapy, and psychoanalysis. In *Psychotherapy and Behavior Change* (Eds Bergin A.E. & Garfield S.L.) pp. 439–73. John Wiley & Sons, Inc., New York.

Stevens S.S. (1946) On the theory of scales of measurement. *Science* **103**, 667–80.

Stevens S.S. (1975) *Psychophysics: Introduction to Its Perceptual, Neural and Social Prospects.* John Wiley & Sons, Inc., New York.

Syrjala K.L. & Chapman C. R. (1984) Measurement of clinical pain: a review and integration of research findings. *Advances in Pain Research and Therapy* **7**, 71–97.

Tearnan B. & Dar R. (1986) Physician ratings of pain descriptors: potential diagnostic utility. *Pain* **26**, 45–51.

Thomas P.K. (1984) Clinical features and differential diagnosis. In *Peripheral Neuropathy*, vol. II (Eds Dyck P.J., Thomas P.K., Lambert E.H. & Bunge R.) pp. 1169–90. W.B. Saunders, Philadelphia.

Thompson K.L. & Varni J.W. (1986) A developmental cognitive-biobehavioural approach to pediatric pain assessment. *Pain* **25**, 283–96.

Turk D.C., Rudy T.E. & Salovey P. (1985) The McGill Pain Questionnaire reconsidered: confirming factor structure and examining appropriate uses. *Pain* **21**, 385–97.

Tursky B., Jamner L.D. & Freidman R. (1982) The pain perception profile: a psychophysical approach to the assessment of pain report. *Behavior Research and Therapeutics* **13**, 376–94.

Wall P.D. (1984) Introduction. In *Textbook of Pain* (Eds Wall P.D. & Melzack R.) p. 15. Churchill Livingstone, Edinburgh.

Walsh T.D. & Bowman K. (1984) Letter to the Editor. *Pain* **19**, 96–8.

65

Psychological Factors in Acute and Chronic Pain

C. R. CHAPMAN

Recently, anaesthetists have moved outside the operating room to become involved in advancing both pain research and therapy. Some anaesthetists work in pain clinics, others treat pain in patients with far advanced cancer and others are involved in postoperative pain.

Those anaesthetists who have had extended experience with pain control outside the immediate surgical setting recognize that pain is a complex psychological experience. However, training in anaesthesia provides little or no background in psychology, and many anaesthetists feel uncomfortable addressing such problems in their role as a pain specialist. This chapter is an introduction to psychological aspects of acute and chronic pain for the anaesthetist. Its purposes are to:

1 Provide an integrated perspective on psychological factors.

2 Offer practical guidelines for patient evaluation and pain management.

Basic definitions

PAIN

Pain is a complex, unpleasant perception associated normally with tissue injury or disease processes. It has sensory, emotional and cognitive aspects and it is manifest as a pattern of behaviour which has social implications.

Acute versus chronic pain

Pain is *acute* when it is linked in time and severity to the healing of an injury or disease. It is *chronic* when it persists beyond the normal healing period for injury or disease. Although many writers have defined 6 months or some other time period as the limit for transition from acute to chronic pain, this distinction cannot be made on the basis of time alone. The fundamental question is whether or not pain is dictated by organic pathology, or exists indefinitely, either in the absence of such pathology or to a degree of severity that cannot be accounted for by physical findings (Bonica, 1983; Chapman & Bonica, 1985).

An exception is made for pain associated with chronic disease conditions. When disease or pathology continues for weeks or years, the associated pain may be called chronic. With time, the causal link of tissue pathology to illness behaviour becomes less clear, and major personality and life-style change occur. Prolonged pain in cancer patients fits this description sometimes, but many acute pain problems occur in this population also (Twycross & Lack, 1983; Foley, 1985; Chapman *et al.*, 1986).

PSYCHOLOGICAL FACTORS

Psychological factors are perceptual or behavioural processes that are components of the experience and expression of human pain. Perceptual processes are subjective; behavioural processes are those which may be observed. These processes include:

1 Sensory/motor.

2 Affective.

3 Cognitive.

4 Behavioural/environmental.

The last factor represents the interaction of the person in pain with the social environment.

Psychological factors are important for the understanding and control of pain (Chapman & Turner, 1986; Keefe & Gil, 1986; Sternbach, 1986; Turk & Rudy, 1986). Certain patients may exaggerate or suppress pain complaints, making medical diagnosis of disease or injury inaccurate or difficult. The physician who fails to recognize and deal appropriately with psychological factors may err by pursuing excessive diagnostic investigation, over- or underprescribing medication, or undertaking inappropriate treatments. With chronic pain patients, unrecognized psychological factors may lead to unnecessary surgery and chronic overmedication. An understanding of basic psychological insights and principles in patient management may help to prevent or limit psychological problems in day-to-day patient care.

A multi-dimensional model for human pain

Because the brain is the organ for perception and behaviour, it is the focal point of theory regarding psychological aspects of pain. The psychology of pain can be presented as a development of MacLean's evolutionary theory for the organization of the brain (MacLean 1973, 1978, 1983). For MacLean, the 'triune' brain has evolved along the lines of three basic formations: reptilian, paleomammalian and neomammalian (Fig. 65.1). These divisions differ anatomically and biochemically and each corresponds to a qualitatively different type of consciousness and a relatively characteristic set of psychological phenomena. The human brain is a hierarchy of organizational levels which act as a system to produce human behaviour.

A full treatise on MacLean's theory and evidence for it lies beyond the scope of this chapter and is described elsewhere (MacLean 1973, 1978, 1983). However, a synopsis is provided below of a psychological model for

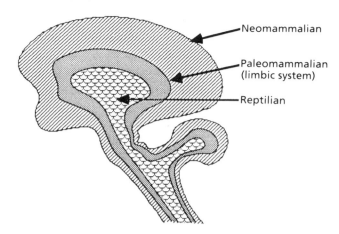

Fig. 65.1 Evolution of the brain as three hierarchically organized basic patterns: reptilian, paleomammalian and neomammalian. (Redrawn from MacLean, 1983.)

human pain perception and pain behaviour derived from this theory. The model provides a framework for examining psychological problems in the clinical setting.

Overview of the model

Figure 65.2 presents a schematic representation of the model. It commences with nociception, progresses through sensory/motor, affective and cognitive functions and culminates in the patient's behavioural interactions with the environment. The model identifies three determinants of pain corresponding to different levels of neurological structure and activity in

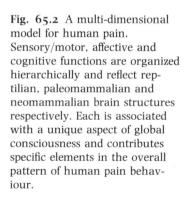

Fig. 65.2 A multi-dimensional model for human pain. Sensory/motor, affective and cognitive functions are organized hierarchically and reflect reptilian, paleomammalian and neomammalian brain structures respectively. Each is associated with a unique aspect of global consciousness and contributes specific elements in the overall pattern of human pain behaviour.

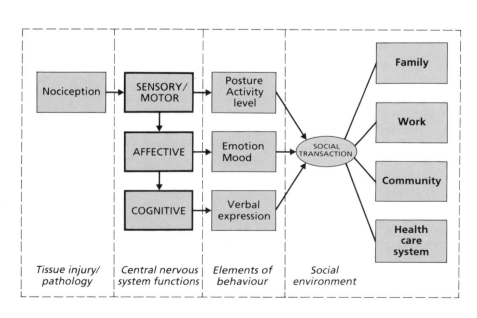

addition to a fourth determinant, the environment. The presentation of the pain patient, his or her dealings with health-care providers and ultimately his or her reaction to treatment, are composite patterns of response which reflect all four determinants.

The four factors are described below. The discussion parallels the hierarchical organization of the brain as described by MacLean (1973, 1978) but employs psychological rather than anatomical terminology.

SENSORY/MOTOR

Pain commences normally with activation of the peripheral nervous system through nociception, the response of injury-sensitive $A\delta$- and C-fibres to a stimulus (Basbaum, 1980; Yaksh & Hammond, 1982; Melzack, 1986). For brevity, the term nociception here will include peripheral neuropathies which may produce pain through ephaptic transmission or other mechanisms not involving receptor end organs (Thomas, 1984). The process of signal generation, centripetal transmission via the spinal cord and brainstem structures and arrival at thalamus, constitutes the sensory aspect of pain. Anatomically, this process and simple behavioural reactions involve the R-complex defined by MacLean (1978) as the reptilian level of the brain, but since peripheral and spinal cord structures are included in the model, it is more inclusive.

The reptilian brain level is responsible for a variety of behaviour patterns which man holds in common with phylogenetically simpler creatures. It is devoid of emotion, empathy or reason, and its role in pain behaviour is very basic. Typical behaviours related to sickness or pain include specific posturing and gait, ritualistic displays, social grouping and the will to wield power over others. General classes of clinically relevant behaviour observed in the actions of the reptilian brain include social withdrawal (return to the nest) after injury, learning by imitating others, perseveration including routine and ritualistic behaviours, displacement activities (e.g. attending to minor sensory stimulation when threatened or stressed), deceptive behaviours and trophic behaviours such as intense attraction to certain objects or events.

The presentation of the chronic pain patient may include strong reptilian components sometimes: exaggerated posturing, ritualistic limitations on daily activity, habitual use of various home therapies or obviously ineffective prescribed medications and decreased activity including excessive bed rest are all manifestations of the reptilian brain. Less obvious are

the subtle imitating of parents and other family members or peers who have suffered the same type of pain in the past. For example, as noted in the companion chapter (Chapter 64) on pain measurement, patients with back pain groan, sigh, brace, rub the affected area and walk with an altered gait (Keefe & Block, 1982).

It may be seen that the sensory/motor aspect of the model includes many behaviour patterns associated normally with injury. When pain is chronic, such behaviours may become responses to stimuli in the social environment through positive reinforcement (Fordyce, 1976). In addition, deception is one of the basic survival skills of the reptilian brain, and the presentation of one's self as injured or sick in the absence of notable organic pathology is consistent with this type of behaviour.

AFFECTIVE

Feeling states such as emotion and mood play a prominent role in pain. Moreover, humans react normally to pain in others with compassion and empathy. These processes originate at the paleomammalian level of the brain. Many of the feeling states that we consider profoundly meaningful in human interactions and religious experiences arise from the paleomammalian brain.

The paleomammalian area of the brain is the limbic lobe which surrounds the brainstem. MacLean (1978) described it as the common denominator in the brains of all mammals and suggested that it be considered the 'limbic system'. Because of connections with hypothalamus, the limbic brain can affect directly autonomic and endocrine functions. Three main limbic subdivisions have been identified by MacLean (1978): the amygdala, the septum and the mammillary bodies. The first is concerned with functions that centre around the mouth such as feeding, fighting and self-protection. The second subserves procreation. The third is associated with nurturing and parental care. The three basic behaviours which distinguish mammals from reptiles are nursing, the isolation call and play.

The emotional dimension of acute pain is limbic in origin, and fears which lead people to evade painful therapeutic encounters (e.g. a visit to the dentist) are also limbic. The expression of extreme distress whilst in pain and the sometimes emotionally florid presentations of chronic pain patients originate in the paleomammalian brain. Similarly, mood disorders such as depression, a frequent concomitant of chronic pain, are limbic disorders.

Behaviour is directed often at fulfilling a need, and the emotional needs of the pain patient can become a motivational force for the expression of pain. In addition, the limbic brain is responsible for the sense of empathy and trust that exists ideally between the physician and patient.

COGNITIVE

The neomammalian level of the brain is the neocortex; it gives humans the unique capacity for language and speech. Although vocalization is a paleomammalian characteristic, the limbic structures produce only expletives which are gross utterances and without refined meaning. The neocortex takes responsibility for defined symbolism and information exchange. It accomplishes logical thought, symbolic reasoning and logical extraction.

It is through the neocortex that humans achieve complex social interactions, and the imprint of society and culture on the brain are only found here. Within the brain, the neocortex performs an executive function. On one hand, it is the agent of the reptilian and paleomammalian levels of brain organization and operates in their service in negotiating with the environment. On the other hand, it holds society's imprint upon the individual, and it imposes standards for conduct, holds moral values and forms beliefs. The tension between these two responsibilities can be great; conflicts between the animal and societal needs of man have been identified by psychoanalytical and other classical theories of psychopathology as the basis for neurosis.

The neocortex is responsible for the social presentation of the self, and it strives normally to create images for others that conform to acceptable social expectations. It has been noted that, amongst chronic pain patients, there is often a difference between what the patient says he or she does and what he or she actually does (Fordyce, 1976; see also the discussion on bias in Chapter 64). Patients exaggerate their activity levels and under-report their medication usage and other socially negative actions. In the more difficult cases of chronic pain, large-scale denial of marital conflicts, difficulties of job adjustment, and antisocial behaviours are common (Pilowsky *et al.*, 1977; Chapman *et al.*, 1979; Pilowsky, 1986). Such inconsistencies are examples of a class of actions termed 'defence mechanisms' by psychoanalytical theorists. They constitute the

protective actions of the cortex on behalf of the reptilian and paleomammalian brains.

Much of the time, the neocortex does not understand the needs of the lower levels of brain and could not report them accurately in language even if it could perceive them clearly. Freud's concept of the 'unconscious' (Freud, 1942) corresponds to the inability of the neocortex to monitor, understand or accept the motives of the lower brain levels. Lack of insight is often implicated in neurosis and many psychotherapies are based on developing the capability for insight. MacLean (1978, 1983) did not postulate an unconscious; he simply emphasized that the consciousness of each of the three brain levels is very different and, in the case of the first two, verbally inexpressible. The theory holds that insight cannot solve complex behavioural pain problems; reptilian and paleomammalian levels of the brain must be addressed directly.

SOCIAL/ENVIRONMENTAL

The brain and the environment together constitute a system; what occurs within this system is the concern of psychology. The neocortex functions within the system in a manner similar to a middle management executive in an organization. The lower levels of the organization are reptilian and paleomammalian brain structures, and the higher levels are social structure and the culture itself. The neocortex is responsible for meeting the needs of those below it in the organization and must negotiate on their behalf and act as their agent towards those above who hold environmental resources and social power. At the same time, it must convey the rules and governance of those above to those below and see to it that the actions of those within its charge conform to the expectations of those in power.

In common with middle management executives, the neocortex can rarely, if ever, satisfy both sides fully, but it is held responsible by both. Persons with limited intrapersonal management skills are seen as neurotic or manipulative by others, are burdened with dysphoria and unfulfilled needs for nurturance by the limbic brain and predisposed to rigidity, ritualistic habits or obsessions by the reptilian brain. For these unhappy persons, life is perpetually a poor compromise.

Adopting the social role of chronic illness is one such compromise. Presenting oneself to family and society as unable to fulfil normal responsibilities owing to sickness was termed *illness behaviour* by Mechanic

(1968). It is, in essence, the adopting of an alternate position in society and an alternative social role.

Psychological manifestations of pain

The four psychological functions offer separate ways of viewing a patient in pain, as described below.

ACUTE PAIN

The sensory/motor aspects are reflected in postural changes, reflexive responses including withdrawal, and reduced levels of activity. For example, the patient with pain from advanced carcinoma of the pancreas assumes typically a characteristic fetal position. A rich variety of postural and motor responses to immediate injury can be seen on the football field.

The affective or emotional dimension of acute pain is apparent readily in most injury situations. LeResche (1982) has demonstrated that there is a human facial expression unique to pain: 'brow-lowering with skin drawn tightly around closed eyes accompanied by a horizontally stretched open mouth, sometimes with deepening of the nasolabial furrow'. In children, acute pain is accompanied almost invariably by emotional display (crying), and in adults, pain is expressed often as an emotion that stimulates emotional reactions in others.

Often, affect can be a problem when patients expect immediate pain, further pain or the worsening of present pain. This problem is called fear when negative anticipatory emotional arousal is present and associated with a clearly defined object or event. For example, the term 'dental fear' describes a focused fear of dental visits. In contrast, when the negative anticipation is a diffuse or global hypervigilance without a specific object or focus, it is termed anxiety. An extreme example is the presentation of a patient in the emergency room with panic disorder and all the signs and symptoms of myocardial infarction. The panic attack can present with dyspnoea, palpitations, smothering sensations, dizziness and extreme chest pain. The patient may tremble, sweat, shake and express a fear of dying. Such problems are more common in patients with enduring depression and those with habitual somatic preoccupation.

The cognitive aspects of pain are related often intimately to fear (Chapman, 1985). Uncertainty feeds fear, and many patients require more information on painful medical events than they receive. Others suffer from inappropriate beliefs or expectations about what

will happen to them or what will be felt (Johnson et al., 1978). At the root of many behaviour problems in the acute care setting is the basic fear of loss of control. In terms of the model, this means that the neocortex fails in controlling the actions of the lower levels of brain. Typically, patients cannot tell you specifically what they fear. It is as though they might abandon themselves to screaming in terror and in so doing lose all social dignity and self-respect.

The social/environmental aspect of pain represents the transaction between the patient and the social environment. Both acute and chronic pain patients show sometimes extreme or exaggerated pain behaviours in the presence of their spouses but not when alone with hospital staff (Block et al., 1980). In some cases the pain may become a vehicle for meeting emotional needs expressing anger or outrage, or burdening someone else with guilt and helplessness.

CHRONIC PAIN

Sensory/motor aspects of chronic pain are manifest behaviourally as excessive bed rest, abnormal posture or gait and a general tendency to withdraw from normal life.

The principal affective theme in chronic pain is depression rather than anxiety (Beutler et al., 1986; Sternbach, 1986; Romano & Turner, 1985). In addition, patients tend to indulge in excessive emotional dependence upon others. They may manipulate family members or others for emotional ends through the expression of pain and performance of the sick role.

Cognitively, pain problems are manifest psychologically by somatic preoccupation. In extreme cases, these patients seem to reject reassurance that the pain does not represent a serious condition. They rationalize their adoption of the sick role and become elaborate in presenting themselves as sick or impaired by pain and other symptoms. One characteristic of this overall behaviour pattern is a tendency to deny all of life's stresses and problems (e.g. marital conflict, vocational maladjustment, financial problems) and to express life as being perfect except for the pain (Pilowsky et al., 1977; Chapman et al., 1979).

The social/environmental aspects of chronic pain are those associated with abnormal illness behaviour. Pilowsky (1978, 1986) defined abnormal illness behaviour as the adoption of the sick role (including chronic pain) to be used as a coping or defence strategy for adjusting to environmental demands. Patients whose claim to illness and the associated social role exceed their organic findings appear with regularity at most chronic pain clinics.

Inappropriate illness-affirming behaviours may be seen as attempts on the part of the neocortex to minimize the tension produced by the conflicting demands of the two lower level brains on the one hand and society (family, community, vocational responsibility) on the other. By taking on the sick role, the neocortex limits the demands of the social environment. In addition, it legitimizes the cravings of the limbic brain for nurture from others, and it may allow the patient to manoeuvre for a position of social dominance within the family, a need originating at the reptilian level of the brain. When successful, all family life becomes organized around the patients and their pain with its associated social limitations.

The sick role is rarely a satisfactory compromise. Such patients are cheerless because the needs of the lower brain levels are unmet, and other people respond with resentment rather than empathy and nurture. Many such patients seek perpetually validation from the health-care system by demanding repetitive medical examinations; some seek surgery and drugs since these actions on the part of physicians help to legitimize a patient's claim to the sick role (Sternbach, 1974).

Guidelines for patient evaluation and management

The evaluation of psychological factors and the use of psychological principles differ for acute and chronic pain, but the parallel evaluation of the four major factors is held in common as shown in Fig. 65.3.

Acute pain

SENSORY/MOTOR

Postoperative pain is complicated sometimes by muscle tension or spasm (Bonica & Benedetti, 1980). Thoracic and abdominal surgery may involve severe muscle splinting that can add to the nociception of the surgical wound. Patients who are able to control muscle tension suffer less than those who cannot (Wells, 1982). With proper guidance, many patients can be taught to relax muscles during recovery from surgery or in other painful situations.

AFFECTIVE

Anxiety and fear including fear of loss of control can exacerbate the misery of the patient (Chapman, 1985). The easiest apparent solution is to use anxiolytic medication, but it is important to remember that such drugs compromise the patient's cognitive ability to cope with pain. Patients who cope badly are likely to be more satisfied with heavy medication than those who cope well. Many patients benefit from instruction in cognitive and other methods for modulating pain.

COGNITIVE

Coping skills often involve controlled mental imagery (Pickett & Clum, 1982); for example, an escape in fantasy to a far away pleasant place. Turk et al. (1983) have described some of the fantasies used by patients to cope with pain. In many cases it is possible to guide a patient's mental imagery through suggestion, to encourage intense concentration on a distant or abstract thought, or to help the patient to relabel uncomfortable sensations as non-painful. These and other coping strategies can relieve patient suffering greatly and help to foster the patient's sense of personal control over the pain (Egbert et al., 1964; Thompson, 1981; Wilson, 1981; Tan, 1982; Tan & Poser, 1982; Taylor, 1983).

SOCIAL/ENVIRONMENTAL

Sometimes a patient may be a problem only in the presence of family members or certain visitors. There

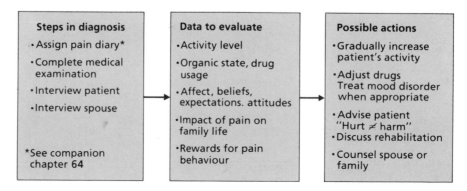

Fig. 65.3 Basic steps in the psychological assessment and management of chronic pain.

are many reasons why patients alter their pain behaviours for their family or other persons and it is rarely cost effective in the acute pain situation to attempt to intervene in this. Ordinarily, it is enough to inform the nursing staff of this relationship, if they have not noted it already, to ensure that the patient is not subjected to overmedication.

Chronic pain

Many patients with chronic pain have had extensive dealings with the health-care system in search of a cure. Specialists who provide yet another unremarkable medical evaluation and pass the patient along to others have not provided a useful service. It is the responsibility of the pain specialist to undertake the long-term management of such patients and to protect them from the risk of potentially harmful surgery and drug toxicity. Psychological principles play a role in such management. Figure 65.3 illustrates some basic steps for assessing and dealing with chronic pain patients.

The first steps in dealing with chronic pain patients are:

1 To form a relationship of trust with the patient.
2 To reassure the general practitioner that the pain does not signal a serious threat to the patient's health and to take on the responsibility of managing the pain.
3 To dissuade the patient from hoping for a rapid or miraculous cure. Patients must abandon this hope in order to initiate a slow, step-by-step process of recovery and rehabilitation. When this basic negotiation has been completed, the four psychological components can be evaluated.

SENSORY/MOTOR

The basic concerns are the lack of normal activity, abnormal posture or gait, and any tendency towards excessive bed rest. When acute injury is present, rest fosters healing; however, when healing has been completed and pain persists, rest only fosters invalid status and contributes to the general degradation of the patient's overall health (Fordyce, 1976). It is important to communicate to the patient that 'hurt does not imply harm' and that activity can be undertaken in the presence of pain without deleterious effects. In general, it is desirable to increase activity levels using graduated quotas and, where necessary, to use physical therapy to help to reactivate the patient.

AFFECTIVE

The key issue is depression (Sternbach, 1986). When in doubt, and when the depression is severe, psychiatric consultation is in order. Depression is a frequent concomitant of chronic pain, and in some cases the depression is masked. Depression linked to grief over the loss of a loved one is an example (Melges & DeMaso, 1980; von Knorring et al., 1983). This must be dealt with directly and may require psychiatric or psychological consultation and psychotherapeutic intervention. Many pain patients benefit from tricyclic antidepressant medications because they restore sleep; markedly depressed patients may benefit from mood elevation.

COGNITIVE

The major concerns are the beliefs and expectations of the patient. Those with extreme hypochondriasis, major patterns of denial of significant life problems or other somatoform disorders can be major frustrations. Once the patient's problem is understood well, the physician may present the patient with information that is fundamentally reassuring and informative. If the patient fails to alter behaviour in accordance with the information, abnormal illness behaviour is present and psychiatric or psychological evaluation should be considered. For patients who are able to handle the information appropriately, the prospects for long-term rehabilitation are favourable.

SOCIAL/ENVIRONMENTAL

Finally, the social environment can perpetuate the pain by rewarding pain expression (Fordyce, 1976, 1986). If performance of the sick role and the display of pain behaviours earns the patient time out from social responsibilities which he or she dislikes or generates much-needed nurturance and attention from others, such factors must be identified and dealt with if the patient is to be rehabilitated. It is often necessary to work with the family by educating them in the nature of these contingencies and enlisting their co-operation in increasing the activity level and social responsibilities of the patient.

In summary, the overall treatment plan for the chronic pain patient should involve increasing activity level, altering the interaction of the patient with his or her social environment where appropriate, dealing with mood disorders, if they exist, and enlisting the co-operation of the patient him- or herself in a step-by-step, long-term process of recovery.

Conclusion

Psychological factors sometimes play a major role in problems of pain management. A simple approach to such problems is presented above as a model based on the neuroanatomical organization of the brain. The model represents a multi-dimensional approach to the diagnosis and management of pain and accounts for sensory/motor, affective and cognitive dimensions of human pain in addition to the influence of the environment. The distinction between acute and chronic pain is emphasized. The model is designed to complement rather than compete with conventional medical management.

Acknowledgement

This work was supported in part by grant number CA 38552 from the National Cancer Institute of the National Institutes of Health, United States Public Health Service.

References

Basbaum A.L. (1980) The anatomy of pain and pain modulation. In *Pain and Society* (Eds Kosterlitz H.W. & Terenius L.Y.) pp. 93–122. Verlag Chemie, Weinheim, Germany.

Beutler L.E., Engle D., Dró-Beutler M.E., Daldrup R. & Meredith R. (1986) Inability to express intense affect: a common link between depression and pain? *Journal of Consulting and Clinical Psychology* **54**, 752–9.

Block A.R., Kremer E.F. & Gaylor M. (1980) Behavioral treatment of chronic pain: the spouse as a discriminative cue for pain behavior. *Pain* **9**, 243–52.

Bonica J.J. (1983) Current status of postoperative pain in therapy. In *Current Topics in Pain Research and Therapy* (Eds Yokota J. & Dubner R.) pp. 169–89. Excerpta Medica, Tokyo.

Bonica J.J. & Benedetti C. (1980) Postoperative pain. In *Surgical Care: A Physiological Approach to Clinical Management* (Eds Condon R.E. & DeCosse J.J.) pp. 394–414. Lea and Febiger, Philadelphia.

Chapman C.R. (1985) Psychological factors in postoperative pain and their treatment. In *Acute Pain*, vol. 1 (Eds Covino B. & Smith G.) pp. 233–55. Elsevier, Amsterdam.

Chapman C.R. & Bonica J.J. (1985) Chronic pain. In *Current Concepts* (Ed. Mann K.M.) p. 68. Upjohn Co., Kalamazoo.

Chapman C.R., Kornell J.A. & Syrjala K.L. (1987) Painful complications of cancer diagnosis and therapy. In *Cancer Pain* (Eds Yarbro C.H. & McGuire D.) pp. 47–67. Grune & Stratton, Orlando.

Chapman C.R., Sola A. & Bonica J.J. (1979) Illness behavior and depression compared in pain center and private practice patients. *Pain* **6**, 1–7.

Chapman C.R. & Turner J.A. (1986) Psychological control of acute pain in medical settings. *Journal of Pain and Symptom Management* **1**, 9–20.

Egbert L.D., Battit G.E., Welch C.E. & Bartlett M.K. (1964) Reduction of postoperative pain by encouragement and instruction of patients. *New England Journal of Medicine* **270**, 825–7.

Foley K. (1985) Medical progress: the treatment of cancer pain. *New England Journal of Medicine* **313**, 84–95.

Fordyce W.E. (1976) *Behavioural Methods in Chronic Pain and Illness.* Mosby, St Louis.

Fordyce W.E. (1986) Learning processes in pain. In *The Psychology of Pain* 2nd edn. (Ed. Sternbach R.A.) pp. 49–65, Raven Press, New York.

Freud S. (1942) *Beyond the Pleasure Principle.* Hogarth Press, London.

Johnson J.E., Rice V.H., Fuller S.S. & Endress M.P. (1978) Sensory information, instruction in a coping strategy, and recovery from surgery. *Research in Nursing and Health* **1**, 4–17.

Keefe F.J. & Block A.R. (1982) Development of an observation method for assessing pain behavior in chronic low back pain patients. *Behaviour Research and Therapeutics* **13**, 363–75.

Keefe F.J. & Gil K.M. (1986) Behavioral concepts in the analysis of chronic pain syndromes. *Journal of Consulting and Clinical Psychology* **54**, 776–83.

LeResche L. (1982) Facial expression in pain: a study of candid photographs. *Journal of Nonverbal Behavior* **7**, 46–52.

MacLean P.D. (1973) A triune concept of the brain and behavior. In *The Hincks Memorial Lectures* (Eds Boag T.J. & Campbell D.). pp. 6–66. University of Toronto Press, Toronto.

MacLean P.D. (1978) A mind of three minds: educating the triune brain. In *Seventy-seventh Yearbook of the National Society for the Study of Education* pp. 308–42. University of Chicago Press, Chicago.

MacLean P.D. (1983) Brain roots of the will-to-power. *Zygon* **18**, 359–74.

Mechanic D. (1968) *Medical Sociology.* Free Press, London.

Melges F.T. & DeMaso D.R. (1980) Grief-resolution therapy: reliving, revising and revisiting. *American Journal of Psychotherapy* **34**, 51–61.

Melzack R. (1986) Neurophysiological foundations of pain. In *The Psychology of Pain* 2nd edn. (Ed. Sternbach R.A.) pp. 1–24. Raven Press, New York.

Pickett C. & Clum G.A. (1982) Comparative treatment strategies and their interaction with locus of control in the reduction of postsurgical pain and anxiety. *Journal of Consulting and Clinical Psychology* **50**, 439–41.

Pilowsky I. (1978) A general classification of abnormal illness behaviours. *British Journal of Medical Psychology* **51**, 131–7.

Pilowsky I. (1986) Psychodynamic aspects of the pain experience. In *The Psychology of Pain* 2nd edn. (Ed. Sternbach R.A.) pp. 181–95. Raven Press, New York.

Pilowsky I., Chapman C.R. & Bonica J.J. (1977) Pain, depression and illness behaviour in a pain clinic population. *Pain* **4**, 183–92.

Romano J.M. & Turner J.A. (1985) Chronic pain and depression. *Psychological Bulletin* **97**, 18–34.

Sternbach R.A. (1974) *Pain Patients—Traits and Treatment.* Academic Press, New York.

Sternbach R.A. (1986) Clinical aspects of pain. In *The Psychology of Pain* 2nd edn (Ed. Sternbach R.A.) pp. 223–39. Raven Press, New York.

Tan S.Y. (1982) Cognitive and cognitive–behavioral methods for pain control: a selective review. *Pain* **12**, 201–28.

Tan S. & Poser E.G. (1982) Acute pain in a clinical setting: effects of cognitive-behavioral skills training. *Behavior Research and Therapeutics* **20**, 535–45.

Taylor S.E. (1983) Adjustment to threatening events: a theory of cognitive adaptation. *American Journal of Psychology* **28**, 1161–73.

Thomas P.K. (1984) Symptomatology and differential diagnosis of peripheral neuropathy: clinical features and differential diagnosis. In *Peripheral Neuropathy*, vol. II (Eds Dyck P.J., Thomas P.K., Lambert E.H. & Bunge R.) pp. 1169–90. W.B. Saunders, Philadelphia.

Thompson S.C. (1981) Will it hurt less if I can control it? A complex answer to a simple question. *Psychological Bulletins* **90**, 89–101.

Turk D.C., Meichenbaum D. & Genest M. (1983) *Pain and Behavioral Medicine: A Cognitive–Behavioral Perspective*. Guilford Press, New York.

Turk D.C. & Rudy T.E. (1986) Assessment of cognitive factors in chronic pain: a worthwhile enterprise? *Journal of Consulting and Clinical Psychology* **54**, 760–8.

Twycross R.G. & Lack S.A. (1983) *Symptom Control in Far Advanced Cancer: Pain Relief*. The Pitman Press, Bath.

von Knorring L., Perris C., Eisemann M., Eriksson U. & Perris H. (1983) Pain as a symptom in depressive disorders. I. Relationship to diagnostic subgroup and depressive symptomatology. *Pain* **15**, 19–26.

Wells N. (1982) The effect of relaxation on postoperative muscle tension and pain. *Nursing Research* **31**, 236–8.

Wilson J.F. (1981) Behavioral preparation for surgery: benefit or harm? *Journal of Behavioral Medicine* **4**, 79–102.

Yaksh T.L. & Hammond D.L. (1982) Peripheral and central substrates involved in the rostrad transmission of nociceptive information. *Pain* **13**, 1–85.

Postoperative Pain

G. SMITH

In common with all other types of pain, acute postoperative pain is an extraordinarily complex sensation which may be described as an integration of three components: afferent nociceptor stimulation, interpretation of these signals by higher centres (involving memory and experiences of painful situations) and an emotive or affective component which generally comprises anxiety and/or depression. It is difficult in the human to identify accurately the extent of each component of pain, and is preferable to regard the patient as a whole who exhibits a spectrum of pain comprising conscious discomfort, autonomic changes and emotional qualities embracing fear, anxiety and depression.

Generally, the factor which separates postoperative pain from other types of pain is the transitory nature of the former, although the intensity of the subjective discomfort may vary from severe to mild or even non-existent. The transitory nature of acute pain renders the condition more easily amenable to therapy than is the case for chronic types of pain.

Treatment of acute pain has failed traditionally to recognize the complex nature of pain. Thus, the standard conventional practice is to prescribe intramuscular administration of fixed dose of opioid on a p.r.n. basis (or as required) i.e. at the discretion of a nurse, on demand by a patient whose pain threshold has been exceeded. This regimen leads to poor control of postoperative pain for the following reasons:

1 Responsibility for management of the patient is delegated from the anaesthetist to junior medical staff, who in turn delegate responsibility to nursing staff.

2 Nursing staff may vary widely in their level of rapport with the patient. In addition, they may withhold strong opioids because of fear of the side-effects of these drugs, notably physical dependence or addiction and respiratory depression. Whilst there is little evidence to suggest that treatment of acute pain with opioids for some 2–3 days in the postoperative period is likely to produce addiction, respiratory depression is a valid concern nonetheless.

3 In the absence of personal experience of the severity of postoperative pain, it is difficult for nursing staff to acknowledge the extent of a patient's suffering in the postoperative period.

Furthermore, there are more fundamental reasons why the management of postoperative pain remains difficult as:

1 Measurement of pain is difficult and it is not possible to titrate the dose of a drug to achieve a measurable end-result.

2 Analgesic requirements vary widely according to the type and severity of surgery.

3 Analgesic requirements vary widely as a result of variations in pharmacokinetics and pharmacodynamics between different patients.

4 Administration of adequate doses of analgesics may be inhibited because of induction of side-effects, notably respiratory depression and nausea and vomiting.

Thus, the disadvantages of the conventional method of administration of intramuscular opioids is that the standard dose prescribed may be too large (side-effects) or too small (no analgesia), the technique results in fluctuating plasma concentrations of the drug, the drug is administered by intramuscular injection which is painful, the onset of analgesia is delayed following the point at which the opioid is administered and the technique induces a feeling of dependency on the nursing staff (see Fig. 68.6, p. 1223). There are, however, some advantages to the conventional method, notably that it represents familiar practice and by and large familiar practices have an inherent

Abdominal		Non-abdominal		Thoracic	
Upper	63.2%	Limbs	26.9%	Cardiac	72.5%
Lower	51.3%	Perineal	24.3%	Non-cardiac	74.6%
Inguinal	22.7%	Body wall	20.0%		
		Neck	11.7%		

Table 66.1 Incidence of patients requiring analgesics. (From Loan & Dundee, 1967)

safety simply because of accumulated experience: the technique is inexpensive, whilst the gradual onset of analgesia permits observation of the gradual onset of possible pharmacological overdose.

Causes of variation in extent of postoperative pain

The degree of discomfort experienced by patients in the postoperative period varies enormously. Thus, following cholecystectomy, it has been reported that some patients require no opioid, whilst others may require as much as 1200 mg of pethidine within the first 24 hr for effective analgesia. This variability reflects the difficulty in quantifying pain (see Chapter 64) and so it is difficult to rank factors in order of importance.

Type of surgery

The site of operation is probably the most important factor determining the presence and severity of postoperative pain. In general terms, thoracic and upper abdominal operations produce the most severe postoperative pain, almost invariably requiring opioid analgesics for control, whereas minor upper limb, cutaneous, or chest-wall surgery may require no opioid for pain relief. This is illustrated in Table 66.1 which details the frequency of need for postoperative opioids found in a study from Belfast, and in Table 66.2 which notes the recorded number of intramuscular injections of analgesic drugs required during the first 48 hr of operation in a study from Oxford. However, it should be noted that in both of these studies, analgesia was prescribed on a conventional on-demand intramuscular basis and these data may not be replicated by studies in which patients are treated by patient-controlled analgesia (PCA; see below).

It is clear that the duration of severe pain after surgery is relatively short-lived. This is reflected by the fact that in traditional UK practice, the administration of opioids continues for up to 48 hr after abdominal surgery, whilst in the USA, it lasts typically for 72 hr.

Table 66.2 Percentage of patients who required various numbers of analgesic injections. (From Parkhouse et al., 1961)

Operation	Proportion of patients who required no postoperative-additional analgesic (%)	Three or more analgesic injections
Minor chest wall	81.7	0
Inguinal hernia	52.4	0
Appendicectomy	25	10%
Lower abdominal surgery	17.6	40% (approx.)
Upper abdominal surgery	10 (approx.)	45–65%

The rapid reduction in opioid requirements after abdominal surgery may be a reflection partly of medical and nursing expectations, as the use of PCA has been shown in several studies to be associated with a relatively constant opioid consumption during the first 24 hr (Gibbs et al., 1982) or even 48 hr (White, 1985).

Age, gender and body weight

It is assumed commonly that age, gender and body weight are important factors in pain perception and response to analgesic drugs.

In respect of gender, all studies have suggested that women exhibit higher pain scores than men in chronic pain and experimental pain (Glynn et al., 1976) and also in postoperative pain (Nayman, 1979). However, it has been suggested that these differences are a result of difference in expression of pain suffering by the two sexes. Recent studies using PCA have demonstrated that there is no sex difference in demand for analgesics (Dahlstrom et al., 1982; Tamsen et al., 1982a,b).

Although it is frequent clinical practice to calculate opioid requirements on a body-weight basis, there is no evidence in adults to suggest that there is any basis for this practice (Cohen, 1980).

Bellville *et al.* (1971) studied the variables of height, weight and age on pain and found that only age correlated with extent of pain and analgesic requirements, confirming the clinical impression that elderly patients require smaller doses of analgesic drugs to achieve adequate pain relief. Although Bellville and his colleagues did not think that pharmacokinetic factors were responsible for age-related differences, several workers have reported higher serum levels of morphine in elderly patients as a result of decreased volume of distribution (Berkovitz *et al.*, 1975). Mather and Meffin (1978) have also reported higher concentrations of free drug in elderly patients. In the elderly patient, trait anxiety tends to increase with age, whilst state anxiety decreases, and these have been shown to correlate with postoperative pain (Scott *et al.*, 1983).

Although the cause of increased sensitivity to opioids has not been elucidated, there seems clear agreement that elderly patients obtain effective analgesia for longer periods of time with smaller doses of opioids than young patients.

Psychological factors

Psychological differences between patients may account for much of the variation in response to surgery and also response to opioid analgesics. The psychological factors in postoperative pain have been discussed in an excellent review elsewhere by Chapman (1985) and are reviewed also by Chapman in Chapter 65 of this book. In brief, he has classified these factors into two types:
1 Predisposing factors. These consist of personality type, intelligence level, social class and family history.
2 Situational factors.

Amongst the predisposing factors, for personality it has been shown that patients with low pain tolerance demonstrate high scores on anxiety and neuroticism personality scales (Austin *et al.*, 1980a). Furthermore, the studies of Parbrook and his colleagues (Parbrook *et al.*, 1973; Boyle & Parbrook, 1977) have shown that there is a correlation between preoperative neuroticism scores and impairment of postoperative vital capacity and increased incidence of postoperative chest infection.

Anxiety may be considered under two headings—anxiety proneness or trait, and anxiety state (tendency to become anxious in response to circumstances). The study by Scott *et al.* (1983) demonstrated that the level of state anxiety was a linear predictor of postoperative pain.

Of the situational factors involved in the psychological response to surgery, the most important variables comprise the attitudes of the nursing and medical staff, the response of other patients to pain and the ward environment (Dodson, 1985).

Pharmacokinetic factors

There are great variations in the plasma opioid concentration profile following intramuscular injection of an opioid. Thus, following the intramuscular administration of pethidine, it has been demonstrated that there may be a two- to five-fold difference in the peak plasma concentrations, and a three- to seven-fold difference in the rate at which they are attained (Austin *et al.*, 1980a,b) (Fig. 66.1). This variability in response to a standard injection of an opioid is the major reason for the inappropriateness of prescribing intramuscular opioids on a p.r.n. basis.

The pharmacokinetic properties of a drug are calculated usually following changes in blood concentrations after an intravenous injection, because of this variability in absorption from an intramuscular injec-

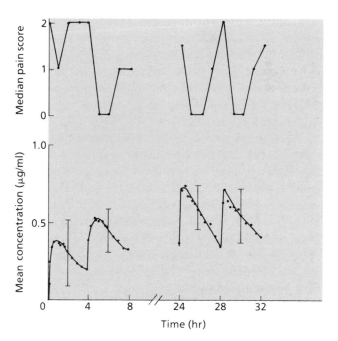

Fig. 66.1 Measured plasma concentration of pethidine (below) and pain score (above) in the postoperative period in response to intramuscular injections of pethidine. Pain score of 0 indicates no pain, while 2 represents very severe pain. (Redrawn from Austin *et al.*, 1980a.)

Table 66.3 Pharmacokinetic and related data for commonly available opioids

Drug	Intravenous potency ratio	Ionized (%) pH 7.4	Plasma protein binding (%) pH 7.4	$t_{\frac{1}{2}}\alpha$ (min)	$t_{\frac{1}{2}}\beta$ (hr)	Clearance (litre/min)	MEAC (ng/ml)
Fentanyl	292	91	83	2.3	2–5	0.8–1.2	1–3
Alfentanil	73	11	91	3	1.3–3.3	0.29	100–300
Sufentanil	4521	80	92	1	2.5	0.73	
Pethidine	0.53	95	65	4.2–11.4	3–7	0.5–1.8	300–650
Morphine	1	76	35	25	1.4–4	0.9–1.5	12–24
Methadone	1	99	85	10	25–45	0.1–0.2	30–70
Buprenorphine	33	91	96	3	2–4.5	1.1–1.5	

MEAC = minimum effective analgesic concentration.

tion. The pharmacokinetic parameters of commonly used opioid drugs are shown in Table 66.3. It may be seen that the pharmacokinetic properties of pethidine, morphine and fentanyl are relatively similar, whilst methadone differs substantially.

Variation in patient characteristics may lead to variations in pharmacokinetic parameters.

In hepatic disease, it has been shown that the β half-life ($t_{\frac{1}{2}}\beta$) of pethidine is approximately doubled because of decreased drug clearance rather than alteration in the volume of distribution. Following viral hepatitis, pharmacokinetics may return to normal. It has been shown also that the oral bioavailability of pethidine in cirrhotic patients is increased greatly, although there is relatively little change for morphine or fentanyl (Bentley et al., 1982).

In renal failure, it has been shown that for morphine the terminal half-life ($t_{\frac{1}{2}}\beta$) is the same for patients with end-stage renal failure as for normal volunteers (Aitkenhead et al., 1983).

Age has a marked effect on pharmacokinetic parameters. The half-life of pethidine in humans ($t_{\frac{1}{2}}\beta$) is considerably longer in neonates than in mothers. In patients over 80 yr of age, clearance is reduced and the volume of distribution is smaller. Bentley et al. (1982) have shown also that the β half-life of fentanyl is more than double in elderly patients as a result of decreased drug clearance, in the presence of an unchanged volume of distribution. This leads to higher fentanyl concentrations in plasma in the elderly. Other factors causing decreased clearance in the elderly may be the result of impaired metabolism and/or a decrease in liver blood flow.

Concurrent drug therapy may have a marked effect also on the pharmacokinetics of opioids. Thus, the concomitant administration of phenytoin increases pethidine clearance considerably and reduces the

terminal half-life. In contrast to enhanced opioid metabolism produced by phenytoin or phenobarbitone, cimetidine impairs the metabolism of both fentanyl and pethidine. Although cimetidine may decrease liver blood flow, it inhibits Phase I reactions in the liver, notably hepatic oxidative metabolism. Thus, cimetidine impairs the metabolism of both pethidine and fentanyl leading to prolongation of β half-life. Interestingly, cimetidine does not affect morphine metabolism which occurs predominantly by glucuronidation, which is not affected by cimetidine.

It has been suggested that under general anaesthesia, a decrease in hepatic blood flow may occur, leading to a decrease in clearance. If the volume of distribution is reduced also, then terminal β half-life may remain unchanged, as was demonstrated by Mather et al. (1975) for pethidine in patients anaesthetized with halothane.

Other factors affecting pharmacokinetics

Hypothermia leads to hypovolaemia and hypotension, resulting in reduced absorption of drugs from injection sites. There is also a reduction in distribution of drug to tissues with a reduced blood flow and a tendency to preserve cerebral blood flow. In addition, hypothermia may lead to a reduction in metabolism causing increased sensitivity to drugs.

In hypothyroidism, metabolism is depressed also, leading to sensitivity to CNS-depressant drugs.

With hyperventilation, there is an increase in pH leading to alteration in the degree of ionization. For morphine, it has been shown that hyperventilation leads to higher concentrations of morphine in CNS with a slower decline in brain concentration.

Enterohepatic circulation may affect also the pharmacokinetics of several drugs including pethidine and fentanyl. Both of these drugs are excreted into the stomach, and then reabsorbed from the lower gastrointestinal tract, leading to a secondary increase in plasma concentration. Such a mechanism has been alleged to contribute to recurrence of respiratory depression following the administration of fentanyl.

Pharmacodynamic factors

For many years, it was held generally that there was no relationship between the plasma concentration of an opioid and analgesia. This belief stemmed from three reasons:

1 The lack of a suitably sensitive and accurate method for measurement of opioids. In recent times, this has been corrected by the development of HPLC and sensitive radioimmunoassay techniques.

2 As the most common method of pain control was intramuscular injections, there resulted a markedly fluctuating plasma concentration of opioid with wide interindividual variations (Fig. 66.1).

3 For an individual patient, there is a very steep concentration–response relationship (Fig. 66.2) and the effective plasma concentration associated with analgesia may vary four- to five-fold between individual patients.

With a constant infusion of an opioid, depending on the drug, steady-state concentrations are reached eventually, at which receptor–drug concentration is in equilibrium with plasma concentration of the drug. The minimum plasma concentration achieved by this means, at which analgesia is produced, is termed the minimum effective analgesic concentration (MEAC)

and values for the commonly available opioids are described in Table 66.3.

The variation of MEAC level between different patients accounts for the widespread variation in drug demand using PCA systems. This varies between 13 and 44 mg/hr for pethidine, 30 and 100 μg/hr for fentanyl, and 0.3 and 9 mg/hr for morphine.

Pharmacodynamic variability includes the variability produced by differences in psychological profile (personality, anxiety and neuroticism; see above). A possible link between personality profile and opioid-receptor sensitivity is that there may be a variation in endogenous opioid levels in patients of different personality. Lim *et al.* (1983) suggested 'that certain psychological parameters may be related to the ease of activating the endogenous pain suppression system' and by analogy Tamsen and colleagues have suggested that 'subjective need for analgesics may also be linked to endogenous pain modulation'. Evidence to support this hypothesis was obtained by Tamsen and his colleagues who demonstrated a relationship between concentrations of pethidine in cerebrospinal fluid (CSF) during PCA and the preoperative concentration of endorphins in CSF (Tamsen *et al.*, 1982c) (Fig. 66.3).

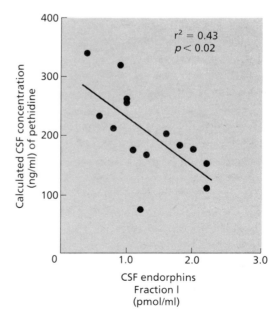

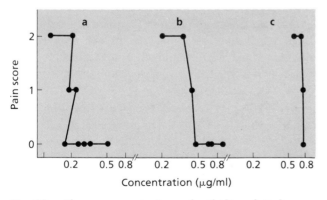

Fig. 66.2 Plasma concentrations of pethidine plotted against pain score for three patients (**a, b, c**). Note that there is a very steep concentration–response relationship for each patient and that the minimum effective plasma concentration (MEAC) varies four-fold between patients. (Redrawn from Austin *et al.*, 1980a.)

Fig. 66.3 Cerebrospinal fluid concentrations of pethidine in patients during PCA plotted against the patient's preoperative concentration of endorphins in CSF. Note that the higher the resting concentration of endorphin, the lower is the amount of pethidine required in CSF to achieve analgesia. (Redrawn from Tamsen *et al.*, 1982c.)

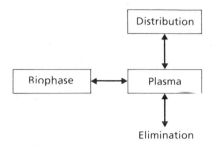

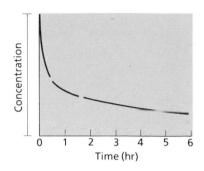

Fig. 66.4 Change in plasma concentration of opioid following bolus intravenous administration. (Redrawn from Hull, 1985.)

RELATIONSHIP BETWEEN PLASMA DRUG CONCENTRATION AND ANALGESIC EFFECTS

Following the intravenous administration of an opioid, there is a rapid decline in plasma concentration as the drug is redistributed into the volume of distribution (where it is inactive) and also into the biophase, and this is followed by a phase of elimination (Fig. 66.4).

In plasma, opioids are bound to plasma protein, usually by hydrophobic forces, and so the extent of binding is dependent on pH and lipid-solubility.

Opioids are weak bases, and thus at physiological pH, they exist in both un-ionized and ionized form. It is only the unbound and un-ionized portion of drug (lipid-soluble) which is free to penetrate lipid membranes and this is termed the diffusible fraction. This amounts to 16% of plasma morphine, 2.5% of pethidine and only 1.4% of fentanyl.

The process of diffusion of the opioid from plasma to receptors in the brain is described in Fig. 66.5.

Free base in plasma diffuses through the blood–brain barrier, the extent of diffusion proportional to the lipid-solubility of the drug and the concentration gradient. Within the brain, the extent of binding to the receptors depends on receptor affinity and the extent of binding to brain lipid, which is again dependent on lipid-solubility.

Thus, for example, morphine possesses a relatively low lipid-solubility, resulting in difficult penetration of the blood–brain barrier. However, within the brain, high receptor affinity and low lipid-solubility result in a large mass of drug reaching the receptor sites in the biophase (Hull, 1985).

Physiological effects of pain

Respiratory function

It is well known that following abdominal and thoracic surgery there is a reduction in tidal volume (V_T), vital

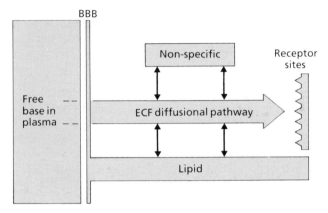

Fig. 66.5 Diagram to administer the diffusion of opioid from plasma to the drug receptors in the brain. BBB = blood–brain barrier; ECF = extracellular fluid. (Redrawn from Hull, 1985.)

capacity (VC), forced vital capacity (FVC), functional residual capacity (FRC) and peak expiratory flow rate (PEFR). This deterioration in respiratory function is greater following upper abdominal surgery than lower abdominal surgery, and greater following thoracic surgery than abdominal surgery.

Following upper abdominal surgery, the reduction in VC is greatest approximately 24 hr after surgery, and thereafter improves gradually but still may not be back to preoperative levels by 10 days after surgery. Similar changes occur also in FRC.

Earlier studies by Spence and Smith (1971) suggested that there was a small but significant difference between the deterioration in pulmonary function in patients undergoing cholecystectomy with extradural postoperative analgesia compared with conventional intramuscular morphine for postoperative analgesia. Thus, for patients receiving morphine for postoperative analgesia, VC diminished from a mean value of 3.8 litre to 1.2 litre at 24 hr, 1.61 litre at 48 hr and 2.45 litre at 5 days. In comparison, the patients receiving postoperative analgesia with extradural bupivacaine exhibited a preoperative VC of 3.92 litre which diminished to 1.07 litre 24 hr postoperatively, 2.04 litre at 48 hr and 2.45 litre at 5 days. The corresponding changes in P_{O_2} were 12.4, 9.2, 9 and 11 kPa (93, 69.3, 68 and 83.5 mmHg) respectively for the morphine group and 12.6, 11, 10.8 and 12.3 kPa (94.8, 82.8, 81.6 and 92.3 mmHg) respectively for the extradural group.

However, in this earlier study by Spence and Smith (1971) the quantity of morphine administered was very modest, and when this study was repeated several years later by Spence and Logan (1975), it was found that there was no significant difference between extradural analgesia and morphine analgesia in terms of FRC, VC or arterial oxygenation.

These two studies suggested, therefore, that poor analgesia is accompanied by a poorer respiration function following abdominal surgery. Nonetheless, the difference in respiratory function between good analgesia and poor analgesia in the later postoperative period is relatively small compared with the extent of reduction in pulmonary function produced by surgery itself.

Extensive studies from this author's department have suggested that of the common respiratory function tests available, those which correlated best with linear analogue pain scores are PEFR, $FEV_{1.0}$ (forced expiratory volume in 1 sec) and VC. Functional residual capacity correlates relatively poorly.

In the early postoperative period, respiratory function tests may be a much more sensitive index of analgesia, and Bromage and his group have used $FEV_{1.0}$ extensively as an index of pain relief (Bromage et al., 1980) (Fig. 66.6).

Neuroendocrine changes

After surgery, there is a variety of neuroendocrine and metabolic responses which are termed collectively 'the stress response' to surgery. The stress response is activated by many factors including emotion, pain, cardiovascular changes, starvation, infection, etc. The extent of the stress response is related to the extent of tissue trauma, but it is evident that the responses may be modified to varying degrees by different techniques of postoperative pain relief. In general terms, those techniques associated with the best degree of postoperative analgesia tend to lead to the greatest suppression of the stress responses. This statement must, however, be modified in respect of spinal or extradural local anaesthesia which, if sufficiently high, blocks the efferent fibres to the adrenal cortex and medulla.

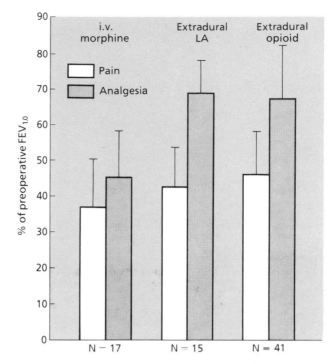

Fig. 66.6 Change in $FEV_{1.0}$ produced by inducing analgesia by three different techniques in patients following abdominal surgery. Note that the improvement in FEV was significantly greater following extradural opioid which produced better analgesia than that following intravenous opioid. LA = local anaesthetic. (Redrawn from Bromage et al., 1980.)

Following abdominal surgery, there is a marked increase in plasma cortisol in patients who receive systemic opioids. However, with an effective high extradural anaesthetic block, there may be no change in plasma cortisol compared with preoperative baseline values. In contrast, extradural morphine which may produce better anaesthesia than extradural local anaesthesia, is associated with intermediate levels of plasma cortisol in the postoperative period (Fig. 66.7).

Similar changes are seen with regard to the effects of local anaesthetic subarachnoid block and extradural morphine on sympatho-adrenal responses. Figures 66.8 and 66.9 illustrate changes in plasma catecholamines following cholecystectomy. In patients receiving intramuscular morphine for postoperative analgesia, there is a marked increase in both adrenaline and noradrenaline plasma concentrations, whilst those patients receiving high extradural block with local anaesthetic exhibited very little change in catecholamine concentrations. In contrast, those with extradural morphine exhibited intermediate levels of catecholamines. Despite this, the quality of analgesia was best with extradural morphine (Fig. 66.10).

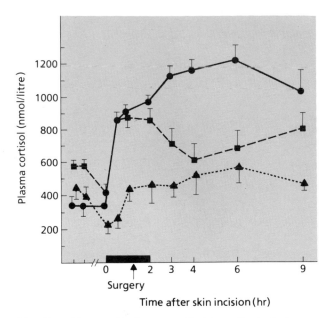

Fig. 66.7 Changes in plasma cortisol in patients during operation (0–2 hr) and the postoperative period (2–9 hr). ● General anaesthesia with systemic opioids (N = 12); ■ general anaesthesia followed by extradural morphine (N = 12); ▲ high extradural block with local anaesthetics both intra- and postoperatively (N = 12). (Redrawn from Christensen *et al.*, 1982.)

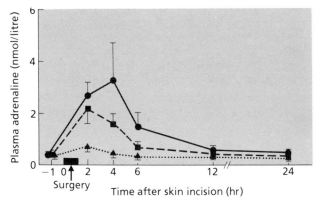

Fig. 66.8 Changes in plasma concentrations of adrenaline in patients following cholecystectomy. ● General anaesthesia; ■ general anaesthesia and extradural morphine; ▲ general anaesthesia and extradural local anaesthesia. Note that blockade of efferent fibres to the adrenals (T8–L1) inhibits the increase in adrenaline which occurs with general anaesthesia, whilst extradural opioid is associated with intermediate levels of catecholamines but optimal postoperative analgesia (Fig. 66.10). (Redrawn from Rutberg *et al.*, 1984.)

Further information on the effect of anaesthesia and postoperative analgesia on the stress responses to anaesthesia and surgery are detailed in Chapter 12 of this book, and are described also in great detail by Kehlet (1986).

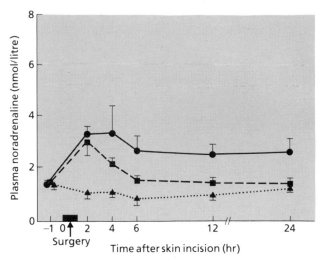

Fig. 66.9 Changes in plasma concentrations of noradrenaline in patients following cholecystectomy. ● General anaesthesia; ■ general anaesthesia and extradural morphine; ▲ general anaesthesia and extradural local anaesthesia. Note that blockade of efferent fibres to the adrenals (T8–L1) inhibits the increase in noradrenaline which occurs with general anaesthesia, whilst extradural opioid is associated with intermediate levels of catecholamines but optimal postoperative analgesia (Fig. 66.10). (Redrawn from Rutberg *et al.*, 1984.)

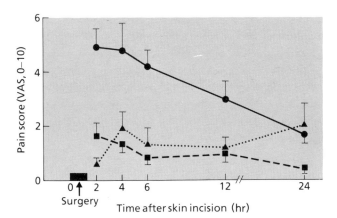

Fig. 66.10 Changes in pain score (visual analogue scale, VAS) in patients following cholecystectomy. ● General anaesthesia; ■ general anaesthesia and extradural morphine; ▲ general anaesthesia and extradural local anaesthesia. Note that extradural morphine produces optimum analgesia followed by extradural local anaesthesia followed by intramuscular morphine. (Redrawn from Rutberg *et al.*, 1984.)

Methods of treating postoperative pain (Table 66.4)

Conventional administration of opioids

The failings inherent in the conventional method of administration of opioids by intramuscular bolus ad-

Table 66.4 Methods of treating postoperative pain

'Conventional administration of opioid'
i.m. on-demand bolus

Newer opioid agonist/antagonist drugs

Newer parenteral routes of administration of opioid
Bolus i.v. administration
Continuous i.v. infusion
Patient-controlled analgesia
   Bolus
   Bolus+infusion } i.v./i.m./s.c.

Non-parenteral administration of opioid
Buccal/sublingual
Oral
Rectal
Transdermal

Respiratory route of administration of volatile/gaseous agents

Local anaesthetic techniques

Spinal/extradural opioids

Non-pharmacological methods
Cryotherapy
TENS
Acupuncture
Psychological methods

with unacceptable side-effects such as nausea, vomiting and respiratory depression.

One of the more simple ways of overcoming the problem of inadequate analgesia is to administer opioids on a regular 4-hourly basis. This has been undertaken in several studies resulting in a quality of analgesia approaching that which may be obtained by the use of PCA (Ellis *et al.*, 1982). However, whilst the regular prescription of opioids may be associated with improved analgesia compared with the infrequent administration associated usually with a p.r.n. regimen, it is clearly likely to be associated with an increased incidence of side-effects.

Another technique which has been promoted vigorously by the pharmaceutical industry, is the development of newer opioid drugs which may possess analgesic properties comparable with those of morphine but possess fewer side-effects. This would permit the administration of drugs on a regular basis, resulting in improved analgesia without the development of respiratory depression.

ministration on demand by the patient have been detailed above. In essence, this technique fails to deliver optimum analgesia for many patients as it results in fluctuating plasma concentrations of opioid. In some patients, the troughs are associated with lack of analgesia, and in some the peaks may be associated

Newer synthetic opioids

The newer synthetic opioid drugs are described elsewhere (Chapter 6) but for completeness a list of agents which have been used for postoperative pain is shown in Table 66.5 with an indication of activity at various opioid receptors. The effect of stimulating such receptors is described in Table 66.6.

Table 66.5 Opioid agonist and agonist/antagonist drugs. (From Rosow, 1985)

Drug	Receptor		
	μ	κ	σ
Morphine	Agonist	Agonist	No activity
Buprenorphine	Partial agonist	No activity	No activity
Profadol	Partial agonist	No activity	No activity
Propiram	Partial agonist	No activity	No activity
Dezocine	Partial agonist	No activity	No activity
Meptazinol	Partial agonist*	No activity	No activity
Nalorphine	Antagonist	Partial agonist	Agonist
Pentazocine	Antagonist	Partial agonist	Agonist
Butorphanol	Antagonist†	Partial agonist	Agonist
Nalbuphine	Antagonist**	Partial agonist	Agonist
Naloxone	Antagonist	Antagonist	Antagonist

* Additional mechanisms appeared to be involved also in the analgesic effect.
† An opioid antagonist in animals but does not precipitate abstinence in humans.
** May also have partial agonist activity.

Test system	Receptor		
	μ	κ	σ
Analgesia	Yes	Yes	No
Respiration	Depression	Depression	Stimulation
Behaviour	Euphoria	Sedation	Dysphoria
Pupil	Miosis	Miosis	Mydriasis
Morphine withdrawal	Suppression	No suppression	No suppression

Table 66.6 Opioid receptor subtypes. (From Rosow, 1985)

Many of these newer agents have been assessed in studies examining their efficacy in postoperative pain. However, for those with a marked 'ceiling' effect to respiratory depression, analgesia has been found usually to be inadequate for severe types of postoperative pain. To date, those with less 'ceiling' effect to respiratory depression have not been found to produce superior analgesia to that obtained with morphine.

Of these recently introduced opioid agonist/antagonist drugs, buprenorphine is perhaps one of the most useful as it may be administered by the sublingual route. Using this route, it has been shown that satisfactory analgesia may be produced for both upper and lower abdominal surgery (Ellis *et al.*, 1982). The major disadvantage of this agent is a considerable degree of sedation which may be undesirable where it is hoped to mobilize patients as soon as possible after surgery.

REVERSAL OF THE EFFECTS OF PARTIAL AGONIST OPIOIDS

Pure agonist drugs, such as morphine, pethidine and fentanyl, are considered to be μ-selective but with significant activity on the δ- and κ-receptor. The receptor specificity of the pure opioid antagonist, naloxone, mirrors closely this profile. Thus, all the effects of the agonists are reversed readily with naloxone in a dose-dependent manner typical of competitive antagonism. It should be remembered, however, that the duration of action of a single intravenous dose of naloxone is only approximately 20 min. Repeated doses or a continuous infusion may be necessary when high doses of a long-acting agonist have been administered.

The situation with the partial agonist drugs is somewhat more complex. Typically, they have agonist properties on some of the opioid receptor types but are antagonistic on others. In general, reversal of effect demands the use of a pure antagonist. Morphine, by contrast, can be reversed with partial agonists with strong antagonistic properties such as nalorphine.

Thus, pentazocine, butorphanol, meptazinol and nalbuphine may all be antagonized with naloxone despite their differing receptor specificities. Buprenorphine, however, has the property of very slow rate of dissociation from the μ-receptor and is not reversed reliably by naloxone. In cases of persisting respiratory depression with this drug, the use of the respiratory stimulant, doxapram, is recommended.

Where adequate analgesia has been produced by a partial agonist drug, it is conceivable that continuing antagonistic action may hinder the effect of a pure agonist drug administered subsequently.

SEQUENTIAL ANALGESIA

Sequential analgesia is the term given to a technique whereby a pure agonist drug may be antagonized by an agonist/antagonist agent. The opioid antagonist properties of pentazocine were exploited in this technique described first by De Castro and Viars in 1968. High-dose fentanyl was used preoperatively and the unwanted respiratory depression was reversed in the postoperative period by high doses of pentazocine. A similar technique, employing lower doses, was described by Rifat in 1972. It was claimed that excellent postoperative analgesia was obtained. Recently, interest has been aroused by the possibility of using buprenorphine following morphine. Although not an antagonist, it is theorized that with a stronger μ-receptor affinity than morphine, buprenorphine would displace the former drug from the μ-receptor, thereby 'antagonizing' respiratory depression and, with a lower receptor activity, would maintain analgesia without signs of opioid overdosage.

In practice, the technique of sequential analgesia does not seem to have found widespread favour.

Newer parenteral methods of administering opioids

From the discussion on p. 1177, it is clear that in order to obtain effective analgesia, the purpose of administering opioids parenterally should be to provide a steady-state plasma concentration of opioid at a level equivalent to the MEAC. However, as the MEAC level varies widely between different patients, it is not possible to define the dosage regimen required in advance of assessing an individual's opioid sensitivity. With the bolus intravenous and continuous intravenous infusion techniques, assessment of the patient's requirements is in the hands of the observer, nurse or medical attendant. With PCA, a servo feedback loop is produced whereby the patient controls his or her own level of plasma opioid concentration.

BOLUS INTRAVENOUS ADMINISTRATION

For many years, it has been common practice to administer small intravenous boluses of opioid in the recovery room to produce analgesia in patients immediately following anaesthesia and surgery. An extension to this practice, which may be undertaken in high-dependency nursing units, is to prescribe small intravenous doses of opioid to be given when necessary by the nursing staff in the later postoperative period. Provided that there is a 1:1 nursing:patient ratio to detect respiratory depression, this technique may be acceptable. However, it does produce widely fluctuating plasma concentrations of opioid, and the advantage of the intravenous infusion and PCA techniques is that these fluctuations are reduced by a considerable extent.

CONTINUOUS INTRAVENOUS INFUSION STRATEGY

Various authors have attempted to assess the patient's opioid requirements by means of small intravenous boluses until adequate analgesia is achieved, and then prescribing arbitrarily a fixed continuous intravenous infusion rate dependent upon the initial quantity of opioid administered. Thus, Rutter et al. (1980) assessed the initial titration dose and then prescribed 3.5 times this dose over 72 hr. Saha (1981) administered papaveretum at a rate of 1 mg/min until analgesia was achieved, and then continued the infusion for 40–50 hr at a rate of 1 mg/hr reducing to 0.83 mg/hr after 24 hr (allowing some flexibility in these rates). Catling et al. (1980) achieved analgesia in a similar manner and then gave an infusion of four times the initial analgesic dose per 24 hr.

There are various problems associated with this technique, the most important of which is the possibility of inducing respiratory depression. Catling et al. (1980) observed in the first 24 hr episodes of apnoea associated with significant arterial desaturation. In addition, patients may notice inadequate analgesia on day 1 for reasons which are explained in Fig. 66.11. This shows that the bolus plus infusion technique leads to inadequate plasma concentrations of opioid in the early period. In order to prevent this early subanalgesic concentration, it is necessary to fill the central compartment and follow this by a maintenance infusion rate equivalent to the rate of elimination of the opioid. However, it may be seen from this theoretical analysis that the initial bolus has to be so large as to produce very high plasma concentrations, which would lead undoubtedly to apnoea (Fig. 66.11).

More complicated infusion regimens have been devised in order to approach rapidly and then maintain a steady-state plasma concentration in the region of the MEAC level. For further information on this complex topic, the reader is referred to the publications by Stapleton et al. (1979), Austin et al. (1981) and Hull (1985).

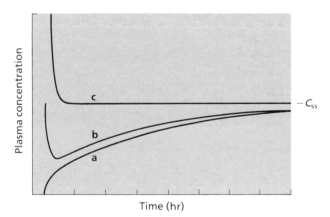

Fig. 66.11 Plasma concentrations of opioid produced by three techniques:
a Following a fixed rate of infusion.
b After a bolus followed by same infusion rate.
c After a bolus designed to fill the volume of distribution followed by the same infusion rate which is identical to the rate of elimination.
Note that (**a**) and (**b**) may be associated with inadequate levels of opioid in the early period, whilst (**c**) is associated with an extremely high plasma concentration. C_{SS} = steady-state plasma concentration. (Redrawn from Hull, 1985.)

The problems inherent in intravenous infusion techniques based on observer control, notably respiratory depression, are so inherently dangerous in the view of this author that such techniques must be confined to patients observed closely in a high-dependency nursing area or intensive therapy unit (ITU).

Patient-controlled analgesia

The concept of PCA was initiated by Sechzer some 15 yr ago (Sechzer, 1971). The concept may be regarded as a simple closed loop control system and it differs from the infusional strategy in that, with the latter technique, it is the observer who determines the plasma concentration of opioid required to maintain analgesia. With PCA it is the patient who determines the plasma concentration of opioid, which represents a balance between the total amount of the drug demanded by the patient to satisfy his or her subjective requirements for analgesia, and avoidance of excessive dosage which would produce either unacceptable side-effects such as nausea/vomiting, or a degree of CNS sedation which would by itself inhibit further activation of the apparatus.

The first commercially available machine, the Cardiff Palliator, was designed to provide the facility for the patient to self-administer a single bolus dose of drug (i.e. 10–30 mg of pethidine). In order to prevent accidental activation of the machine, the patient was required to press the control button twice within 1 sec. Administration of an overdose is rendered unlikely by the clinician setting the dose size (bolus size) and the minimum time interval between doses (the period during which the machine is rendered inactive—this is termed the lock-out time). Thus, the maximum possible dose over a period is controlled at a safe level by the clinician.

Two other parameters can be controlled by the clinician, namely the rate of infusion of each individual dose and the dilution factor.

Provided that the patient has not received a large initial loading dose from the clinician, the changes in plasma concentration produced in a conscious patient are likely to resemble those depicted in Fig. 66.12. However, if the patient goes to sleep and stops demanding the drug, the plasma concentration may fall below the analgesic threshold, leading to arousal and discomfort until the plasma concentration has attained the analgesic level once again (Fig. 66.13).

Because of this theoretical disadvantage of the PCA technique delivering a bolus alone, other workers have devised apparatus which provides a continuous, low-dose background infusion, on which the patient superimposes patient-activated boluses.

The problem with continuous infusion strategies is the possibility of overdosage leading to development of respiratory depression. This was overcome in the original on-demand analgesic computer (ODAC) developed by Hull (1985) by the use of a stethograph, which reduced the infusion rate if the respiratory rate diminished below a preset level. The original ODAC (Newcastle prototype) was adapted subsequently and a commercially available equipment marketed by Janssen Scientific Instruments. The device was designed initially for fentanyl, as pain would be relieved more rapidly after each bolus than with pethidine or

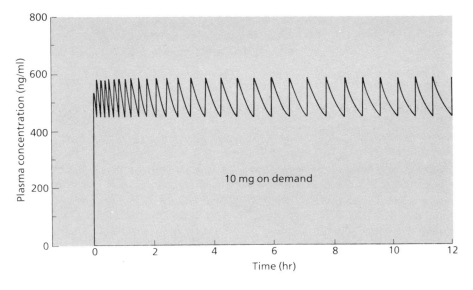

Fig. 66.12 Simulated plasma concentrations of pethidine in a pharmacokinetic model for pethidine whereby 10 mg of pethidine is given as a bolus to maintain the plasma concentration in the region of the mean MEAC level. Note that initially, frequent boluses are given and later the frequency of administration becomes relatively constant. (Redrawn from Tamsen et al., 1982a.)

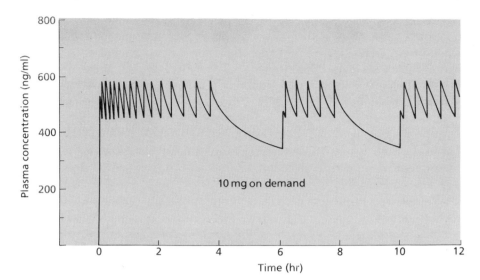

Fig. 66.13 The model shown in Fig. 66.12 in which two periods of sleep are simulated, thereby requiring an increased frequency of administration to restore plasma concentration to the MEAC level. (Redrawn from Hull, 1985.)

morphine and, in addition in later versions, a continuous infusion rate was delivered, computed upon the previous hour of dosage. The infusion rate is computed as 50% of the present hourly rate, which of course diminishes as patient-activated demand diminishes.

A similar philosophy was developed by Tamsen in Sweden leading to the production of the Prominject apparatus. This apparatus has three separate modules, only one of which is active at a time:

1 Patient control.
2 Consecutive infusions.
3 Constant infusion.

In the constant infusion mode, the apparatus functions as a straightforward motor infusion syringe.

Patient-controlled analgesia equipment currently available is shown in Table 66.7, which indicates features of each type of apparatus.

PRACTICAL EXPERIENCE WITH PCA APPARATUS

To date, the use of PCA has been confined largely to a few centres. As there has not been widespread use of the technique in routine clinical practice in district general hospitals, it is therefore difficult to evaluate fully the usefulness and potential side-effects of the technique. Nonetheless, there are sufficient data to suggest that it represents one of the most significant advances in the treatment of postoperative pain in the last one to two decades.

The experiences of investigators in different centres have revealed relatively similar findings. By and large, patients find the use of the PCA technique very acceptable, and they tend to maintain a relatively constant plasma concentration of opioid (although there may be a four- to five-fold difference in concentrations between different patients). The dose requirements are generally smaller than the maximum which may be administered on a p.r.n. basis and for an individual patient, the dose requirement is relatively constant.

There is no suggestion that PCA with intravenous opioids leads to more side-effects such as sedation, nausea or respiratory depression than conventional intramuscular analgesia and, if anything, the technique is likely to be associated with less respiratory depression than conventional methods. Respiratory

Table 66.7 Apparatus available for patient-controlled analgesia. (From Harmer *et al.*, 1985)

Apparatus	Manufacturer	Infusion strategy	Patient demand signal	Battery power
ODAC	Janssen	Bolus + infusion	Two presses in 1 sec	Yes
Prominject	Pharmacia, Sweden	Bolus + infusion	Two presses in 1 sec	Yes
Harvard PCA 2000	CR Bard, USA	Bolus dose	Single press	Yes
Abbott Lifecare	Abbott Laboratories, USA	Bolus dose	Single press	Yes
Palliator MS 402	Graseby Medical, UK	Bolus + infusion	Two presses in 1 sec	Yes

depression has occurred in postoperative patients, associated particularly with advanced age, hypovolaemia or large bolus doses. Buprenorphine may be a less desirable drug to use with PCA as it has a relatively long onset time and unless the lock-out time is adjusted appropriately, it may be possible for the patient to administer a larger dose than is desirable.

Most workers, with one or two exceptions, suggest that PCA provides superior analgesia to conventional intermittent intramuscular injection. There have been very few comparisons of PCA equipment delivering bolus alone with PCA equipment delivering bolus plus low-dose infusion, but a recent study (Vickers *et al.*, 1987) suggested that the latter technique provided marginally superior analgesia than bolus alone, as might be predicted on theoretical grounds. To date, no studies have been devised to determine if the sense of autonomy and placebo effect produced by the PCA apparatus are responsible for any of the perceived benefits of this technique.

ROUTE OF ADMINISTRATION

The PCA technique may be used to administer opioids intravenously, intramuscularly or subcutaneously.

For the intramuscular route, a cannula is inserted into the deltoid muscle immediately postoperatively and the site covered with an occlusive dressing. It has been shown that injection is relatively painless and virtually free from local and inflammatory complications.

As the rates of absorption of opioid by the intramuscular route and subcutaneous routes are much slower than that following the intravenous route, it is necessary to increase the lock-out time. The slower onset time of analgesia compared with the intravenous route would seem to detract from some of the advantages offered by the PCA intravenous technique.

The PCA technique has been used also to administer opioids via the extradural route, with both morphine and pethidine. To date, this can be regarded only as an investigative technique and should be confined to the high-dependency unit.

Non-parenteral administration of opioids

ORAL ADMINISTRATION

The oral route of administration of drugs is the most widely used for all types of medication and most acceptable to the patient. However, apart from minor ambulatory surgery and in the late postoperative period following inpatient surgery, the oral route of administration of opioid analgesics possesses major disadvantages:

1 Absorption occurs from the small intestine and following surgery there is frequently delay in gastric emptying. Not only will the administration of oral drugs in this situation lead to non-absorption, but there is a danger of dumping of a large bolus of drug into the small intestine when gastric motility resumes, leading to the possibility of overdosage. Studies conducted by the author on MST (morphine sulphate tablets) following abdominal surgery suggest that absorption is delayed within the first 24 hr. This is illustrated in Fig. 66.14. Thus, MST is *not* recommended for use within the first 24 hr following surgery.

2 Oral administration of drugs may be prevented by nausea and vomiting which are common accompaniments of anaesthesia and surgery.

3 Oral administration of opioids leads to metabolism in the gut wall and also in the liver (first-pass metabolism). Thus, the bioavailability of opioids is reduced greatly. Oral bioavailability ratios for commonly available opioids are shown in Table 66.8.

It is concluded, therefore, that the oral route is unsuitable for administration of strong opioids to

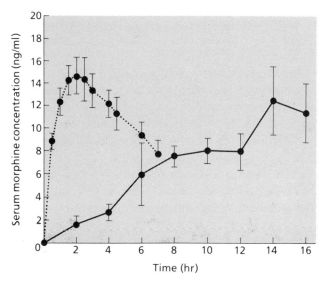

Fig. 66.14 Plasma concentrations of morphine following single administration of MST 20 mg to volunteers (dotted line) and also following regular 4-hourly administration of MST 20 mg to patients following peripheral vascular surgery (solid line). Note that there is a marked delay in the absorption of morphine in patients, and that the peak concentration attained by 16 hr is relatively low. (Redrawn from Pinnock *et al.*, 1986).

Table 66.8 Oral/parenteral bioavailability ratios of some commonly available opioid drugs. (From Hanning, 1985)

Drug	Onset of action (min)	Peak action (min)	Duration of action (hr)	Oral/parenteral bioavailability	Oral dose equal to 10 mg morphine intramuscularly (mg)
Morphine	60	60–90	4–5	0.17–0.33	60
MST	60	180	8	0.18	20
Hydromorphone	15–30	30	4–5	0.2	7.5
Pethidine	40–60	60–120	2–4	0.25–0.71	300
Levorphanol	20–60	60–120	8–14	0.5–1.0	4
Methadone	30–60	30–120	4–8	0.45	20
Pentazocine	40–60	60–180	3–4	0.25–0.3	180
Buprenorphine	60–120	120–240	6–8	0.1	4
Meptazinol	60–120	180	5–6	0.2	300
Nefopam	30–60	60–180	6–8	0.3	90

patients in the early postoperative period, despite the fact that several reports have indicated that satisfactory analgesia may be achieved using this route.

When the need for strong analgesics has decreased, however, after 1, 2 or 3 days following surgery it is common practice to prescribe a mild opioid (such as codeine, dihydrocodeine, or dextropopoxyphene), one of the minor analgesic agents such as acetylsalicylic acid or one of the large number of non-steroidal drugs available currently. Many of these types of drugs have been shown to be quite effective in relieving pain following minor orthopaedic surgery.

SUBLINGUAL ROUTE

The sublingual route possesses two important safety features compared with the oral route of administration; firstly, the tablets may be removed from the mouth in the event of overdosage, and secondly, for drugs with high first-pass metabolism, accidental swallowing of tablets will not result in toxicity. The disadvantages of the sublingual route relate to patient tolerance, and absorption may be affected by the rate of production of saliva, chewing or sucking.

The major advantage of the sublingual route is that absorption occurs directly into the systemic circulation and there is no first-pass metabolism (de Boer *et al.*, 1984).

The drug which has been used most commonly by this route for postoperative pain is sublingual buprenorphine, which has a sublingual/parenteral bioavailability of approximately 30% which is far greater than that by the oral route. Thus, swallowing results in considerable deactivation of the tablet and lessens any possibility of toxicity.

Absorption of sublingual buprenorphine is relatively rapid, and blood concentrations 3 hr after administration are similar following both sublingual and parenteral administration.

Sublingual buprenorphine (as 0.4 mg on a regular 6-hourly basis) has been used successfully as the sole analgesic for major abdominal surgery and it has been shown to produce analgesia comparable to that following PCA with pethidine or regular 4-hourly intramuscular morphine. The major disadvantages of buprenorphine are a relatively high degree of sedation and nausea (Ellis *et al.*, 1982).

RECTAL ROUTE

The rectal route possesses the following advantages:
1 Absorption from the lower part of the rectum bypasses first-pass metabolism, although in the upper part, absorption through the superior rectal vein leads to first-pass metabolism. In general, therefore, bioavailability is higher than that following the oral route although there may be considerable interindividual variations depending on siting of the suppository in the rectum.
2 Absorption is unaffected by gastric emptying, nausea and vomiting, and administration may be discontinued by removal of the suppository.

The major disadvantages are that the rate of onset of analgesia is slow, and aesthetic considerations render the technique relatively unpopular in the UK and North America.

The rectal route of administration has been used with sustained-release preparations impregnated with morphine, and it has been suggested that this may be a suitable technique for maintenance of relatively low levels of analgesia i.e. it might be useful for producing a low sustained plasma concentration of morphine, which may be augmented by further systemic administration (Hanning *et al.*, 1988).

TRANSDERMAL ROUTE

The transdermal route of administration is now an accepted technique for administration of hyoscine and nitroglycerin, utilizing rate-control delivery vehicles. Currently, studies are in progress evaluating the use of fentanyl by similar rate-control delivery systems in the treatment of postoperative pain (Duthie *et al.*, 1988).

RESPIRATORY ROUTE OF ADMINISTRATION OF VOLATILE/GASEOUS AGENTS

The volatile anaesthetic agents trichlorethylene and methoxyflurane have been used in draw-over vaporizers, suitably calibrated and temperature compensated, to provide analgesia in labour. These agents have been superseded to a large extent by the use of Entonox (50% nitrous oxide/50% oxygen in a premix cylinder) dispensed to the patient through a demand valve. This is a popular technique for obstetric analgesia.

Entonox has been found to be extremely useful for treating acute pain in other situations, particularly in acute trauma. It has been used (in the field) by ambulance men or first-aid workers, and it may be used also for the initial treatment of trauma patients in accident and emergency departments.

However, there are few indications for the use of Entonox in the treatment of postoperative pain. Spence and Wallace (A.A. Spence, personal communication) showed in a double-blind study on intermittent self-administration, that nitrous oxide 50% in oxygen was not superior to nitrogen in oxygen. Furthermore, increasing concern regarding the potentially toxic effects to staff of exposure to low concentrations of nitrous oxide suggest that the technique has very limited application.

Local anaesthetic techniques (Table 66.9)

In recent years, there has been increased enthusiasm for the use of somatic nerve blocks to provide postoperative analgesia. Using bupivacaine, useful postoperative analgesia may be produced for 8–12 hr following injection. Thus, a single administration is particularly useful for outpatient anaesthesia, especially in children.

Table 66.9 Local analgesic techniques used for postoperative pain relief

Upper extremity	Axillary brachial plexus Interscalene or supraclavicular
Lower extremity	Femoral nerve block Sciatic nerve block Femoral/sciatic/obturator 'three-in-one' Lumbar extradural Caudal
Thoracic	Extradural Intercostal
Abdominal	Extradural Intercostal
Penis	Caudal Block of dorsal nerve of penis

In paediatric practice, it is now common to administer a local anaesthetic somatic nerve block, or extradural block, following induction of general anaesthesia. The type of blocks which are particularly useful in paediatric day-case surgery (Dodson, 1985) include:
1 Ilioinguinal block (for herniotomy and orchidopexy).
2 Penile dorsal nerve block (for circumcision).
3 Caudal block (for circumcision in outpatients, or repair of hypospadias for inpatients) (Dodson, 1985).

In children, bupivacaine is used usually in a concentration not exceeding 0.25%, in a dose not exceeding 2 mg/kg and a total volume not exceeding 20 ml in older children (Dodson, 1985).

However, other blocks may be used for appropriate surgery including brachial plexus block, ulnar nerve block, etc.

In adults, 'single-shot' somatic nerve blocks with bupivacaine are used frequently to provide postoperative analgesia for 8–12 hr, by brachial plexus block for upper limb surgery, caudal block for haemorrhoidectomy and intercostal nerve blocks for thoracotomy or cholecystectomy.

Whilst these techniques may provide excellent analgesia for 10–12 hr after surgery, further prolongation of analgesia is required for the majority of patients. One of three approaches may be used to achieve this end:
1 Prolongation of the local anaesthetic agent—so far no satisfactory drug has been produced which will provide prolonged sensory blockade.
2 Repeated somatic nerve blockade.

3 Placing a catheter close to the nerves which require blockade.

For detailed information on this subject, the reader is referred to earlier chapters in this book and also to an excellent article by Buckley in *Acute Pain* (1985). The following represents a synopsis of Buckley's article.

Repeated somatic nerve blocks

An example of this method would include intercostal or paravertebral blocks for upper abdominal incisions or thoracotomies, and the constraints of this method are enumerated in Buckley's article (1985).

CATHETER TECHNIQUES

Insertion of catheters for prolonged anaesthesia has been advocated for the following situations:

Axillary blocks. It has been suggested that a catheter is placed into the brachial plexus sheath following identification by use either of a stimulator or tactile perception of penetration of the sheath. Initial doses administered through the catheter are similar to those using a single injection technique (40–50 ml) and repeated doses using slightly smaller volumes. The problems of this technique include systemic toxicity, nerve injury, haematoma (all very small) and a relatively high incidence of kinking of the catheter.

Interscalene and supraclavicular perivascular blocks. Several authors have described the insertion of catheters into the brachial plexus sheath via the supraclavicular route or the interscalene route. Intermittent injections of 20–30 ml of bupivacaine 0.25% are administered at 6–8-hourly intervals.

Lower limb blocks. Peripheral nerve blocks for the lower extremity are less popular because extradural and caudal blocks are much easier technically. However, various authors have described femoral nerve blocks, lumbar plexus blocks via the psoas compartment and sciatic nerve blocks. It is unlikely that these techniques will be utilized by any other than local analgesia enthusiasts.

Intercostal nerve blocks. Although techniques have been described for placing cannulae percutaneously into intercostal nerve spaces, such techniques have not superseded that of intermittent administration of individual intercostal nerve blocks.

For upper paramedian incisions, intercostal bilateral blocks from T5 to T11 are necessary and, because the major complication of intercostal nerve block is pneumothorax, such a technique is not advocated. However, for subcostal incision, unilateral block of T5 to T11 is required.

Paravertebral block. This technique is a useful alternative to multiple intercostal blocks because it requires only a single injection of 15 ml of bupivacaine to block up to four intercostal nerves. For more information, the reader is referred to Eason and Wyatt (1979).

Extradural and subarachnoid local anaesthetic techniques

Subarachnoid and extradural local analgesic blocks have been described in detail elsewhere (Chapter 58).

Because single-shot extradural and subarachnoid injections produce analgesia of only a relatively short duration of action (4–8 hr and 2–4 hr respectively with bupivacaine) these techniques are seldom employed for postoperative pain relief. However, the insertion of a catheter into the subarachnoid or extradural space permits continuous extradural analgesia to be provided for 2–3 days postoperatively. Whilst the use of catheter techniques for the subarachnoid space has been described in US practice, in the UK the fear of introduction of infection has rendered this technique virtually unacceptable. Thus, for all practical purposes, extradural techniques for postoperative analgesia are confined to:

1 Thoracic extradural catheters.
2 Lumbar extradural catheters.
3 Caudal extradural catheters or single-shot techniques.

Details of the physiological effects, and description of insertion of extradural catheters are provided in excellent accounts by Bowler *et al.* (1986) and Stanton-Hicks (1985). The following is a brief summary of these accounts and for more information the reader is referred to the original articles.

PHYSIOLOGICAL EFFECTS OF EXTRADURAL BLOCK

For practical purposes, extradural blocks may be categorized into high blocks (above T5) or low blocks (below the level of T5). The heart receives sympathetic innervation from T1 to T5, the lower limbs from T10 to L2, the adrenal medulla from T8 to L1, abdominal visceral T6 to L2, liver T7 to T9, and kidneys T10 to L1.

With high sympathetic blocks, there is very little change in cardiac output and mean arterial blood pressure in the conscious normovolaemic patient but a reduction in systemic vascular resistance (SVR). With low blocks there is a reduction in blood flow in the upper limbs accompanied by vasoconstriction and an increase in blood flow in the lower limbs as a result of vasodilatation, leaving central venous pressure (CVP), cardiac output and SVR, and mean arterial pressure more or less unchanged. With hypovolaemia, however, high blocks are associated with dramatic reductions in cardiac output and mean arterial pressure. In contrast, the patient with a low block is capable of compensating for small reductions in blood volume.

In patients free from respiratory disease and pain-free, low extradural blocks have little effect on lung volumes, FRC, expiratory reserve volume (ERV), residual volume (RV) and V_T remaining more or less unchanged. With high blocks, there is a decrease in ERV with little change in inspiratory capacity.

In contrast, for patients in pain, extradural blockade improves VC, FRC and Pao_2. However, there is little difference in the improvement produced by extradural blockade or optimum administration of systemic opioids. High extradural blockade causes a reduction in pulmonary artery pressure, with an increase in alveolar deadspace leading to slight hyperventilation and maintenance of $Paco_2$. Perhaps the greatest benefit of extradural blockade is the maintenance of respiratory function in the absence of respiratory depression or sedation, thus permitting improved patient co-operation with physiotherapy.

TECHNIQUES FOR POSTOPERATIVE PAIN CONTROL

For post-thoracotomy pain, a catheter should be inserted at the level of incision, for upper abdominal surgery at T6–10, for lower abdominal surgery T10–L1 and for the lower limbs at L3–4. Low concentrations of local anaesthetic solution should be used in order to obviate motor block; thus, bupivacaine is used normally in a concentration of 0.25%, although the lumbar region may require higher concentrations because the nerve routes are of larger diameter.

For bolus administration, the volume of solution infused varies from 4 to 7 ml but by continuous infusion from a motor syringe pump, a rate of 7–22 mg/hr may be utilized (Stanton-Hicks, 1985).

The contra-indications and potential complications of extradural catheter techniques are described in Chapter 58.

Wound infusions

The technique of injecting local anaesthetic solution into the edges of a surgical incision was described in 1935, but there has been recently a resurgence of interest in this technique.

Single injections of bupivacaine may be placed into the wound edges at the end of surgery but, in addition, catheters may also be placed, particularly in the sheath posterior to the rectus muscle.

Intermittent injections of local anaesthetic maintain somatic analgesia for a considerable period after surgery.

Provided that bacterial filters are used, there would appear to be little danger of wound infection. Adrenaline should be avoided as, theoretically, it may reduce blood supply to the tissues.

The technique abolishes only somatic pain and has little effect on visceral pain but, nonetheless, good results have been claimed for this technique following abdominal surgery.

Spinal and extradural opioids

Following the identification of opioid receptors in the brain by Pert and Snyder in 1973 and the isolation of endogenous opioids by Hughes and colleagues in 1975, there has been enormous interest in the administration of opioids by the subarachnoid and extradural routes for the relief of postoperative pain and the reader is referred to reviews by Cousins and Mather (1984), Yaksh (1984) and Cousins and Bridenbaugh (1986).

Following injection into CSF, morphine dispersion occurs as follows:

1 Morphine is taken up into the region of the substantia gelatinosa in the spinal cord close to the point of injection. Within the dorsal horn, there are opioid inhibitory systems which act both presynaptically and postsynaptically. It is thought that morphine acts predominantly on the presynaptic enkaphalin receptors.

2 Dispersion within the CSF occurs as a result largely of diffusion which may be helped by movements such as coughing or change in position. This may account for the difference in respiratory depression seen in patients receiving extradural morphine in different positions (greater respiratory depression in the supine and semi-supine than sitting positions).

Some drug may reach the brain and be taken up by lipid.

3 Absorption from CSF into the circulation.

Following extradural administration of opioids, it has been demonstrated clearly that diffusion through the dura occurs into CSF. The more lipid-soluble drugs may gain more rapid access to the spinal fluid, via the arachnoid granulations in the dural cuff region and also by diffusion across the dura. In addition, opioids in the extradural space are absorbed directly into the circulation via the rich supply of vessels in the extra-dural space.

Consequently, following injection of opioid into the extradural space, there is a rapid increase in both CSF and blood concentrations of the drug (Fig. 66.15).

It may be seen, therefore, that the most important physical property of the opioid is its lipid-solubility which determines both the rate of onset of action of analgesia following either subarachnoid or extradural injection, and also duration of action.

Delayed respiratory depression is also a feature of the lipid-solubility of the drug. For a lipid-insoluble drug such as morphine, there is relatively little uptake

into extradural fat and thus a larger bolus resides in the extradural space for passage into the CSF. Uptake locally into the spinal cord is relatively small because of low lipophilicity, thereby permitting rostral spread of drug. Comparison of the lipid-solubilities of commonly available agents is shown in Table 66.10.

CLINICAL USE OF SUBARACHNOID OPIOIDS

This route of administration is less popular than the extradural route, as it may induce spinal headaches and the incidence of respiratory depression and other side-effects is higher than that following the extradural route. The only advantage of the intrathecal route is that, generally, much smaller doses are required than those with the extradural route and therefore systemic concentrations are lower.

Most experience has been gathered with morphine which has been injected in doses ranging from 0.25 to 0.5 mg or higher.

The quality of analgesia does not approach that which may be achieved using local anaesthetic agents in the subarachnoid space, but there are many studies in which excellent analgesia has been demonstrated in the postoperative period, for example following open-heart surgery.

As with the extradural route, it would appear that the quality of analgesia in obstetric patients is poorer than that in non-obstetric patients.

CLINICAL USE OF EXTRADURAL OPIOIDS

Considerable experience has now been gained using a variety of opioids injected into the extradural space by either intermittent or continuous infusion techniques.

The reasons for the enthusiastic use of opioids by the extradural route are that it is possible to achieve analgesia without producing the motor or autonomic block produced by local anaesthetic injected into the

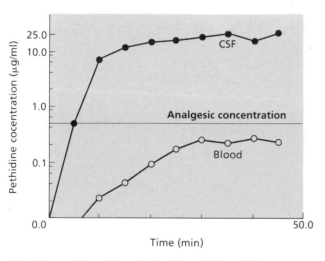

Fig. 66.15 Absorption of opioid into CSF and the circulation from an extradural infection.

Table 66.10 Characteristics of the use of opioids by the extradural route

Drug	Lipid-solubility	Dose	Onset time (min)	Duration of analgesia (hr)	Comments
Morphine	Low	25 mg	35	20+	Late respiratory depression common
Pethidine		50 mg	15	7	Late respiratory depression infrequent
Fentanyl		25–100 µg	10	5	Slight respiratory depression in early stages Late respiratory depression not reported
Methadone	High	4–6 µg	17	7	Respiratory depression rare but reported in one patient

extradural space. Thus, postural hypotension and changes in heart rate do not occur whilst the patient retains the ability to vasoconstrict in response to hypovolaemia. Early respiratory depression may occur as a result of systemic absorption of the drug (i.e. within 1–2 hr) but, provided the dose of the drug is kept low, this effect should be minimal. However, the development of late respiratory depression (6–24 hr) is a result of the rostral spread of opioid in the CSF to the brain. This side-effect has not been described with fentanyl, but is a feature of the hydrophilic drug, morphine. Rostral spread of the hydrophilic agents may give rise also to late CNS sedation, which may be extremely marked.

In obstetric practice, extradural opioids are frequently ineffective for the pain of second stage: this is probably because of the increased vascularity of the extradural space with absorption of drug directly into the circulation.

The doses of opioid should be kept relatively low. Studies have suggested that doses of 1–2 mg may be satisfactory, although a dose of 4–5 mg of morphine in 10 ml of saline is used commonly.

SIDE-EFFECTS OF EXTRADURAL OPIOIDS

The side-effects produced by opioids are shown in Table 66.11. The most significant side-effect produced by opioids injected into either the subarachnoid or extradural space is respiratory depression. This occurs most commonly following morphine. Early respiratory depression from vascular absorption has been described with fentanyl, but late respiratory depression is so far unrecognized.

With all opioids, depending on the dose, early respiratory depression may occur as a result of vascular absorption. Late respiratory depression, produced by rostral spread in the CSF, is unpredictable and may occur at any time from 4 to 5 hr onwards. Because of this unpredictability, it is highly advisable that all patients receiving extradural opioids be nursed in a high-dependency area.

Late respiratory depression, and also coma, can be reversed by naloxone (occasionally this may require very large doses). However, because the duration of action of naloxone is relatively short, patients may relapse back into respiratory failure and coma, and naloxone may require administration in repeated dose or by continuous infusion.

In general, it is possible to give naloxone in such a dosage as to reverse respiratory depression without

Table 66.11 Complications associated with the use of extradural opioids

Respiratory depression
Early: from systemic absorption
Late: from rostral spread in CSF augmented by:
    Dose
    Age
    Posture
    Aqueous solubility
    Additional systemic opioid

Nausea/vomiting
Similar incidence to that following i.m. administration

Itching
More common with morphine than fentanyl/diamorphine
Mechanisms possibly central and only relieved potentially by naloxone, antihistamine

Urinary retention
Incidence varies from 0 to 20%
Diuretic drug lasts from 2 to 20 hr
Improved by naloxone

Sedation
Associated invariably with the severe late form of respiratory depression

reversing analgesia. For an infusion, the recommended doses of naloxone range from 0.6 mg/hr to $5 \, \mu g \cdot kg^{-1} \cdot hr^{-1}$.

There are several factors which are known to increase the likelihood of respiratory depression following extradural morphine:

1 Posture. Rostral spread may be encouraged by the supine posture, particularly if there is a large element of coughing or straining.
2 The administration of further systemic opioids.
3 Increasing age of the patient. In the elderly, the dosage of morphine given via the extradural route should be reduced greatly and should be restricted to 0.5–1 mg.
4 Dosage of drug. Clearly, the higher the initial bolus dose of drug placed in the extradural space, the higher will be the CSF concentration.
5 Lipophilicity of drug; as discussed above.

Other methods of treating postoperative pain

Cryoanalgesia

Because the intercostal nerves are readily accessible during thoracotomy, it has been common practice for the thoracic surgeon to perform intercostal block with

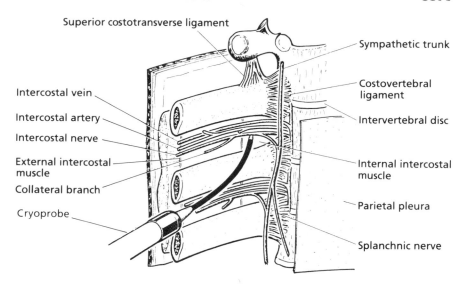

Fig. 66.16 Application of a cryo-probe to the intercostal nerve at thoracotomy to produce post-operative somatic analgesia. (Redrawn from Maiwand *et al.*, 1986.)

local anaesthetics, before closing the thoracotomy incision. With the advent of the cryoprobe, many units now employ routinely cryotherapy of the intercostal nerves at the time of surgery (Fig. 66.16).

Depending on the duration of freezing, numbness in the distribution of the intercostal nerves can be produced for a period of 30–200 days after application.

Excellent postoperative analgesia may be achieved by this technique, comparable if not superior to the use of opioids, although there are some disadvantages. The posterior primary rami of the intercostal nerves are not blocked and therefore back pain may be severe in the early postoperative period. In addition, prolonged analgesia in the region of the nipple of younger women is subjectively distressing (Maiwand *et al.*, 1986).

The technique does not eliminate totally the need for opioids in the early postoperative period, or the use of oral analgesics in the later postoperative period, but nonetheless it is an extremely useful technique.

NON-PHARMACOLOGICAL METHODS OF PAIN CONTROL

Stimulation-produced analgesia (transcutaneous nerve stimulation)

The modes of action of transcutaneous nerve stimulation (TNS or TENS) and acupuncture are probably similar. The techniques act probably by stimulation of non-pain afferent fibres (Aα-fibres) which activate directly modulation systems at spinal cord level.

For postoperative pain control, TENS is used frequently in the form of two electrodes placed on each side of the incision. However, electrodes may be placed also over the dermatome where pain is perceived. It has been suggested that the more effective sites for TENS electrodes correspond to established acupuncture points.

It is agreed generally that TENS does not produce satisfactory postoperative analgesia. However, it may produce a modest reduction in the overall requirements for systemic opioids, although this effect is not apparent in every patient. Its advantages are that it is non-invasive and drug-free.

Acupuncture

There have been relatively few studies of the use of acupuncture in the treatment of postoperative pain in Western Europe and its use is confined largely to the chronic pain clinic.

Psychological methods

A variety of psychological methods has been described in the management of acute postoperative pain and these have been shown to be associated with improvement in the postoperative experience. The reader is referred to articles by Chapman (1985) and Chapter 69, p. 1230. It would be true to say that good doctors have always employed such methods in the treatment of pain. In essence, a patient's surgical experience will be rendered much more pleasant and less distressing if he or she is encountered by a courteous and kindly doctor, who provides a full and rational explanation of the surgical experience, and who will reassure the patient that all his or her anxieties and somatic pain will receive prompt, immediate and effective therapy. In addition, the patient should be looked after by highly trained nursing staff of a similar disposition to that of the attending doctor and receive similar support and encouragement from friends and relatives. Positive encouragement from patients who have been through the same experience provides further reassurance and support.

This overall description of what constitutes good medical practice has been analysed into several components:

1 Cognitive techniques. This comprises the provision of adequate explanations and coaching.

2 Social modelling. This term is applied to the technique whereby patients are introduced to others who have coped successfully with the same procedure.

3 Biofeedback. This term describes the use of distraction, suggestion and relaxation, which can help to reduce analgesic requirements. The technique requires considerable training, whereby the patient learns to relax muscles and reduce tension by providing cognitive and behavioural help.

Hypnosis

This technique has been used to only a small extent in acute postoperative pain, with claims for reduced analgesic requirements postoperatively.

References

Aitkenhead A.R., Vater M., Cooper C.M.S. & Smith G. (1983) Pharmacokinetics of single dose i.v. morphine in normal volunteers and patients with end-stage renal failure. *British Journal of Anaesthesia* **55**, 905.

Austin K.L., Stapleton J.V. & Mather L.E. (1980a) Multiple intramuscular injections: a major source of variability in analgesic response to meperidine. *Pain* **8**, 47–62.

Austin K.L., Stapleton J.V. & Mather L.E. (1980b) Relationship between blood meperidine concentrations and analgesic response: a preliminary report. *Anesthesiology* **53**, 460–6.

Austin K.L., Stapleton J.V. & Mather L.E. (1981) Pethidine clearance during continuous intravenous infusions in postoperative patients. *British Journal of Clinical Pharmacology* **1**, 25–30.

Bellville J.W., Forrest W.H., Miller E. & Brown B.W. jr (1971) Influence of age on pain relief from analgesics. *Journal of the American Medical Association* **217**, 1835–41.

Bentley J.B., Borel J.D., Nenad R.E. & Gillespie T.J. (1982) Age and fentanyl pharmacokinetics. *Anesthesia and Analgesia* **61**, 968–71.

Berkowitz B.A., Ngai S.H., Yang J.C., Hempstead J. & Spector S. (1975) The disposition of morphine in surgical patients. *Clinical Pharmacology and Therapeutics* **17**, 629–35.

Bowler G.M.R., Wildsmith J.A.W. & Scott D.B. (1986) Epidural administration of local anaesthetics. In *Acute Pain Management* (Eds Cousins M.J. & Phillips G.D.) pp. 187–235. Churchill Livingstone, Edinburgh.

Boyle P. & Parbrook G.D. (1977) The interrelation of personality and postoperative factors. *British Journal of Anaesthesia* **49**, 259–64.

Bromage P.R., Camporesi E.M. & Chestnut D. (1980) Epidural narcotics for postoperative analgesia. *Anesthesia and Analgesia* **59**, 473.

Buckley F.P. (1985) Somatic nerve block for postoperative analgesia. In *Acute Pain* (Eds Smith G. & Covino B.G.) pp. 205–27. Butterworths, London.

Catling J.A., Pinto D.M., Jordon C. & Jones J.G. (1980) Respiratory effects of analgesia after cholecystectomy: comparison of continuous and intermittent papaveretum. *British Medical Journal* **281**, 478.

Chapman C.R. (1985) Psychological factors in postoperative pain. In *Acute Pain* (Eds Smith G. & Covino B.G.) pp. 22–41. Butterworths, London.

Christensen P., Brandt M.R., Rem J. & Kehlet H. (1982) Influence of extradural morphine on the adrenocortical and hyperglycaemic response to surgery. *British Journal of Anaesthesia* **54**, 23–7.

Cohen F.L. (1980) Postsurgical pain relief: patient's status and nurses' medication choices. *Pain* **9**, 265–74.

Cousins M.J. & Bridenbaugh P.O. (1986) Spinal opioids and pain relief in acute care. In *Acute Pain Management* (Eds Cousins M.J. & Phillips G.D.) pp. 151–85. Churchill Livingstone, Edinburgh.

Cousins M.J. & Mather L.E. (1984) Intrathecal and epidural administration of opioids. *Anesthesiology* **61**, 276.

Cousins M.J., Mather L.E., Glynn C.J., Wilson P.R. & Graham J.R. (1979) Selective spinal anaesthesia. *Lancet* **i**, 1141.

Dahlstrom B., Tamsen A., Paalzow L. & Hartvig P. (1982) Patient-controlled analgesic therapy. part IV: pharmacokinetics and analgesic plasma concentrations of morphine. *Clinical Pharmacokinetics* **7**, 266–79.

De Boer A.G., De Leede L.G.J. & Breimer D.D. (1984) Drug absorption by sublingual and rectal routes. *British Journal of Anaesthesia* **56**, 69–82.

De Castro J. & Viars P. (1968) Anesthesie analgesique sequentielle *Ars Medici* **23**, 121.

Dodson M.E. (1985) *The Management of Postoperative Pain* p. 274. Edward Arnold, London.

Duthie D.J.R., Rowbotham D.J., Wyld R., Henderson P.D. & Nimmo W.S. (1988) Plasma fentanyl concentrations during transdermal fentanyl delivery to surgical patients. *British Journal of Anaesthesia* **60**, 614–8.

Eason M.J. & Wyatt R. (1979) Paravertebral thoracic block—reappraisal. *Anaesthesia* **34**, 638–42.

Ellis R., Haines D., Shah R., Cotton B.R. & Smith G. (1982) Pain relief after abdominal surgery—a comparison of intramuscular morphine, sublingual buprenorphine and self-administered intravenous pethidine. *British Journal of Anaesthesia* **54**, 421.

Gibbs J.M., Johnson H.D. & Davis F.M. (1982) Patient administration of intravenous buprenorphine for postoperative pain relief using the 'Cardiff' demand analgesia apparatus. *British Journal of Anaesthesia* **54**, 279.

Glynn C.J., Lloyd J.W. & Folkard S. (1976) The diurnal variation in perception of pain. *Proceedings of the Royal Society of Medicine* **69**, 369.

Hanning C.D. (1985) Non-parenteral techniques. In *Acute Pain* (Eds Smith G. & Covino B.G.) pp. 180–204. Butterworths, London.

Hanning C.D., Vickers A.P., Smith G., Graham N.B. & McNeil M.E. (1988) The morphine hydrogel suppository: a new sustained release rectal preparation. *British Journal of Anaesthesia* **61**, 221–8.

Harmer M., Rosen M. & Vickers M.D. (1985) *Patient Controlled Analgesia*. Blackwell Scientific Publications, Oxford.

Hughes J., Smith T.W., Kosterlitz H.W., Fothergill L.A., Morgan B.A.

& Morris H.R. (1975) Isolation of two related pentopeptides from brain with potent opiate activity. *Nature* **258**, 577.

Hull C.J. (1985) The pharmacokinetics of opioid analgesics with special reference to patient controlled administration. In *Patient Controlled Analgesia* (Eds Harmer M., Rosen M. & Vickers M.D.) pp. 7–17. Blackwell Scientific Publications, Oxford.

Kehlet H. (1986) Pain relief and modification of the stress response. In *Acute Pain Management* (Eds Cousins M.J. & Phillips G.D.) pp. 49–75. Churchill Livingstone, Edinburgh.

Lim A.T., Edis G., Kranz H., Mendelson G., Selwood T. & Scott D.F. (1983) Postoperative pain control: contribution of psychological factors and transcutaneous electrical stimulation. *Pain* **17**, 179–88.

Loan W.B. & Dundee J.W. (1967) The clinical assessment of pain. *Practitioner* **198**, 759–68.

Maiwand M.O., Makey A.R. & Rees A. (1986) Cryoanalgesia after thoracotomy. *Journal of Thoracic and Cardiovascular Surgery* **92**, 291–5.

Mather L.E. & Meffin P.J. (1978) Clinical pharmacokinetics of pethidine. *Clinical Pharmacokinetics* **3**, 352–68.

Mather L.E., Tucker G.T., Pflug A.E., Lindop M.J. & Wilkerson C. (1975) Meperidine kinetics in man. Intravenous injection in surgical patients and volunteers. *Clinical Pharmacology and Therapeutics* **17**, 21–30.

Nayman J. (1979) Measurement and control of postoperative pain. *Annals of the Royal College of Surgeons* **61**, 419.

Parbrook G.D., Steel D.F. & Dalrymple D.G. (1973) Factors predisposing to postoperative pain and pulmonary complications: a study of male patients undergoing elective gastric surgery. *British Journal of Anaesthesia* **45**, 21–33.

Parkhouse J., Lambrechts W. & Simpton B.R.J. (1961) The incidence of postoperative pain. *British Journal of Anaesthesia* **33**, 345.

Pert C.B. & Snyder S. (1973) Opiate receptors: demonstration in nervous tissue. *Science* **179**, 1011.

Pinnock C.A., Derbyshire D.R., Achola K.J. & Smith G. (1986) Absorption of controlled release morphine sulphate in the immediate postoperative period. *British Journal of Anaesthesia* **58**, 868–71.

Rifat K. (1972) Pentazocine in sequential analgesic anaesthesia. *British Journal of Anaesthesia* **44**, 175–82.

Rosow C.E. (1985) Newer synthetic opioid analgesics. In *Acute Pain* (Eds Smith G. & Covino B.G.) pp. 68–103. Butterworths, London.

Rutberg H., Hakanson E., Anderberg B., Jorfeldt L., Martensson J. & Schildt B. (1984) Effects of the extradural administration of morphine, or bupivacaine, on the endocrine response to upper abdominal surgery. *British Journal of Anaesthesia* **56**, 233–8.

Rutter P.C. Murphy F. & Dudley H.A.F. (1980) Morphine: controlled trial of different methods of administration for postoperative pain relief. *British Medical Journal* **1**, 12–13.

Saha S.K. (1981) Continuous infusion of papaveretum for relief of postoperative pain. *Postgraduate Medical Journal* **57**, 686–9.

Scott L.E., Clum G.A. & Peoples J.B. (1983) Preoperative predictors of postoperative pain. *Pain* **15**, 283.

Sechzer P.H. (1971) Studies in pain with the analgesic-demand system. *Anaesthesia* **50**, 1–10.

Spence A.A. & Logan D.A. (1975) Respiratory effects of extradural nerve block in the postoperative period. *British Journal of Anaesthesia* **47**, 281–3.

Spence A.A. & Smith G. (1971) Postoperative analgesia and lung function: a comparison of morphine with extradural block. *British Journal of Anaesthesia* **43**, 144–8.

Stanton-Hicks M.J. (1985) Subarachnoid and extradural analgesic techniques. In *Acute Pain* (Eds Smith G. & Covino B.G.) pp. 228–56. Butterworths, London.

Stapleton J.V., Austin K.L. & Mather L.E. (1979) A pharmacokinetic approach to postoperative pain: continuous infusion of pethidine. *Anaesthesia and Intensive Care* **7**, 25–32.

Tamsen A., Bondesson U., Dahlstrom B. & Hartvig P. (1982b) Patient-controlled analgesic therapy, part III: pharmacokinetics and analgesic plasma concentrations of ketobemidone. *Clinical Pharmacokinetics* **7**, 252–66.

Tamsen A., Hartvig P., Fagerlund C. & Dahlstrom B. (1982a) Patient-controlled analgesic therapy, part II: individual analgesic demand and analgesic plasma concentrations of pethidine in postoperative pain. *Clinical Pharmacokinetics* **7**, 164–75.

Tamsen A., Sakurada T., Wahlstrom A., Terenius L. & Hartvig P. (1982c) Postoperative demand for analgesics in relation to individual levels of endorphins and substance P in cerebrospinal fluid. *Pain* **13**, 171–83.

Twycross R.G. & Lack S.A. (1983) *Symptom Control in Far-advanced Cancer: Pain Relief*. Pitman, London.

Vickers A.P., Derbyshire D.R., Burt D.R., Bagshaw P.F., Pearson H. & Smith G. (1987) Comparison of the Leicester Micropalliator and the Cardiff Palliator in the relief of postoperative pain. *British Journal of Anaesthesia* **59**, 503–9.

White P.F. (1985) Use of a patient controlled analgesia infuser for the management of postoperative pain. In *Patient Controlled Analgesia* (Eds Harmer M., Rosen M. & Vickers M.D.) pp. 140–8. Blackwell Scientific Publications, Oxford.

Yaksh T.L. (1984) Multiple opioid receptor systems in brain and spinal cord. *European Journal of Anaesthesiology* **1**, 171 (Part I), 201 (Part II).

67

Common Conditions in the Pain Clinic and Their Management

H. J. McQUAY

This chapter describes the clinical management of conditions which occur commonly in the pain clinic. The technical details for drug management, nerve blocks and alternative measures are described elsewhere; this chapter suggests which of these measures is appropriate and when. A safe and conservative view (hopefully) is presented.

Which are the common pain conditions? The prevalence of chronic pain (pain resistant to one month of treatment) in the population at large is not known. Within the pain clinic population, 25% of all patients have pain associated with malignancy, whilst 75% have 'non-malignant' pain.

An outline of the commoner causes of pain associated with malignancy is given on p. 1202. However, the simple distinction between malignant and non-malignant is not very practical because the treatment methods may be the same, and also because the differential diagnosis for many pain conditions includes both malignant and non-malignant causes (cf. back pain and facial pain, p. 1204 and 1210). Therefore, the common pain conditions (prevalence greater than 3%; Table 67.1) are described after discussing separately the pain of malignant and non-malignant origin.

PAIN ASSOCIATED WITH MALIGNANCY
(p. 1202 and Chapter 68)

Not all patients with cancer have pain, but the prevalence increases with the progression of disease, so that, with advanced disease, 60–90% of patients have significant pain (Twycross & Lack, 1983; Foley, 1985).

Management of *acute* cancer-related pain associated with diagnosis or treatment involves identifying the cause, and treating the pain, which is often self-limited. The methods needed are often analogous to those used in postoperative pain.

Chronic cancer-related pain may be related to tumour progression (62%), tumour treatment (25%), or may be a pre-existing chronic pain (10%) (Foley, 1985) unrelated to the tumour. Transient relief in malignant pain may be achieved by the same blocks which are used in non-malignant pain, such as extradural local anaesthetic, and by using a catheter the duration of relief may be extended if necessary. These 'simple' measures are often forgotten. Longer-term relief may be provided by injections using neurolytic solutions, cryoanalgesia or radiofrequency, percutaneous cordotomy or hypophysectomy (see Chapter 70 for technical details). Pain produced by malignancy is managed often on a co-operative basis between general practitioner, the oncology/radiotherapy department, hospice and pain clinic. While the specific role of the pain clinic is to provide pain-relieving nerve blocks, most patients benefit from the combination of these procedures with skillful analgesic management, radiotherapy and appropriate control of symptoms other than pain.

The pattern of referral of malignant pain problems to pain clinics may be allocated to two main categories. The first relates to problems which are thought to be amenable to nerve-blocking procedures; the referral may come at an early stage in the patient's illness, or when they are terminally ill. The educative role of pain clinics is important here, because others involved in the patient's care are sometimes unaware of what is possible. The second category is the despairing referral, often at a late stage in the illness, when the pain is not responding well to drug management alone. The commoner pain conditions associated with malignancy are discussed later. Analgesic management, and

Table 67.1 Data from 1115 patients with chronic non-malignant pain

Pain condition*	Percentage of total	Sex ratio (M:F)	Age (yr) (mean and range)	Duration of pain (yr) (mean and range)
Low back pain	26.2	1:1.7	51.8 (23->80)	8.8 (0.5-32)
Postherpetic neuralgia	10.8	1:1.6	73.0 (35->80)	2.6 (0.5-20)
Post-traumatic neuralgia	8.6	1:1.2	50.0 (19->80)	4.8 (0.5-36)
Atypical facial neuralgia	5.9	1:2.0	48.2† (22-79)	4.3 (0.5-17)
Intercostal neuralgia	5.2	1:1.5	55.0† (25->80)	4.3 (0.5-30)
Trigeminal neuralgia	4.6	1:2.4	64.3 (32->80)	9.3 (0.5-52)
Perineal neuralgia	3.9	1:1.9	64.5 (32->80)	6.8 (0.5-35)
Abdominal neuralgia	3.7	1:1.2	56.2 (26->80)	5.6 (1-24)
Stump/phantom pain	3.0	1:0.4	62.6** (28->80)	12.5 (1-61)
Osteoarthritis hip	2.8	1:1.2	74.4 (30->80)	4.3 (0.5-15)
Sympathetic dystrophy	2.4	1:1.1	59.1 (27->80)	4.2 (1-6)
Coccydynia	2.3	1:4.2	53.8 (26-73)	5.7† (0.5-31)
Cervical spondylosis	2.1	1:1.5	52.6 (37->80)	5.9 (0.5-17)
Other conditions	18.5			

* All conditions with >2% incidence.
† Significant difference ($p<0.05$) in mean age or mean pain duration (female >male).
** Significant difference ($p<0.01$) in mean age or mean pain duration (female >male) (student's 't' test).
  'Other conditions' includes osteoarthritis (unspecified), osteoarthritic spine, causalgia, other nerve neuralgia, cord damage, thalamic syndrome, disseminated sclerosis, occipital neuralgia, claudication and neuroma.

the special case of the dying patient, are described in Chapter 68.

NON-MALIGNANT PAIN

The prevalence of the various pain conditions at the Oxford Unit is shown in Table 67.1 (McQuay *et al.*, 1985). The population served by the Oxford region is 2.3 million. The table summarizes the information (age, sex, duration of pain at first attendance) for diagnostic categories with a prevalence greater than 2%. The pain condition with the highest prevalence (26%) is low back pain; only postherpetic neuralgia had a prevalence which was also greater than 10%. For the purposes of this chapter, 'common' non-malignant pain conditions are those with a prevalence greater than 3% as shown in Table 67.1; clinical features and an outline of management of these conditions are provided on p. 1204.

The list of conditions shown in Table 67.1 is long; the doctor must therefore be able to manage a variety of conditions which are not common. The length of the list of diagnostic categories means that no one clinic will see large numbers of patients with conditions of low prevalence. Management strategy is then necessarily empirical because such small numbers make controlled studies very difficult to perform.

Non-malignant pain management presents great resource problems, because for many conditions there is no cure, but treatment may provide short-term relief. Many of these patients have normal life expectancy, and continue to seek such short-term relief because it improves their quality of life. The ethos of the pain clinic, often the last medical resort, is very important to these patients and to their management (Editorial, 1982).

EXAMINATION OF THE PATIENT

The most important principle is that the patient and the physician are served best if the physician believes the patient's report (Foley, 1985). Pain is necessarily subjective, and there are few objective signs which the doctor can use to judge the severity of reported pain. Many patients have no visible handicap, and their problems may not be understood well, and may even be disbelieved at work and at home. Much time and energy is wasted on procedures designed to 'catch the patient out'. Chronic pain changes people, affecting their personal and working lives, and ultimately their personalities. Often such changes are reversible with successful treatment. Labelling patients as malingerers or the pain as psychogenic may be easier than admitting that there is no successful treatment.

The pain history

The extra emphasis of a pain history compared with a 'normal' medical history is summarized in the following series of questions.

Site of pain. Where do you feel this pain? Does it go anywhere else? Is it numb where you feel the pain?

Character of pain. What sort of a pain is it? (Burning/shooting/stabbing/dull, etc.)

History of pain. How long have you had this pain? How did it start? Did it come on out of the blue or was it triggered by something?

Relieving factors. Does anything make it better? (Position, drugs, distraction, alcohol, etc.)

Accentuating factors. Does anything make it worse? (Position/exercise/weather, etc.)

Pattern. Is there any pattern to the pain? (frequency/severity.) Is it worse at any particular time of day?

Sleep disturbance. Do you go to sleep with no trouble? Does the pain wake you up?

Activities. What activities does the pain stop you doing which you would otherwise do?

Some index of function is necessary as a base-line so that improvement or deterioration may be monitored. Outcome measures in the pain clinic have been notoriously lacking; the Burford pain thermometer, combining a simple visual analogue pain intensity score with a record of analgesics taken (on the same record) has worked well for both in- and outpatients (Burford Nursing Development Unit, 1984).

Previous treatments. What methods have been tried already? Did they help the pain?

It is important to be sure if nerve blocks used previously were technically effective (e.g. did the patient have any numbness after an extradural which included local anaesthetic?), before dismissing them as of no help to this patient. Equally, other measures, such as transcutaneous nerve stimulation, may not have been used correctly, and may succeed if the patient receives correct instructions in their use.

Drug history. It is important to enquire specifically regarding the efficacy of each particular drug class (major and minor analgesics, anticonvulsants, etc., cf. Table 67.2). This information prevents the inept prescription of drugs which have failed previously, and may give important clues as to the type of pain and its sensitivity to different classes of drug.

It is important also to ascertain the dose size, frequency, duration of prescription and side-effects for each drug which has been prescribed. Dose–response relationships apply in analgesic management, and therapeutic failure should not be presumed if the dosage was inadequate (cf. carbamazepine in trigeminal neuralgia, see below).

It is important to ascertain if the patient is receiving drugs other than analgesics. Anticoagulants, for instance, are not only an (almost) absolute contraindication to pain management by injection procedures, but also interact with some anti-inflammatory drugs.

Examination and investigations. Specific features of physical examination and investigations are noted with the pain conditions. As patients may be seen over many years in a pain clinic, an accurate serial record of physical signs is important in deciding if a new pathology has developed or if new or repeat investigations are required.

TREATMENT OPTIONS

The major options are shown in Table 67.2.

Nerve blocks

The common nerve-block procedures which the pain clinic should provide are summarized in Table 67.3. Many of these blocks may be performed 'diagnostic-ally', with local anaesthetic drugs as a preliminary to making a more permanent block as with cryoanal-gesia, radiofrequency lesions, phenol or surgery. The use of steroids may convert the diagnostic block to a therapeutic block, as with an extradural for low back pain. Repeated blocks with local anaesthetic drugs may be therapeutic *per se* (e.g. repeated stellate ganglion blocks for causalgia).

Table 67.2 Treatment options

Nerve block or surgery	Reversible	e.g. Local anaesthetic $\pm$ steroid, cryoanalgesia
	Irreversible	e.g. Ablative nerve blocks, surgical procedures, radiofrequency
Analgesics	*Conventional* Minor non-opioid	Aspirin, paracetamol, non-steroidal, anti-inflammatory (NSAI), nefopam
	Minor opioid and combination	Codeine, dihydrocodeine, dextropro-poxyphene, alone or in combination with minor non-opioid
	Major opioid	Morphine, buprenorphine, etc.
	Unconventional Anticonvulsant	Carbamazepine, valproate, phenytoin, clonazepam
	Antidepressant	Amitriptyline, dothiepin, mianserin
Alternatives	Transcutaneous nerve stimulation, hypnosis, acupuncture, etc.	

Table 67.3 Common nerve blocks. (From Foley, 1985)

Block	Common indications
Trigger point	Focal pain (e.g. in muscle)

Peripheral	Pain in dermatomal distribution
	    Intercostal
	    Sacral nerves
	    Rectus sheath

Extradural	Uni- or bilateral pain (lumbosacral, cervical, thoracic, etc.) Midline perineal pain
Intrathecal	Unilateral pain (neurolytic injection for pain from malignancy, limbs, chest, etc.) (Midline perineal pain)
Autonomic Stellate ganglion	Reflex sympathetic dystrophy Arm pain Brachial plexus nerve compression
Lumbar sympathetic	Reflex sympathetic dystrophy Lumbosacral plexus nerve compression Vascular insufficiency lower limb
Coeliac plexus	Abdominal pain

The technical aspects and the potential morbidity of these blocks are familiar to most anaesthetists. The rectus sheath, intercostal and lumbar sympathectomy blocks are described well in Mackintosh and Bryce-Smith (1962). 'Modern' lumbar sympathectomy has the advantage of image intensification and the current technical controversies are discussed by Boas (1983). Stellate ganglion and 'blind' coeliac plexus blocks are described well by Bryce-Smith (1976), and sacral nerve blocks by Labat (1924).

Many of these procedures are performed on an outpatient basis, and the period between performance of the block and when the patient goes home should be sufficient for any complications (most of which are 'early', viz. pneumothorax after intercostal or stellate blocks) to become apparent *before* the patient leaves. Two complications present particular problems. Hypotension occurs during the first few hours after coeliac plexus block, so that patients should be admitted to hospital for the procedure. Lumbar sympathectomy with neurolytic agents may cause troublesome neuralgic pain, often in the groin or on the anterior aspect of the thigh. Although this may be severe, occurring in as many as 10% of patients, it is self-limiting (6–8 weeks), and transcutaneous nerve stimulation may produce very effective relief.

Analgesic drugs

Anaesthetists used to treating postoperative pain assume rightly that most acute pain can be managed satisfactorily with conventional analgesics. One of the many differences between acute and chronic pain is that the latter may not be so amenable to satisfactory therapy. At the Oxford Unit, one-third of patients in both malignant and non-malignant categories have pains which respond poorly, if at all, to conventional analgesic drugs, major or minor. For example, carbamazepine is a classic 'unconventional' analgesic but it is used successfully in the management of trigeminal neuralgia; opioid-resistant pain was described well by Tolstoy in *The Death of Ivan Ilyich*. Clinically, pains in numb areas (deafferentation e.g. phantom limb pain), nerve compression, postherpetic neuralgia and many abdominal pains) do not respond well to opioids. Their use may make the patient feel better, but the analgesic effects may be poor.

Pain conditions associated with malignancy

The specific role of the pain clinic in pain associated with malignancy is the provision of nerve-blocking procedures. However, the role of these blocks is very ill-defined, because, despite widespread use of the techniques, careful studies of quality and duration of relief and morbidity compared with other methods are lacking. Nonetheless, those expert in the use of these techniques have no doubt of their value (Wood, 1984). However, improvement in pain control generally, with better use of oral opioids, has reduced the numbers of blocks performed. This carries the danger that the expertise required to perform techniques which may be of great value, particularly in pain responding poorly to opioids, may be lost.

Pharmacological management

Drug therapy is discussed in Chapter 68. In the pain clinic, many patients are not terminal, and patients referred for a specific nerve block may be helped also by sensible use of analgesics (in addition to other supportive measures). Thus, the pain clinic doctor must be familiar with the use of oral opioid analgesics in the ambulant patient in addition to the terminal case.

It is important to remember that not all pains are sensitive to opioids (see above). A careful history (noting response of the pain at *each* site of pain to analgesics) is required. Any increase in dose required to sustain analgesia should be noted, with the time intervals. Patients may be referred to the pain clinic for therapeutic trial of opioids given spinally, and selection of patients for extradural or intrathecal catheterization for opioids requires careful attention to these details for the procedures to be worthwhile (Editorial, 1986).

Lack of response to pharmacological management and/or unacceptable side-effects are major indications for nerve-blocking techniques in pain resulting from malignancy. The anticonvulsant and antidepressant drugs (Table 67.2) may be useful alternatives if a block is impossible, or for the management of pain at other sites.

Simple remedies, such as the short-term use of extradural local anaesthetic, may be of inestimable value in allowing correct assessment of those patients who have not had analgesic benefit from 'industrial' doses of opioids. The opioids may be withdrawn under the cover of the local anaesthetic, and appropriate therapy may be instituted.

Nerve blocks

Technical details of ablative nerve blocks are discussed in Chapter 70.

HEAD AND NECK

Pain in the distribution of the trigeminal nerve, accompanied at worst by trismus, dysphagia or halitosis, may be helped by blocking the relevant nerve branch; mandibular or maxillary blocks are the most useful (Churcher, 1983). Dysphagia may limit the intake of opioids orally, and in this group, subcutaneous opioid infusions and more recently intracerebroventricular opioids have been used (Lobato *et al.*, 1984).

CHEST WALL

Intercostal diagnostic blocks with local anaesthetic may be used, and to extend duration of relief, cryoanalgesia has superseded the use of neurolytic agents. If the pain does not respond to intercostal block, an intrathecal neurolytic block may be used. Extradural neurolytic agents possess limited efficacy. Whilst claims have been made that the paravertebral approach is preferable, patchy results may be attributed to unpredictable spread of the injectate.

ABDOMEN

Abdominal pain associated with pancreatic cancer responds well to coeliac plexus block (Jones & Gough, 1977), and this block may also help those with abdominal or perineal pain from tumour in the pelvis. In general, abdominal pain from tumour is not easy to manage with opioids alone, and these drugs in conjunction with coeliac plexus block (if feasible) may provide better pain control. The splanchnic approach, placing the solutions dorsal rather than ventral to the diaphragmatic crura, has been claimed to enhance the technical precision of the block (Boas, 1983). The good results with the classic method [technically improved by use of image intensification or computerized tomography (CT) scan imaging] are unlikely to be improved by the newer approaches but the existing low technical morbidity may be reduced further.

Sympathetic blocks (lumbar sympathectomy) may be useful also for rectal pain. Rectal 'phantom' pain following resection is not uncommon, and both this phantom pain and tenesmus may respond to sympathectomy.

Pain in the distribution of the sacral nerves may respond to sacral extradural block with local anaesthetic and steroid, and individual sacral nerves may also be blocked diagnostically at the foramina (Labat,

1924). Cryoanalgesia may be used to extend the duration of relief.

For severe pelvic or perineal pain, intrathecal neurolytic block can be most rewarding (Wood, 1984). The limitation is the presence of bilateral pain requiring bilateral blocks with the attendant higher risk of bladder dysfunction.

PAIN FROM BONY METASTASES

Isolated metastases which occur in areas already irradiated maximally, or unresponsive to radiation, may respond to 'simple' blocks, such as extradural local anaesthetic and steroid for spinal metastases. Intrathecal neurolytic blocks may be necessary for pain in arm or leg long bones. Cordotomy may be most useful for unilateral pelvic, hip or leg pain.

Hypophysectomy in pain management of multiple bony metastases works by unknown mechanism, but it may produce worthwhile relief in hormone-dependent tumours.

PAIN FROM NERVE PLEXUS COMPRESSION

Local spread of tumour, metastases or the treatment of tumour may result in compression of either the lumbosacral or brachial plexus. Pelvic tumour (cancer of colon, rectum, cervix, etc.) may produce direct nerve compression or compress the lumbosacral plexus at various levels. Carcinoma of the breast (and radiotherapy), together with carcinoma of the lung (Pancoast's) are the commonest causes of brachial plexus involvement seen in the pain clinic.

The pain which results may be the most difficult pain of all to treat. In an advanced stage the pain occurs often in a numb (deafferented) area.

The breast-cancer patient may present with a swollen painful arm. Initial investigation should determine if tumour spread has occurred (potentially treatable) or if radiation fibrosis is the cause. In its early stages, the swelling may be reduced by simple techniques used to control lymphoedema; results in late cases are poor. The pain from Pancoast's tumour may be more restricted to a particular dermatome(s).

In both conditions, poor management with conventional analgesics may be improved by using an anticonvulsant and antidepressant regimen. Intrathecal neurolytic blocks for the relevant dermatome may be required. Cordotomy is often not feasible if the pain is higher than the C6 level, and extradural neurolytic injection gives poor results. The response to intrathecal neurolytics is better for tumour damage than for radiation fibrosis.

Lumbosacral plexus involvement may present as root pain, pain from peripheral nerve involvement, or pain in widespread areas of numbness. Successful peripheral diagnostic nerve blockade with local anaesthetic may be extended (as with cryoanalgesia). Cordotomy is practicable in this region for root or more widespread pain, and again intrathecal neurolytic blocks are a major option, restricted to unilateral pain when it is imperative to preserve bladder function.

Common pain conditions

Chronic back pain

Chronic back pain is the commonest condition seen in the pain clinic (approximately 25% of non-malignant cases). The patients may be allocated to three main categories:
1 Pain from malignancy.
2 Pain which has not responded to conservative measures.
3 Pain recurring despite previous surgery.

The major pitfall is to miss a treatable cause of pain in the urgency to treat symptoms. With failed conservative management, the most difficult problem may be to decide what changes in signs and symptoms warrant further investigation. Pain despite surgery should become less common as awareness increases that pain alone may not justify laminectomy, as 40% of these patients had recurrent pain after 1 yr (Martin, 1981; Benzon, 1986). Whilst such patients are still being referred, it is important to remember that some may *still* have a surgically remediable lesion.

The next section outlines some common and some obscure causes of back pain. There are many different ways of classifying back pain; the following uses the common categories presenting at the pain clinic. For more general purposes, the fundamental distinction of three main presenting problems (mechanical back pain, possible spinal pathology, nerve root pain) should be used (Waddell, 1982). Management of the pain is discussed subsequently.

CAUSES OF BACK PAIN (Table 67.4)

Prolapsed intervertebral disc

Site: pain in the back (lumbago) with pain down the leg (sciatica) if severe.

Table 67.4 Causes of back pain in the pain clinic

Major
Prolapsed intervertebral disc
Facet joint degeneration
Pain recurring after previous surgery
Arachnoiditis
Pitfalls
Cauda equina claudication
Cauda equina tumours
Pelvic lesions
Arteriovenous malformations of the cord
Tumour
Primary e.g. myeloma
Secondary (breast, prostate, melanoma, etc.)
Compression of lumbosacral plexus
Tuberculosis, osteomyelitis, ankylosing spondylitis

Features: often occurs once or twice a year, with or without a history of provocation, and often settles spontaneously (conservative management). The pain is thought to arise from swollen nerve roots, and subsequently the disc retracts with the development of scarring after months.

A herniated disc compressing a nerve root may produce limitation of one specific movement only, and straight leg raising of the normal leg may produce crossed pain in the affected leg.

Facet joint degeneration

Site: back pain with or without leg pain.

Features: the pain arises from degeneration of the facet joints. Some distinction from disc disease may be possible from the history. Facet joint degeneration may produce pain on sitting which may be relieved by standing up and walking (the opposite of the usual history for disc problems). On examination, pain from the facet joints may be elicited by lying the patient prone and extending the facet joints by lifting the legs.

Pain recurring after previous surgery on the back

Patients referred to the pain clinic because of back pain recurring after surgery on the back present special diagnostic problems. The causes of such recurrent pain include the following.

Recurrent prolapsed intervertebral disc. Does the patient have a recurrent disc? The patient may have a good original story with a positive myelogram, and a disc protrusion removed at operation and have done well for several months or indeed years. Then history repeats itself (Martin, 1981), and the pain (and any radiation) may be the same as that before the operation.

The disc which was causing the pain was not removed at operation. Straight X-ray of the lumbar spine reveals the level of the operation.

The disc removed was not the cause of the pain. If a prolapsed intervertebral disc *was* found on myelography, and was removed at operation, and yet the pain persisted, that disc may not have been the cause of the pain. Original investigations (myelography) must include the conus in order to exclude other causes of pain co-existing with a disc lesion.

Patients in this category may respond to facet joint procedures, suggesting that this may have been the cause of the original pain.

Postoperative complications causing pain. Such complications include dural damage, arachnoid hernia, nerve root pressure, sciatica and sterile osteitis. Patients referred soon after operation (6 weeks) may have this sterile osteitis, which presents as severe lumbar back pain induced by the slightest movement. Translucency at the upper and lower margins of the adjacent vertebral bodies, raised erythrocyte sedimentation rate (ESR) and white cell count confirm the diagnosis. The condition settles with rest and leads spontaneously to bony fusion at which time the pain does not recur.

Arachnoiditis

Intrathecal adhesions which occur after a variety of intrathecal insults may result in the clinical syndrome of arachnoiditis, which can cause serious chronic problems (Shaw *et al.*, 1978). The causes include:
1 Myelography.
2 Bleeding.
3 Poor or recurrent surgery.
4 Infection.
5 Idiopathic.

Approximately 50% of patients develop symptoms and/or signs within 1 yr; in a small number (15%), 10 yr may elapse before problems develop (Shaw *et al.*, 1978). In Shaw's series of 80 patients, 43 had undergone myelography, and in many this had been difficult technically. Fifty-one had undergone spinal surgery.

Approximately 25% of the patients had progressive disease. In a clinic with a high proportion of 'failed-surgery' back-pain patients, arachnoiditis may be a common problem.

Site: back pain, with root signs in 50%.

Features: classically the pain of arachnoiditis is a burning constant pain with sciatic distribution to one or both legs, with signs of gradual and progressive loss of leg reflexes. In reality, the pain may be difficult to distinguish from that caused by other back problems and the signs may be unconvincing. The diagnosis rests on the history, examination and myelographic evidence, where at least two of the following changes should be sought (Shaw *et al.* 1978) to support the diagnosis:
1 Partial or complete block.
2 Narrowing of the subarachnoid space.
3 Obliteration of the nerve root sleeves and thickening of the nerve roots.
4 Irregular distribution and loculation of the contrast medium.
5 Fixity of previously inserted contrast medium.
6 Pseudocyst formation.

The pitfalls

Cauda equina claudication, caused by spondylosis producing narrowing of a pre-existing narrow lumbar canal, occurs mainly in those over 60-yr old, and there is often a long history. The pain is sciatic in type with paraesthesiae on standing and walking, relieved by sitting and lying down. The pain is often made worse by bending forward (flexion presumably accentuating the narrowing). It may be distinguished from claudication *per se* because resting relieves claudication, but may not do so in the cauda equina condition. Some patients may be able to walk further by bending forward. Cycling often does not induce pain. On examination, one or both ankle jerks may be absent. On investigation, myelography shows complete block or marked stenosis.

Cauda equina tumours have the reputation of being classic diagnostic pitfalls (Fearnside & Adams, 1978). The patients are often labelled hysterical personalities. The site of pain is in the back with a sciatic component in 50%. There is a progressive history characteristically, and the pain is worse at night. The patient *has* to get out of bed and then sit in a chair for the rest of the night. The pain may be made worse by jolting or jarring rather than by the twisting or bending which elicits pain from disc problems. There may be difficulties with micturition some time before motor or sensory signs are found. The clinical diagnosis rests largely on the history because there may be few neurological signs.

Primary or secondary malignancy in the pelvis may produce back pain with or without leg pain. This may arise from the disease mass or from invasion of the lumbar plexus invasion.

Arteriovenous malformation of the spinal cord can produce back pain, with or without leg pain. The pain may be worse on walking. Neurological signs appear progressively, and myelography may be reported as normal.

Tumour and infection around the spine can produce back pain: causes include primary myeloma, bony secondaries, extradural tumour, tuberculosis, osteomyelitis and ankylosing spondylitis. The symptoms, signs and investigations to distinguish these diagnoses are discussed by Waddell (1982).

MANAGEMENT OF BACK PAIN

History

In taking the pain history, the most useful questions potentially for distinguishing the causes of the pain are those relating to potentiating and relieving factors (Fig. 67.1).

It is useful to have some idea of which activities are limited by the pain; improvement in such indices may be the best guide on efficacy of treatment.

The drug history may indicate the type of pain. The patients have usually tried non-opioid analgesics, and often report that 'they just take the edge off the pain'. They may have distinct preferences for certain drugs because of differential incidence of side-effects. This information is important when choosing the most effective drug and particularly when injections fail to help, leaving analgesic drugs as the last resort. Some patients with arachnoiditis obtain little benefit from conventional analgesics and this may indicate a deafferentation type of pain.

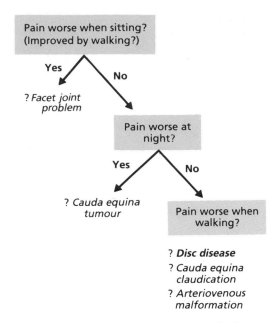

Fig. 67.1 Causes of back pain—clues from the history.

Examination

The serial measurement and recording of neurological signs is important in these patients so that change may be monitored objectively.

For sensory innervation it is simple to remember that L1, L2 and L3 supply the anterior aspect of the thigh, L4 the medial malleolus and toes, and S1 the lateral malleolus. More emphasis should be placed on numbness with tingling than on the finding of numbness alone.

For motor innervation, one may remember that L2 and L3 are involved in hip flexion, L3 and L4 in knee extension (knee jerk), other hip and knee movements being L5. Ankle movements involve S1 and S2 (ankle jerk S1).

Gauging the limitation of straight leg raising (SLR) may require common sense. Gross limitation of SLR is incompatible with the ability to sit comfortably at 90° with legs outstretched.

Investigations

Straight X-ray of spine; check facet joints (exclude e.g. tumour, infection, spondylolisthesis).

There is disagreement as to whether myelography or CT scans are most useful in helping to decide if surgery is indicated. The lowest rate of false-positive findings occurs with myelography with screening. If abnormality at the conus is suspected, radiculograms are inadequate. The combination of myelography and CT scanning may be the final arbiter in problem cases.

Type and timing of treatment (Fig. 67.2)

The philosophy presented is to use the low morbidity outpatient facet joint and extradural (lumbar or sacral) steroid injections (where these are appropriate; Fig. 67.2) as first-line treatment. This is justified for the back-pain sufferer because even short-term benefit from injections may be better than poor relief with drugs. Drugs often cause more side-effects than the injections.

There are some careful studies of the efficacy of *extradural steroids* (for reviews see Kepes & Duncalf, 1985; Benzon, 1986), which justify this technique. Better results may be achieved if the patient is treated earlier (Benzon, 1986), and when there is good evidence that the pain results from nerve root irritation. Used as a first-line treatment for back pain in the Oxford Unit (mean duration of pain 9 yr at first visit, Table 67.1), approximately 50% of patients have short-term (4–8 weeks) benefit, and 10% have pain relief for 6 months or more. These figures improve in direct relation to the duration of the pain and are better in patients who have not had back surgery.

It may take up to 1 week for benefit to occur from the steroid (Benzon, 1986), so it is unwise to dismiss the injection as a failure after 1 hr. If the injection produced incomplete or short-lived relief, it is worth repeating, and a course of three injections is recommended. No additional benefit accrued from more than three injections.

The steroid should be diluted in 5–10 ml diluent to prevent toxicity from the glycol or phenol derivatives in the ampoule of steroid. The use of local anaesthetic with the steroid provides a 'marker' for correct extradural injection, so that failure of the technique is not attributed to technical failure in placement.

Facet joint injection with local anaesthetic and steroid as a diagnostic/therapeutic procedure may be indicated from a history of pain worsened on sitting, and pain on lateral rotation and spine extension. Transient improvement (less than 6 weeks) may be produced by cryoanalgesia or radiofrequency blocks to the nerves to the joints. Careful outcome studies are required, comparing these two techniques and to confirm that while cryoanalgesia may be superior initially (6 weeks), radiofrequency lesions provide relief for much longer.

If sciatic pain is the predominant feature, *sacral foramen block* may be the best type to use. Some patients

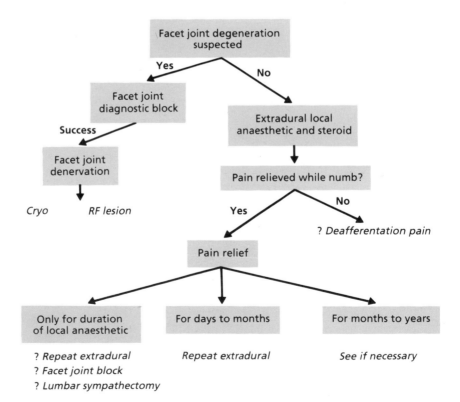

Fig. 67.2 The type and timing of treatment.

with long histories of back pain, particularly where arachnoiditis is suspected, may have symptoms and signs suggestive of deafferentation. Diagnostic *lumbar sympathectomy* with local anaesthetic may help such pains. Temporary improvement may be prolonged with chemical sympathectomy.

Drug therapy of back pain is often unsatisfactory. The pain may be both sufficiently severe and sufficiently sensitive to justify the use of strong opioid analgesics, but this is rarely a socially acceptable solution. Non-opioid analgesics may be used in conjunction with injections, or if injections have failed to help. In many patients such drugs provide inadequate relief even at their maximum permitted dosage (Moore *et al.*, 1986). Effervescent paracetamol, ibuprofen (fewest NSAI side-effects) and mefenamic acid are the most useful. Where the pain is clearly a deafferentation pain, the unconventional analgesic combination of anticonvulsants and antidepressants should be used (valproate 200 mg b.d. and amitriptyline 25 mg *nocte* as first-line).

Those who do not respond

Some back pain patients, particularly those who have had back surgery, respond poorly, which is disheartening for both patient and doctor. It is important that they receive honest advice and treatment, and that patients who still have surgically remediable disease are identified (a minority). Those with arachnoiditis are at risk of progressive disease.

Alternative methods such as transcutaneous nerve stimulation, acupuncture or psychological/behavioural therapies are often tried at this point which is probably an unfair test of any treatment, and all may produce temporary relief in a subgroup, but again this is not sustained. There is no simple way to manage these 'failed' back-pain patients. It may be difficult to protect them from the worst excesses which may be offered as they go seeking help desperately. Their heterogeneity suggests that no single new treatment or drug is likely to be the complete answer.

Postherpetic neuralgia

BACKGROUND

Postherpetic neuralgia (PHN), in common with other neuralgias, is a pain in the distribution of a nerve. It follows an acute herpetic (shingles) attack, the pain of PHN resulting from destruction of cells in the posterior nerve root. If enough are destroyed there is sensory loss and this is directly proportional to the degree of dysaesthesia. The natural history of PHN is intriguing and important for management.

Shingles

Shingles is an infection with the varicella zoster DNA virus. Some 90% of the urban population have had chickenpox by early adulthood, and a prolonged carrier state results with intracellular latency in the dorsal root ganglion. Reactivation of the latent virus causes shingles. The overall incidence of three to four per 1000 masks a difference related to increasing age; it is rare in children (less than one per 1000 up to the age of 9 yr) and much commoner in those over 80 yr old (10 per 1000) (Hope-Simpson, 1975). While adults do not acquire zoster by contact, children can obtain chickenpox by contact with zoster. In the general population shingles is most common in the thoracic region (more than 50%), with 10–15% of cases occurring in the trigeminal distribution (most common in first division).

Incidence and natural history of postherpetic neuralgia

The incidence of PHN in general practice is 10–15% of patients who had pain which lasted more than 1 month and 5–7% who had pain for more than 3 months. One-third of patients who are more than 80 yr old when they contracted shingles then developed PHN (Hope-Simpson, 1975). Postherpetic neuralgia is thus more common in the elderly, but so also is the incidence of shingles; it is unclear whether or not the elderly have an increased risk of PHN independent of their increased risk of shingles.

Postherpetic neuralgia in the pain clinic reflects the increased incidence with increasing age (Table 67.1), so that 90% of pain clinic PHN patients are more than 60 yr old. Postherpetic neuralgia in the trigeminal nerve distribution is more likely to be referred to the pain clinic than PHN affecting other sites (30% trigeminal PHN in the pain clinic, 10–15% in general practice).

The 'classic' accounts of the natural history of PHN claimed that it did not last more than 6 months (Burgoon *et al.*, 1957). However, median pain duration at the first clinic visit is more than 2 yr (Table 67.1), and 15% of patients attending have had PHN for more than 5 yr, so that these early accounts are incorrect.

PAIN OF POSTHERPETIC NEURALGIA

There is rarely difficulty in diagnosing PHN. The site of the pain is in the distribution of the shingles, and the scarring is often visible to confirm the diagnosis if this is in doubt. Postherpetic neuralgia patients are not usually wakened at night by their pain.

Four qualities of pain may be distinguished, and this may be helpful in management.

1 Burning pain; a dysaesthetic pain which is initiated by light touch, clothing, etc., 'hypersensitive'. Seen in approximately 25% of pain clinic PHN patients.

2 Constant deep aching pain with no dysaesthesia (50% incidence).

3 Crawling or scratching pain, just under the skin surface.

4 Stabbing or shooting pain (30% incidence).

In the acute attack, there may be involvement of the viscera supplied with afferent fibres by the posterior nerve roots corresponding to the affected skin areas (Wyburn-Mason, 1957). Symptoms akin to PHN may persist such as constipation, indigestion, frequency or dysuria, depending on the affected nerve.

MANAGEMENT

The depressing statement that 'the good results reported by one author are not confirmed subsequently by others, and no single method of therapy has produced more than temporary enthusiasm' (de Moragas & Kierland, 1957) is unfortunately still true for PHN. There is a strong feeling that the success of any remedy is in inverse relation to the duration of the pain. Claims for putative remedies must be examined in this light.

Does treating the pain of shingles prevent PHN?

It has long been held that effective management of the pain of the attack of acute shingles reduces the incidence of PHN. While sympathetic blocks (stellate, lumbar sympathetic or extradural) may undoubtedly be effective in relieving the pain of acute zoster (Courtin, 1981; Harding *et al.*, 1986), as yet there is no controlled evidence to show if such pain relief prevents the development of PHN. A control group in whom the intervention is *not* made is required.

The use of antiviral agents such as topical idoxuridine 35 or 40% in DMSO or acyclovir 800 mg 4 hourly orally may help to 'abort' the acute zoster attack if given early (McKendrick *et al.*, 1986). It is not known yet if curtailing the acute attack in this way results in a lower incidence of PHN.

Injections to relieve PHN

There is little evidence from controlled studies to support particular remedies. While sympathetic, regional or even local nerve blocks may provide temporary relief, there is little evidence that they alter the natural history of the disease process. If the affected area still has sensation, diagnostic nerve blocks with local anaesthetic may produce short-term relief, and this may be extended by measures such as cryoanalgesia. Neurolytic agents are not indicated, because initial short-term relief may be followed by pain worse than that which the patient had initially. The relevant blocks include:

1 Sympathetic system: stellate ganglion block for head and neck, lumbar sympathetic or extradural for trunk and lower limb.

2 Peripheral nerve: subcutaneous infiltration of local anaesthetic and steroid, repeated weekly for 3 weeks.

The subcutaneous infiltration may be most effective in treating hyperaesthetic burning pain.

Pharmacological management

Conventional analgesics have a limited role in PHN. The pain does not appear to be sensitive to opioids.

Of the unconventional analgesics, widespread use of the tricyclic antidepressants in PHN is supported by the positive results obtained in a controlled study (Watson *et al.*, 1982). Amitriptyline 25 mg *nocte* is the drug of choice, reducing the dose to 10 mg in the elderly or infirm. Its use may be made difficult in elderly men by prostatic problems.

Persistent shooting or stabbing pain may respond to anticonvulsants, and valproate 200 mg b.d. or clonazepam 500 μg *nocte* (increasing to b.d.) may be helpful.

Local anaesthetic creams or topical non-steroidal agents are of limited benefit, but they may reduce the hyperaesthetic pain.

Alternative methods

Transcutaneous nerve stimulation may be useful in the dysaesthetic pain, as indeed may a simple vibrator

Table 67.5 Common causes of facial pain

Trigeminal neuralgia
Atypical facial pain
Postherpetic neuralgia
Post-traumatic neuralgia
Malignancy
Temperomandibular dysaesthesia

applied to the junction of the skin areas with normal and abnormal sensation.

Facial pain

The most common causes of facial pain in the pain clinic are shown in Table 67.5.

Postherpetic neuralgia affecting the trigeminal division is not uncommon but it presents difficulties with diagnosis rarely. Two other neuralgias affecting the face, trigeminal neuralgia and atypical facial pain, are relatively common in the pain clinic. Distinguishing these should not be difficult, but often cases of atypical facial pain are referred to the clinic as trigeminal neuralgia resistant to carbamazepine.

TRIGEMINAL NEURALGIA

Background

This is the prototypic cranial neuralgia. It is a primary neuralgia although many attempts have been made to explain its pathology on the basis of a somatic cause. Tumour, vascular malformations, dental disease, sinusitis or multiple sclerosis (3%) may cause trigeminal neuralgia, but the aetiology of the majority of the cases is unknown (White & Sweet, 1969). An abnormality in the pattern of the afferent transmission to the trigeminal nucleus is one explanation. Vascular elongation, local demyelination with age, local compression or cross-axonal discharges have all been proposed as causes of the abnormal transmission.

The condition occurs more often in the middle-aged, and is twice as common in females as in males. This pattern of incidence is the same in the pain clinic; the striking feature is the long duration (mean 9 yr) of pain prior to the first visit.

Patients may be referred to a pain clinic with trigeminal neuralgia because the diagnosis is in doubt, because straightforward management with carbamazepine has failed, because of tolerance, side-effects or allergy, or because previous invasive measures have failed.

Pain: site and features

For practical purposes the pain is strictly unilateral (White & Sweet, 1969); multiple sclerosis patients constitute the majority of the 2% of patients with bilateral disease. Trigeminal neuralgia is twice as common on the right side. Combining published figures (8124 cases), the most common (32%) pain referral was to both the mandibular and maxillary divisions. The frequency for divisions 1, 2 and 3 separately were 4%, 17% and 15% respectively. Seventeen percent had pain in all three divisions (White & Sweet, 1969). The pain may remain unchanged, but there is usually spread to involve another division.

The pain in the face is characteristically *sharp*, severe (paroxysmal) and brief, lasting no more than a few seconds. Tic douloureux describes the facial contortions which may accompany the pain. A high frequency of these attacks may lead to a persistent pain which is duller in nature.

The pain may be induced by thermal, tactile or proprioceptive stimuli, but not by nociceptive stimuli. These intermittent attacks may last for 6–8 weeks. Long spontaneous remissions of months or even years may occur in the early stages, but tend to be shorter as the disease progresses. The severity and frequency of the attacks thus increase with the passage of time.

The history and examination should exclude other potential pathology. There should be no abnormal neurological signs in trigeminal neuralgia, and pain relief with carbamazepine is taken to be diagnostic.

Pharmacological management

Patients are often taking (or have already tried) the anticonvulsant carbamazepine on arrival in the pain clinic. If the drug is tolerated well but is ineffective, increasing the dose (in divided doses) to a maximum of 1500 mg daily should be tried. If the drug is tolerated poorly (nausea and vomiting, ataxia, skin rash or blood dyscrasia), phenytoin 100 mg t.d.s. may be tried instead, or in addition to the lowest tolerated dose of carbamazepine.

Peripheral nerve blocks

The role of nerve blocks is to provide pain relief when pharmacological management is unsuccessful, or as an adjunct to allow reduction in dose. Individual divisions of the fifth nerve may be blocked with local anaesthetic where they leave the skull and enter the face and mouth (infraorbital, supraorbital, inferior dental and mental nerves).

In addition to their diagnostic value, it is not uncommon for these blocks to break a cycle of pain. Relief may be obtained subsequently for much longer than the duration of the local anaesthetic. Because the natural history of the disease is one of spontaneous remissions, it is difficult to quantify this relief in the absence of untreated controls; when such relief occurs, the patient and the doctor accept it gratefully.

Temporary relief from local anaesthetic may be prolonged with cryoanalgesia (Barnard *et al.*, 1981). In Barnard's study of 24 patients, the median duration of relief was 186 days (range 0–1236), contrasting with a median duration of sensory loss of 67 days (range 14–80) which indicates the 'reversible' nature of the cryoanalgesia lesion. There were no complications in that series.

Cryoanalgesia, 'peripheral' radiofrequency lesions, neurolytic injections or avulsion and/or nerve section should not be regarded as curative; they are ineffective long-term. Relapse rates are higher as the follow-up lengthens. The advantage of cryoanalgesia is that the patient is no worse off if the pain returns, and the cryoanalgesia may be repeated successfully. This is not always the case with the other measures.

Surgical and other more central procedures

Many surgical procedures have been used to treat trigeminal neuralgia. However, it takes many years to establish the success of a novel procedure, because of the extended follow-up required to assess recurrence rate. Procedures should be judged also on operative morbidity and mortality and long-term morbidity (sensory or motor loss, anaesthesia dolorosa, damage to other cranial nerves). This is a difficult balance to achieve. A patient referred for such procedures may rightly expect to be cured but, unfortunately, the operations with the lowest recurrence rates are likely to be those with the highest complication rates. Some of the procedures are listed in Table 67.6. Of these, probably the most predictable manoeuvre to ablate tic douloureux is sensory root rhizotomy, performed usually in the middle cranial fossa, and although there may be some sparing of sensation, corneal ulceration, drooling and trophic lesions of the skin may occur. The recurrence rate with this procedure is low (4% at 4 yr).

Table 67.6 Nerve block and surgical procedures for trigeminal neuralgia

Peripheral nerve section or injection
Middle fossa
    Section
    Injection
    Decompression
    Radiofrequency

Posterior fossa
    Section
    Decompression

Medullary tractotomy

The most serious morbidity is anaesthesia dolorosa, a constant burning pain in the numb area. The incidence of this complication is probably 5–10%, and the only treatment is symptomatic.

Vascular decompression procedures are fashionable currently, but it is too early to determine if the low complication rate is balanced by a high recurrence rate (?50% at 4 yr). If that proves to be the case, such major surgery may not be justified. Radiofrequency lesions at the Gasserian ganglion, where the electrode is inserted through the foramen ovale under X-ray control, use controlled temperatures to destroy smaller pain fibres selectively. If sensation is preserved, recurrence rates for the first division may be as high as 25%, and there is also a risk of anaesthesia dolorosa (0.3–3%).

The injection of glycerine into Meckel's cave appears not to have been as successful as early reports claimed. Equally, the clinical utility of alcohol block of the Gasserian ganglion (Churcher, 1983) (less predictable than rhizotomy and carrying a higher risk of the same complications) is limited in the light of the alternatives.

Different pain clinics have varying views on management, usually held very firmly, but trigeminal neuralgia is a condition where the medical aphorism that the patient should not be made worse is particularly appropriate. The strategy proposed is that failed medical management is an indication for peripheral nerve diagnostic injection, with sustained relief if necessary provided by cryoanalgesia. If these peripheral measures fail, radiofrequency lesion of the Gasserian ganglion or rhizotomy should be considered.

ATYPICAL FACIAL PAIN

The diagnosis of atypical facial pain is made often by exclusion of other causes of facial pain. Classically, it affects middle-aged women (Miller, 1968). Pain-clinic patients in whom this is the ultimate (correct) diagnosis may have been referred because they were thought to have trigeminal neuralgia which failed to respond to carbamazepine, or because their facial pain was associated wrongly with dental problems, and had continued despite extraction(s). It should not be a difficult diagnosis to make, but the major differential diagnosis is trigeminal neuralgia.

Pain: site and features

Whilst the site of pain is in the face, it may not coincide with the distribution of any particular nerve and it may cross the midline.

The features are that it is a *dull* pain (cf. the *sharp* pain of trigeminal neuralgia), which may be persistent or recurrent, uni- or bilateral, in the absence of muscular or joint problems and with no abnormal neurological signs, akin to those of trigeminal neuralgia. Although the pain is episodic, it is unlike that of trigeminal neuralgia in that it builds up gradually to a climax and it may last for hours and even days. It is anatomically imprecise and covers a much larger territory than that supplied by an individual cranial nerve. The pain is never 'electric' and is described usually as tearing or crushing.

The pain may be associated with other symptom complexes, such as spastic colon, dysfunctional uterine bleeding, headaches and low back pain. These complexes may recur sequentially or simultaneously in response to stress.

It is wise to look for a hidden cause; teeth, sinuses and eyes may be incriminated. At least three 'parallel' conditions may be associated with atypical facial pain.

Temperomandibular dysaesthesia (facial arthromyalgia) may be difficult to distinguish from atypical facial pain but there is usually a history of pain in muscles and/or joints, clicking, sticking or trismus, and a feeling of buzzing or fullness in the ear. On examination, there may be ridged buccal mucosa, crenated tongue or masseteric hypertrophy, and arthritic change may be seen on X-ray of the condylar surface.

Atypical odontalgia may be distinguished from atypical facial pain because the continuous or throbbing pain is felt in the teeth (tooth), is hypersensitive to all stimuli and may move from tooth to tooth.

Glossodynia or oral dysaesthesia is the sensation of a dry mouth, burning tongue and gums, with denture intolerance, disturbance of taste and salivation and no organic pathology.

Management and course

The pathogenesis remains mysterious, but the patients should be reassured that it is a 'real pain' and is best managed medically rather than by surgery, which may make it more refractory. The association with adverse life events (80% of patients) emphasizes that this condition may affect the otherwise emotionally healthy as a stress response.

Tricyclic antidepressants are the treatment of choice. Dothiepin is recommended because it has been shown to be tolerated best in this patient group (Feinman *et al.*, 1984). Treatment (75–150 mg *nocte*) should be maintained for 3 months. Trifluoperazine 2–4 mg *mane* may then be prescribed in addition if relief is poor. Thirty percent of patients require short courses (3 months or less) in response to stress, and 40% need 18–24 months maintained therapy. Four yr after diagnosis, 70% of patients are pain-free, but 50% need intermittent medication and 10% still need continuous treatment (Feinman *et al.*, 1984).

Post-traumatic neuralgia (including postoperative wound pain)

Pain after trauma and pain in or near the operative scar, occurring for months and even years after surgery, may be extremely difficult to manage. Because the principles of management are similar, they are discussed together.

Post-traumatic neuralgia may occur in a context where the patient is seeking compensation for the accident. Much has been made of the intransigence of the neuralgia until the compensation is settled; unfortunately, for many patients the pain remains long after compensation is paid. The aetiology of postoperative wound pain is unknown to the extent of why some patients are affected and others not. As usual when this is the case, doctors may ascribe a psychogenic overlay.

SITE AND FEATURES OF THE PAIN

Post-traumatic neuralgia

The pain may occur in any part of the body, and may be associated with damage to bone, nerve, muscle or other tissue. Specific information should be sought in the history and examination of nerve damage to the affected area at the time of injury and the current neurological status of the painful area. Is it numb? Are there painful paraesthesiae? Is there any difference in temperature between affected and unaffected areas?

Postoperative wound pain

Three particular situations seem most likely to result in postoperative wound pain: thoracotomy (particularly thoraco-abdominal incisions), nephrectomy and inguinal herniorrhaphy, but pain at or around scars from other operations is seen also.

The quality of the pain is described often as burning, even if the area still has normal sensation (unusual). Commonly, there is no hyperaesthesia. The aura of the pain (the extent of the area affected) may increase as time elapses.

MANAGEMENT

Pharmacological

Conventional analgesics may have a very limited role in both post-traumatic and postoperative neuralgias referred to the pain clinic. Indeed, the patient may be referred because such regimens have failed to help significantly.

The use of antidepressants and anticonvulsants is more likely to help, particularly if the pain is burning and occurring in an area of altered sensation. Amitriptyline 25 mg *nocte* with valproate 200 mg b.d. may be a useful starting combination. An alternative anticonvulsant is clonazepam, beginning with 500 μg *nocte*, and increasing the dose in the absence of side-effects to 1.5 or 2 mg t.d.s.

Peripheral nerve blocks

Diagnostic blocks with local anaesthetic should be tried when appropriate in these conditions. For postoperative pains, intercostal blocks for thoracotomy or nephrectomy and ilioinguinal blocks for herniorrhaphy may produce relief. If the relief is transient, the duration may be extended by repeating the block with cryoanalgesia. This may be achieved best (especially for the ilioinguinal nerve) with surgical exposure under direct vision rather than with a percutaneous approach.

Autonomic nerve blocks

Stellate ganglion (for head, neck, upper limbs and upper chest wall) or lumbar sympathectomy may be the first line of management, particularly in post-traumatic neuralgia. The greatest chance of success is if the pain is in an area of altered sensation.

Extending the duration of pain relief with successful 'single-shot' stellate ganglion block may be achieved by repeating the block every 3–7 days on up to 10 or more occasions. Reports that infusion of local anaesthetic via a catheter to the stellate ganglion for 7 days produces better results still require confirmation. If there is undoubted success with local anaesthetic blocks but this cannot be sustained despite repeated injections, surgery may be appropriate. Perhaps the best results may be achieved with a transthoracic approach using the operating microscope.

Transient relief from lumbar sympathectomy with local anaesthetic may be prolonged by using phenol.

Perineal neuralgia

Perineal neuralgia with no malignant cause occurs most commonly in women, often postmenopausal, and it is a most difficult pain to treat successfully. The aetiology is unknown, but pelvic varicosities are thought to be a cause of pelvic pain (Beard *et al.*, 1986), although the symptoms and signs (or lack of) in perineal pain would seem to be distinct from the pelvic pain syndrome (Beard *et al.*, 1986).

SITE AND FEATURES OF THE PAIN

The pain is described variously as a 'tugging', 'pulling' or 'crawling' sensation, commonly in the clitoral area. Many women with this condition prefer to stand, because the pain is worse when they sit.

MANAGEMENT

Pharmacological

Conventional analgesics are rarely effective, and unfortunately antidepressants and anticonvulsants do not help most patients. Women are often prescribed local hormone therapy; few seem to be helped.

Nerve blocks

Sacral extradural with local anaesthetic may be tried diagnostically. Many of these patients still have pain even when the relevant area is numb from the local anaesthetic. If the local anaesthetic does help the pain, duration of relief may be prolonged with sacral extradural cryoanalgesia.

Lumbar sympathectomy may be a logical procedure if the cause is pelvic varicosities, but this has not proved to be successful.

Phantom and stump pain

BACKGROUND

Phantom pain

The proportion of amputees suffering from phantom pain is high (78 % of the 55% responding to a survey of 5000 amputees; Sherman *et al.*, 1984), although previous reports had suggested a lower incidence of pain. There seem to be few predictors of disabling phantom pain; age at amputation, years since amputation, reason for amputation, site of amputation and pain before surgery were similar in those with and without problematic phantom pain (Sherman *et al.*, 1984).

The aetiology of the pain is unknown, but the mechanism is presumed to be central, the lack of sensory input causing decreased tonic inhibition.

Stump pain

Pain in the stump may occur early after surgery as a result of surgical postoperative complications, but pain-clinic patients with stump pain tend to be late referrals with well-healed stumps, and the origin of the pain is attributed to neuroma development.

MANAGEMENT

Phantom pain

At least 50 different methods of treating phantom limb pain are in use currently, but only 1% of patients have long-term benefit from any (Sherman *et al.*, 1984). Best results are achieved with early treatment whichever method is used.

Pharmacological. Neither minor (including NSAID agents) nor major conventional analgesics are of great benefit, but opioids may make the patient feel better. The use of anticonvulsants has been more successful, but with no controlled evidence to support their use.

Severe shooting or lancinating pains are most likely to respond, and clonazepam 500 μg *nocte* increasing to 1.5–2 mg t.d.s. if the drug is tolerated well may be the most effective of this group.

Nerve blocks. Sympathetic blocks with local anaesthetic may be used diagnostically, and transient relief may be prolonged with repeat local anaesthetic blocks or chemical sympathectomy. Despite pain-clinic claims for the efficacy of these procedures, there is little evidence for long-term benefit.

Surgery. Surgical procedures seem to be the least successful.

Stump pain

Stump pain co-exists often with phantom pain (Sherman *et al.*, 1984), and treatment of the phantom pain with anticonvulsants may help also the stump pain. A purely 'local' stump pain with neuroma development may benefit from local anaesthetic injection to the site, repeated if required, and with either percutaneous or direct vision cryoanalgesia to extend the duration of relief.

Conclusion

What function is served by pain clinics? There are those who argue that a good doctor, whatever his or her speciality, should be able to treat pain. The reality is that this does not always happen, and the pain clinic provides a focus, a 'critical mass' of experience, where, by combining pharmacological means, nerve blocks and other measures, patients may be helped. Pain management is not an exact science, but it will become more rational when underlying mechanisms are elucidated (cf. phantom pain), and as the methods used to provide a rational basis for treatment in other branches of medicine are applied.

What is the role of the anaesthetist in chronic pain management? Many patients benefit from their skills with nerve-blocking procedures, and many anaesthetists enjoy the contrast between pain-clinic work and theatre sessions.

How do we progress? It is unfortunate that, at a time when basic scientists are fascinated by pain mechanisms and pharmacology, clinical progress with chronic pain control has been limited largely to better use of oral opioids, attributable to the teaching of the hospice movement. Nerve-blocking procedures, which are the historical reason why anaesthetists became involved in pain control, are unfashionable. The reason for this is the lack of careful data comparing quality and duration of relief, both between different nerve-blocking techniques and between nerve blocks and other measures. Without such data, not only is management necessarily empirical, but the spectre of litigation may deprive patients of potentially beneficial treatment. It is incumbent on pain clinics which use blocks to gather this information.

Acknowledgement

The constructive advice of Dr J.W. Lloyd is acknowledged gratefully.

References

Barnard D., Lloyd J. & Evans J. (1981) Cryoanalgesia in the management of chronic facial pain. *Journal of Maxillofacial Surgery* 9, 101–2.

Beard R.W., Reginald P.W. & Pearce S. (1986) Pelvic pain in women. *British Medical Journal* 293, 1160–2.

Benzon H.T. (1986) Epidural steroid injections for low back pain and lumbosacral radiculopathy. *Pain* 24, 277–95.

Boas R.A. (1983) The sympathetic nervous system and pain relief. In *Relief of Intractable Pain* (Ed. Swerdlow M.) pp. 215–37. Elsevier, Amsterdam.

Bryce-Smith R. (1976) Local analgesia of the trunk. In *Practical Regional Analgesia* (Eds Lee J.A. & Bryce-Smith R.) pp. 81–110. Excerpta Medica. Amsterdam.

Burford Nursing Development Unit (1984) Nurses and pain. *Nursing Times* 18, 94.

Burgoon C.F., Burgoon J.S. & Baldridge G.D. (1957) The natural history of herpes zoster. *Journal of the American Medical Association* 164, 265–9.

Churcher M. (1983) Peripheral nerve blocks in relief of intractable pain. In *Relief of Intractable Pain* (Ed. Swerdlow M.) pp. 147–74. Elsevier, Amsterdam.

Courtin R. (1981) The treatment of herpes zoster from the algologist's point of view. *Dallas Medical Journal* 67, 132–5.

de Moragas J.M. & Kierland R.R. (1957) The outcome of patients with herpes zoster. *Archives of Dermatology* 75, 193–5.

Editorial (1982) Pain clinics. *Lancet* i, 486.

Editorial (1986) Spinal opiates revisited. *Lancet* i, 655.

Fearnside M.R. & Adams C.B.T. (1978) Tumours of the cauda equina. *Journal of Neurology, Neurosurgery and Psychiatry* 41, 24–31.

Feinman C., Harris M. & Cawley R. (1984) Psychogenic facial pain: presentation and treatment. *British Medical Journal* 288, 436–8.

Foley K.M. (1985) The treatment of cancer pain. *New England Journal of Medicine* 313, 84–95.

Harding S.P., Lipton J.R., Wells J.C.D. & Campbell J.A. (1986) Relief of acute pain in herpes zoster ophthalmicus by stellate ganglion block. *British Medical Journal* 292, 1428.

Hope-Simpson R.E. (1975) Postherpetic neuralgia. *Journal of the Royal College of General Practitioners* 25, 571–5.

Jones J. & Gough D. (1977) Coeliac plexus block with alcohol for relief of upper abdominal pain due to cancer. *Journal of the Royal College of Surgeons* 59, 46–9.

Kepes E.R. & Duncalf D. (1985) Treatment of backache with spinal injections of local anesthetics, spinal and systemic steroids. A review. *Pain* 22, 33–47.

Labat G. (1924) Blocking of spinal nerves. In *Regional Anesthesia* pp. 260–72. W.B. Saunders, Philadelphia.

Lobato R.D., Madrid J.L., Fatela L.V., Rivas J.J., Gozalo J. & Barcena A. (1984) Analgesia elicited by low-dose intraventricular morphine in terminal cancer patients. *Pain* (Suppl. 2), S342.

Macintosh R. & Bryce-Smith R. (1962) *Local Analgesia Abdominal Surgery*. Churchill Livingstone, Edinburgh.

McKendrick M.W., McGill J.I., White J.E. & Wood M.J. (1986) Oral acyclovir in acute herpes zoster. *British Medical Journal* ii, 1529–32.

McQuay H.J., Machin L. & Moore R.A. (1985) Chronic non-malignant pain: a population prevalence study from the Oxford Regional Pain Relief Unit. *Practitioner* 229, 1109–11.

Martin G. (1981) The management of pain following laminectomy for lumbar disc lesions. *Annals of the Royal College of Surgeons* 63, 244–52.

Miller H. (1968) Pain in the face. *British Medical Journal* 2, 577–80.

Moore R.A., McQuay H.J., Carroll D., McMahon C. & Allen M.C. (1986) Single and multiple dose analgesic studies of mefenamic acid in chronic back pain. *Clinical Journal of Pain* 2, 29–6.

Shaw M.D.M., Russell J.A. & Grossart K.W. (1978) The changing pattern of spinal arachnoiditis. *Journal of Neurology, Neurosurgery and Psychiatry* 41, 97–107.

Sherman R.A., Sherman C.J. & Parker L. (1984) Chronic phantom and stump pain among American Veterans: results of a survey. *Pain* 18, 83–95.

Twycross R.G. & Lack S.A. (1983) *Symptom Control in Far Advanced Cancer: Pain Relief*. Pitman, London.

Waddell G. (1982) An approach to backache. *British Journal of Hospital Medicine* 28, 187–233.

Watson C.P., Evans R.J., Reed K., Merskey H., Goldsmith L. & Warsh J. (1982) Amitriptyline vs placebo in postherpetic neuralgia. *Neurology* 32, 671–3.

White J.C. & Sweet W.H. (1969) *Pain and the Neurosurgeon* pp. 123–78. Thomas, Springfield.

Wood K.M. (1984) Peripheral nerve and root chemical lesions. In *Textbook of Pain* (Eds Wall P.D. & Malzack R.) pp. 577–80. Churchill Livingstone, Edinburgh.

Wyburn-Mason R. (1957) Visceral lesions in herpes zoster. *British Medical Journal* i, 678–81.

68

The Management of Pain in Cancer

R. G. TWYCROSS

Cancer is a major world problem. Each year more than 6 million new patients are diagnosed and more than 4 million die (World Health Organization, 1986). This amounts to 10% of all deaths. Pain is a major symptom in 70% of patients with far-advanced cancer, and in 50% of patients still undergoing anticancer treatment. This means that there are 3.5 million people suffering from cancer pain at any one time. Data from 11 reports covering nearly 2000 patients in developed countries suggests that the majority of these do not receive satisfactory relief (World Health Organization, 1986).

Of the many potential reasons for inadequate pain control, the following are among the more important (World Health Organization, 1986):

1 A lack of recognition that established methods exist for cancer pain management.
2 Fears concerning 'addiction' in both cancer patients and the wider public if strong opioids are more readily available for medicinal purposes.
3 A lack of systematic teaching of medical students, doctors, nurses and other health-care workers on management of cancer pain.
4 Non-availability of necessary relief drugs in many parts of the world.

Caring for cancer patients is emotionally demanding. This is for several reasons; notably an instinctive fear of death and, in consequence, a reluctance to care for those who remind us of our common destiny. A failure to understand this and to take corrective measures also hinders good pain control.

Pain in cancer

Pain is a complex 'somatopsychic' experience (Chapter 65, p. 1166). In advanced cancer, a sense of hopeless-

ness and the fear of impending death add to the total suffering of the patient. In these circumstances, the concept of 'total pain' is helpful (Saunders & Baines, 1983; Mount, 1984). This takes account of psychological, spiritual, social and financial factors in addition to the underlying physical component.

The physical causes of pain in cancer may be allocated to four categories:

1 Cancer related.
2 Treatment related.
3 Debility related.
4 Concurrent disorder.

In other words, a diagnosis of cancer does not necessarily imply that the malignant process is the cause of pain.

A prospective survey of 100 cancer patients with pain illustrates the pattern of pain in advanced cancer (Fig. 68.1). The number of anatomically distinct pains totalled 303, an average of three per patient. All but 20 had more than one pain; 34 had four or more. Cancer was the sole cause of pain in 41 patients. Cancer was

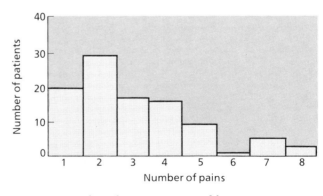

Fig. 68.1 Number of pains experienced by 100 consecutive cancer patients with pain on admission to Sir Michael Sobell House. (Redrawn from Twycross & Fairfield, 1982.)

not responsible for any of the pains in nine patients; these had a total of 17 pains, nine of which were musculoskeletal. Four of these nine patients had only one pain—postoperative, pulmonary embolus and, in two, constipation.

Of the pains caused by cancer, bone and nerve compression were the most common (Table 68.1). Soft tissue infiltration and visceral pains also occurred frequently. Pain caused by muscle spasm secondary to underlying bone disease occurred in 11 patients. Postoperative pain was the most common pain related to treatment and constipation the most common debility-associated pain. Six of the eight postoperative pains related to the incisional scar (three postmastectomy, two postlaparotomy and one after a biopsy of a supraclavicular node). In all but one, the pain was chronic i.e. not attributable to recent surgery. Of the other two, one was an aching pain in the axillary portion of a postmastectomy scar linked with a superficial burning pain and hyperaesthesia on the inner aspect of the upper arm. This pattern of pain, which tends to develop 1–2 months after mastectomy, is caused by section of the intercostobrachial nerve (T1–2) close to the lateral chest wall (I. Granek, R. Ashikari & K.M. Foley, personal communication). The other chronic postoperative pain was a deep ache in the right upper thigh. This was caused by a Thompson's hemi-arthroplasty inserted 6 months before.

Twenty-seven patients recorded a total of 43 musculoskeletal pains of non-malignant origin. Of those with non-malignant low back pain, it had been long-standing in six. Of the other two, the pain appeared to be related to a large abdominal mass in one case (cf. pregnancy) and in the other by a compensatory lumbar scoliosis associated with a pelvis tilt caused by necrosis of the femoral head. Two other patients had vague but troublesome pain in relation to both ischial tuberosities and around both ankles respectively.

The most common muscular cause was myofascial trigger-point (TP) pain. This occurred in 12 patients and accounted for 24 pains. Five of these patients had one myofascial pain and seven had two or more. The maximum number in any one patient was five. Although classified as unrelated, the incidence of myofascial pains is almost certainly higher in cancer patients, particularly in those who are anxious, exhausted or cachectic. Miscellaneous, unrelated pains included tension headache, pain in one or both pinnae, several abdominal complaints, urinary retention, coccydynia, restless legs syndrome and artherosclerotic claudication.

Table 68.1 Causes of pain in 100 cancer pain patients. (From Twyross & Fairfield, 1982)

Cause	Number of pains	Number of patients
Caused by cancer		
Bone	58	31
Nerve compression	56	31
Soft-tissue infiltration	35	31
Visceral involvement	33	31
Muscle spasm	14	11
Lymphoedema	4	3
Raised intracranial pressure	2	2
Myopathy	2	2
Total	204 (67%)	91
Related to treatment		
Postoperative	8	7
Colostomy	2	2
Nerve block	2	1
Postoperative adhesions	1	1
Postradiation fibrosis	1	1
Oesophageal	1	1
Total	15 (5%)	12
Related to debility		
Constipation	11	11
Capsulitis of shoulder	4	4
Bedsore	1	1
Postherpetic neuralgia	1	1
Pulmonary embolus	1	1
Penile spasm/catheter	1	1
Total	19 (6%)	19
Concurrent disorders Musculoskeletal		
Myofascial	24	12
Low back	8	8
Spinal osteoporosis	4	3
Ischial tuberosity	2	1
Ankle	2	1
Traumatic	2	1
Sacroiliac	1	1
Total	43	27
Other		
Osteoarthritis	4	3
Migraine	2	2
Miscellaneous	16	13
	65 (22%)	39
Overall total	303 (100%)	100

Assessment

Doctors caring for cancer patients, need, as far as possible, to acquire the skill of determining the cause of the pain on the basis of diagnostic probabilities. Invasive investigations are contra-indicated increasingly as patients become more terminally ill. A comprehensive list of possible causes of pain is unnecessary because, inevitably, it would be too long to be helpful. What is required is an informed imagination, making use of the data presented above. An awareness of the common muscular pain syndromes is necessary to prevent many erroneous conclusions. Similarly helpful is some knowledge of the patterns of metastatic spread (Fig. 68.2 and 68.3).

THURSDAY   **Sleep** 11 p.m. – 6 a.m. No disturbance
            Awoke 6 a.m.

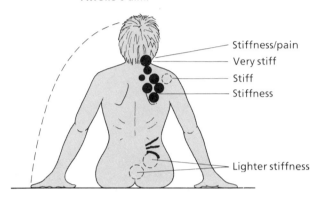

Fig. 68.2 Pain self-portrait by 65-yr old male patient with pancreatic cancer. Sites of pain indicate that pain was probably muscular/myofascial in origin. Explanation, massage and diazepam at night prescribed. (Redrawn from Twycross & Lack, 1986.)

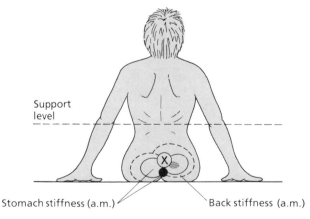

Fig. 68.3 Second pain-portrait by patient with pancreatic cancer. Myofascial pains have now resolved. New pain probably also non-malignant, related to lying in bed for long periods. Again analgesics were not prescribed. Explanation, sheepskin and progressive mobilization resulted in relief. (Redrawn from Twycross & Lack, 1986.)

If assumed wrongly to be cancerous in origin, the pain tends to be invested with all the negative implications of cancer pain. Such investment makes the pain much worse.

Case history

A 63-yr old woman complained of weight loss, epigastric pain and insomnia of several months duration. At laparotomy, a carcinoma in the tail of the pancreas was found, with liver metastases. When seen 10 days postoperatively by a hospice doctor, she was receiving 25 mg of morphine sulphate by mouth every 4 hr. This failed to provide adequate relief (Fig. 68.4). She was drowsy, distressed mentally and complained of continued insomnia. It was explained that some of her pains were muscular and that she probably had pain from a cracked rib also. She was advised that an abdominal incision (particularly with deep tension sutures) could be uncomfortable on movement for several weeks, but that it would improve progressively. It was pointed out that certain pains respond better to aspirin and non-drug measures than to morphine. She was told also that some of the abdominal pain was caused probably by constipation. She was prescribed aspirin regularly every 4 hr, and the nurses advised on the nature of the rib pain. The morphine dosage was reduced and a specific hypnotic introduced at night. A laxative was prescribed and rectal measures planned for the following day. The next day she had improved dramatically following a good night, and had much less pain. Her morphine was reduced further and after 3 days she was taking only 5 mg every 4 hr with 15 mg at night.

This case history reinforces the following points:
1 Not all pains in cancer are malignant in origin.
2 Cancer patients with pain often have more than one pain.
3 Muscular pains may be as severe as (or even more severe than) much cancer-caused pain.
4 Some pains, however intense, do not benefit by the use of increasing doses of morphine.
5 Careful clinical assessment is necessary before commencing treatment.
6 Explanation is an essential modality of treatment.
7 Reassessment after initiating treatment is necessary to confirm or modify the initial assessment.
8 Reassessment may lead also to changes in treatment in the light of initial results and/or side-effects.

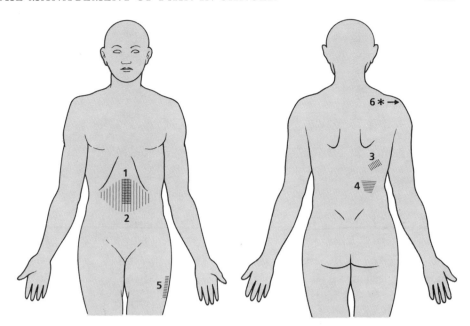

Fig. 68.4 Pain chart of 63-yr old woman with cancer of tail of the pancreas, 10 days postoperatively. (Redrawn from Twycross & Lack, 1986.)

Management of pain

The use of analgesics and pain management are not synonymous. Not only is pain a complex somatopsychic experience, but all pains do not respond equally to analgesics. Thus, the use of analgesics may be regarded only as part of a multi-modality approach to treatment (Table 68.2). Even so, it must be emphasized that most cancer patients with pain do require analgesics, often for several months.

Table 68.2 Pain control in cancer. (From Twycross & Lack, 1986)

Examination	To establish trust	
Explanation	To reduce psychological impact of pain	
Modification of pathological process	Radiation therapy Hormone therapy Chemotherapy Surgery	Correction of hyper-calcaemia Pituitary fossa injection of alcohol
Elevation of pain threshold	Relief of other symptoms Sleep Rest Sympathy Understanding Companionship	Diversional activity Reduction in anxiety Elevation of mood Relaxation Analgesics Anxiolytics Antidepressants
Interruption of pain pathways	*Local anaesthesia* Lignocaine Bupivacaine	*Neurolysis* Chemical Alcohol Phenol Chlorocresol Cold (cryotherapy) Heat (thermocoagulation)
Modification of lifestyle	Avoid pain-precipitating activities	
Immobilization	Rest Cervical collar Surgical corset	Moulded plastic splints Slings Orthopaedic surgery

From a pharmacological point of view, pain in cancer may be allocated into four categories:

1 Opioid-non-responsive pains.
2 Opioid-partially responsive pains.
3 Opioid-responsive pains—but do *not* use opioids.
4 Opioid-responsive pains—do use opioids.

The term 'opioid-responsive pain' is used to describe pains that respond increasingly well to increasing doses of opioid analgesics. In other words, if moderately severe, the pain responds to codeine and, if very severe, to morphine. The importance of this classification lies in the fact that it reminds doctors that opioids are of limited value for certain pains, and that sometimes they are contra-indicated (Table 68.3).

Opioid-non-responsive pains

MUSCLE PAIN

A severe muscle cramp is a universal experience. The pain is extremely intense for a short time. It is coped with partly by saying; 'it is only cramp'. Muscle pain in cancer patients—unless recognized for what it is—conveys a different message, namely; 'my God, it's the cancer!'. Such a response inevitably magnifies and perpetuates the pain.

Muscle spasm pain secondary to underlying bone pain with or without skeletal deformity is common in cancer patients. Myofascial, TP-related pains occur also. Explanation, physical therapies (local heat and massage), diazepam and relaxation therapy, injection of TPs with local anaesthetic and a corticosteroid (corticoid) constitute the correct approach (e.g. bupiva-caine 0.5% and depot methylprednisolone). However severe, *morphine is not indicated for muscle spasm and TP pains.*

DEAFFERENTATION PAIN

This is caused by nerve destruction (Chapter 5, p. 60). Typical examples include causalgia and postherpetic neuralgia. In cancer, deafferentation pain results usually from infiltration of a nerve by the malignancy. The pain is characteristically dermatomal in distribution, and resembles a superficial burning or scalding. There is often associated allodynia (i.e. light touch causes exacerbation of the pain). Stabbing pain may be a feature also. Sometimes stabbing is predominant. *This type of pain does not respond to opioids.* It is, however, helped greatly by an antidepressant for burning pain and/or an anticonvulsant for stabbing pain (Gerson *et al.*, 1977; Raftery, 1979).

Amitriptyline is often too toxic for the elderly and the debilitated, although it is probably the best drug for younger, more robust patients. The author generally uses dothiepin. A 25 mg capsule is given at bedtime as an initial test dose. This is increased to 50 mg (25 mg × 2) the following night if the initial dose does not cause significant untoward side-effects. After a few nights, the dose is increased to a single 75 mg tablet and then reviewed again following a further week or 10 days. Concurrent night sedation may often be 'trimmed'. For patients intolerant of dothiepin, mian-serin is used, commencing with 10–30 mg *nocte*, and increasing step by step to 60–120 mg *nocte*.

If stabbing is the main problem, sodium valproate is prescribed, also at night. In the elderly and the debilitated, the dose should be 200–500 mg *nocte*. As it

Type of pain	Treatment	
Somatic (nociceptive)		
Muscle spasm	Physical therapy	
	Diazepam	
Tissue distortion	Analgesics	
Nerve compression	Analgesics	
	Corticosteroids	
	Nerve blocks	
Deafferentation (nerve destruction)	Antidepressants	
	Anticonvulsants	
	Opioids	If peripheral nerve lesion, occasionally useful
	Corticosteroids	
	Nerve blocks	If spinal cord lesion, of no benefit
	Cordotomy	

Table 68.3 Types of pain and implications for treatment

cumulates, or causes daytime drowsiness, it may be necessary to reduce the dosage. Alternatively, if there is no response, the dose may need to be increased to 1000–1500 mg *nocte*. Carbamazepine is a well-tried alternative. It is given two or three times a day, commencing with a dose of 100–200 mg b.d. The dose is built up *each week* until a good response is obtained, or until side-effects such as dizziness, unsteadiness and drowsiness occur. Both sodium valproate and carbamazepine may cause nausea.

Opioid-partially responsive pains

BONE PAIN

Pain caused by bone metastases is often only partially responsive to opioids. Best results are obtained with a combination of aspirin, or an alternative non-steroidal, anti-inflammatory (NSAI) agent, and morphine. Many osseous metastases produce or induce the production of a prostaglandin (PG) which causes osteolysis (Galasko, 1981). The PG lowers also the 'peripheral pain threshold' by sensitizing the nerve endings (Ferreira, 1972). Aspirin and other NSAI agents inhibit the synthesis of PGs and thereby alleviate pain.

Response to PG inhibitors is variable. Even so, aspirin or an alternative strong NSAI agent should be used routinely when seeking to relieve bone pain with drugs, either alone or in combination with an opioid. Aspirin in a dose of between 3 and 4 g per day is very useful. If a twice daily preparation is considered preferable, one of the newer strong NSAI agents should be prescribed e.g. flurbiprofen 100 mg b.d., diflunisal 500 mg b.d., naproxen 500 mg b.d. For patients who have difficulty with tablets, benorylate suspension 10 ml b.d. is a useful option. This dose provides approximately 4 g of aspirin and 4 g of paracetamol each 24 h. Patients of low body weight and/or who are hypoproteinaemic may complain on this dose of deafness resulting from a toxic free salicylate plasma concentration. In such patients, the dose should be reduced to 7 ml b.d. (or 5 ml t.d.s.).

NERVE COMPRESSION PAIN

Neuralgic pain caused by nerve compression is often not controlled with morphine alone. In this situation a corticoid should be prescribed (e.g. dexamethasone 4 mg daily or b.d.). Commonly, a marked improvement is seen within 48 hr. If the nerve compression relates to an identifiable bone metastasis or soft tissue mass,

radiotherapy should be considered. It is normally possible to reduce the dose of morphine and dexamethasone after radiotherapy. For patients who do not respond adequately to the combined use of morphine and dexamethasone, a neurolytic or neuro-ablative procedure should be considered (Chapter 70, p. 1243). In a report from Italy on the treatment of more than 1200 cancer patients, neurolytic procedures were used in 29% (Ventafridda *et al.*, 1987). At most centres in the UK, however, such procedures are used less frequently, probably in no more than 5% of all cancer-pain patients.

OTHER CORTICOID-RESPONSIVE PAINS

A corticoid should be considered as a 'co-analgesic' whenever there is a large tumour mass within a relatively confined space (Table 68.4). A tumour is surrounded often by inflamed oedematous tissue, and pressure on neighbouring veins and lymphatics may lead to further local or regional swelling. Corticoids reduce the inflammation and thereby reduce the total tumour mass (Fig. 68.5). The classical situation is that of headache caused by raised intracranial pressure in association with a cerebral neoplasm. There may be other CNS symptoms or signs, and patients often show improvement which lasts for weeks or months after commencing treatment with dexamethasone 4 mg b.d. to q.d.s. Analgesics are often necessary also (e.g. paracetamol or co-proxamol). Sleeping in a propped up position with three to five pillows or elevating the head

Table 68.4 Indications for corticosteroids in patients with terminal cancer

Non-specific uses	Specific uses
Improve appetite	Hypercalcaemia
Enhance mood	Carcinomatous neuropathy
Improve strength	Spinal cord compression
Reduce fever ± sweats	Superior vena cava obstruction
Use as a co-analgesic	Airways obstruction
Raised intracranial pressure	Carcinomatous lymphangitis
Nerve compression	Haemoptysis
Spinal cord compression	Leucoerythroblastic anaemia
Head and neck tumour	Pericardial effusion
Hepatomegaly	Adjunct to chemotherapy
Intrapelvic tumour	Minimization of radiation-induced reaction oedema
Metastatic arthralgia	Discharge from rectal tumour (use locally)

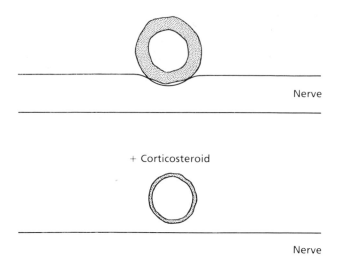

Fig. 68.5 Presumed mechanism of action of cortico-steroids in relief of nerve compression pain. Total tumour mass = neoplasm + surrounding hyperaemic oedematous tissue. General anti-inflammatory effect of corticosteroid reduces total tumour mass, resulting in reduction of pain. (Redrawn from Twycross & Lack, 1983.)

of the bed may be helpful if the headache is particularly troublesome on waking.

Corticoids prevent the release of PGs by exerting a 'stabilizing' effect on cell membranes. They do not inhibit PG synthesis as such but modify the inflammatory process in other ways. As a bonus, corticoids may stimulate appetite and elevate mood also. There is, therefore, a theoretical case for using both corticoids and NSAI agents in the management of certain pains (e.g. bone metastasis). However, more tablets may lead to reduced compliance and increased side-effects. Sometimes, though, maximal relief is obtained only by using an opioid, a NSAI agent, and a corticoid concurrently (e.g. pelvic malignancy invading bone and compressing nerves). If such a combination is considered, the effect of each agent should be assessed separately by adding one preparation at a time rather than prescribing all three simultaneously.

Metastatic arthralgia (Table 68.4) refers to the pain caused by metastatic involvement of the acetabulum or glenoid fossa. It occurs mostly in patients with cancer of the breast, bronchus or prostate. In addition to radiation therapy, here too, maximum relief may be obtained only by the combined use of an opioid, a NSAI agent and a corticoid. Injection into the joint space of a depot preparation of either methylprednisolone or triamcinolone should be considered also.

Opioid-responsive pains—but do *not* use opioids

FUNCTIONAL BOWEL PAINS

Although these may be ablated with opioids, it is clearly a second-best approach. Colic associated with constipation should be managed by treating the constipation, and so too should rectal spasm caused by faecal impaction. A third pain syndrome associated with constipation is that of right iliac fossa pain. In this, the descending colon (and sometimes the transverse colon) is easily palpable as it is full of hard faecal lumps. The caecum feels distended and is tender on palpation. The pain is that of gaseous caecal distension secondary to constipation. Identical caecal symptoms and signs are seen also in obstruction of the colon. Careful history-taking and assessment indicates normally which is the more likely of the two diagnoses. Sometimes, because of the intensity of the discomfort, a weak opioid preparation (e.g. co-proxamol) may be necessary for several days whilst the constipation is corrected.

Intestinal colic associated with obstruction responds to opioids. Sometimes, however, an antispasmodic is preferable. Mild recurrent colic responds often to agents such as mebeverine 135–270 mg q.d.s., propantheline 15 mg b.d. to t.d.s and hyoscine *butylbromide* (Buscopan) 10–20 mg p.o./i.m. q.d.s. Unpredictable, occasional severe colic is treated better perhaps with sublingual hyoscine *hydrobromide* (Quick Kwells) 0.3 mg as required. This acts within minutes of administration.

Irritable bowel syndrome occurs in approximately 10% of cancer patients (as in the general population) and, likewise, demands appropriate measures (Read, 1985).

SQUASHED-STOMACH SYNDROME

This is seen frequently in advanced cancer and warrants special mention. In this syndrome, epigastric pain is caused by relative gastric distension. This occurs often in patients with a grossly enlarged liver, whether or not there is associated gastric abnormality. It is important to recognize this cause of postprandial discomfort because explanation to the patient is crucial in management. Some patients, particularly those with a Celestin tube, experience also retrosternal pain resulting from acid-induced oesophagitis. The aim of treatment is to prevent distension. This requires a combination of dietary and pharmacological measures (Table 68.5).

Table 68.5 'Squashed-stomach syndrome'

Symptoms	Treatment
Early satiation	Explanation
Epigastric fullness	Dietary advice
Epigastric discomfort/ pain Flatulence	Antiflatulent (e.g. Asilone 10 ml after meals and bedtime)
Hiccup Nausea	Metoclopramide (after meals and bedtime or 4-hourly if also receiving morphine)
Vomiting (especially postprandial) Heartburn	Cyclizine 50 mg 8-hourly is occasionally also necessary

Opioid-responsive pains—do use opioids

Three important concepts govern the use of analgesics in the management of opioid-responsive pains, namely:
1 'By the mouth'.
2 'By the clock'.
3 'By the ladder'.

'BY THE MOUTH'

Morphine and other strong opioids are effective by mouth. Thus, apart from the last 2–3 days of life, few patients require injections to control their pain. How-ever, because of reduced bioavailability, the doses are 2–3 times larger than when given by injection. Patients with intractable vomiting in addition to pain need parenteral medication—both antiemetic and analgesic. When the vomiting has been controlled, it is usually possible to revert to the oral route.

'BY THE CLOCK'

To allow pain to re-emerge before administering the next dose causes unnecessary suffering and encourages tolerance. 'As required' medication has no place in the treatment of persistent pain (Fig. 68.6). Whatever the cause, *continuous pain requires regular preventive therapy*. The next dose is given before the effect of the previous one has terminated and, therefore, before the patient may think it necessary.

For codeine and morphine, a 4-hourly regimen is optimal. If a strong analgesic other than morphine is used, the doctor should be familiar with its pharmacology. For example, pethidine—effective for an average of only 2 or 3 hr—is given commonly every 4 or 6 hr, leaving the patient in pain for as many as 3 of every 6 hours. On the other hand, levorphanol and phenazocine are satisfactory when given every 6 hr, and buprenorphine and methadone every 8 hr. With methadone (plasma half-life of over 2 days when taken regularly by mouth) there is a real danger of cumulation with worsening side-effects, particularly in the elderly and debilitated.

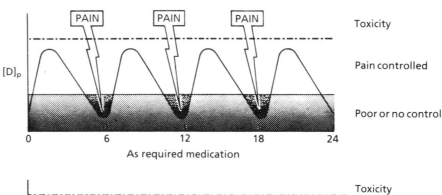

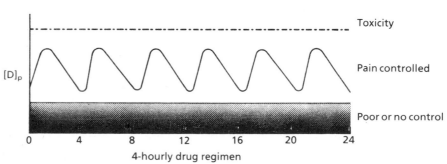

Fig. 68.6 Diagram to illustrate the results of 'as required' compared with regular 4-hourly morphine sulphate. [D]p = plasma concentration of drug. (Redrawn from Twycross & Lack, 1983.)

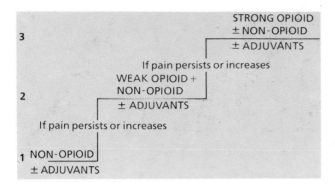

Fig. 68.7 The analgesic ladder for cancer pain management. (Redrawn from the World Health Organization, 1986.)

'BY THE LADDER' (Fig. 68.7)

The archetypal analgesics are aspirin, codeine and morphine. Other analgesics should be considered alternatives of fashion or of convenience. It is necessary, though, to be familiar with one or two alternatives for patients who cannot tolerate the standard preparations. Aspirin has two alternatives: paracetamol (which has no anti-inflammatory effect) and NSAI agent. The author uses dextropropoxyphene in preference to codeine. It is less constipating and in the UK, the compound tablet with paracetamol (co-proxamol) has a considerably greater 'codeine-equivalent' content than other weak opioid-compound tablets.

If one weak opioid preparation given regularly does not control the patient's pain, rather than attempting to control the pain with a drug from a different group, morphine should be prescribed. The use of morphine is determined by analgesic need and not, for example, by the doctor's estimate of life expectancy—which is often incorrect. A patient should not be forced to remain in pain because 'he is not ill enough for morphine yet'. The correct dose of morphine is that which gives adequate relief for 4 hr without unacceptable side-effects. 'Maximum' or 'recommended' doses, derived mainly from postoperative, parenteral, single-dose studies, are not applicable in cancer.

Morphine may be given either as an aqueous solution of morphine sulphate or as MST-Continus tablets. The latter are available as 10, 30, 60 and 100 mg strengths. Most patients changing from a weak opioid, commence on *60 mg a day* i.e. aqueous morphine sulphate 10 mg every 4 hr or MST-Continus 30 mg every 12 hr. As the effective dose of oral morphine sulphate ranges from as little as 5 mg to more than 1 g every 4 hr, the top of the ladder is not reached simply by prescribing morphine. Most patients, however, never require more than 100 mg every 4 hr; the majority continue to be controlled well on doses as small as 10–30 mg (or MST-Continus 30–100 mg b.d.).

When increasing the dose of morphine from an initial low level, increments tend to be greater in percentage terms than when adjusting a higher dose. With aqueous morphine sulphate, for example:

$$5\,mg \rightarrow 10\,mg$$

is a 100 per cent increase. Whereas

$$10\,mg \rightarrow 15\,mg$$
$$40\,mg \rightarrow 60\,mg$$

are 50% increases, and

$$30\,mg \rightarrow 40\,mg$$
$$60\,mg \rightarrow 80\,mg$$

are increases of 33%.

A change from 20 to 25 mg or from 40 to 50 mg is not advised. Each adjustment takes time and, if an adjustment yields little or no benefit, time and confidence are lost.

Increments tend to be more stereotyped at home as the patient has only one strength of morphine sulphate solution. Almost all increments are 50% in the first instance with the possibility of a second increment of 33% before a new stronger supply of morphine sulphate is issued. For example, 10 ml → 15 ml (50%) → 20 ml (33%).

It is important to be equally bold when increasing the dose of MST-Continus. Patients treated initially with aqueous morphine may be converted readily to MST-Continus if a twice-daily regimen seems preferable, for example, for the elderly patient living alone at home. The total daily dose is summed and divided by two (Hanks *et al.*, 1987). It may be necessary to round up (or down) the dose to fit a convenient tablet regimen.

The following points should be noted also:
1 It is pharmacological nonsense to prescribe simultaneously two weak opioids or two strong opioids.
2 It is sometimes justifiable for a patient on a strong opioid to be given another weak or strong opioid as a second 'as required' analgesic for occasional, troublesome pain. Generally though, if pain breaks through the 'analgesic cover', patients should be advised to take an extra dose of their regular medication.

3 Short-acting preparations should be avoided e.g. pentazocine (weak opioid), pethidine/meperidine (intermediate), and dextromoramide (strong opioid).

4 Opioid agonist/antagonists should not be prescribed (e.g. pentazocine, buprenorphine) with an opioid agonist (e.g. codeine, morphine).

Adjuvant medication

PSYCHOTROPIC DRUGS

If a patient is very anxious, an anxiolytic should be prescribed (e.g. diazepam 5 mg stat and 5–10 mg *nocte*). If a patient remains depressed after 2 or more weeks of improved pain relief and psychological support, an antidepressant may be used. This should be introduced in the same way as for deafferentation pain (p. 1214).

In some centres, morphine is prescribed premixed with a second drug, either cocaine (a stimulant) or a phenothiazine (a tranquillizer), or both. Increasing the dose of morphine may be hazardous if the dose of the adjuvant medication is automatically increased also, leading to agitation and restlessness on the one hand or somnolence on the other. It is preferable to give adjuvant medication separately. The dose of each pharmacologically active substance may then be adjusted separately in relation to the patient's need. Cocaine is no longer recommended (Melzack *et al.*, 1979; Twycross, 1979).

INSOMNIA

Discomfort is worse at night when the patient is alone with the pain and his or her fears. The cumulative effect of many sleepless, pain-filled nights is a substantial lowering of the patient's pain tolerance threshold with a concomitant increase in pain intensity. Temazepam is a useful hypnotic and may be given in doses ranging from 10 mg to 60 mg. If this results in morning somnolence, triazolam 125–500 μg may be used instead. Some patients fare better on dichloralphenazone, chlormethiazole or a sedative phenothiazine. In others, an antidepressant is useful. Sometimes, it is necessary to use a larger dose of morphine at bedtime to relieve pains that are particularly troublesome during the night (e.g. up to three times the daily dose).

It is now the general rule in many centres to administer a double dose of aqueous morphine at bedtime in order to obviate the need for a dose in the middle of the night. The larger bedtime dose causes added somnolence which is clearly of benefit in this situation. Published data confirm that there is no additional risk when a larger bedtime dose is given (Regnard & Badger, 1987). On the other hand, if the patient wakes regularly between 1 a.m. and 3 a.m. to micturate, it may be better to adhere to a 4-hourly regimen even overnight.

Analgesic side-effects

CONSTIPATION

A laxative is almost always necessary for patients receiving an opioid. The author uses co-danthrusate (Normax) capsules as the preparation of choice. These contain a colonic peristaltic stimulant (danthron) and a faecal softener (docusate). The median daily dose is three capsules. Some patients require as many as eight or 12. Smaller quantities are given generally as a single dose at bedtime. Approximately 30% of patients continue to require rectal measures (suppositories, enemas or manual evacuations).

Some patients do not respond well to co-danthrusate, possibly because they have a relatively greater ileal component to the constipation. In these, a small bowel flusher should be tried e.g. lactulose 20–40 ml b.d. or t.d.s. It is, of course, necessary to optimize the dose of co-danthrusate before discarding it in favour of lactulose.

Many patients are severely constipated when referred to a hospice or pain clinic, sometimes sufficient to cause symptoms and signs of partial ('subacute') obstruction. These patients require rectal measures—suppositories, enemas, manual disimpaction—for up to 2 weeks, in addition to commencing an appropriate dose of an oral laxative. Frequently, the management of constipation is harder (sometimes far harder) than the control of pain. The doctor who cares for cancer pain patients must understand how to use laxatives scientifically and methodically (Twycross & Lack, 1986).

NAUSEA AND VOMITING

Nausea and vomiting is common in cancer, particularly in those receiving strong opioids. At Sobell House, 60% of patients receiving morphine require an antiemetic.

If the patient is eating well and has been taking weak opioids or an alternative strong opioid without experiencing nausea or vomiting, an antiemetic is probably not necessary. It may, however, be wise to supply outpatients with a small number of haloperidol 1.5 mg tablets. If nausea develops, the patient can take one tablet stat and then one at bedtime thereafter for 7 days. For some, nausea is only an initial side-effect and resolves spontaneously after a few days. For others, it is necessary to continue the antiemetic indefinitely.

In approximately 10% of patients receiving morphine, haloperidol is ineffectual. This is because the morphine causes delayed gastric emptying of sufficient degree to induce nausea and vomiting ('pseudopyloric stenosis'). If a patient does not respond to haloperidol and the pattern of vomiting is suggestive of gastric stasis, a gastrokinetic antiemetic (metoclopramide or domperidone 10 mg 4-hourly) should be substituted.

In patients with raised intracranial pressure or with intestinal obstruction, cyclizine is the drug of choice. In approximately 10% of patients, it is necessary to use two different antiemetics concurrently. As with laxatives, it is necessary to be both scientific and methodical (Twycross & Lack, 1986).

RESPIRATORY DEPRESSION

Pain is the physiological antagonist to the central depressant effects of morphine. Thus, respiratory depression is not a problem when using morphine or other strong opioids regularly by mouth to relieve pain in cancer. In contrast to postoperative use of opioids, the cancer patient in pain:

1 Has usually been receiving a weak opioid for some-time (i.e. is *not* opioid-naive).
2 Takes medication by mouth (slower absorption; lower peak concentration).
3 Titrates the dose upwards step by step. (Much less likelihood of an excessive dose being given.)

Moreover, the fact that a double dose of morphine at bedtime causes no excess night-time mortality indicates that there is a reasonable safety margin (Regnard & Badger, 1987).

On the other hand, if the patient's pain is treated successfully by neurolytic or neuro-ablative techniques, life-threatening respiratory depression can occur if the dose of morphine is not reduced equally dramatically (Hanks *et al.*, 1981). *A reduction to 25% is recommended.* If the nerve block is totally successful, it will be possible to tail off the morphine completely over the next week or so. However, if only partly successful,

it may be necessary to increase the dose again to 50–60% of the original dose, or even more.

In short, morphine is a safe drug, provided a patient is not dying from exhaustion as a result of weeks or months of intolerable pain associated with insomnia and poor nutrition. In this circumstance, almost anything which eases the patient's mental or physical distress is likely to 'tip the scales' further in the direction of death. Circumstantial evidence suggests, however, that the correct use of morphine *prolongs* the life of a cancer-pain patient, as he or she is free of pain, better able to rest, sleep and eat, and is more active generally.

DROWSINESS

This is comparable to nausea; in the majority of patients, it is an initial side-effect which clears after 3–7 days on a steady dose. Elderly patients and their families, in particular, should be warned, as it may be associated with an element of confusion and/or unsteadiness. If severe, it may be an indication that the dose of morphine is excessive and a trial reduction should be made. Alternatively, it may be a matter of changing from a night sedative such as nitrazepam (with a prolonged half-life) to temazepam; or discontinuing a concurrently prescribed phenothiazine (particularly chlorpromazine) and using haloperidol if a neuroleptic or an antiemetic is needed.

After the first few days, some less physically active patients continue to experience drowsiness when sitting or reclining in a chair or bed. This inactivity drowsiness is usually not a problem. It helps pass what might otherwise be a long day and conserves limited energy for when other family members are home or friends visit.

Review

All cancer patients receiving analgesics need close supervision to achieve maximum comfort with minimal side-effects. Review of treatment is sometimes necessary within hours; certainly, after 1–2 days; and always at the end of the first week. Subsequent follow-up varies according to psychological and therapeutic needs. New pains may develop and old pains re-emerge. A fresh complaint of pain demands reassessment; not just a message to increase pain medication, although this may be an important short-term measure.

Alternative routes of administration

INJECTION

When injections are necessary, freeze-dried dia-morphine hydrochloride should be used, preferably subcutaneously:

1 mg injected diamorphine =
2 mg oral diamorphine =
3 mg oral morphine.

Some patients with inoperable bowel obstruction need parenteral medication for several days or weeks. The use of a battery-driven, portable syringe-driver facilitates the continuous subcutaneous infusion of diamorphine and antiemetic medication (Oliver, 1985; Jones & Hanks, 1986).

SUPPOSITORIES

Morphine sulphate suppositories provide another alter-native mode of administration. Fifteen mg and 30 mg suppositories are available commercially in the UK, and one pharmaceutical company makes suppositories of other strengths on receipt of a special order from a local pharmacy or hospital. Assessment of the plasma morphine concentration after oral and rectal routes suggests that the oral:rectal potency ratio for mor-phine sulphate is 1:1 (Pannuti et al., 1982). Oxyco-done pectinate suppositories (30 mg) are made by Boots. These need be given only every 8 hr. Oxycodone and morphine are equipotent (i.e. oxycodone pectinate 30 mg 8-hourly is equivalent to aqueous morphine sulphate 15 mg 4-hourly).

EXTRADURAL MORPHINE

Extradural morphine has been used in selected patients in recent years (Ventafridda et al., 1986). It is indicated occasionally in patients with localized regional pain who cannot tolerate morphine systemically, because of excessive sedation and/or dysphoria.

Alternatives to morphine

The regular use of aqueous morphine sulphate solu-tions (every 4 hr) or long-acting MST-Continus (every 12 hr) is regarded by the author as the treatment of choice for cancer patients in pain who require a strong opioid. Other strong opioids are available but none has any clear advantage over morphine (Twycross & Lack, 1983). It is necessary to have an alternative for the small minority of patients who literally cannot stom-ach morphine because of a functional gastric outflow obstruction that is not responsive to gastrokinetic agents (i.e. metoclopramide; domperidone).

Traditional formulations of morphine such as Ne-penthe and the Brompton Cocktail have no place in modern practice. Nepenthe, at one time a standardized solution of opium, is now essentially a solution of morphine hydrochloride. The Brompton Cocktail ap-peared in early editions of the British National Formu-lary (New Series) but is not included now. It has nothing to commend it (Twycross & Lack, 1983).

PHENAZOCINE

The author uses phenazocine in morphine-intolerant patients. Each 5 mg tablet is equivalent to 20–25 mg of morphine sulphate by mouth. Thus 'one tablet every 4 hr' may well be excessive. The tablets may, however, be halved and need not be taken more than four times a day. Thus 2.5 mg q.d.s. is equivalent approximately to 10 mg of morphine sulphate every 4 hr. In some centres, phenazocine is used successfully every 8 hr (Baines, personal communication). Although not manufactured specifically for sublingual use, the tab-lets dissolve readily in the mouth. Phenazocine appears to be equipotent whether swallowed or taken sub-lingually. Phenazocine is useful also in the patient who has deeply rooted irrational fears regarding morphine, and who declines firmly to take it.

BUPRENORPHINE

Sublingual buprenorphine is used widely in the UK. For this reason, it is important to be familiar with its properties. It is a morphine-type agonist/antagonist. It causes psychotomimetic side-effects only rarely. In this, it is similar to morphine and unlike pentazocine (a nalorphine-type agonist/antagonist). It should be stressed that it is an alternative to morphine, and not codeine (Table 68.6).

The author maintains patients on buprenorphine if pain is controlled well, and adjusts the dose sub-sequently if the need arises. Apart from the fact that it is not a controlled drug, there are no other advantages. In common with morphine, a proportion of patients experience troublesome nausea and vomiting, and virtually all become constipated with regular use.

Table 68.6 Guide to the use of sublingual buprenorphine

A semi-synthetic thebaine derivative with both agonist and antagonist properties

An alternative to oral morphine sulphate in the low–medium part of morphine's dose range

In very low doses, buprenorphine and morphine are additive in their effects but, at high doses, antagonism by buprenorphine may occur

Buprenorphine is available as a buccal ('sublingual') tablet. Ingestion reduces bioavailability and efficacy

Should be given only every 8 hr: to give more often is to make life unnecessarily harder for a hard-pressed patient

Exception to 8-hr rule: at upper dose limit, patients may find it easier to take 1.2 mg q.i.d. rather than 1.6 mg t.i.d

Effective dose range = 0.2 mg 8-hourly to 1.2 mg 6-hourly

Analgesic ceiling at a daily dose of approximately 5 mg; this is equivalent to approximately 50 mg of morphine sulphate by mouth every 4 hr

Buprenorphine is *not* an alternative to codeine or detropropoxyphene. As with morphine, it should be used only when a weak opioid has failed

Assuming previous regular 4- to 6-hourly use of codeine or dextropropoxyphene, most patients should commence on 0.2 mg sublingually every 8 hr with the proviso that 'if it is not more effective than your previous tablets take a further 0.2 mg after 1 hr, and 0.4 mg 8-hourly thereafter'

When changing to morphine because of unrelieved pain, multiply total daily dose by 100 and convert to a convenient 4-hourly morphine regimen i.e. divide by six and round to nearest 10 mg

When changing because of unacceptable side-effects (pain controlled well), use a conversion ratio of 60–70

Side-effects—nausea and vomiting, constipation, drowsiness—need to be monitored as with morphine

Prescribing should be simple: there is never any need for a patient to take both buprenorphine and morphine. Use one or the other. In this circumstance, unintended antagonism cannot occur

Expectations

Two surveys indicate the degree of success that may be anticipated. In the first, 156 patients were treated according to the 'three-step' analgesic ladder popularized by the World Health Organization (Takeda, 1987). Eighty-seven percent of the patients had complete relief, 9% had 'acceptable relief' and 4% had partial relief. The second survey covered more than 1200 patients (Ventafridda *et al.*, 1987). The analgesic ladder alone proved efficacious in 71% of patients. In the remainder, neurolytic procedures were used also. These data suggest that expectations for relief should be high.

However, whereas relief is obtained within 2 or 3 days in some patients, in others (particularly those whose pain is made worse by movement and in the very anxious and depressed) it may take 3–4 weeks of inpatient treatment to achieve satisfactory control. Even so, it should be possible to achieve some improvement within 24 to 48 hr in all patients. Although the ultimate aim is complete freedom from pain, there will be less disappointment but, paradoxically, more success if in practice the aim is 'graded relief'. Further, as some pains respond more readily than others, improvement must be assessed in relation to each pain.

The initial target should be a night free of pain with adequate sleep. Many patients have not had a good night's rest for weeks or months and are exhausted and demoralized. To sleep through the night pain-free and wake refreshed is a boost to both the doctor's and the patient's morale. Next, one aims for relief at rest in bed or chair during the day; finally, for freedom from pain on movement. The former is always eventually possible; the latter is not. However, the encouragement that relief at night and when resting during the day brings, gives the patient new hope and incentive and enables him or her to begin to live again despite limited mobility. Freed from the nightmare of constant pain, the patient's last weeks or months begin to take on a new look.

Conclusion

In the majority of cancer patients it is *not* difficult to achieve good or even complete relief. It does, however, require a doctor who:

1 Appreciates that pain is a somatopsychic experience.

2 Evaluates carefully the cause(s) of pain.

3 Adopts a multimodality approach, combining non-drug with drug measures.

4 Differentiates between 'opioid-responsive' and 'opioid-non-responsive' pains.

5 Uses the correct drug in the correct dose at the appropriate time intervals.

6 Recognizes that the effective dose of a strong opioid varies widely.

7 Monitors closely patients receiving strong opioids, and controls carefully any side-effects, particularly constipation.

8 Works closely with, and listens to, the nurses and other care-givers.

References

Ferreira S.H. (1972) Prostaglandins, aspirin-like drugs and analgesia. *Nature New Biology* **240**, 200–3.

Galasko C.S.B. (1981) The development of skeletal metastases. In *Bone Metastasis* (Eds Weiss L. & Gilbert H.A.) pp. 83–113. G.K. Hall, Boston, Massachusetts.

Gerson G.R., Jones R.B. & Luscombe D.K. (1977) Studies on the concomitant use of carbamazepine and clomipramine for the relief of postherpetic neuralgia. *Postgraduate Medical Journal* **53** (Suppl. 4), 104–9.

Hanks G.W., Twycross R.G. & Bliss J.M. (1987) Controlled-release morphine tablets: a double-blind trial in patients with advanced cancer. *Anaesthesia* **42**, 840–4.

Hanks G.W., Twycross R.G. & Lloyd J.W. (1981) Unexpected complication of successful nerve block. *Anaesthesia* **36**, 37–9.

Jones V.A. & Hanks G.W. (1986) New portable infusion pump for prolonged subcutaneous administration of opioid analgesics in patients with advanced cancer. *British Medical Journal* **292**, 1496.

Melzack R., Mount B.M. & Gordon J.M. (1979) The Brompton mixture versus morphine solution given orally: effects on pain. *Canadian Medical Association Journal* **120**, 435–9.

Mount B.M. (1984) Psychological and social aspects of cancer pain. In *Textbook of Pain* (Eds Wall P.D. & Melzack R.) pp. 460–71. Churchill Livingstone, Edinburgh.

Oliver D.J. (1985) The use of the syringe driver in terminal care. *British Journal of Clinical Pharmacology* **20**, 515–16.

Pannuti F., Rossi A.P., Iafelice G., Marraro D., Camera P., Cricca A., Strocchi E., Burroni P., Lapucci L. & Fruet F. (1982) Control of chronic pain in very advanced cancer patients with morphine hydrochloride administered by oral, rectal and sublingual route. Clinical report and preliminary results on morphine pharmacokinetics. *Pharmacological Research Communications* **14**, 369–80.

Raftery H. (1979) The management of postherpetic pain using sodium valproate and amitriptyline. *Irish Medical Journal* **72**, 399–401.

Read N.W. (1985) *Irritable Bowel Syndrome*. Grune & Stratton, London.

Regnard C.F.B. & Badger C. (1987) Opioids, sleep and the time of death. *Palliative Medicine* **1**, 107–10.

Saunders C. & Baines M. (1983) *Living with Dying. The Management of Terminal Disease*. Oxford University Press, Oxford.

Takeda F. (1987) Preliminary report from Japan on results of field testing of WHO draft interim guidelines for relief of cancer patients. *The Pain Clinic* **1**, 83–9.

Twycross R.G. (1979) Effects of cocaine in the Brompton Cocktail. In *Advances in Pain Research and Therapy*, vol. 3 (Eds Bonica J.J., Liebeskind J.C. & Albe-Fessard D.) pp. 927–32. Raven Press, New York.

Twycross R.G. & Fairfield S. (1982) Pain in far-advanced cancer. *Pain* **14**, 303–10.

Twycross R.G. & Lack S.A. (1983) *Symptom Control in Far-Advanced Cancer: Pain Relief*. Pitman, London.

Twycross R.G. & Lack S.A. (1986) *Control of Alimentary Symptoms in Far-Advanced Cancer*. Churchill Livingstone, Edinburgh.

Ventafridda V., De Conno F., Tamburini M. & Pappalettera M. (1986) Clinical evaluation of chronic infusion of intrathecal morphine in cancer pain. In *Advances in Pain Research and Therapy*, vol. 8 (Eds. Foley K.M. & Inturrisi C.E.) pp. 391–405. Raven Press, New York.

Ventafridda V., Tamburini M., Caraceni A., De Conno F. & Naldi F. (1987) A validation study of the W.H.O. method for cancer pain relief. *Cancer* **59**, 851–6.

World Health Organization (1986) *Cancer Pain Relief*. World Health Organization, Geneva.

69

Acupuncture, TENS, Hypnosis and Behavioural Therapy

J. E. CHARLTON

Drug therapy is the chief method of pain relief for both acute and chronic pain. Problems with drugs in the form of side-effects or lack of appropriate response have led to some disenchantment and a search for other methods of pain relief. Destructive procedures such as neurolytic blockade or neurosurgery may provide an answer for certain carefully selected patients but carry serious risks of morbidity and mortality and are inappropriate for acute pain relief.

There is a variety of relatively non-invasive methods of pain relief which provide alternatives to conventional therapy. Examples include acupuncture, transcutaneous electrical nerve stimulation (TENS), hypnosis, biofeedback and various psychological and psychiatric techniques. All these techniques are important in the management of chronic pain and may have some application to acute pain relief.

Acupuncture

Throughout history, man has learned to fight pain with pain. As a rule, brief moderate pain tends to abolish severe prolonged pain. Procedures such as cupping, cauterization and the application of 'counter-irritants' are found in most cultures. The fact that they have survived thousands of years suggests that they must be more effective than placebo. None of these therapies has been subjected to clinical trial, but work with acupuncture and TENS suggests that there is every reason to believe that they have survived because they are effective. They have the advantage that they do not need necessarily to be administered by a physician but may be carried out by less highly trained personnel or by the patient and family. In addition, they do little harm.

Classical acupuncture

Acupuncture has been practised in China for at least 2000 yr, and it is linked inextricably with classical ideas of health and disease. The ancient Chinese believed that the universe was permeated with a vital life-force or energy (called Ch'i) which circulated continuously through all living organisms. In man the energy was thought to follow specific pathways or meridians upon which the acupuncture points lie. Classically, there are 12 bilaterally symmetrical meridians and two non-paired midline control meridians, each representing internal organs as visualized by traditional Chinese medicine.

If the circulation of Ch'i along the meridians was altered by any disease process, either physical or emotional, an increase or deficit of Ch'i resulted. The resultant imbalance revealed itself eventually as pain or disease. This imbalance could be corrected by the insertion of acupuncture needles into specific points along the meridians near the surface of the body. The selection of the appropriate acupuncture points was made after studying the patient and by taking into account various philosophical and theoretical concepts. Many years of study are required to master all the subtleties of traditional acupuncture.

Modern acupuncture

The meridians are unrelated to any known nervous, circulatory or lymphatic system. However, many acupuncture points are close to branches of cutaneous nerves, nerves to muscles and main nerve trunks (Kaada, 1976). In addition, more than 60% of acupuncture points correspond to known trigger points and it has been suggested that they may represent the same phenomenon and may be explained in terms of the same underlying neural mechanisms (Melzack *et al.*, 1976). This does not seem likely as trigger points have a physical existence whereas acupuncture points do not.

Acupuncture points have a functional electrical existence in that they are sites of low skin resistance (and therefore high conductivity) and they may be identified using a skin resistance meter. It has been suggested that the low skin resistance is a result of local changes in sympathetic tone (Nakatani & Yamashita, 1977). The most effective acupuncture points are located often where nerves enter muscle (Gunn, 1978). Acupuncture points are stimulated generally with fine, 30 gauge, solid stainless-steel needles. There are no convincing data to show that variations in gauge or in the type of metal make any difference to the clinical effect. Methods of stimulating acupuncture points range from simple digital pressure, through the spectrum of high technology to lasers. None has been shown to be better than electrical stimulation alone.

Once the appropriate acupuncture point has been selected, the needle is inserted deep into the muscle. In the author's experience this is achieved best by holding the needle at the mid-point of the shaft between thumb and forefinger and using a quick twirling motion. The needle is advanced subsequently into the muscle until the point is reached and the patient experiences the sensation of 'Teh Chi'. This is a feeling, described variously as tingling, soreness, numbness or heaviness, which is essential if acupuncture is to be successful. If it is not obtained, the needle should be re-inserted, and it should be noted that this characteristic sensation is almost impossible to obtain at non-acupuncture points.

ELECTRO-ACUPUNCTURE

Modern acupuncture practice utilizes electrical stimulation of the needle with a pulse generator. Most generators deliver pulsed direct current with a square wave and have the options of varying frequency, pulse width and voltage. Most modern practitioners prefer to use low-frequency stimulation (2–4 Hz) (Omura, 1975), and it is alleged that this produces much longer-acting pain relief than that provided by high-frequency stimulation, albeit at the cost of a slower onset time. The intensity of stimulus is usually of the order of 200 μA, but this may vary widely. Stimulation is applied for approximately 20 min and, when effective, treatment may have to be repeated on several occasions to produce an effect of prolonged duration.

MECHANISMS OF ACTION

The gate-control theory of pain (Melzack & Wall, 1965) may explain some of the effects of acupuncture, but not others. It explains why stimulation in the same dermatome may be effective, but it does not explain why stimulation at distant sites may be equally as effective. However, it does offer a theoretical explanation for why acupuncture is frequently unsuccessful in relieving pain characterized by large fibre destruction such as trigeminal or postherpetic neuralgia.

Acupuncture has been shown to release endorphins and other peptides and to be reversed by naloxone (Melzack, 1973), but this does not imply that this is the mechanism of action of acupuncture; it may represent only a small part.

Animal studies

In a study using mice, naloxone has been shown to block acupuncture analgesia, whilst sham electro-acupuncture produced no analgesia, and naloxone infusion alone had little effect (Pomeranz & Chiu, 1976). The same authors have shown a similar effect in anaesthetized cats (Cheng & Pomeranz, 1979).

Human studies

A double-blind study of experimental tooth pain showed that acupuncture analgesia could be produced by manual stimulation of needles in the hand, and that this could be reversed by intravenous naloxone (Mayer *et al.*, 1977).

It has been shown in other studies that acupuncture does not induce significant analgesia in all human volunteers and may cause temporary hyperalgesia in some individuals. Only 42% of subjects are able to increase their pain threshold by 20% or more above baseline after 20 min of acupuncture (Benedetti & Murphy, 1985). Practical experience would suggest that similar results are obtained in treatment of both acute and chronic pain, and it is this lack of a predictable, uniform and intense analgesia which leads to ambivalence by Western physicians and their patients with regard to its use.

INDICATIONS

Acupuncture is used in the treatment of acute and chronic pain of musculoskeletal and neurogenic origin. Neck and back problems, myofascial pain and acute strain/sprain injuries have been treated successfully with acupuncture. There have been reports also of the successful treatment of postoperative pain, although in general this has been disappointing. There are theoretical grounds for its use in patients in whom opioids are contra-indicated or where conventional analgesia might diminish the level of consciousness.

RESULTS

It is impossible to provide accurate figures on the success of acupuncture analgesia in either acute or chronic pain. Many claims have been exaggerated which leads to cynicism on the part of physicians who do not practice acupuncture therapy.

In order for acupuncture to be successful, several important points must be borne in mind. Firstly, the patient must be motivated psychologically for the acupuncture therapy to be successful. This appears to be essential, as several studies have shown total failure of acupuncture analgesia for acute pain in unmotivated patients and in chronic pain patients with associated depression (Frost et al., 1976; Hossenlopp et al., 1976). Secondly, only a small percentage of patients respond to acupuncture treatment. Acupuncture may not produce anaesthesia or true analgesia but only a modest reduction in painful sensations. Finally, the physician should have no false illusions or hopes on the efficacy of acupuncture and should communicate his or her doubts beforehand to the patient.

Acupuncture has large limitations and it is unrealistic to expect good results in severe pain from acupuncture therapy except in a few individuals. The difficulties of assessing the results of acupuncture therapy have been summarized by one of its protagonists (Lewith, 1984). Many of the reports cited by Lewith are unconvincing, and a more recent attempt has been made to improve the standards by which clinical studies of acupuncture are studied (Vincent & Richardson, 1986). The same authors have reviewed the clinical use of acupuncture where adequate controls are available (Richardson & Vincent, 1986). Practical experience and further information is obtained best by attending a good practical course.

COMPLICATIONS

Acupuncture treatment has few complications provided adequate care is taken in sterilizing skin and equipment. The patient may have a syncopal attack and a haematoma may occur at the site of needle insertion. However, more serious complications have occurred including pneumothorax and damage to the spinal cord.

Physiotherapy

Physiotherapy plays a vital role in the management of both acute and chronic pain. The restoration of normal function is the most important goal of any pain-management programme, and analgesic measures are directed usually at making it possible for the patient to begin the necessary activity. It may be argued that many of the techniques used in physiotherapy will eliminate or reduce pain.

A comprehensive list of the various treatments available is beyond the scope of this chapter, but obvious examples include the use of heat and cold, massage, traction, manipulation and electrical stimulation. For a review of this topic, the reader is referred to Lehmann and de Lateur (1985).

Heat and cold

Heat treatment may be given by superficial or deep heat. Most patients with chronic pain are aware of the effects of superficial heat, applied locally in the form of a hot water bottle, or generally in the form of a hot bath or shower. Deep heat may be applied by one of three methods: shortwave diathermy, microwave diathermy or ultrasound. The energy of shortwave diathermy is transferred into the deeper tissue layers by a high-frequency, electromagnetic current (27.12 MHz), whereas microwave diathermy energy is propagated by means of electromagnetic radiation at a frequency of 2456 and 915 MHz. Under optimal conditions, shortwave diathermy causes an increase in tissue temperature to a depth of 3 cm, whereas microwave diathermy causes an increase to a depth of 5 cm (Griffin & Karselis, 1978). Ultrasound comprises the use of high-frequency acoustic vibration at 0.8–1.0 MHz. All three methods may produce valuable pain relief in both acute and chronic pain states, particularly in musculoskeletal pain.

Local heat produces many different responses including changes in neuromuscular activity, blood flow, capillary permeability, enzymatic activity and pain. Distant heat causes less marked changes, but nonetheless alters muscular function, blood flow and local reflexes. The mode of action of heat has not yet been demonstrated clearly but would appear to include improved blood supply and suppression of sympathetic overactivity.

Cold therapy has been used for the relief of pain since ancient times. In recent years, it has become used increasingly in the form of ice packs, vapocoolant sprays and ice massage. It is most useful in acute musculoskeletal pain associated with sports injuries or trauma. Pain can be alleviated frequently and to some extent prevented by early application of cold in the form of an ice pack. Not only may this help pain, but it also reduces bleeding and oedema by causing vasoconstriction.

Massage, traction and manipulation

Massage has also been used for centuries in many different cultures for the purpose of pain relief. There are many different types of massage, but all are essentially a form of stimulation technique aimed at muscle relaxation and improvement in local blood flow. It is not clear if benefit is produced by local reflex activity or by mechanical stimulation.

Lumbar and cervical traction are used frequently for musculoskeletal disorders and problems arising from discs and degenerative joint disease. The purpose of traction is to distract the vertebrae and relieve muscle spasm; by doing so it is believed that pain arising from nerve-root compression and from the facet joints may be relieved.

Similar properties are claimed for the manipulation which has also been employed for many centuries in the successful treatment of acute and chronic pain. Manipulative medicine takes many forms; osteopathy, chiropractice in addition to 'orthodox' medical manipulation. For a helpful introduction to this subject, the reader is referred to Paterson and Burn, 1985.

Electrical stimulation

Therapeutic electrical stimulation in physiotherapy is usually either low-frequency, alternating or faradic current, or direct current of a wide range of frequencies, termed galvanic current. These are distinct from TENS with portable stimulating units which are considered separately below.

The same conditions that benefit from treatment by ultrasound or short-wave diathermy may be expected to improve with electrical stimulation techniques. Galvanic stimulation with high-voltage, high-peak current generators is alleged to provide better results as the current is believed to penetrate deeper and to cause less painful contractions during stimulation.

Transcutaneous electrical nerve stimulation

There are historical precedents extending back to the Ancient Greeks for the therapeutic use of electricity. The first clinical report was that of Scribonius Longus who used the electrical discharge of the torpedo fish to treat headache and arthritis. Electrostatic generators and Leyden jar condensers reawakened an interest in electrotherapy in the late Middle Ages, and the invention of the battery provided another impetus in Victorian times. However, little work that was of clinical use emerged until two decades ago.

The use of TENS in clinical pain relief is a direct result of the publication in 1965 of Melzack and Wall's 'Spinal gate-control theory'. This theory suggested that the dorsal horn of the spinal cord was an important modulator of pain transmission. One of the most important predictions of the gate-control theory was that signals in the large primary afferent fibres (the A-fibres) would, by stimulating inhibitory circuits in the dorsal horn, suppress the onward transmission of signals in the small unmyelinated primary afferent fibres (the C-fibres).

This supposition was put to the test by Wall and Sweet (1967) who showed that clinical and experimental pain could be reduced by prolonged stimulation of peripheral nerves by percutaneous electrodes, without untoward effects. Since then, a great deal of research has been performed on the clinical application of electrical stimulation, which now includes not only TENS but also direct peripheral nerve stimulation, extradural and direct spinal stimulation, and even direct stimulation of the pain-regulating areas of the brain. However, the discussion in this chapter is confined to TENS.

Theory

Peripheral nerve stimulation utilizes the large myelinated afferent nerve fibres to activate local inhibitory circuits within the dorsal horn of the spinal cord. These inhibitory circuits reduce the transmission of painful impulses through the spinal cord. Transcutaneous electrical nerve stimulation produces non-painful paraesthesiae and is used usually in a segmental fashion as inhibition of nociception mediated by the large A-fibres is segmental. This is in contrast to acupuncture and similar counter-irritant techniques which are extrasegmental and use painful stimuli. Polysegmental inhibitory circuits do exist, but require generally much higher intensity stimuli to become activated, as they are usually mediated by the smaller Aδ- and C-afferents (Woolf, 1985).

The long-term relief of pain produced by TENS is more difficult to explain. Melzack (1973) has suggested two mechanisms. Firstly, a painful joint relieved of pain by stimulation becomes more mobile and is able to undergo more activity, thus restoring large-fibre input and 'closing the gate'. Secondly, pain may form part of a central 'memory', with self-perpetuating neural circuits in the periaqueductal grey region forming the 'central biasing mechanism'. Electrical stimulation may break into this closed loop system and allow a reduction in the pain experienced.

Equipment

The equipment required for electrical stimulation is a pulse generator, an amplifier and a system of electrodes. Most modern stimulators are small and relatively inexpensive. They use rechargeable batteries and may power up to four electrodes.

In most stimulators, the frequency range is from 1 to 100 Hz. Most patients find that stimulation at a fairly high frequency (70 Hz) is the most comfortable and effective. Stimulation at low frequency (2 Hz) requires a higher intensity and may produce painful muscle contractions. There appear to be fundamental differences between high- and low-frequency stimulation. High-frequency stimulation produces fast onset of pain relief, which lasts only a short period of time and is not reversed by naloxone. Low-frequency stimulation has a slow onset of pain relief, a long after-effect and is reversed by naloxone. An attempt has been made to utilize both forms of stimulation with the 'burst' stimulator which delivers short trains of high-frequency bursts repeated at low frequency. This method of delivery makes it possible to use higher intensities of stimulation without distress to the patient (Erikssen et al., 1979).

There has been much research claiming to identify the optimal waveform, but in practice, rectangular pulses are easiest to generate and are quite satisfactory for clinical use. It has been suggested that those waveforms that have the most influence on circulation are the most effective in relieving chronic pain. The standard pulse width varies between 0.1 and 0.5 msec. A higher pulse width than this may stimulate motor or Class III fibres, producing unwanted activity and unpleasant sensations for the patient.

The output intensity control on most TENS units provides an output up to 50 V. Although only 20 mV or so are necessary to excite large myelinated fibres, TENS units can produce at least 1000 times this level. This is necessary, as a large amount of current is distorted and lost in the tissues between the electrode and the target nerve. In the normal configuration of electrode, electrode gel and skin, resistance is of the order of 1 kohm and the peak current 50 mA if the maximal output is 50 V.

The most important principle is that the current density produced by the apparatus should be able to excite the target nerve in a controllable fashion and without damage to the skin. Many types of electrode have been used, the most common being soft, carbonized, silicone rubber. These are strong, inert and conform to most of the body contours. Electrodes should be at least 4 cm^2 in area, as too high a current density in a small electrode may cause skin irritation. Conversely, large electrodes may not deliver sufficient current to stimulate the nerves effectively because of decline in current density with length (Brennan, 1976). Electrolyte gel should always be used to lower the high skin impedance and obtain a good contact, thus minimizing the possibility of skin damage.

Clinical use

The basic aim of TENS is to stimulate the large sensory myelinated fibres without discomfort to the patient and without muscle contraction. This is achieved most readily by positioning the electrodes proximally over the nerve supplying the painful area. This is not always possible, nor is it always successful and it is important to realize that it may take some time to find the most effective site for stimulation. It is best to work in a logical fashion, commencing along the length of the appropriate sensory nerve and following with stimulation at the point of maximum intensity of the pain, then dermatomally, over trigger points and on the contralateral side.

It is important to choose a site where the stimulus can be felt by the patient. The aim is to produce what is termed the 'maximum comfortable paraesthesia' and the patient is asked to increase the level of stimulation until it is frankly painful; the highest intensity below that which is not painful is the maximum comfortable paraesthesia. It is most unlikely that the patient will gain any benefit if an adequate paraesthesia is not experienced. It is equally important to allow the patient sufficient time to become familiar with the apparatus. Many patients are overawed by the machine and do not use it unless they have received a comprehensive explanation and demonstration. It has been argued that patients should be admitted to hospital for an adequate trial to be carried out (Wynn-Parry, 1980).

Patients should be encouraged to experiment with electrode positions and with the settings on the machine. For chronic pain a minimum of 3 hr stimulation per day is recommended, and this should be continued for 4–6 weeks. With chronic pain there is frequently a gradual development of pain relief which may not be noticeable immediately and the patient should be encouraged to persevere with treatment even though the initial response is unfavourable. There is also a small group of patients who find the sensation produced by the stimulator unpleasant and who cannot tolerate it. There are neither predictors of the type and intensity of stimulus that is effective, nor predictors for the type of condition or patient that responds. Some patients obtain pain relief only while using the stimulator; others may gain none whatsoever during stimulation but experience long periods of relief after stimulation.

ACUTE PAIN

Transcutaneous electrical nerve stimulation has been used to treat a wide variety of acute pains, with varying degrees of success. Probably the most appropriate and successful use of TENS is in acute musculoskeletal injuries. Outstanding pain relief may be obtained in many conditions where there is associated muscle spasm, such as acute low back pain, whiplash injuries and sports injuries. It has been reported that TENS is highly effective in the management of fractured ribs (Myers et al., 1977), acute orofacial pain (Hansson & Ekblom, 1983) and childbirth (Augustinsson et al., 1977). Subsequent work suggests that whilst it may be effective for the early part of labour it is ineffective for the pain of the second stage of delivery.

The majority of studies of TENS in acute pain have been undertaken on postoperative pain. However, there are few really good studies of its effect. There are technical problems with the structure of controlled double-blind trials with a treatment method that requires a comprehensive explanation to be effective and produces also a characteristic sensation that has to form part of the explanation. Nonetheless, TENS has been shown to be effective in several reasonable studies (Pike, 1978; Rosenberg et al., 1978; Schuster & Infante, 1980; Ali et al., 1981; Tyler et al., 1982). Not only did the patients complain of less pain, but also postoperative opioid requirements were reduced.

Other studies have demonstrated a reduction in postoperative ileus (Ledergerber, 1978), but this was not seen by others (Vanderark & McGrath, 1975, Rosenberg et al., 1978). Patients receiving TENS for postoperative pain relief showed also less depression of Pao_2, vital capacity and functional residual capacity (Ali et al., 1981).

There is still a need for further controlled studies of TENS in postoperative pain. Despite the obvious advantages of TENS in that it is simple to use, cheap, portable, continuously available and non-addictive, it has not gained a great deal of acceptance, and the suspicion is that this is because it is not effective. There is some evidence that if opioids have been used preoperatively, TENS is ineffective (Solomon et al., 1980).

CHRONIC PAIN

There is no doubt that TENS is an effective way to treat a wide variety of painful conditions. It is most useful in the control of pain of neurogenic origin such as peripheral nerve damage, plexus injuries (Wynn-Parry, 1980), causalgia (Meyer & Fields, 1972), phantom limb pain (Miles & Lipton, 1978), postherpetic neuralgia (Nathan & Wall, 1974) and post-thoracotomy neuralgia. In addition, root compression, radiculopathies, postlaminectomy syndrome and many other forms of low back pain respond to TENS (Procacci et al., 1982). Chronic pain states that are unlikely to respond to TENS include psychogenic pain (Nielzen et al., 1982), pain with multiple sites and aetiologies, and those that are difficult to localize, such as visceral pain.

Transcutaneous electrical nerve stimulation becomes less effective with the passage of time. Various authors have noted a high initial success rate of the order of 70%. This declines to approximately 60% after 1 month and a stable long-term success rate of the order of 20–30% is achieved usually. Some of the early success may be attributed to a placebo effect, but this is usually transient, and the results are more impressive when the wide variety of clinical conditions that have been treated successfully is considered. Woolf (1985) has reviewed the literature and lists those conditions where TENS has been of benefit and of little or no help.

COMPLICATIONS

There are few side-effects. The most common problems are associated with an allergic response to either tape or electrode gel and, less commonly, the electrode itself. It is possible to produce superficial erythema with overzealous stimulation over a partially denervated area or where insufficient gel has been applied. Some patients experience an increase in pain when TENS is used.

The use of stimulators in patients with cardiac pacemakers is an absolute contra-indication. Theoretical risks may be present if stimulation is applied over the carotid sinus or the gravid uterus, although no problems have been reported so far. Stimulators are relatively contra-indicated where the patient may have difficulty either understanding or using the machine, for example, at the extremes of age or where mental or physical handicap prevent full control. The most common problem is for a patient to fall asleep wearing a stimulator and to change position, with a consequent improvement in the electrical contact which may prove quite a shock to the system.

Hypnosis

Hypnosis has been used for the control of acute and chronic pain for more than 100 yr. Despite some widely publicized successes, it remains little used except by a small number of talented practitioners. In the past, proponents of hypnotherapy tended to present their findings in an overenthusiastic and uncritical way, which led to indiscriminate use and inevitable disappointment with the results. However, many practitioners may use hypnotic techniques unknowingly; for example, during induction of anaesthesia or during dentistry.

Definitions

The nature of hypnosis cannot be defined readily. It has been described as an altered state of awareness during which the patient experiences increased suggestibility, and during which the patient's conscious and unconscious mind is more likely to accept ideas uncritically (Hilgard & Hilgard, 1975). Another description suggests that hypnosis is a communication of ideas and understanding to a patient in such a way that he or she will be more receptive to suggestions, thereby becoming motivated to explore their ability to control

psychological or physiological responses and behaviour (Erikson, 1968).

Although hypnosis is an altered state of consciousness, the hypnotized individual does not lose consciousness and control. The patient is aware all the time, sometimes in a heightened fashion. As the patient is in control, it is possible to terminate the hypnotic state at any time if so desired, and contrary to popular belief, the patient does not begin spontaneous recitals of personal and intimate information. Hypnotic susceptibility is the subject of continuing debate. Approximately 60% of the population have some hypnotic capacity, whilst approximately 10% is extremely susceptible. To assess this, there are several standard scales for predicting the subject's susceptibility. Difficulties in predicting susceptibility and variability in effect are two of the biggest problems that occur in the clinical use of hypnosis.

Clinical use in acute pain

Hypnosis has been used in a very wide range of medical and behavioural problems. Among the best known use for hypnosis is pain relief. There is reasonable evidence that hypnosis may modify experimental pain (Orne, 1974). However, such pain relief is usually transient, and this is frequently so where acute pain is concerned, such as that of an operation. In general, it is not feasible to use hypnosis predictably to permit painful surgery. However, there are many anecdotal reports of major procedures being performed, and the only analgesia provided is that by hypnosis. The author has witnessed a patient use autohypnotic techniques whilst undergoing an intramedullary nailing of a fractured femur, a procedure that included reduction of the fracture and intramedullary reaming. At no stage during or after this procedure was there any complaint of pain or demand for analgesia.

Hypnosis may be most useful in the susceptible individual for less painful procedures such as dentistry and where frequent painful procedures are necessary such as dressing changes or the debridement of burns.

Clinical use in chronic pain

By definition, chronic pain lasts for a prolonged period, and for hypnosis to have a useful role it must form part of a broader co-ordinated approach that uses conventional therapy in addition to psychotherapeutic interventions. Various hypnotic control strategies have been described and the following are examples.

Suggestions of deep relaxation are frequently effective in pain control, as anxiety and pain are usually inter-related and relaxation produces reduction in anxiety and accompanying muscle tension. This technique is utilized in relaxation training (p. 1168).

Direct suggestions of decreased pain may be given; for example, 'your unconscious mind will now help you to become more comfortable'. Suggestions may be given to the patient that the pain is decreasing slowly or diminishing.

Displacement of pain to another part of the body may often help. For instance, a pain in the chest may be relocated to a hand or finger where it is less trouble-some.

Dissociation may be used to separate the patient from painful circumstances. They may be asked to imagine themselves floating above the pain or being in a different place and observing the procedure from afar.

Transformation of the pain into a sensation that may be tolerated such as a feeling of warmth or tingling.

Time distortion enables a painful procedure to pass by more quickly.

It is most likely that the hypnotized patient experiences benefit by entering a deep state of relaxation, which may short-circuit the continuum of stress/anxiety/pain. In addition, there may be other advantages such as involving the patient in their own care which, in turn, may lead to the patient developing a sense of control over the pain. Other benefits may accrue from the necessarily close relationship between patient and hypnotherapist, whereby hidden factors that have a significant influence upon the pain may be brought out, such as the influence of family and workmates, or fears regarding security and health (Chapter 65, p. 1166).

If hypnosis is to be used successfully, the patients must be assessed thoroughly and the expectations of both patient and physician must be realistic. Scepticism on the part of pain-clinic staff is an obstacle to successful treatment (Finer, 1979). As it is not easy to attain an uncritical acceptance of any treatment in most pain clinics, especially when there is more and more emphasis on the 'scientific' approach, it is unsurprising that hypnotherapy forms only a small part of their work (Pilowsky, 1986).

Motivation and compliance are important if success is to be achieved, but once a patient derives some benefit from hypnosis, continuation is not a problem usually. In addition, once success has been experienced, these techniques are learned easily by the patient and may be applied at any time without the need for professional help. Finally, it should be emphasized that hypnosis is used best as part of an overall treatment strategy that involves other methods of pain relief, and that hypnosis does not produce changes in pain or behaviour that the patient is not willing to modify (Orne & Dinges, 1984).

Relaxation training

The object of relaxation training is to decrease levels of stress, anxiety and muscle tension. It is customary to begin with an attempt at educating the patient on his or her condition and the technique to be employed, with an emphasis upon positive results. The next step is to have the patient assume a comfortable position in a comfortable environment (quiet room and lighting, non-restrictive clothing). Relaxation is taught by a cognitive technique such as by having the patient repeat silently words, sounds or images. These focus the attention upon the differences in sensation from alternatively relaxed and contracted muscle groups and lead to the patient being able to relax tense muscle groups by following simple steps. These manoeuvres may be used by the patient at home with the aid of prerecorded tapes.

Biofeedback

This treatment method is analogous to that of other behavioural approaches and is used rarely in isolation. Biofeedback has been used most commonly to treat headache.

There are four types of biofeedback being used at present. Electromyographic feedback is used to reduce muscle tension. Electroencephalographic feedback is used to increase α-wave activity in the brain as this is thought to be incompatible with pain. Skin temperature feedback is used to alter sympathetically mediated blood flow, and temporal artery blood flow feedback is used to control temporal artery flow in migraine.

There are many reports of benefit, but at least one excellent review has cast doubt upon what, if anything, biofeedback may achieve (Turner & Chapman, 1982a, b).

Meditation techniques

Meditation techniques are quoted frequently as being of value in the management of pain (Choi, 1987). Unfortunately, science has not yet found any method of measuring the validity of meditation as a treatment method.

Behavioural therapy

Basic concepts

When dealing with pain, it is important to recognize that pain is a subjective phenomenon, whatever its cause. The pain that is suffered by patients with psychiatric or psychological problems is no different from that described by patients with purely organic disease. The concept of 'psychogenic' pain should be discarded, as it implies that somehow the pain is not genuine, yet the distress suffered by the patient with psychiatric or behavioural problems is as bad as that experienced by the patient with purely organic disease.

It is important to recognize and look for psychiatric and psychological problems in any patient presenting with pain. Anxiety regarding the cause of pain is a natural response, as is depression when faced with the prospect of unrelieved or partially relieved pain associated with either acute or chronic disease. Anxiety and depression are expressed frequently in terms of physical illness of which pain is a common symptom. Failure to recognize this may lead to misdiagnosis and consequent mistreatment.

Emotional components of pain

The gate-control theory of pain (Melzack & Wall, 1965) has recognized the influence that higher centres may have upon the appreciation of pain and has superseded previous pain models that emphasized sensory physiology alone. There is now an established neurophysiological basis for the different psychological components of pain, and the neurophysiological mechanisms for many emotional states are becoming delineated. Attention has been directed to the unpleasant affective qualities of pain and the roles of anxiety in acute pain and depression in chronic pain. In general, these affective qualities vary with the chronicity of the pain.

Acute versus chronic

Acute pain is characterized usually by tissue damage, and this causes action to minimize the damage, which itself has strong affective qualities such as fear and anxiety. The greater the pain, the greater the anxiety. By definition, acute pain is transient and reduces as healing takes place.

Chronic pain is sometimes defined as pain that serves no useful purpose and is quite capable of destroying the physical and emotional well-being of the individual, with further malign effects upon the patient's family and friends. It is important to recognize the difference between acute and chronic pain, as treatment of an individual with chronic pain by methods that are suitable only for acute pain relief may lead to further problems. For example, if strong analgesics are prescribed for long periods of time, and the individual is recommended to undergo extensive periods of inactivity and convalescence, this leads inevitably to cessation of normal activity such as work or caring for the family.

Pain expression

Pain is an intensely personal experience, and methods of evaluating pain accurately are still being developed. One of the most well-known attempts to measure pain systematically is the McGill pain questionnaire (Chapter 63, p. 1156). This method permits the patient to describe pain in three dimensions: sensory, affective and evaluative. By including the emotional aspects of pain, this questionnaire contributes to the accuracy of diagnosis, as recognizing the way certain pains are described may suggest the diagnosis.

In addition, it is important to recognize pain behaviour, and note that behaviours that occur for one set of reasons may persist for a different set of reasons. For example, when an injury is followed by a period of rest, freedom from work and household responsibilities, sympathetic attention and a continuation of income in the form of sickness benefit, there is a strong risk that the patient may become trapped in the role of the invalid (Fordyce, 1984).

Psychiatric/psychological considerations

Most patients presenting in a chronic pain-relief clinic have an organic problem with some evidence of emotional disturbance. The task is to decide which is the more important component. The bulk of psychiatric disease seen in pain clinics comprises one of two major categories: reactive depression or a larger group with essentially neurotic conditions such as anxiety, often with hysterical symptoms or personality abnormalities (Merskey, 1984). Both these groups of conditions present with pain frequently, as it is much more acceptable for the patient to complain of pain than to say that depression and anxiety are overwhelming his or her life.

Psychiatric or psychological screening tests are useful in establishing a diagnosis. However, a positive result on a screening test does not suggest that the patient has anxiety or depression, it implies merely that further help should be sought from an appropriately trained individual to determine the contribution of anxiety or depression to the whole problem. No matter what diagnosis is reached eventually, the pain is always 'real' pain to the individual and every effort should be made to communicate to the patient that the physician believes that this is so. There can be little worse than the all too commonly held belief that pain is 'imaginary' or 'all in the mind'.

Placebo

It has been considered generally since the work of Beecher (1955) that a placebo effect can be found in 35% of patients with postoperative or acutely painful conditions. This is rarely so in patients with chronic pain. However, it should be emphasized that a placebo responder is no more than that; an individual who responds to placebo. This is a normal response, and not evidence of psychiatric or psychological problems.

Acute pain

Factors affecting the appreciation of acute pain
(Chapter 66, p. 1175)

There do not seem to be any predictors for the amount of pain that an individual experiences postoperatively. It is likely that psychological variables may account for some of the puzzling differences in the response of patients to surgery. These may be classified into two groups: predisposing factors and situational factors. The former are factors over which physicians have no control such as personality type, intelligence level, social class and family history. These have been reviewed well by Bond (1980).

Situational factors may have a great impact on the pain response and may be modified by appropriate therapeutic intervention. Chapman (1977) has proposed a multi-dimensional model for acute pain that takes into account the emotional and social aspects of the response to pain in addition to other factors.

Examples of factors that influence the perception of pain are previous experience, the meaning of the surgery, present social circumstances and cultural background. Techniques that can be used to control or lower the amount of pain are social modelling, relaxation training and the provision of information to the patient in the preoperative period.

Hospital stress

Stress is a pattern of responses which occur when the individual is threatened. These responses may be both physiological and psychological. There is no doubt that the simple act of being admitted to hospital is extremely stressful as it entails vast changes in social routines, diet and surroundings. There may be confusion and uncertainty regarding the intended procedure with an associated helplessness. This is even worse if there are language difficulties or if the patient is from a very different cultural background.

Anxiety is a very complex phenomenon which plays a major role in the perception of pain postoperatively. In general, there is a direct relationship between preoperative anxiety and the amount of distress suffered after operation. Anxiety may be measured easily with standard questionnaires and can be related to pain (Speilberger et al., 1973). The concept of state and trait anxiety is a useful one. State anxiety measures the response to a specific event such as surgery, whereas trait anxiety is the patient's predisposition to become anxious in any stressful situation. Patients with high trait anxiety scores preoperatively may be expected to show high state anxiety and high levels of pain and distress postoperatively.

Any individual who has undergone major surgery may find him- or herself physically helpless. Helplessness is a well-known source of stress and if the condition is prolonged for any length of time may lead to depression. It has been estimated that a hospital stay of 3 weeks or more predisposes to depression and a prolonged period of helplessness is a potent factor in inducing this state.

The reasons for the surgery and the postoperative consequences are powerful stressors. Surgery may be associated with benefit, such as the delivery of a baby, or the cure of painful condition. However, there are circumstances when the surgery may have catastrophic consequences such as the confirmation of an inoperable malignancy or the loss of a limb. Preoccupation with the effects of surgery upon future life, work or recreation may lead easily to great distress which must be anticipated and handled in a sympathetic and speedy fashion.

Psychological preparation for surgery

There is excellent evidence that preoperative psychological preparation reduces the pain and anxiety associated with surgery. Several methods are available, of which the commonest are cognitive, behavioural and social modelling. Cognitive methods require the presentation of information regarding the operation and its likely effects, coupled with instructions on methods of coping with the pain. Examples of this are the preoperative visit by the anaesthetist or explanations by ward or intensive therapy staff on what the patient may expect on return from their operation. Behavioural methods utilize relaxation training and breathing exercises.

Social modelling is used commonly in paediatric patients and involves the use of film or videotape to show children what they may expect on admission to hospital. Other examples are self-help groups in which patients who have undergone a particular procedure provide practical advice on the proposed operation and its long-term effects to those awaiting the same type of surgery.

Chronic pain

Many patients with chronic pain present with a confusing combination of organic and emotional problems. This is made worse frequently by other difficulties relating to excessive treatment and medication, and these in turn may be related to associated problems regarding family, work, compensation or legal action. No single therapeutic approach is appropriate for all these problems, and behavioural management of chronic pain problems forms merely part of an overall strategy that may include other methods of treatment such as drug therapy, nerve blocks or neurosurgery.

Specific techniques for the psychological management of pain

Analytical psychotherapy of the 'notebook and couch' variety is used rarely in the treatment of chronic pain. It is more common to use what may be described as 'support psychotherapy' (Pilowsky & Bassett, 1982). This treatment seeks to maximize the patient's own coping mechanisms and is coupled with cognitive strategies aimed at increasing the patient's insight into his or her condition and the various treatments that have been offered, or are about to be offered. There are extensive reviews of these therapies by Tan (1982) and Turner and Chapman (1982).

The development of behavioural programmes for the management of chronic pain results largely from the work of Fordyce (1976). These 'operant' programmes stem from the belief that chronic pain patients display or operate 'pain behaviours' that they use to manipulate their own lives and those of close relatives and friends. For example, moaning, limping or grimacing make it more likely that they are believed to be in pain, and thus sympathy, time away from work and household tasks, prescription of medicines and financial reward in the form of sickness benefit are all easier to obtain and maintain. These positive benefits tend therefore to reinforce these behaviours and make them more frequent.

Equally, such behaviours tend to make it easy to avoid aversive situations such as unpleasant tasks or undesired responsibilities. Thus, the goal of operant programmes is to decrease the number and frequency of learned pain behaviours and replace them with behaviours that are incompatible with the sick role: well behaviours. For these programmes to be effective, inpatient admission for up to 16 weeks is required. The treatment consists of a structured programme of therapy designed to maximize the patient's activities and minimize pain behaviour.

Thus, when the patient displays pain behaviour either by movement or complaint, this is ignored by the staff; when patients are indulging in well behaviour, by taking part in exercise classes or occupational therapy, they are rewarded by attention and support. This part of the programme is associated usually with the setting of targets to increase the amount of activity undertaken by the patients, vocational training, counselling sessions with the family and the systematic reduction of the amount of medicines taken (Buckley et al., 1986). Incentives are given to encourage participation and the achievement of targets in the form of passes for weekend leave or visits from family and friends.

Doubts have been cast on the value of operant programmes (Merskey, 1984). It has been suggested that it is unlikely that the pain may be alleviated merely by ignoring pain behaviour, especially if there is a physical basis for it, and that it requires a change in the physical status of the patient for improvement to occur. This may be produced by improvements in the patient's fitness following an increase in activity. However, there is no doubt that patients complain of less pain, take less medicine and are able to do more after treatment on an operant programme. Long-term results seem to indicate that although the patient's complaints of pain tend to recur, the long-term gains are maintained in terms of higher activity levels, decreased drug intake and better work records than similar patients who were treated by conventional means. The overall results are a little difficult to assess, as the majority of programmes include other treatment methods in addition, such as TENS, biofeedback or relaxation training. It would appear that operant programmes, when coupled with other non-invasive therapy, represent a most effective, if costly, way of improving the life of the patient with chronic pain.

References

Ali J., Yaffe C. & Senette C. (1981) The effect of transcutaneous electric nerve stimulation on postoperative pain and pulmonary function. *Surgery* **89**, 507–12.

Augustinsson L., Bonlin P., Bundsen P., Carlsson C.A., Forssman C., Sjoberg P. & Tyreman N.D. (1977) Pain relief during delivery by transcutaneous nerve stimulation. *Pain* **4**, 59–65.

Beecher H.K. (1955) The powerful placebo. *Journal of the American Medical Association* **159**, 1602–5.

Benedetti C. & Murphy T.M. (1985) Non-pharmacological methods of acute pain control. In *Acute Pain* (Eds Smith G. & Covino B.) pp. 260–1. Butterworths, London.

Bond M.R. (1980) Personality and pain: the influence of psychological and environmental factors upon the experience of pain in hospital patients. In *Persistent Pain*, vol. 2 (Ed. Lipton S.) pp. 1–25. Academic Press, London.

Brennan K.R. (1976) The characterization of transcutaneous stimulating electrodes. *IEEE Transactions on Biomedical Engineering* **23**, 337–40.

Buckley F.P., Sizemore W.A. & Charlton J.E. (1986) Medication management in patients with chronic non-malignant pain. A review of the use of a drug withdrawal protocol. *Pain* **26**, 153–65.

Chapman C.R. (1977) Psychological aspects of pain: patient management. *Archives of Surgery* **112**, 767–72.

Cheng R. & Pomeranz B. (1979) Electroacupuncture analgesia is mediated by stereospecific opiate receptors and is reversed by antagonists of Type I receptors. *Life Sciences* **26**, 631–9.

Choi J.J. (1987) Meditation. In *Pain Management. Assessment and Treatment of Chronic and Acute Syndromes* (Eds Wu W. & Smith L.G.) pp. 216–44. Human Sciences Press, New York.

Erickson M.H. (1968) An introduction to the study and application of hypnosis for pain control. In *Hypnosis and Psychosomatic Medicine* (Ed. Lassner J.) pp. 125–40. Springer-Verlag, New York.

Erikssen M.B.E., Sjolund B.H. & Nielzen S. (1979) Long term results of peripheral conditioning stimulation as an analgesic measure in chronic pain. *Pain* **6**, 335–47.

Finer B. (1979) Hypnotherapy in pain of advanced cancer. In *Advances in Pain Research and Therapy*, vol. 2 (Eds Bonica J.J. & Ventafridda V.) pp. 223–30. Raven Press, New York.

Fordyce W.E. (1976) *Behavioural Methods for Chronic Pain and Illness*. Mosby, St Louis.

Fordyce W.E. (1984) Behavioural science and chronic pain. *Postgraduate Medical Journal* **60**, 865–8.

Frost E.A.M., Hsu C.Y. & Sadowsky D. (1976) Acute and chronic pain: a study of the comparative values of acupuncture therapy. In *Advances in Pain Research and Therapy*, vol. 1. (Eds Bonica J.J. & Albe-Fessard D.G.) pp. 823–9. Raven Press, New York.

Griffin J. & Karselis T. (1978) *Physical Agents for Physical Therapists*. Charles C. Thomas, Springfield, Illinois.

Gunn C.C. (1978) Motor points and motor lines. *American Journal of Acupuncture* **6**, 55–8.

Hansson P. & Ekblom A. (1983) Transcutaneous electrical nerve stimulation (TENS) as compared to placebo-TENS for the relief of acute orofacial pain. *Pain* **15**, 157–65.

Hilgard E.R. & Hilgard J.R. (1975) *Hypnosis in the Relief of Pain*. William Kaufman, Los Altos.

Hossenlopp C.M., Leiber L. & Mo B. (1976) Psychological factors in the effectiveness of acupuncture for chronic pain. In *Advances in Pain Research and Therapy*, vol. 1 (Eds Bonica J.J. & Albe-Fessard D.G.) pp. 803–9. Raven Press, New York.

Kaada B. (1976) Neurophysiology and acupuncture: a review. In *Advances in Pain Research and Therapy*, vol. 1 (Eds Bonica J.J. & Albe–Fessard D.G.) pp. 733–41. Raven Press, New York.

Ledergerber C.P. (1978) Postoperative electro-analgesia. *Obstetrics and Gynecology* **151**, 334–8.

Lehmann J.F. & de Lateur B. (1985) Ultrasound, shortwave, microwave, superficial heat and cold in the treatment of pain. In *Textbook of Pain* (Eds Wall P.D. & Melzack R.) pp. 717–24. Churchill Livingstone, Edinburgh.

Lewith G.T. (1984) Can we assess the effects of acupuncture? *British Medical Journal* **288**, 1475–6.

Mayer D.J., Price D.D. & Raffii A. (1977) Antagonism of acupuncture analgesia in man by the narcotic antagonist naloxone. *Brain Research* **121**, 368–73.

Melzack R. (1973) *The Puzzle of Pain*. Penguin, Harmondsworth.

Melzack R., Stilwell D.M. & Fox E.J. (1976) Trigger points and acupuncture points for pain: correlations and implications. *Pain* **3**, 3–23.

Melzack R. & Wall P.D. (1965) Pain mechanisms—a new theory. *Science* **150**, 971–9.

Merskey H. (1984) Psychological approaches to the treatment of chronic pain. *Postgraduate Medical Journal* **60**, 886–92.

Meyer G.A. & Fields H.L. (1972) Causalgia treated by selective large fibre stimulation of peripheral nerves. *Brain* **95**, 163–7.

Miles J. & Lipton S. (1978) Phantom limb pain treated by electrical stimulation. *Pain* **5**, 373–82.

Myers R.A.M., Woolf C.J. & Mitchell D. (1977) Management of acute traumatic pain by peripheral transcutaneous electrical stimulation. *South African Medical Journal* **52**, 309–12.

Nakatani Y. & Yamashita K. (1977) *Ryodoraku Acupuncture*. Ryodoraku Research Institute, Tokyo.

Nathan P.W. & Wall P.D. (1974) Treatment of post-herpetic neuralgia by prolonged electrical stimulation. *British Medical Journal* **iii**, 645–7.

Nielzen S., Sjolund B.H. & Eriksson B.E. (1982) Psychiatric factors influencing the treatment of pain with peripheral conditioning stimulation. *Pain* **13**, 365–71.

Omura Y. (1975) Electro-acupuncture: its electro-physiological basis and criteria for effectiveness and safety. Part 1. *Acupuncture and Electrotherapy Research* **1**, 157–81.

Orne M. (1974) Pain suppression by hypnosis and related phenomena. In *Advances in Neurology*, vol. 4 (Ed. Bonica J.J.) pp. 563–72. Raven Press, New York.

Orne M.T. & Dinges D.F. (1984) Hypnosis. In *Textbook of Pain* (Eds

Wall P.D. & Melzack R.) pp. 806–16. Churchill Livingstone, London.

Paterson J.K. & Burn L. (1985) *An Introduction to Medical Manipulation.* MTP Press, Lancaster.

Pike P.M. (1978) Transcutaneous electrical stimulation: its use in management of postoperative pain. *Anaesthesia* 33, 165–71.

Pilowsky I. (1986) Current views on the role of the psychiatrist in chronic pain. In *The Therapy of Pain* (Ed. Swerdlow M.) pp. 31–55. MTP Press, Lancaster.

Pilowsky I. & Bassett D. (1982) Individual dynamic psychotherapy for chronic pain. *In Chronic Pain: Psychosocial Factor in Rehabilitation* (Eds Roy R. & Tunks E.) pp. 107–24. Williams and Wilkins, Baltimore.

Pomeranz B. & Chiu D. (1976) Naloxone blockade of acupuncture analgesia: endorphin implicated. *Life Sciences* 19, 1757–62.

Procacci P., Zoppi M. & Maresca M. (1982) Transcutaneous electrical stimulation in low back pain: a critical evaluation. *Acupuncture and Electrotherapy Research* 7, 1–6.

Richardson P.H. & Vincent C.A. (1986) Acupuncture for the treatment of pain: a review of evaluative research. *Pain* 24, 15–40.

Rosenberg M., Curtis L. & Bourke D.L. (1978) Transcutaneous electrical nerve stimulation for the relief of postoperative pain. *Pain* 5, 129–35.

Schuster G.D. & Infante M.C. (1980) Pain relief after low back surgery: the efficacy of transcutaneous electrical nerve stimulation. *Pain* 8, 299–302.

Solomon R.A., Viernstein M.R. & Long D.M. (1980) Reduction of postoperative pain and narcotic use by transcutaneous electrical nerve stimulation. *Surgery* 87, 142–6.

Speilberger C.D., Gorsuch R. & Lushene R. (1973) *The State–Trait Anxiety Inventory.* Consulting Psychologists Press, Palo Alto.

Tan S-Y. (1982) Cognitive and cognitive behavioural methods for pain control. *Pain* 12, 201–28.

Turner J.A. & Chapman C.R. (1982a) Psychological interventions for chronic pain: a critical review. I. Relaxation training and biofeedback. *Pain* 12, 1–21.

Turner J.A. & Chapman C.R. (1982b) Psychological interventions for chronic pain: a critical review. II. Operant conditioning, hypnosis and cognitive–behavioural therapy. *Pain* 12, 23–46.

Tyler E., Caldwell C. & Ghia J.N. (1982) Transcutaneous electrical nerve stimulation: an alternative approach to the management of postoperative pain. *anesthesia and Analgesia* 51, 449–56.

Vanderark G. & McGrath K. (1975) Transcutaneous electrical stimulation in treatment of postoperative pain. *American Journal of Surgery* 130, 336–40.

Vincent C.A. & Richardson P.H. (1986) The evaluation of therapeutic acupuncture: concepts and methods. *Pain* 24, 1–14.

Wall P.D. & Sweet W.H. (1967) Temporary abolition of pain in man. *Science* 155, 108–9.

Woolf C.J. (1985) Transcutaneous and implanted nerve stimulation. In *Textbook of Pain* (Eds Wall P.D. & Melzack R.) pp. 679–90. Churchill Livingstone, Edinburgh.

Wynn-Parry C.B. (1980) Pain in avulsion lesions of the brachial plexus. *Pain* 9, 41–53.

70

Ablative Nerve Blocks and Neurosurgical Techniques

K. BUDD

In the treatment of chronic pain, it may seem reasonable to suppose that destruction of the afferent sensory pathways from the area in which the pain is produced would have the desired effect of preventing access of nociceptive impulses to the sensorium and its appreciation as pain. Many techniques both surgical and non-surgical have been introduced during the past 50 yr for this purpose, and whilst some remain in contemporary use, none has achieved universal popularity. Although ablative techniques in general are used less frequently, for some well-defined indications they retain major clinical usefulness and may be the treatment of choice. The patient only benefits significantly, however, when such techniques are performed with care following well-established procedural guidelines.

Because the side-effects of many of these techniques include conditions worse than the original painful state, every effort should be taken to avoid not only these complications for the patient but also the possibility of consequent litigation against the practitioner.

Neurolysis

Interruption of nerve pathways (neurolysis) may be achieved using a variety of methods. These may induce either temporary or permanent cessation of nervous transmission; the former is utilized mainly for diagnostic procedures, the latter is the main therapeutic modality used in the treatment of chronic pain as an alternative to drug therapy. Neurolytic methods include:

1 Pressure applied to the nerve ⎫ for
2 Local anaesthetic applied to ⎬ temporary
the nerve ⎭ neurolysis.

3 Application of chemicals to the nerve ⎫
4 Application of cold to the nerve ⎪ for
5 Application of heat to the nerve, ⎬ permanent
nerve root or tract ⎪ neurolysis.
6 Surgical section of the nerve, ⎪
nerve root or tract ⎭

In the majority of cases, permanent neurolysis should be preceded by a temporary block with local anaesthetic in order that the degree of pain relief and its extent may be appreciated by both patient and doctor, and potential side-effects such as numbness and muscle weakness may be experienced by the patient. In the light of all these factors, informed discussion may take place between patient and doctor before the decision is taken to produce permanent neurolysis.

Neurolytic agents

CHEMICAL AGENTS

The commonly used neurolytic chemicals are phenol, alcohol and chlorocresol.

Phenol

Phenol is a weak acid with both bactericidal and neurolytic properties. Even in concentrations as low as 1%, neurolysis may be achieved, but in clinical practice the concentration used varies between 5 and 10% in aqueous solution. The neurolytic effect is more pronounced on small $A\delta$- and C-fibres which conduct pain, whereas the larger fibres with motor function are affected much less. This differential action is valuable, as pain may be relieved without disturbance of motor function and sensory modalities other than pain (Nathan & Sears, 1960).

Clinically, the effect of phenol appears to be exclusively on small fibres, but histological evidence shows that the effect is exerted on fibres of all sizes although a larger proportion of the smaller diameter ones are affected. The eventual outcome is dictated, however, by the concentration of solution, nature of solvent and duration of contact with nervous tissue. As a neurolytic agent, phenol is quicker in action than alcohol but less predictable in its spread and effect. A significant advantage is that it is less likely to produce chemical neuritis than is alcohol.

Phenolic solutions are thought to spread along the perineural sheath and nerve destruction is followed by gradual regeneration of the fibres over 5–20 weeks (Khalili & Ditzler, 1968). If phenol is placed inadvertently on a mixed somatic nerve, transient evidence of complete nerve block is seen, but appreciable reversal occurs within 1–2 weeks, and there is a high likelihood of complete motor function being restored. This is not usually the case with alcohol when motor function returns rarely to pretreatment values.

Toxic effects with phenol are seen infrequently with the small doses used in clinical practice. However, following inadvertent intravascular injection, patients may complain of faintness and dizziness accompanied by excitement. This progresses rapidly to depression of the vital centres leading to loss of consciousness, circulatory and respiratory collapse.

In the adult, the toxic dose for phenol is 8–15 g (Esplin, 1970) but in normal clinical practice this figure is never approached. Bryce-Smith (1966) recommends that the maximum amount injected in one bolus should be 66 mg. In doses less than this, patients may experience tenderness at the site of injection for several days and may exhibit also mild, influenzal-like symptoms for 48 hr, but serious complications are rare. When used intrathecally, phenol is dissolved in glycerine or a radio-opaque medium in order to render the resulting solution hyperbaric (SG 1025 compared with cerebrospinal fluid SG 1005–1009). Phenol produces an immediate local anaesthetic effect with recovery occurring over the subsequent 15–30 min followed by permanent nerve destruction (Nathan & Scott, 1958; Editorial, 1964). Patchy degeneration occurs in nerve fibres of all sizes, the principle site of action being the nerve roots between the cord and the dural cuff. The cord itself is undamaged, but degeneration in the posterior columns has been reported following repeated injections.

Ethyl alcohol

This is the most reliable agent for the production of peripheral nerve neurolysis (Dam & Larsen, 1974). It was used first to treat the pain of trigeminal neuralgia in 1888 (Pitres & Vaillard, 1888) and although its popularity has waned because of a high incidence of postinjection neuritis, some authorities advocate its use as the treatment of choice for the blockade of autonomic ganglia (Mehta, 1973).

When ethyl alcohol is injected intra- or perineurally, coagulation necrosis occurs characterized by diffuse eosinophilic staining with complete loss of detail in axons, myelin sheath, nodes of Ranvier and Schwann cells (Pizzolato & Mannheimer, 1961). Under similar conditions, phenol produces almost identical damage but regeneration of the axon occurs within 2 months. By injection, alcohol is extremely irritating to tissues, and causes pain, burning and local tenderness. In order to minimize these effects, the injection should be placed accurately so that the minimum volume is used. Nevertheless, the incidence of postinjection neuritis is significant and has resulted in loss of popularity of this agent.

When injected either peripherally or intrathecally, alcohol is used undiluted. As it has a lower specific gravity than cerebrospinal fluid (0.805 compared with 1.005) in the intrathecal space, the hypobaric alcohol floats upwards onto the specific nerve roots thereby allowing the patient to be positioned with the painful side uppermost.

Dilute solutions of alcohol are used occasionally for ablation of the coeliac plexus. Fifty percent alcohol in saline or bupivacaine is used commonly, but, as the injection is painful, it is necessary to perform this block under general anaesthesia or heavy sedation. With the dilute solutions, chemical neuritis is seen in up to 15% of patients (Brown, 1981).

Chlorocresol

Chlorocresol is a more potent agent than phenol and has been used only in the extradural and intrathecal spaces (Maher, 1963) as a 2% solution in glycerine and a 5% solution in glycerine respectively. It is one of the more effective agents for the treatment of cancer pain and has a greater ability to penetrate cancerous tissue surrounding nerve roots than does phenol or alcohol.

After injection of chlorocresol into the extradural or subarachnoid spaces, pain relief is delayed usually for up to 24 hr and, unlike phenol, it is not associated with immediate sensory changes or the onset of para-esthesiae. Until the full effect has been produced, the patient may complain of dull pain, sluggish limb movement and diminished sensitivity to heat and cold in the affected segments.

In the intrathecal space, chlorocresol appears to diffuse more widely than phenol, and is used therefore in a smaller dose, 0.35 ml of 2% solution in glycerine being equivalent to 0.5 ml of 5% phenol solution in the same solvent. Localization of the block with chloro-cresol is more difficult than with alcohol or phenol because of the absence of immediate sensory changes but the neurolysis is of a more intense nature after it has developed.

OTHER NEUROLYTIC AGENTS

Ammonium chloride

This agent has been used intrathecally in concentra-tions varying from 0.5 to 20%. Although excellent neurolysis is obtained with the higher concentrations, the injection is painful and the active agent may require dilution with local anaesthetic (Dam, 1965). Reduction in concentration produces adequate results in terms of neurolysis without discomfort (Mehta, 1973). After intraneural injection, severe injury and degeneration is produced, but regeneration may be complete within 60 days (Pizzolato & Mannheimer, 1961).

Silver nitrate

In resistant cancer patients, silver nitrate may be added to solutions of phenol in glycerine to increase penetra-tion. Maher (1957) has recommended the addition of 0.6 mg silver nitrate to 1 ml of a 4% solution of phenol in glycerine. Because of apparent lack of damage to sacral outflow and consequent sphincter sparing, the main uses are in the lower thoracic and lumbosacral areas. Excellent penetration may be achieved although it may take up to 5 days for the peak effect to become established (Maher, 1969). The use of silver nitrate in cervical and upper thoracic regions is not advocated because of the toxic properties of the agent. Based on pathological studies, Nathan and Scott (1958) sugges-ted that siver nitrate is dangerous at all levels.

Glycerine

The injection of glycerine into the trigeminal cistern may abolish completely typical trigeminal pain. In many patients, this pain relief is accompanied by very little disturbance of facial sensation (Hakansen, 1981). Long-term follow-up of this treatment shows a relapse rate of 31%, suggesting that this is safe and effective therapy (Hakansen, 1983). Glycerine does not appear to have the same neurolytic action when injected around a peripheral nerve or intrathecally.

Hypertonic saline

This has been used intrathecally to treat the pain of both benign and malignant disease, with claims for a 50% permanent improvement (Hitchcock & Pradinin, 1973). However, pain, hypertension and muscle fasci-culations produced on injection make the concomitant use of general anaesthesia necessary.

Sclerosant solution

This solution has been used for injection into strained ligaments and joint capsules for the relief of pain. It acts by destruction of fine nerve endings. It is claimed also to tighten flaccid ligaments, possibly by the formation of scar tissue. The solution contains: phenol 2%, dextrose 20%, glycerine 25% and water to 100%. As the solution is an irritant to tissues and may produce pain on injection, it may be combined with local anaesthetic agents prior to use or its injection preceded by infiltrat-ion of the tissue with local anaesthetic solution (Barber, 1971).

The application of cold: cryotherapy

Although the principle of using extreme cold to pro-duce insensibility to pain has been known and used for centuries (Armstrong-Davison, 1965), its clinical application to produce analgesia was not introduced until 1976 (Lloyd et al., 1976).

The cryoprobe comprises a fine needle probe with built-in thermocouple. It utilizes the Joule–Thompson effect with either nitrous oxide or carbon dioxide as the expanding gas, thereby reducing the temperature at the tip of the probe to $-70\,°C$ (Fig. 70.1). When introduced into the body, by freezing tissue water the iceball formed at the tip of the probe grows to encompass the selected nerve (Fig. 70.2), thereby dis-rupting the neural tissue but with minimal effects on endoneurium and other connective tissue. This lesion produces a break in the functional continuity of the nerve and hence analgesia which may last up to 6 months. The incidence of postlesion neuralgia is less

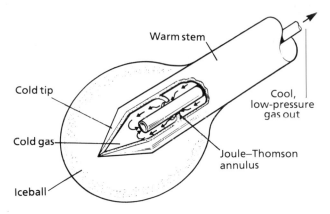

Fig. 70.1 Principle of cryoprobe. (Courtesy of Spembly Ltd.)

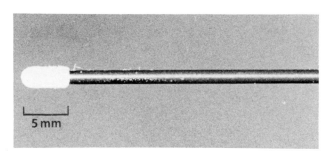

Fig. 70.2 Cryoprobe tip with iceball. (Courtesy of Spembly Ltd.)

with cryotherapy than with other neurolytic techniques (Carter *et al.*, 1972; Loyd *et al.*, 1976; Barnard, 1980).

A lesion may be produced either by picking up the exposed nerve on the tip of the probe (e.g. when the nerve is exposed at surgery) for postoperative analgesia (Katz *et al.*, 1980; Maiwant & Make, 1981; Orr *et al.*, 1983) or percutaneously using the stimulator built into the probe to locate the probe tip on or close to the selected nerve (Fig. 70.3). The lesion is made using two, 2-min freeze cycles separated by a 1-min warming period. This technique appears to give better results both in terms of degree and duration of analgesia than a single freeze of equivalent duration (Jones & Murrin, 1987).

There are few side-effects following cryotherapy, and these are limited usually to soreness at the site of insertion of the probe and occasional neuritic pain along the course of the nerve. On the rare occasion that the latter does not resolve spontaneously, infiltration of the site of the cryolesion with bupivacaine and methylprednisolone is beneficial. Alternatively, oral medication with an anticonvulsant (carbamazepine or sodium valproate) in combination with a tricyclic antidepressant (amitriptyline or nortriptyline) may produce remission within 2 weeks (Budd, 1981).

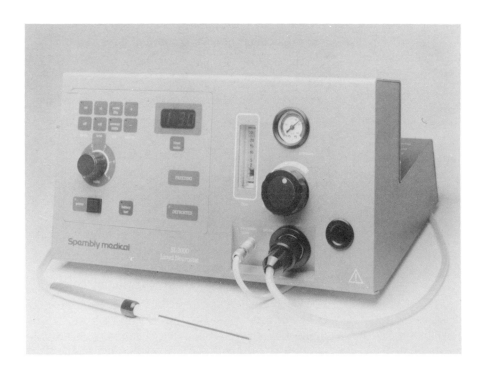

Fig. 70.3 Cryotherapy apparatus. (Courtesy of Spembly Ltd.)

The application of heat

Cautery was used by the ancient Egyptians to coagulate tissue and was favoured also by the Arab school of surgery (Ellis, 1984).

Electrocautery was introduced in 1896 and was used first in 1926 for neurosurgical operations by Harvey Cushing.

In spite of various refinements in surgical diathermy, it was not until 1965 that radiofrequency current was used to produce therapeutic lesions in appropriate areas of the CNS (Mullan et al., 1965).

Nervous tissue is resistant to temperatures up to 42.5 °C. At 42.5–44 °C there is temporary disturbance of function, and above 45 °C there are irreversible changes. This effect is not spread uniformly and the initial lesions at temperatures above 45 °C tend to be confined to the smaller nerve fibres including Aδ- and C-fibres. Consequently, a heat lesion has a central area of total destruction surrounded by a zone that is damaged selectively. If the central temperature is high, the central area of the lesion is large in comparison with the peripheral zone. If the central temperature is low, the extent of the selectively damaged zone is relatively more important.

For any given electrode current, thermal equilibrium is established in approximately 60 sec. Lesion size may be controlled by limiting the current to an exposure of approximately 60 sec or by generating higher currents for periods shorter than 30 sec. The most satisfactory method of controlling the size of lesion is by maintaining a constant electrode tip temperature for a period of 1–2 min. By doing so, time-dependent factors are eliminated as thermal equilibrium is established, and lesion size depends directly on the measured temperature (Fig. 70.4).

The electrode current required to produce a given tip temperature depends on tip diameter and area and on the thermal characteristics of the target site. Consequently, accurate measurement of temperature is the single most important requirement of a lesion generator. This is achieved by building a thermistor or thermocouple into the tip of the electrode. Lesion generators deliver an alternating current with a frequency above 250 kHz to avoid the unpleasant sensory responses which occur at lower frequencies (Alberts et al., 1972). A wide power range and fine output resolution are provided to give accurate temperature control. Variables which may be measured include temperature, current, voltage and impedance. Facilities are inbuilt also for electrical stimulation

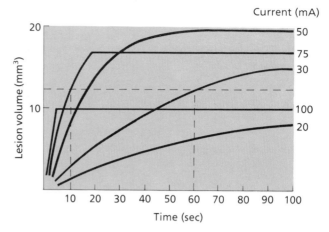

Fig. 70.4 Relationship between lesion size, current and duration of current flow. The horizontal dotted line represents the volume of optimal lesion. The vertical dotted line indicates the time taken to achieve this at varying levels of current. At 75 and 100 mA the tissue boiled; this insulation caused cessation of current flow.

(Fig. 70.5). In general, the technique for producing a lesion in either a peripheral or central structure consists of positioning the insulated cannula in or close to the target area under X-ray control. The electrode is inserted through the cannula and the position of its tip determined finally both radiologically and by electrical stimulation (Fig. 70.6). An increase in tissue electrical impedance may be used also during percutaneous cordotomy to indicate passage of the electrode from cerebrospinal fluid (CSF) into the cord. Because of the need for patient co-operation, such procedures are undertaken using local anaesthesia, neuroleptanalgesia or intermittent general anaesthesia.

The most common side-effects caused by radiofrequency lesions are neuritic pain and hyperaesthesia in the treated dermatome. Fortunately, this tends to resolve spontaneously within 4–5 weeks and needs treatment rarely. Specific side-effects related to the site of lesion are discussed later in this chapter.

The use of surgery

Since the introduction of new therapeutic agents and techniques, particularly radiofrequency lesions, the need for surgical interruption of nerve pathways has diminished greatly. However, there is still occasionally a need for surgical neurectomy, applied usually to peripheral nerves when all other forms of neurolytic manoeuvres have failed to relieve pain. Even in such cases, surgery may fail.

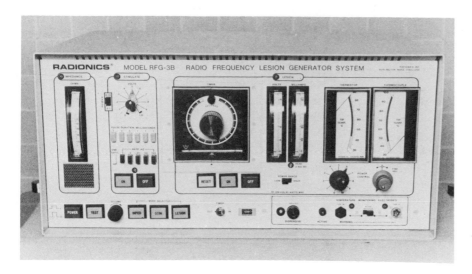

Fig. 70.5 Radiofrequency lesion generator. (Courtesy of Radionics Ltd.)

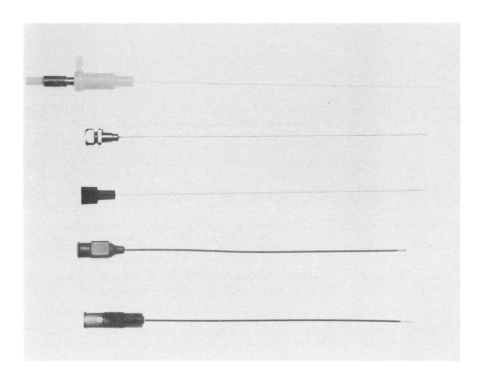

Fig. 70.6 Radiofrequency needle and electrode. Top: electrode. Centre: two stilettes. Bottom: two needles. (Courtesy of Radionics Ltd.)

Common neuroablative techniques (Table 70.1)

Peripheral nerve

The entrapment of a perforating cutaneous nerve in the abdominal wall may occur spontaneously or following previous surgical intervention. In the former case, compression of the nerve takes place in the posterior rectus sheath as a result of scar formation following a small herniation of the fatty plug through which the nerve passes (Applegate, 1972). In such a case, the patient presents with constant or intermittent abdominal pain which may be localized or widespread. Often it radiates into the loin or chest wall along the segmental distribution of the nerve. Diagnosis is made by locating a discrete, tender area, deep in the rectus muscle at its outer border and confirmed by the abolition of pain temporarily following injection of local anaesthetic.

Permanent cure may be obtained by the injection of a neurolytic agent e.g. phenol 5% aqueous solution, 2–3 ml. This may require repeated injections and if

Table 70.1 Possible levels of neuroablation

Peripheral nerve
Receptor containing tissue or end-organ
Nerve trunk
Nerve plexus
In the paravertebral space
Extradurally
Subdurally or within the subarachnoid space

Nerve root
Intra- and extradurally
Dorsal root ganglion

Cord
Ascending tracts
Spinal decussation

Intracranial
Brainstem
Thalamus
Hypothalamus
Pituitary
Sensory cortex
Frontal lobes
Cranial nerves intra- or extracranially

Autonomic system
Sympathetic chain
Parasympathetic outflow

pain persists, cryotherapy or radiofrequency lesions should be instituted. Occasionally, some cases are resistant to these treatments and are referred for surgical exploration and open neurectomy; the rectus muscle is reflected and the nerve sectioned as it passes forward through the posterior rectus sheath.

Surprisingly, a few patients obtain only a short period of relief. Permanent relief may be obtained by the insertion of an extradural catheter behind the rectus muscle and the infusion by pump of aqueous phenol over the course of 48 hr (phenol 7% aqueous, 20 ml in 48 hr).

Intercostal neuralgia may be treated following an initial diagnostic block with local anaesthetic using a neurolytic subcostal block with either phenol 7% aqueous or absolute alcohol or by a direct cryo- or radiofrequency lesion following electrical stimulation to confirm the diagnosis and correct placement of the probe.

Following the use of any of these neurolytic techniques, there may be intermittent pain and hyperaesthesia in the distribution of the lesioned nerve for several days after treatment. This settles invariably without further treatment. Rarely, the neuritis may

persist for several months before settling spontaneously.

Nerve plexus

Apical tumours of the lung (Pancoast tumour) spread occasionally to involve the adjacent brachial plexus with consequent pain in the arm, reduced mobility and lymphoedema.

In many of these patients, the prognosis is poor and pain relief is extremely important. It is essential to explain to the patient that neurolytic techniques result in the loss of both sensation and mobility in the arm and it is important to ensure that the patient understands and consents to this.

Phenol 5% aqueous, 15 ml, may be injected into the brachial plexus, usually by the supraclavicular route. Repeated injections may be required until adequate analgesia is obtained; alternatively, an extradural catheter may be inserted into the plexus to enable multiple injections to be given.

If the tumour involves only the lower cords of the plexus, a percutaneous cervical cordotomy or multiple dorsal root ganglion lesions should be considered (see below).

Other alternatives include the use of neurolytics (either alcohol or phenol) intrathecally or extradurally via a catheter.

Side-effects of the intraplexus neurolytic include failure to relieve pain, with or without motor impairment, and chemical neuritis with increased pain or pain of a different nature—a burning dysaesthesia—that may be unresponsive to oral or parenteral analgesics.

Pneumothorax is a complication of the technique, and the production of a persistent sinus along the track of the needle or catheter may be seen occasionally.

Nerve root

DORSAL ROOT GANGLION LESION

This procedure is used mainly for pain in the distribution of one or possibly two nerve roots on one side of the body. Destruction of the cell bodies of the neurones avoids regeneration and produces analgesia in the distribution of the nerve.

Following a prognostic block using local anaesthesia, a radiofrequency probe is introduced under X-ray control into the appropriate intervertebral foramen. The dorsal root ganglia (DRG) are situated posteriorly in the intervertebral foramina and on an anteroposterior view are at the level of a line joining the articular spaces of the facet joints.

Radio-opaque dye is injected to outline the nerve root (Fig. 70.7) and correct localization checked by electrical stimulation (100 Hz at 1.0 V or less) which causes paraesthesiae in the area affected by the pain or reproduces the pain itself. Local anaesthetic is instilled through the probe and the lesion made (80 °C for 60 sec).

Basically, the technique is similar at all spinal levels (Figs 70.8 and 70.9), but below L5 it may be necessary to make burr holes to obtain access to the ganglia of the sacral roots.

The main side-effect is neuritis which may be severe and require medication with anticonvulsant drugs. If untreated, the condition abates within 6–8 weeks.

POSTERIOR PRIMARY RAMUS

The medial branch of the posterior primary ramus provides the articular branches to the facet joints (Fig. 70.10). These joints may undergo similar degenerative and post-traumatic changes affecting any synovial joint. This results in pain not only in the back in the

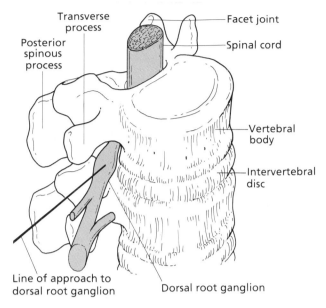

Fig. 70.8 Approach to the DRG.

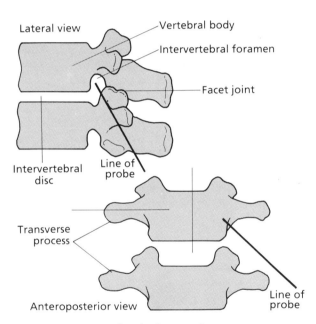

Fig. 70.9 Position of probe for DRG lesion. Diagrammatic representation taken from X-rays.

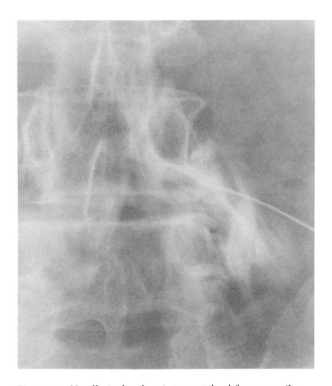

Fig. 70.7 Needle in lumbar intervertebral foramen. Contrast is seen outlining nerve root, dorsal root ganglion (DRG) and flowing into the extradural space.

distribution of the posterior ramus but also in part or all of the distribution of the anterior primary ramus.

Radiofrequency denervation of these joints may be undertaken if local anaesthetic diagnostic block caused temporary pain relief. Under X-ray control, the probe is inserted to a position at the cephalad or caudad (Fig. 70.11) end of the joint in order to lesion the nerve supply to both aspects. Alternatively, the probe is

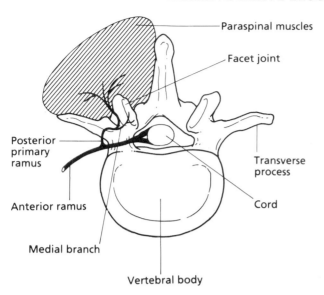

Fig. 70.10 Nerve supply to a lumbar facet joint.

inserted in the groove at the base of the transverse process in which the nerve runs before supplying the joint.

The radiofrequency probe is adjusted to produce a temperature in the range 80–90 °C for 60–160 sec. With the standard probe of 4 mm tip, the longer lesion time at the higher temperature produces a lesion of 5 mm in its longer diameter (Sluijter & Mehta, 1981).

Side-effects are rare; transient back ache is the most common.

EXTRADURAL

The use of extradural neurolytics is restricted usually to those patients who have malignant disease causing pain. The technique has been advocated for patients with severe postherpetic neuralgia but the results do not confirm early optimism for this therapy.

The neurolytic agent may be administered as a single injection using aqueous phenol if spread over several segments is required, or phenol in glycerine if a localized effect is required at one segmental level (Swerdlow, 1974). Catheterization of the extradural space is recommended for repeated injections until optimal results are produced; slow, constant infusion of neurolytic using a syringe-driver may also be useful.

In the lower lumbar or sacral regions, the minimum quantity of neurolytic should be used to obviate spread onto the sacral roots subserving sphincter control to avoid rendering the patient incontinent.

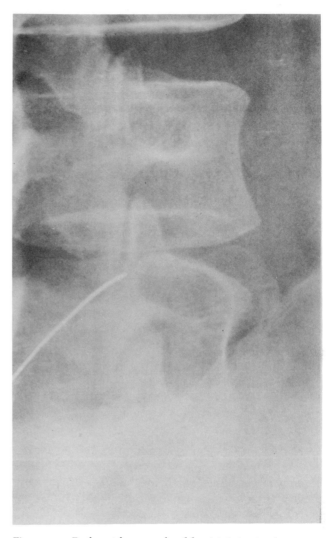

Fig. 70.11 Probe at lower pole of facet joint prior to performing a lesion.

Following resection of rectal cancer, the presacral plexus may have been damaged and urinary sphincter control may be affected readily by small amounts of neurolytic. The most common presentation is with urinary retention which settles usually after a few days.

Other side-effects include painful neuritis, burning dysaesthesia in the affected nerves together with distressing numbness which, in some patients, may be worse than the original pain.

SUBDURAL AND SUBARACHNOID

The extra-arachnoid subdural space has been used as the site of deposition of neurolytic solutions in patients with malignant disease (Maher & Mehta, 1977). The technique described was for use in the cervical spine with phenol 5% in glycerine, but it appears to have no advantages compared with the easier subarachnoid block.

The aim of subarachnoid block is destruction of segmental nerves at the dorsal roots but there may be damage to ventral roots and cord also. The indication for its use is malignant disease where life expectancy is short and pain is severe.

Hyperbaric phenol in glycerine is used if the patient is able to lie with the painful side dependent; if not, hypobaric alcohol is used to float in the CSF.

Following dural puncture, the position of the patient is adjusted with the aid of small amounts of contrast medium injected into CSF. The position of the patient is altered until the correct flow pattern is achieved. The neurolytic is injected, but the patient must remain motionless until the agent fixes to tissues.

The maximum volumes of agents recommended to prevent undue spread (Swerdlow, 1974) are phenol 0.5 ml and alcohol 1.0 ml. It may be necessary to repeat this procedure several times to cover all the segments involved, especially if the pain is bilateral. This technique is more suitable, therefore, for unilateral, sacral or perineal pain caused by malignant disease infiltrating the pelvis or lower lumbar and sacral spine. Lumbar puncture is performed with the patient sitting, and before instillation of hyperbaric neurolytic solution, the patient is tilted backwards to 45° so that the agent runs down the posterior dural wall, investing only the dorsal sensory roots. During this manoeuvre the sacral motor roots are at risk; sphincter disturbances may occur—frequently transient but occasionally permanent. Perineal numbness and paraesthesiae may be unpleasant particularly if unanticipated because of failure to perform a previous local anaesthetic block.

The most common side-effects are related to sensory root damage and include numbness, paraesthesiae and hyperaesthesiae, all of which are usually temporary. Motor paralysis and sphincter disturbances occur rarely, usually with lower lumbar and sacral blocks. Uncommonly, anterior and posterior spinal artery thrombosis may occur causing partial or profound neurological damage. Direct damage to nerve roots by the needle used for the injection may also cause motor and sensory deficit but this persists rarely for more than a few days. Neuritis has been reported following the use of subarachnoid alcohol and headache and neck stiffness have been experienced particularly after cervical neurolytic injections (Swerdlow, 1983).

Cord

PERCUTANEOUS CERVICAL CORDOTOMY

Surgical section of the anterolateral quadrant of the spinal cord was introduced at the beginning of this century. The open method has been superseded almost entirely by the percutaneous cervical radiofrequency heat lesion in the relevant area of the lateral spinothalamic tract (Rosomoff et al., 1965) (Fig. 70.12) to produce analgesia on the contralateral side to the lesion.

There are three approaches to the anterolateral aspect of the cervical cord: laterally through the C1–2 intervertebral space (Rosomoff et al., 1965) (the most common), through a cervical intervertebral disc space (Linn et al., 1966), and a posterior approach between the base of the skull and C1 (Hitchcock, 1969).

Percutaneous cervical cordotomy is suited ideally for patients who have a life expectation not exceeding 2 yr, as the average duration of effect of the technique is 2 yr (Nathan, 1963). It is not a stressful procedure and can be used even in very ill or frail patients. All patients suffering inoperable malignant conditions with pain below the L5 dermatome should be considered for treatment by this method. For those with a normal life expectancy the only patients suitable for cordotomy are the elderly with severe pain in the lower half of the body (Lipton, 1984).

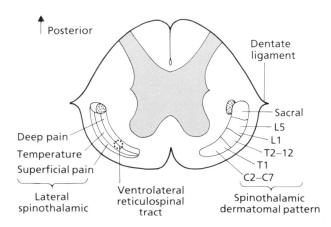

Fig. 70.12 Cross-section of human spinal cord at C2 level.

With the supine patient sedated sufficiently to produce comfort, immobility and ability to respond to questions, the needle (Fig. 70.13) is inserted under X-ray image intensification control through the C1–2 interspace until its tip lies anterior to the dentate ligament (Fig. 70.12). Contrast medium is injected to outline the anterior surface of the cord, the dentate ligament and the posterior dura. A position of the needle 1–2 mm anterior to the dentate ligament and 2–3 mm posterior to the anterior cord surface is ideal. The electrode is inserted through the needle and connected to the impedance meter. When the uninsulated tip of the electrode is in CSF, impedance is low; on entering cord tissue the change in impedance is in the order of 300–1000 ohm. When there is a satisfactory impedance recording, the lesion generator is switched to the stimulus mode. As the voltage is increased, pulsations at 2 Hz are seen in the neck and trapezius muscles on the ipsilateral side. Stimulation at 100 Hz produces sensory hallucinations at approximately one-tenth of the voltage used at 2 Hz stimulation. When all conditions are satisfied i.e. X-ray position, correct impedance measurement and stimulation producing sensations in the painful part of the body, a small test lesion is made using a current of no more than 20 mA for 30 sec. The degree of tract ablation is checked by careful mapping of the hyperaesthetic region on the contralateral body surface. During the passage of current it is essential that corticospinal tract function of the ipsilateral side is evaluated by testing grip strength, etc.

In general, the lesion is produced gradually as a series of bursts of radiofrequency current each no longer than 30 sec until the hypalgesic area corresponds to that in which pain is felt. Once the area of analgesia is achieved, the final power and time of coagulation used are repeated three times with intervals of 1 min to allow heat to dissipate. Horner's syndrome occurs on the ipsilateral side and transitory weakness of the ipsilateral leg develops, returning to normal in a few days.

Decreased or absent thermal sensation occurs also over the whole of the analgesic area and may extend for a few segments beyond.

The main side-effects are motor weakness (40% of these patients have to alter their lifestyle; 2% have permanent weakness), late developing dysaesthesia in the treated area, and occasional disturbance of respiration in patients who have pre-existing respiratory problems, particularly in carcinoma of lung. Impotence, headache, ataxia, hemiparesis and micturition disturbance have been described following cordotomy, but are rare. The frequency of all side-effects and complications is increased dramatically if the cordotomy is bilateral.

Cranial nerves

TRIGEMINAL NERVE

The classical facial pain experienced in the distribution of one or more of the divisions of the trigeminal nerve is trigeminal neuralgia or 'tic douloureux'. The pain is usually transient and described often as 'lancinating'. It is felt mainly in the second and third divisions of the nerve. The pain radiates frequently from one or more trigger points, one of which is often the nasolabial fold. The pain may be induced by touching the trigger area, eating and drinking, talking, and cold winds.

Many patients respond to therapy with anticonvulsant drugs, but destructive therapy of peripheral branches of the nerve or the ganglion may be necessary

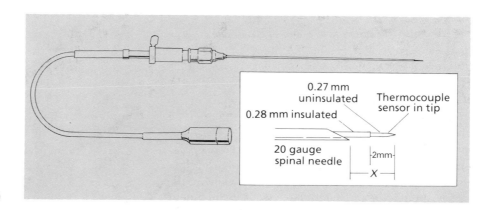

Fig. 70.13 Cordotomy cannula and electrode with details of tip. X = variable electrode extension depending on sizing clamp setting. (Courtesy of Radionics Ltd.)

because of lack of drug efficacy, inability of the patient to tolerate the drug, drug-induced blood dyscrasias and breakthrough pain. If ablative therapy is considered, investigations must be undertaken to exclude defined pathology. These include plain X-rays of the skull including a submentovertical projection and computerized tomography (CT) scan to exclude tumours of the base of skull and some vascular lesions.

If the patient is young, a neurological opinion should be sought to exclude multiple sclerosis or other possible CNS pathologies, particularly if remote neurological signs are evident on routine examination.

Ablative procedures should be considered also if the trigeminal pain results from inoperable malignant disease.

There are two main approaches to the treatment of trigeminal neuralgia: ablative lesions of the peripheral branches or direct approach to the ganglion within the skull. The former may be achieved mainly at the exit foramina of the three divisions of the nerve from the skull using neurolytic chemicals (alcohol, phenol), cryolesions, radiofrequency lesions or surgical neurectomy. These produce not only analgesia in the selected division but also complete anaesthesia which may be extremely distressing.

Lesions of the ganglion may be induced with either glycerine or radiofrequency. The use of glycerine has an advantage that it is a relatively minor procedure giving pain relief in approximately 65% in the long term with only slight disturbance of facial sensation (Hakanson, 1983).

Under X-ray control the trigeminal cistern is punctured percutaneously by the anterior route via the foramen ovale. Following drainage of CSF, a small (0.5 ml) volume of contrast medium (metrizamide) is injected to verify the position of the tip of the needle within the cistern. Glycerine, 0.2–0.3 ml, is injected and the patient maintained in the sitting position for at least 1 hr (Fig. 70.14).

The most common side-effect is headache, occurring almost immediately after the injection of glycerine. This usually resolves rapidly with the use of simple analgesics e.g. paracetamol.

The radiofrequency coagulation technique utilizes the same approach as that for the instillation of glycerine, but is performed usually under general anaesthesia. After insertion through the foramen ovale, the probe (Fig. 70.15) is advanced under or through the ganglion into the sensory roots in the subarachnoid space of the trigeminal cave. The patient is allowed to waken, a 100 Hz stimulating current is

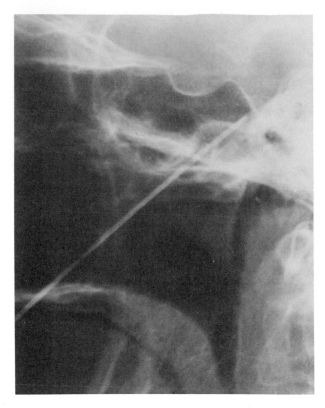

Fig. 70.14 Needle in Gasserian ganglion.

applied to the probe and its position adjusted until the patient experiences paraesthesiae in the area of the face in which the neuralgia is experienced. Brief sleep is induced whilst the first lesion is made (usually 60 sec at 65 °C). The patient is wakened and the face tested with pin prick and cotton wool. The ideal is to produce diminution of sensation in the area over which pain is felt, and further lesions may be made by increasing the temperature of the probe tip to 80 or 90 °C until this is achieved. If pain is experienced mainly in the first division, it may be difficult to angle the probe through the foramen ovale to reach the specific root fibres. To overcome this problem, a side extension tip probe has been developed which, when inserted through the cannula, curves to one side allowing the relevant fibres to be lesioned (Fig. 70.16).

The side-effects of thermocoagulation include numbness in the treated portion of the face and, rarely, keratitis if the first division is treated. Anaesthesia dolorosa may occur also, but the radiofrequency technique is less likely to produce this complication than open surgical rhizotomy or neurolytic injection into the ganglion (Miles, 1980; Rizzi et al., 1985; Schrotter, 1985).

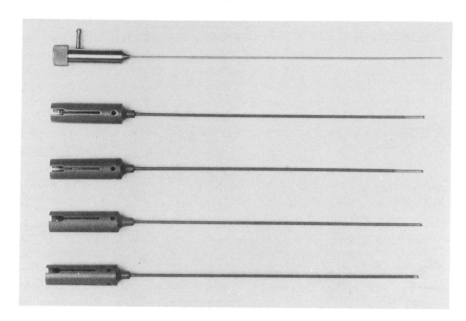

Fig. 70.15 Trigeminal probes with 2 mm, 5 mm, 7 mm and 10 mm uninsulated tips.

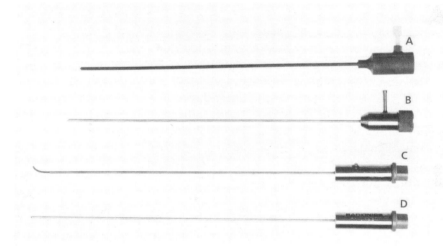

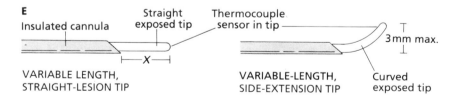

Fig. 70.16 Trigeminal lesion unit with side-extension tip. (A) Cannula (insulated); (B) stilette; (C) variable-length, side-extension tip; (D) variable-length, straight tip; (E) details of (C) and (D).

E
Insulated cannula Straight exposed tip Thermocouple sensor in tip

VARIABLE LENGTH, STRAIGHT-LESION TIP
├─*X*─┤

VARIABLE-LENGTH, SIDE-EXTENSION TIP

3 mm max.

Curved exposed tip

GLOSSOPHARYNGEAL NERVE

Glossopharyngeal neuralgia is an episodic pain of marked intensity, described as hot, burning, sharp or knife-like. Pain is felt in the base of the tongue, larynx, tonsillar region, face, neck or scalp. Constant, dull, aching sensations may persist between attacks which may be triggered by eating, swallowing, chewing or talking (Rushton *et al.*, 1981). A variety of other symptoms may accompany attacks including hiccups, cardiac arrythmias, laryngeal stridor and coughing. Initially, treatment comprises therapy with anticonvulsant drugs, but in unresponsive cases, ablation of the nerve may be produced in the post-tonsillar space.

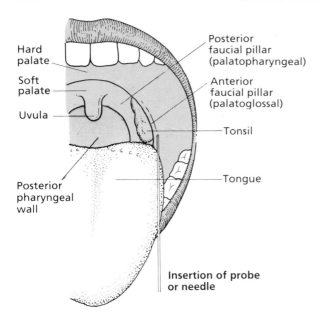

Fig. 70.17 Glossopharyngeal nerve lesion through tonsillar pillar.

Following initial diagnostic block with local anaesthetic, nerve ablation may be carried out using either cryotherapy or radiofrequency coagulation.

The needle or probe is introduced through the anterior pillar or the tonsil on the affected side to a depth of 5 mm, and the lesion made using either two 2-min freeze cycles for a cryolesion or a 90 °C × 80 sec thermal lesion (Fig. 70.17). The procedure is relatively free from side-effects with the exception of occasional transient neuritis and sore throat.

Pituitary ablation

Pituitary ablation has been used to treat patients with pain produced by advanced malignant disease, especially those with bone metastases from breast, prostate and renal tumours unresponsive to drug therapy.

The gland has been subject to destruction by surgery, ionizing radiation, radioactive implants, injection of alcohol and, more recently, by cryo- or radiofrequency lesions.

All techniques produce pain relief in 70% of cases for approximately 3–4 months although some patients have freedom from pain at 1 yr. The exact mechanism of analgesia is unknown, but as pain relief is experienced immediately after the ablative procedure, it is unlikely to be mediated hormonally.

For chemical, thermal or cryodestruction of the pituitary gland, the cannula or probe may be passed through the nose and through the sphenoid bone into the pituitary fossa, under biplanar X-ray control (Moricca, 1977; Duthie, 1983).

The incidence of side-effects and the need for hormone replacement vary according to the operator and technique used. The most dangerous complication is visual blindness which is the main reason for loss of popularity of this technique.

There is a suggestion that pituitary ablation may have a small role in the treatment of pain from non-cancerous sources (Gallimore & Duthie, 1987).

Autonomic system

There is a sound clinical basis for the use of autonomic blockade in the treatment of many specific painful disorders (Table 70.2).

In general terms, ablation should be preceded always by a diagnostic block with local anaesthetic.

Ablative procedures should be performed always with the aid of X-ray image intensification, and the use of contrast medium. Full resuscitation facilities should be available.

The most commonly used ablative agents are alcohol and phenol. The former is more painful on injection and causes significantly more neuritis.

More recently, both cryolesions and radiofrequency lesions have been used, particularly in the lumbar sympathetic chain. The areas in which the sympathetic chain may be ablated are:

Table 70.2 Clinical objectives of sympathetic blockade. (From Boas, 1983)

Sympathetic dystrophy
Diagnostic confirmation
Treatment
Improvement in blood flow
Vasospastic disorders
Acute cold trauma, thromboembolic ischaemia
Postsurgical vasodilatation
Arteriosclerotic disease
Visceral pain
Diagnosis
Long-term treatment
Differential diagnosis
Sympathetic pain or peripheral neuralgia
Somatic or visceral pain
Hyperhydrosis and postherpetic neuralgia
Treatment

Stellate ganglion. This is approached most readily from the front using a paratracheal approach. The sympathetic chain lies on both C6 and C7 transverse processes and can be reached easily using a short 3 cm needle (Boas, 1983).

Upper thoracic chain. This may be approached posteriorly with the patient in the prone position. The levels destroyed most frequently are T2, T3 and T4 (Wilkinson, 1984).

Splanchnic nerve ablation. This provides good analgesia for upper abdominal malignant disease and chronic pancreatitis with an efficacy equal to that of coeliac plexus block but it utilizes less neurolytic solution and produces much less neuritis and hypotension (Fig. 70.18).

Coeliac plexus block. This is the traditional technique for upper abdominal malignant disease (with alcohol or phenol). Large volumes of neurolytic are required and this may be associated with a high incidence of side-effects. The procedure should be performed under general anaesthesia.

Lumbar sympathectomy. This is the standard ablative procedure for the treatment of ischaemic rest pain in the lower limbs, and is used also for pelvic malignancy or causalgia in the perineum. The use of neurolytic solutions is being replaced gradually by thermal lesioning of the sympathetic chain at L2, 3, 4. (Figs 70.19 and 70.20).

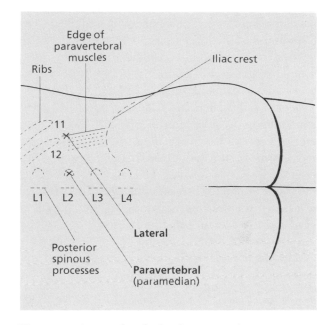

Fig. 70.19 Approaches for lumbar sympathectomy.

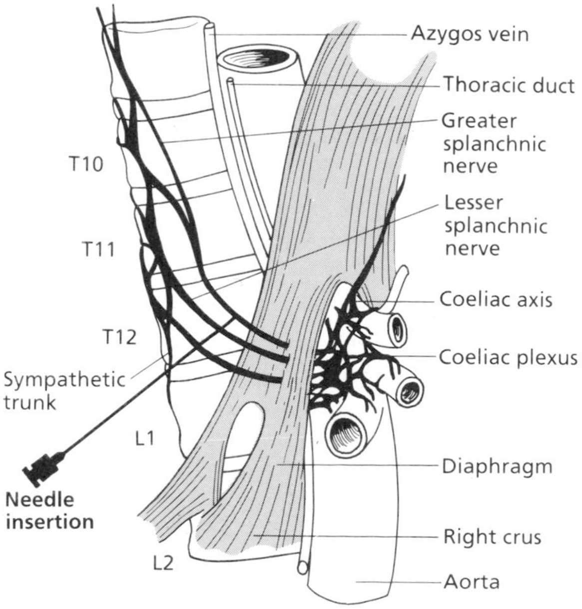

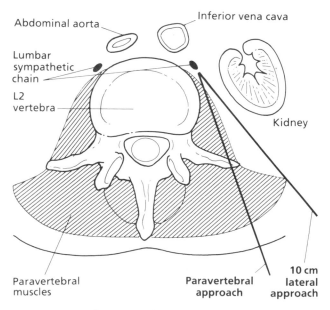

Fig. 70.18 Splanchnic nerve block—anatomy and approach.

Fig. 70.20 Lumbar sympathectomy—anatomy and approaches.

Surgery

Surgery for the relief of pain should be considered only when all other appropriate therapies have been utilized appropriately. The risks of destructive surgery include neurological deficit and incapacity; in time, the pain is likely to return but residual dysfunction may persist. It is possible to attempt further destruction of nervous tissue on a second occasion, but pain recurs usually following a shorter period of remission, and the degree of residual dysfunction may be increased.

These risks are often acceptable in patients in the terminal stages of malignant disease. In those with a normal life expectancy, surgical techniques should be considered only when the relatively non-destructive techniques have failed and the patient has become desperate. Operative intervention may take place at three levels of the pain transmission system (Fig. 70.21).

1 In the region of the first-order neuron. This includes the area of the receptor apparatus of the peripheral nerve and the afferent spinal nerve root.

2 In the region of the second-order neuron. This includes the dorsal horn, spinal decussation, cord and mid-brain up to the synapse in the thalamus.

3 In the region of the third-order neuron. This includes the postsynaptic thalamic regions to the sensory cortex, frontal lobes, limbic system, pituitary and hypothalamus.

In addition to the above neuronal pathways, the autonomic system may be subjected to surgical ablative procedures for the relief of certain chronic painful conditions, hyperhydrosis, etc.

Surgery has a higher success rate for neuronal destruction than other forms of ablation, but it possesses also greater morbidity and mortality. It cannot be performed at many intracranial sites.

First-order neuron

EXCISION OF SKIN

The removal of damaged peripheral sense organs has been practised in such conditions as postherpetic neuralgia and following burns. Re-innervation of the subsequent scarred tissue results frequently in a patchy, dysaesthetic area which is more painful than the original lesion. Because of this poor long-term prospect, the technique is performed rarely.

SECTION OF THE PERIPHERAL NERVE

Peripheral nerves may be exposed and sectioned easily. However, there are few indications for this intervention mainly because of the speed at which regeneration occurs, resulting in restoration of the pain. The commonest indication is when ablation of another modality such as muscle tone is required, and sectioning of the peripheral nerve produces analgesia and loss of tone e.g. multiple sclerosis with painful muscle spasms responds to nerve ablation. Nerve section may be employed also when other forms of neurolysis have failed. Nerve injection, cryotherapy and radiofrequency lesions may not alleviate the pain of abdominal wall nerve entrapment, and section of the segmental nerves as they perforate the posterior rectus sheath produces pain relief. In the debilitated patient who cannot tolerate intracranial surgery for relief of trigeminal neuralgia, section of the appropriate nerve under local anaesthesia as it emerges from the skull e.g. via the supraorbital or infraorbital foramina, is the treatment of choice.

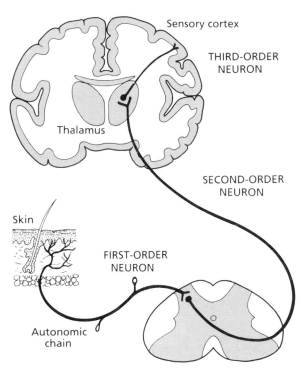

Fig. 70.21 Levels of surgical intervention in the CNS for the relief of pain.

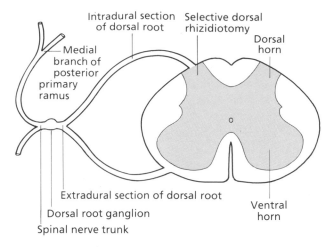

Fig. 70.22 Locations for root surgery.

ROOT SECTION

Surgery on the root may be performed in a number of locations (Fig. 70.22).

Posterior primary ramus

The innervation of the posterior articular facet joints of the spine is by the medial branch of the posterior primary ramus. Attempts to denervate these structures were described first in 1971 by Rees using a long scalpel blade percutaneously to sever the articular branches. This technique has been replaced by the use of either radiofrequency or cryotherapy (Shealy, 1975; Sluijter & Mehta, 1981). Occasionally, during surgery for disc exploration, the nerve supply to degenerate facet joints may be sectioned under direct vision rather than perform a facetectomy.

Spinal nerve root

If a painful dermatome requires denervation, an extra-dural approach is probably the most logical. Thirty percent of afferent sensory fibres enter the spinal cord via the ventral root, even though their cell bodies are in the DRG (Coggeshall *et al.*, 1974).

From a technical aspect, intraspinal approaches are easier and may be undertaken through the standard laminectomy exposure. The surgical approach has been replaced almost entirely by percutaneous radiofrequency lesions which carry fewer side-effects.

Dorsal root ganglionectomy

The DRG may be sectioned or excised following exposure at laminectomy. The dura overlying the ganglion is incised and the ganglion removed, thereby preventing regeneration. The technique suffers from the problems of all sensory root sections; apart from single root-pain syndromes such as chronic disc prolapse, at least two nerve roots above and below the painful segments should be sectioned in addition to the painful segment innervation, as there is considerable sensory overlap. The anaesthesia accompanying division of many roots (especially when involving a limb) makes the operation unattractive.

Extradural root section

The dorsal root may be sectioned proximal to the ganglion through an intraspinal, extradural approach. A hemilaminectomy and facetectomy are performed to expose the relevant root sheath. After identification of the root sheath, it is opened for 5–8 mm just proximal to the ganglion, thereby exposing the dorsal and ventral fibres separated by the dural septum. The ventral roots may be identified by electrical stimulation and the production of muscle contractions. If a 'wake-up' anaesthetic technique is used, stimulation of the dorsal fibres in the awake patient confirms the contribution that the root is making to the pain.

Following accurate identification, the dorsal fibres are cut.

Intradural root section

Intradural roots are conveniently sectioned in the cervical and thoracic segments as the nerve roots exit at levels corresponding to cord level. For intradural section, the correct vertebral level must be ascertained by radiography. After hemilaminectomy, the dura is opened together with the arachnoid and the dorsal rootlets at the correct level identified, sometimes by electrical stimulation in doubtful cases. The relevant rootlets are then divided.

Six adjacent thoracic roots may be sectioned without significant loss of function, but in the cervical and lumbar regions, the number of roots sectioned is governed by the potential loss of limb function.

After the section of a single dorsal root of brachial or lumbar plexus, no proprioceptive deficit and only minimal hypoaesthesia was seen in a series of spinal rhizotomies (White & Kjellberg, 1973). It was recommended also that in the cervical plexus C6 or C7 or else both C5 and C8 should be spared to protect proprioception in the upper limb, and at least one root of L2–4 in cases of extensive lumbosacral rhizotomy. Section of both L5 and S1 may interfere with proprioception in the foot.

Selective dorsal rhizidiotomy

At the junction of each dorsal rootlet with the spinal cord, small afferent fibres tend to cluster in the ventrolateral section of the junction, and they may be divided here by a small incision where they penetrate Lissauer's Tract (Sindov et al., 1974). There are no major limitations to the number and levels of rootlets which may be treated. Identification of rootlets may be made easier particularly in the lumbosacral region by electrical stimulation of the corresponding ventral roots observing for muscle contractions.

Spinal root surgery is useful often for pain associated with tumours of the apex of the lung with involvement of the brachial plexus. Selective rhizidiotomy may be used to prevent total denervation of the arm. It is also the procedure of choice in patients with pelvic malignant disease causing perineal and leg pain as useful afferent function may be preserved.

In general terms, spinal root surgery produces better results in malignant disease than in non-malignant situations, although the long-term results are not good in both groups.

In benign conditions, the most consistent results are obtained with root surgery in occipital neuralgia which may be relieved often permanently by section of the first three cervical dorsal roots.

Postsurgical incisional pain, circumscribed post-traumatic pain and idiopathic intercostal neuralgia may often be managed effectively by either root section or ganglionectomy. Two roots above and below those involved should be sectioned.

Idiopathic coccydynia responds well to bilateral sacrococcygeal root section; the long-term results are good unless there is also pain in the back and/or leg (Albrektsson, 1981).

Conspicuous failures for root surgery include postherpetic neuralgia, postlumbar disc surgery pain and arachnoiditis.

Side-effects of root surgery include failure to achieve adequate analgesia, loss of proprioceptive facility in arms or legs after multiple root sections, loss of sphincter control and impotence after sacral root operations (in addition to the usual complications of open surgery) (Dubuisson, 1984).

After rhizotomy, numbness may be a problem in patients who have not been exposed previously to this by a local anaesthetic block. Genital hypoaesthesiae occur after sacral root surgery and may be made even more distressing if accompanied by impotence or sexual dysfunction.

Severe pain in deafferented dermatomes (anaesthesia dolorosa) may occur following rhizotomy or, more frequently, following ganglionectomy. Transitory paraplegia may follow bleeding into extradural or subarachnoid spaces but irreversible damage to the cord may be produced if this is not diagnosed early or if there is devascularization of the cord–spinal artery syndrome.

Because of the major nature of the surgery and the high failure and complication rate, open surgery to the spinal roots is being replaced almost completely by the use of radiofrequency lesioning of structures.

CRANIAL NERVE SURGERY

Trigeminal nerve

Surgical treatment for trigeminal neuralgia is reserved for patients who fail to respond to anticonvulsant drug therapy or who are unable to tolerate these drugs. There also is a small group of patients whose pain relief following other forms of interventional therapy is transient (radiofrequency lesions, glycerine injections and pressure applied to the Gasserian ganglion by balloon). In such patients, the operation of suboccipital craniectomy with microvascular decompression of the trigeminal nerve is appropriate (Jannetta, 1976). The procedure is performed under general anaesthesia using a small, lateral suboccipital craniectomy and the trigeminal nerve exposed by retracting the cerebellum. Up to 90% of patients have impingement by a small artery or vein upon the nerve, and in 1–3% a tumour or bony abnormality is found. Approximately 5–10% have no apparent pathology. Any tumour is removed and a vessel is eased from the nerve and kept separate by the insertion of a piece of sponge or muscle.

In the group of patients without pathology, a subtotal rhizotomy is performed on the main sensory root preserving some touch sensation over the face and the corneal reflex. The small fibres carrying touch and corneal sensation diverge from the main sensory root just before its entry into the pons and are identified at this point. Following rhizotomy, long-term success rate is 80%, morbidity 5–10% and mortality 1–2% (Loeser, 1984). Peripheral nerve avulsions should be offered only when gangliolysis has failed and the patient cannot or will not tolerate the intracranial procedure. They result in dense sensory loss and provide pain relief for only 1–2 yr. Repeated avulsions are even less likely to be successful.

Patients who have failed to obtain relief from any of these techniques may be offered descending trigeminal tractotomy. This is performed through a C1–2 laminectomy and results in loss of pain and temperature sensation on the ipsilateral side of the face but does not alter touch perception.

Geniculate neuralgia

Geniculate neuralgia has characteristic paroxysms of pain felt deep within the ear. This may be relieved by severing the fibres of the nervus intermedius through a posterior fossa approach (Sachs, 1968).

Glossopharyngeal neuralgia

Glossopharyngeal neuralgia is a severe tic-like pain experienced in the tonsillar region and back of the tongue or larynx. It is induced by swallowing or talking. On rare occasions, the pain may be associated with syncopal attacks, presumably because of involvement of branches from the carotid sinus.

This condition responds frequently to anticonvulsant drug therapy. Resistant cases may be treated surgically by severing the ninth nerve in the neck near the styloid process. The best results are obtained using a posterior fossa exposure and section of the glossopharyngeal rootlets intracranially after separation of these from the vagus.

Autonomic faciocephalgia

Autonomic faciocephalgia (or, as it is more commonly termed, sphenopalatine neuralgia) is a diffuse pain experienced often in the upper half of the face and associated with unilateral lacrimation and nasal discharge. Many cases respond to ergotamine preparations (as does migraine) but intractable cases may be treated by trigeminal nerve section or section of the petrosal nerves through an extradural temporal approach (Gardner *et al.*, 1947). Section of the nervus intermedius may be more effective (Sachs, 1968).

Second-order neuron

ANTEROLATERAL CORDOTOMY

The cord is exposed by laminectomy at either the upper thoracic level for lower trunk and leg pain or in the upper cervical segment for pain extending up to the fifth cervical dermatome.

Access to the contralateral anterolateral quadrant is obtained by gripping and dividing a digitation of the dentate ligament and using it to rotate the cord. The anterolateral tract is cut between two consecutive roots. In this quadrant, the spinothalamic tract exhibits some somatotopic stratification with lower sacral and coccygeal dermatomes being represented superficially and posteriorly whilst higher dermatomes are represented more deeply (Fig. 70.23).

The analgesia produced is always temporary and lasts for a maximum of 2 yr. Consequently, anterolateral cordotomy is reserved usually for patients with a life expectancy limited by malignant disease.

Repeated cordotomy is associated with progressively reduced analgesia both in level and duration. There is an increase also in the risk of neurological morbidity.

Even in the best series, ipsilateral hemiparesis occurs in approximately 15%, postoperative dysaesthesia in 5% and disturbance of sphincter control and sexual function in 5% of patients. These disturbances increase to approximately 20% if bilateral cordotomy is performed; in addition this carries the risk of damage to respiratory function and the possible emergence of 'Ondine's syndrome'.

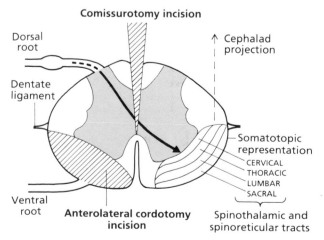

Fig. 70.23 Direct surgical approaches to the cord in the cervical and upper thoracic regions.

The introduction of the percutaneous radiofrequency procedure has replaced the surgical method almost totally.

Spinal commisurotomy is the division of the spinothalamic fibres as they cross the midline of the cord prior to their ascent in the anterolateral tract (Fig. 70.23).

As the fibres cross only gradually, often taking several segments, it may be difficult to determine the length of incision required to produce adequate analgesia. Consequently, a long, multiple laminectomy must be performed. This may explain why the duration of effect does not equate with that following cordotomy (King, 1977).

BRAINSTEM TRACTOTOMIES

These are major operations designed to section the spinothalamic tract at various locations in the midbrain to obtain analgesia without the additional anaesthesia seen with other destructive procedures. Medullary spinothalamic tractotomy involves exposing the medulla between the superior roots of the accessory nerve and the inferior olive at which point the tract is deep to the spinocerebellar tract. Trigeminal tractotomy is designed to divide the descending spinothalamic tract of the trigeminal nerve in the medulla. The operation is a posterior fossa exploration with division of the tract which is within the medullary substance lateral to the line of the cuneate nucleus and behind the line of exit of the spinal accessory nerve rootlets.

Brainstem tractotomy is designed to section the spinothalamic tract in the dorsolateral tegmentum between the superior and inferior colliculi. Morbidity is high with many persistent side-effects including dysaesthesia and diplopia. These operative procedures are rarely performed because of the high morbidity and failure rates.

Third-order neuron

The use of surgery in the region of the third-order neuron is confined almost entirely to the thalamus where stereotactically controlled heat lesions, radiofrequency lesions or cryolesions are induced.

At least part of the spinothalamic tract ends in the region of the ventral posterolateral nucleus of the thalamus and lesions of this locus do not produce analgesia but rather sensory deficits. Indirect pain pathways via the reticular formation connect with the more medial areas of the thalamus and lesions in the centremedian, parafascicularis and intralaminar areas tend to relieve pain without producing sensory deficit. Lesions in the more posterior parts such as the pulvinar, produce analgesia also without sensory deficit but often produce hemiparesis.

Spiegel has summarized the value of thalamic lesions (Spiegel & Wycis, 1966):
1 Pain may be relieved by lesions in either the medial or the lateral pain-conducting systems.
2 Improved results occur by attacking both systems.
3 Successful procedures should produce analgesia for more than 5 yr.
4 If long-lasting analgesia is required, these procedures should be undertaken only as a last resort in view of extensive lesions.

There remain three types of surgery on the third neuron for which certain claims have been made but which are used rarely.

Leucotomy

Frontal leucotomy consists of the interruption of the frontothalamic pathways in the basomedial frontal lobe. The greater the degree of interruption, the greater is the likelihood of pain relief but, at the same time, the greater the modification of affect. This latter effect has rendered the procedure of debatable value and ethically dubious.

Hypothalamotomy

The hypothalamus has numerous direct connections with the thalamus and direct and indirect connections with many parts of the sensory system. Stereotaxic lesions in the posterior medial hypothalamus have been claimed (Sano, 1973) to produce good results in painful malignancy. Ipsilateral lesions were found to be effective in head and neck pain whilst contralateral lesions appeared better for pain relief below that level.

Cortical ablation

Cortical ablation of the parietal sensory cortex followed reports of analgesia being associated with pathological lesions of this area. Long-term results have not been encouraging but Lebal (1973) claims the technique is useful when applied to the frontal cortex.

Surgery to the autonomic system

Surgery of the autonomic system is confined mainly to situations where repeated percutaneous attempts at neurolysis by chemical, cryo- or radiofrequency lesion have failed to produce lasting analgesia.

References

Alberts W.W., Wright E.W., Feinstein B. & Gleason C.A. (1972) Sensory responses elicited by subcortical high frequency electrical stimulation in man. *Journal of Neurosurgery* **36**, 80–2.

Albrektsson B. (1981) Sacral rhizotomy in cases of anococcygeal pain. *Acta Orthopaedica Scandinavica* **52**, 187–90.

Applegate W.V. (1972) Abdominal cutaneous nerve entrapment syndrome. *Surgery* **71**, 118–24.

Armstrong-Davison M.H. (1965) Refridgeration anaesthesia. In *The Evolution of Anaesthesia* pp. 162–70. Sherratt, London.

Barber R. (1971) Sclerosant therapy. In *Textbook of Orthopaedic Medicine*, vol. 2, 8th edn. (Ed. Cyriax J.) p. 286. Cassell, London.

Barnard J.D.W. (1980) The effect of extreme cold on sensory nerves. *Annals of the Royal College of Surgeons of England* **62**, 180–7.

Boas R.A. (1983) The sympathetic nervous system and pain relief. In *Relief of Intractable Pain* (Ed. Swerdlow M.) pp. 215–38. Elsevier, Amsterdam.

Brown A.S. (1981) Current views on the use of nerve blocking in the relief of chronic pain. In *The Therapy of Pain* (Ed. Swerdlow M.) pp. 111–34. MTP Press Ltd., Lancaster.

Bryce-Smith R. (1966) Local and regional analgesia. *Postgraduate Medical Journal* **42**, 367.

Budd K. (1981) Non-analgesic drugs in pain management. In *Persistent Pain*, vol. 3 (Eds Lipton S. & Miles J.) pp. 223–40. Academic Press, London.

Carter D.C., Lee P.W.R., Gill W. & Johnson R.J. (1972) The effect of cryosurgery on peripheral nerve function. *Journal of the Royal College of Surgeons of Edinburgh* **17**, 25–31.

Coggeshall R.E., Applebaum M.L., Fazan M., Stubes T.B. & Sykes M.T. (1974) Unmyelinated axon in human ventral roots, a possible explanation for the failure of dorsal rhizotomy to relieve pain. *Brain* **98**, 157–61.

Dam W.H. (1965) Therapeutic blocks. *Acta Chirurgica Scandinavica* **343S**, 89.

Dam W.H. & Larsen J.V.V. (1974) Peripheral nerve blocks in the relief of intractable pain. In *Relief of Intractable Pain* (Ed. Swerdlow M.) p. 133. Excerpta Medica, Amsterdam.

Dubuisson D. (1984) Root surgery. In *Textbook of Pain* (Eds Wall P.D. & Melzack R.) pp. 590–600. Churchill Livingstone, London.

Duthie A.M. (1983) Pituitary cryoablation. *Anaesthesia* **38**, 495–7.

Editorial (1964) *Lancet* **2**, 896.

Ellis H. (1984) *Famous Operations*. Harwal, Pennsylvania.

Esplin D.W. (1970) Antiseptics and disinfectants; fungicides; ectoparasiides. In *The Pharmacological Basis of Therapeutics* 4th edn. (Eds Goodman L.S. & Gilman A.) p. 1036. Macmillan, London.

Gallimore A.P. & Duthie A.M. (1987) Pituitary cryotherapy; its use in the treatment of chronic non-malignant pain. *The Pain Clinic* **1**, 259–60.

Gardner W.J., Stowell A. & Dutlinger R. (1947) Petrosal nerve section for facial pain. *Journal of Neurosurgery* **4**, 105.

Hakanson S. (1981) Trigeminal neuralgia treated by injection of glycerol into the trigeminal cistern. *Neurosurgery* **9**, 638.

Hakanson S. (1983) Retrogasserian glycerol as a treatment of tic douloureuy. In *Advances in Pain Research and Therapy*. vol. 5. (Ed. Bonica J.J. *et al.*). New York, Raven Press.

Hitchcock E.R. (1969) An apparatus for stereotactic spinal surgery. *Lancet* **1**, 705.

Hitchcock E.R. & Pradinin M.N. (1973) Hypertonic saline in the management of intractable pain. *Lancet* **1**, 310.

Jannetta P.J. (1976) Microsurgical approach to the trigeminal nerve for tic douloureux. *Progress in Neurological Surgery* **7**, 180–200.

Jones M.J.T. & Murrin K.R. (1987) Intercostal block with cryotherapy. *Annals of the Royal College of Surgeons of England* **69**, 261–2.

Katz J., Nelson W., Forest R. & Bruce D.L. (1980) Cryoanalgesia for post thoracotomy pain. *Lancet* **2**, 512–13.

Khalili A.A. & Ditzler J.W. (1968) Neurolytic substances in the relief of pain. *Medical Clinics of North America* **52**, 161.

King R.B. (1977) Anterior commissurotomy for intractable pain. *Journal of Neurosurgery* **47**, 7–12.

Lebal J. (1973) Limited frontal lesions, open and stereotactic. *Symposium sur la Doleur*. pp. 24–5. Paris.

Linn P.M., Gildenberg P.L. & Polakoff P.P. (1966) An anterior approach to percutaneous lower cervical cordotomy. *Journal of Neurosurgery* **25**, 553–60.

Lipton S. (1984) Percutaneous cordotomy. In *Textbook of Pain* (Eds Wall P.D. & Melzack R.) pp. 632–8. Churchill Livingstone, Edinburgh.

Lloyd J.W., Barber J.D.W. & Glynn C.J. (1976) Cryoanalgesia; a new approach for pain relief. *Lancet* **2**, 932.

Loeser J. (1984) Face pain. In *Textbook of Pain* (Eds Wall P.D. & Melzack R.) pp. 426–34. Churchill Livingstone, Edinburgh.

Maiwant O. & Make A.R. (1981) Cryoanalgesia for relief of pain after thoracotomy. *British Medical Journal* **282**, 1749–50.

Maher R.M. (1957) Neurone selection in relief of pain; further experiences with intrathecal injections *Lancet* **i**, 16.

Maher R.M. (1963) Intrathecal chlorocresol in the treatment of pain in cancer. *Lancet* **1**, 965.

Maher R.M. (1969) Some aspects of the management of cancer pain. *Update* **1**, 751.

Maher R.M. & Mehta M. (1977) Spinal (intrathecal) and extradural analgesia. In *Persistent Pain*, vol. 1 (Ed. Lipton S.) pp. 61–99. Academic Press, London.

Mehta M. (1973) Pharmacology of neurolytic agents. In *Intractable Pain* p. 55. W.B. Saunders, London.

Miles J. (1980) Trigeminal neuralgia. In *Persistent Pain*, vol. 2. (Ed. Lipton S.) pp. 203–22. Academic Press, London.

Moricca G. (1977) Pituitary neuroadenolysis in the treatment of intractable pain from cancer. In *Persistent Pain*, vol. 1 (Ed. Lipton S.) pp. 149–73. Academic Press, London.

Mullan S., Hekmapatnah J., Dobson G. & Beckman F. (1965) Percutaneous intramedullary cordotomy utilising the unipolar anodal electrolytic lesion. *Journal of Neurosurgery* **22**, 531–8.

Nathan P.W. (1963) Results of anterolateral cordotomy for pain in cancer. *Journal of Neurology, Neurosurgery and Psychiatry* **26**, 353–62.

Nathan P.W. & Scott P.G. (1958) Intrathecal phenol for intractable pain; safety and dangers of the method. *Lancet* **1**, 76.

Nathan P.W. & Sears T.A. (1960) Effects of phenol on nerve conduction. *Journal of Physiology* **150**, 565.

Orr I.A., Keenan D.J., Dundee J.W., Patterson C.C. & Greenfield A.A. (1983) Post thoracotomy pain relief: combined use of cryoprobe and morphine infusion technique. *Annals of the Royal College of Surgeons of England* **65**, 366–9.

Pitres A. & Vaillard L. (1888) Des nevrites provoques par le contact de l' alcool pur ou dilue avec les nerfs vivant. *C.R. Societee Biologique* **5**, 550.

Pizzolato P. & Mannheimer W.H. (1961) *Histopathologic Effects of Local Anaesthetic Drugs*. Thomas, Illinois.

Rees W.E.S. (1971) Multiple bilateral subcutaneous rhizolysis of segmental nerves in the treatment of the intervertebral disc syndrome. *Annals of General Practice* **26**, 126–7.

Rizzi R., Terrvoli A. & Visentin M. (1985) Long term use of alcoholization and thermocoagulation of the trigeminal nerve for cancer pain. *The Pain Clinic* **1**, 223–33.

Rosomoff H.L., Carroll F., Brow J. & Sheptak P. (1965) Percutaneous radiofrequency cervical cordotomy technique. *Journal of Neurosurgery* **23**, 639–44.

Rushton J.G., Stevens T.C. & Millar R.H. (1981) Glossopharyngeal (vagoglossophryngeal) neuralgia. *Archives of Neurology* **38**, 201–5.

Sachs E. (1968) Posterior fossa approach to nervus intermedius section. *Journal of Neurosurgery* **28**, 54.

Sano K. (1973) Thalamotomy and hypothalamotomy. *Symposium de la doleur*. pp. 24–5. Paris.

Schrotter O. (1985) Results of thermocoagulation in trigeminal neuralgia. Comparison of preoperative treatment with carbamazepine alone versus additional denervation procedures. *The Pain Clinic* **1**, 233–9.

Shealy C.N. (1975) Percutaneous radiofrequency denervation of spinal facets. *Journal of Neurosurgery* **43**, 448–51.

Sindov M., Fischer G., Goutelle A. & Mansuy L. (1974) La radicellotomie posterieurre selective. Premiers resultata dans la chirurgie de la doleur. *Neurochirurgie* **20**, 391–408.

Sluijter M.E. & Mehta M. (1981) Treatment of chronic back and neck pain by percutaneous thermal lesions. In *Persistent Pain*, vol. 3 (Eds Lipton S. & Miles J.) pp. 141–79. Academic Press, London.

Spiegel E.A. & Wycis H.T. (1966) Present status of sterioencephalotomies for the relief of pain. *Confinia Neurologica* **27**, 7–17.

Swerdlow M. (1974) Intrathecal and extradural block in pain relief. In *Relief of Intractable Pain* (Ed. Swerdlow M.) pp. 148–75. Excerpta Medica, Amsterdam.

Swerdlow M. (1983) Intrathecal and extradural block for pain relief. In *Relief of Intractable Pain* (Ed. Swerdlow M.) pp. 175–214. Elsevier, Amsterdam.

White J.C. & Kjellberg R.W. (1973) Posterior spinal rhizotomy; a substitute for cordotomy in the relief of localized pain in patients with normal life expectancy. *Neurochirurgica* **16**, 141–70.

Wilkinson H.A. (1984) Radiofrequency percutaneous upper thoracic sympathectomy. *New England Journal of Medicine* **311**, 34–6.

SECTION V
INTENSIVE CARE

71

Principles of Intensive Care

A. R. AITKENHEAD

Intensive care is the term used to describe the greatest available level of continuing patient management. In addition to nursing care, observation and monitoring, this usually involves active treatment; thus, in some centres the term intensive therapy is used. The intensive therapy unit (ITU) is an area where facilities are concentrated for treatment of the critically ill patient and exceed those available in an ordinary ward. Some hospitals contain a high-dependency unit (HDU), which is an area of care intermediate between that available in a general ward and the high level in an ITU. In addition, some theatre recovery wards provide a standard of care for postoperative patients similar to that provided in an HDU. In some centres, a number of separate ITUs exist for specialized fields of medicine e.g. cardiothoracic surgery, neurosurgery, paediatrics, transplant surgery. However, in the majority of hospitals in the UK, one general ITU deals with critically ill patients of many types.

This chapter discusses administration, patient monitoring, infection and methods of sedation in relation to the general ITU, although many aspects are applicable also to more specialized units.

Administration

Intensive therapy unit design

LOCATION AND SIZE

The siting of an ITU is determined by both building and clinical considerations. The Department of Health and Social Security (DHSS) guidelines (1970) suggest that the ITU should be situated near the operating theatres in order to share engineering services. This is also convenient clinically, as many patients are admitted directly from the operating theatre. However, the unit should be readily accessible also to other areas from which admissions are common, especially the accident and emergency department, medical and surgical wards, and the theatre recovery area. It is also preferable if the ITU is situated close to laboratories and imaging departments so that appropriate investigations may be performed with the minimum of delay.

It is recommended that 1–2 % of the total number of acute beds in a hospital should be allocated to the general ITU, in addition to regional or subregional specialized units for cardiothoracic, neurosurgical and burns patients. Small units (less than four beds) may not be viable, and large units (more than 10 beds) are difficult to manage (Ledingham, 1977). If more beds are required, it may be desirable to divide the unit into more specialized areas (e.g. paediatric, neurological), although it is useful to group these units close to each other in order to share medical, technical, laboratory and engineering services. Normally, it is best to keep the ITU separate from the coronary care unit, although in smaller hospitals it may be necessary to combine them in order to make efficient use of available resources.

ACCOMMODATION (Intensive Care Society, 1984)

The patient area should consist of a large open ward containing four to 10 beds, with at least one side room. Side rooms make efficient nursing difficult, but are essential for patients who require isolation. A floor area of at least 20 metre² is recommended for each bed in the open patient area in order to accommodate the bed, essential equipment and storage cupboards; a floor area of 30 metre² is required in each side room. Ideally, each single room should be equipped with reversible ventilation, to minimize cross-infection. Facilities for renal dialysis should be available in one side room.

In addition to the area available for patient care, space should be allocated for storage, offices and other facilities (Table 71.1).

A management base is required within or immediately adjacent to the patient area. This should be positioned so that all patients are visible. It should house telephones, an intercom connecting it with the offices and rest room, a central monitoring station and computer terminal. Drug cupboards and refrigerator, blood refrigerator, emergency trolley and defibrillator should be within easy reach.

The entire area should be ventilated with air filtered to extract particles larger than 5 μm. Because of the heat generated by equipment, air conditioning should be provided, and temperature and humidity should be adjustable. Windows should be provided in the patient area and in the staff rest area, as lack of natural daylight has adverse psychological effects on both patients and staff (Wilson, 1972). The type of artificial light should be appropriate for ready recognition of cyanosis.

SERVICES

Each bed station should be equipped with wall outlets for vacuum, oxygen and medical air; nitrous oxide or Entonox (50% nitrous oxide/50% oxygen) may be desirable also. The recommended supply pressures and minimum flow rates are shown in Table 71.2. At least two vacuum outlets should be provided in order to accommodate the potential need for low-pressure continuous drainage and high-pressure intermittent suction e.g. for tracheal aspiration. There should be at least three outlets for both oxygen and medical air in order to power ventilators and to supply both flowmeters and gas-mixing devices. Only one nitrous oxide or Entonox outlet is required per bed, but each must be accompanied by an active scavenging point for waste gas.

Table 71.1 Space allocation for intensive therapy unit facilities

Purpose	Floor area	Notes
Storage for consumables	> 30 metre²	Should include shelves, cupboards, drawers
Storage for equipment	> 30 metre²	Should include shelves, cupboards, drawers, bins
Storage for linen	> 10 metre²	
Dirty utility sluice		
Nurses' office	> 15 metre²	Telephone, intercom, notice boards
Medical office	> 15 metre²	Telephone, intercom
Staff restroom		Telephone, intercom, facilities for beverages
Staff changing rooms		Lockable lockers, showers, toilets
Doctor's bedroom	> 15 metre²	Bed, wash basin, shower, toilet, wardrobe, telephone, intercom
Laboratory	> 15 metre²	Power points, sink, specimen fridge
Workshop	> 10 metre²	Bench, compressed gas outlets, power points, sink
Relatives' rooms		At least two waiting areas, one suitable for interviews
Kitchen		
Reception area		
Cleaners' room	> 4 metre²	
Procedures room		All facilities, screened walls if image intensifier to be used
Seminar room	> 30 metre²	Projection facilities
Computer room/technician's office	> 10 metre²	Bench, electrical sockets
Receptionist's office	> 15 metre²	Filing cabinets, typewriter

Table 71.2 Recommended supply pressures and flow rates for piped medical gases and vacuum

Facility	Pressure (kPa)	Pressure should be maintained when all outlets are being used at a flow rate of (litre/min)
Oxygen	414	20
Air	414	20
Nitrous oxide, (Entonox)	414	10
Vacuum	−67	40

A spotlight or Anglepoise lamp and at least 16 electric sockets are required at each bed station. In order to minimize electrical accidents, all electrical outlets in the patient area should be on the same phase and should have a common ground earth. All electrical power to the patient area should be supplied by a standby power source which should be tested monthly. The delay between mains failure and restoration of supply from the standby generator should be no more than 5 sec. Emergency lighting and electrical sockets for ventilators, computers and other equipment sensitive to power failure should be protected by a battery power source which restores power immediately if the mains voltage fails; these emergency sockets must be marked clearly.

A television aerial socket and radio outlet should be provided at each bed. Many patients in the ITU are alert mentally but immobile.

One hand-wash basin should be available for each bed to minimize cross-infection; heated water traps are recommended to sterilize water in the effluent pipe.

BED LAYOUT

Much of the equipment required is located at the head of the bed, and this can create problems of access. The traditional bed position is with the head of the bed located in close proximity to the wall. Equipment is mounted on or close to the wall so that electrical and gas supplies can be obtained from wall sockets or outlets. However, there are several disadvantages associated with this arrangement. In modern hospitals, the wall may have to be reinforced before heavy equipment e.g. physiological monitors, can be supported. The attendants must walk around the foot of the bed in order to move from one side of the patient to the other, and there is a tendency for the nurse to make observations and recordings from the foot of the bed thereby reducing verbal and visual contact with the patient. In addition, access to the head of the bed e.g. for resuscitation, insertion of venous catheters or tracheal intubation, requires the bed to be moved away from the wall.

An alternative layout employed in some units offers significant advantages in terms of access, but is more expensive and requires a larger floor area. The bed is situated with the head approximately 1 metre from the wall, allowing free access to the patient's head (Kerr et al., 1985). All services are supplied from the wall along a boom, or run under the floor to a 'bollard' situated at the side of the bed; a similar arrangement, which permits even greater access than the 'bollard', can be achieved using a 'stalactite' structure attached to the ceiling, although plugs and sockets may be beyond the reach of smaller members of staff. Access for all nursing and medical procedures is improved, and the nurse may observe the patient from a position close to the head, improving communication and contact. In addition, a work surface and storage area can be situated behind the bed.

Storage space is essential at each bedside. Shelves are required for syringes, needles, suction catheters, disposal bins, etc., and cupboards or drawers may be used to store linen, sterile packs for eye and mouth care and other items of equipment which are in frequent use. If these items are readily available, the nurse has to leave the patient less frequently.

A degree of privacy is necessary, and some form of screening must be provided during bedbaths and other intimate nursing procedures.

Charts for recording the patient's observations and results of laboratory investigations should be easily accessible to the nurse and visiting medical staff, but not visible to the patient.

Staffing

NURSING STAFF

Nurses are the most important staff in the ITU. Although it is appropriate for student nurses to receive some training in intensive care nursing, they should attend only in a supernumerary capacity.

The number of trained nurses on the establishment depends on several factors (Intensive Care Society, 1984).

Dependency categories

The most seriously ill patients e.g. those with multiple organ failure or multiple injuries, may require more than one nurse. All patients requiring mechanical ventilation, those with an insecure airway or those receiving continuous drug infusions, should have one nurse in attendance at all times. Patients who are 'recuperating' from more serious illness, or those admitted for routine monitoring, parenteral nutrition or correction of fluid and electrolyte imbalance, require less nursing care, and one nurse may be able to care for two patients simultaneously. The pattern of admissions varies from unit to unit, and calculation of an average 'dependency score' (average number of nurses required for each patient) for an individual unit is based on careful record keeping.

Occupancy

It is clearly impractical to calculate the number of nursing staff on the basis of maximum bed occupancy. The demand varies for general ITU beds, and at times of low bed occupancy, nurses are underoccupied, and may be assigned to other parts of the hospital. This is generally poor for morale. The calculation must therefore take account of the average bed occupancy in conjunction with the average 'dependency score' of each occupied bed. A calculation based on these average values results in a sufficient number of nurses to cope with demand for 50% of the time. In order to meet demand for 95% of predicted needs, the calculation should be based on values of mean + 2 standard deviations.

Effective working time

Allowances must be made for the limited hours worked by nurses (currently 37.5 hr per week in the UK), and for annual and study leave, and predicted sickness leave.

Support nurses

If each nurse at the bedside is to stay with the patient, additional nurses are required to undertake administration, teaching, relief for meal breaks, to collect drugs and equipment from stores and to assist with lifting and turning. One additional nurse is required normally on each shift for three nurses at the bedside.

For an average general ITU, with a 'dependency weighted occupancy (DWO)' (average dependency score × average bed occupancy) of 50–75%, the total number of nurses required to ensure that bedside demand is met on 95% of occasions is:

$$\text{Total beds} \times (\text{mean DWO} + 2\text{SD}) \times 5.5.$$

To allow for support nurses, this value should be multiplied by 1.33.

The nursing establishment should include no less than one sister per bed to ensure that at least one is available to work each day.

OTHER STAFF

Auxiliary nurses may be employed to assist trained staff in lifting, changing linen, and running errands. A ward clerk/receptionist is invaluable, and cleaning staff are required.

In addition, other categories of staff should be available as required. There should be permanent cover by technical staff, who are responsible for maintenance and cleaning of equipment, and a technician, or a member of laboratory staff, to ensure quality control of on-site biochemical analyses. Physiotherapy is required for all patients in the ITU, and this should be provided by those experienced in this type of work. A dietician and radiographer must also be on call at all times, and it is helpful if a pharmacist with knowledge of the special requirements of an ITU is available. Additional staff may be called upon for electrocardiography, ultrasound imaging, electroencephalography, etc.

MEDICAL STAFF

Consultant staff

Consultant medical staff with responsibility for the ITU require a combination of enthusiasm, medical knowledge, technical expertise and diplomatic skill. The consultant's parent specialty is relatively unimportant, provided that he or she has sufficient experience and training. Most ITU consultants in the UK are anaesthetists, probably because of flexibility of sessional commitments, experience in ventilation and cardiovascular monitoring techniques and the fact that anaesthesia is the only specialty which provides currently ITU training for all junior staff. Critically ill patients develop frequently a pattern of progressive organ failure, irrespective of the initial pathology. Treatment therefore involves management of multi-system failure, and consequently an important role of the ITU consultant is to co-ordinate treatment by identifying each patient's requirements and to call upon the services of appropriate specialists for advice.

A consultant experienced in ITU should be on call for the unit at all times. In many units, between three and five consultants share responsibility; a larger number dilutes the experience gained, whilst a smaller number results in an unacceptable on-call commitment, particularly during holiday absences. One consultant should be in administrative charge. It is important that a working relationship is established with referring consultants. In some centres, the latter retain 'control' over patients admitted to the unit, although they may visit the patient only once or twice each week. This is unsatisfactory as it results in time wasted in contacting the consultant and causes confusion among the nurses. Whilst the referring team must be consulted on major policy decisions, diagnosis and management, it is more efficient if the ITU consultant is able to undertake the general management of the patient, and to deal immediately with sudden changes in the patient's condition without recourse to the referring consultant. In general, this policy becomes acceptable to most consultants from other specialties after confidence has been gained in the management of patients by the ITU team.

Junior staff

Junior medical staff should be responsible only for the ITU and should be resident on the unit. They may be drawn from any specialty, but previous experience in maintenance of the airway and in resuscitation is desirable. In many units, the ITU resident post is part of the anaesthetic department rotation. Junior staff should spend a block of at least 3 months working on a unit to become proficient.

The ITU resident is responsible for examination of each patient on admission, and at least once each day. With appropriate guidance, he or she should be responsible also for all aspects of treatment, and all requests for investigations and changes in treatment prescribed by visiting medical teams should be channelled through the resident.

In larger units, a senior registrar may be a member of the ITU team. Although most ITU senior registrars at present are undertaking higher professional training in anaesthesia, this may change in future. The senior registrar assumes a higher degree of responsibility than the ITU resident. He or she should be involved in policy decisions and administration.

Other medical staff

Even the most experienced ITU consultant cannot manage all the possible conditions with which the critically ill patient may present. Thus, he or she should seek advice from a wide variety of specialists when the need arises.

MEDICAL STAFF TRAINING

Currently, there is no accepted standard of training in the UK for the ITU consultant. In the USA, a multi-disciplinary approach to ITU training has been adopted whilst two independent types of ITU have emerged in Australia, one managed by anaesthetists and the other by physicians.

In the UK, intensive care is not recognized by the DHSS as an independent specialty. The majority of new consultant posts in general intensive care are appointed within departments of anaesthesia, although 25% of units have a surgeon or physician in charge. In addition, there are several specialist units (e.g. cardiothoracic, neurosurgical, poisons, burns).

In order to rationalize intensive care training, an interfaculty/collegiate liaison group has considered the problems (Hanson, 1985). It was suggested that full-time intensive-care specialists should not evolve, but that intensive care should be conducted by consultants of different backgrounds after completion of a recommended pattern of training. The liaison group proposed a minimum training period of 7 yr after registration. At the level of Senior House Officer or Registrar, training in intensive care should be incorporated into general professional training (GPT) programmes of anaesthetists, physicians and surgeons, who would proceed to take the appropriate higher qualifications in their parent specialty. A total of 2 yr would be spent in recognized posts in intensive care; in many cases, this would require extension of the GPT period. Overseas experience in appropriate units would be recognized. Research projects would be encouraged, and it has been suggested that presentation of a dissertation should be an essential part of training. At some time during training, a period of 1 yr would be spent in medical training by anaesthetists, and 6 months in an anaesthetic training post by physicians.

The mechanism by which the necessary posts would become available has yet to be decided. The proposed scheme is a source of controversy; some critics believe that anaesthetists should continue to predominate in intensive care (Stoddart, 1986), whilst others suggest that the ITU should be managed by full-time specialist 'intensivists' (Dudley, 1987).

Admission policy

The purpose of the ITU is to provide a level of care unattainable in other areas of the hospital for patients who are suffering an acute illness from which they have a realistic chance of recovery. In many cases, these criteria are met when request is made for admission. For example, a patient with Guillain–Barré syndrome who develops ventilatory failure can be treated only where facilities for long-term artificial ventilation are available, but is likely to recover after the acute illness and should then return to a normal life. Difficulties may arise, particularly if there is pressure for ITU beds, when patients are referred only for 'high-dependency' care, or when a request for admission is made for a patient with severe chronic disease.

The admission policy for high-dependency patients is determined usually by the average demand for ITU beds. Some units admit high-dependency patients routinely, whilst others are seldom able to do so. High-dependency patients require relatively little nursing care, and it may be appropriate to admit patients routinely after major surgery (particularly if a facility for 24-hr recovery is not available), for simple monitoring (e.g. central venous pressure), for supervision of parenteral nutrition, etc. However, nurses in the general wards become progressively less experienced in the management of this type of patient, and are less able to cope satisfactorily on occasions when the unit is busy and admission is not possible.

The admission of patients with severe chronic disease and with a limited life expectancy generates major moral and ethical questions. It is possible in a very small number of patients to predict that there is virtually no chance of survival (see 'Scoring systems' below), although in these circumstances many doctors find it difficult to withhold treatment. The overall mortality of unstable patients is high. In one study, it was found that mortality within 1 month was 56%, and a further 17% died within 1 yr; less than 50% of the 27% who survived returned to a normal life 1 yr after their illness (Cullen, 1977). Patients who

present with an acute illness, but whose life expectancy is limited e.g. patients with incurable malignant disease or chronic incapacitating respiratory or cardiac disease, have a high mortality, and may require treatment for many days or weeks. Only a small proportion survive to return home; their remaining life may be short and its quality severely impaired. For the remainder, the suffering and indignity are unnecessary, and the stress on relatives is enormous (Jennett, 1984).

A similar dilemma is presented by patients with acute complications of severe but potentially curable diseases, particularly in the younger patient. The mortality in patients with autoimmune deficiency syndrome (AIDS) who require admission to ITU is 80% (Deam et al., 1988). At present, the survivors are thought to have limited life expectancy.

In the past, admission policy in some units was based primarily on age. There is conflicting evidence on the relationship between age and outcome from ITU admission. Cullen (1977) found an inverse relationship, although the quality of life for ITU survivors was not influenced by age; in a more recent study, age was not found to have influenced outcome significantly among patients admitted to a medical ITU (Fedullo & Swinburne, 1983).

The decision to admit a patient is influenced also by attitudes towards the termination of treatment in those who fail to progress. Patients who do not improve despite continuing high levels of therapeutic intervention over many days have a very high mortality (Cullen, 1977).

In the USA, it has become necessary to resolve many of these very difficult decisions in courts of law. In some states, only a court can decide that treatment can be terminated. In the UK, decisions regarding termination of treatment are taken usually by all the consultants involved with the care of the patient, and after consultation with relatives. Admission of patients who may benefit little from ITU treatment may be determined also by discussion among all parties involved. As health-care resources become more limited, and medical and technological advances decrease the number of patients deemed 'incurable', less flexible guidelines may become necessary in future.

Scoring systems

General ITUs admit patients with a wide variety of conditions and complications. Thus, it is difficult to compare morbidity and mortality among different units. Many of the new forms of treatment and apparatus used are enormously expensive. In the USA, intensive-care budgets amount to over 20% of total hospital costs, and 1% of the gross national product (Berenson, 1984).

Almost no information is available on the efficiency of ITUs. Although individual units may maintain records of admissions, brief details of therapeutic manoeuvres and patient outcome, these figures are seldom published. In addition, because of differences in admission policies and treatment regimens and the wide variation in the type of illness precipitating admission to a general ITU, results from a small number of units cannot be extrapolated to provide figures representing the country as a whole.

Many of the newer forms of therapy and some invasive monitoring techniques, have not been evaluated adequately for a number of reasons:

1 Many units are small, and most general units admit patients with a wide variety of pathologies.
2 Because of differences in the severity of disease, the patient's individual response, the presence of concurrent chronic disease and the stage of the illness at which the patient is referred for treatment, it is difficult to compare patients with the same disease process.
3 There may therefore be a variety of methods of treatment for each disease within a single unit.
4 Multi-centre trials necessary to obtain sufficient numbers of patients for adequate controlled clinical trials, have proved impractical for the above reasons.

Finally, there is concern that the advanced technology and expertise which is able to maintain life by artificial support of the pulmonary, cardiovascular and renal systems may be used to prolong life in an undignified manner in patients whose prognosis is hopeless (Jennett, 1984). The lack of information available regarding outcome and response to treatment makes prognostic predictions impossible.

Scoring systems have been used for some years for patients with certain types of illness e.g. Glasgow coma score for patients with severe head injury, injury severity score and trauma score for patients with severe trauma. These have proved useful in defining relationships between treatment and outcome. For example, Watt and Ledingham (1984) demonstrated that increased mortality among trauma patients in ITU was related to the introduction of etomidate for sedation rather than to differences in severity of illness.

Three scoring systems applicable to patients in a general ITU have been described.

THERAPEUTIC INTERVENTION SCORING SYSTEM (TISS)

This measures the type and quantity of treatment and monitoring required for an individual patient (Keene & Cullen, 1983). Eighty different nursing or medical tasks are recorded. However, the system assumes that the quantity of treatment initiated is proportional to the severity of illness, which is not always the case. Nursing and medical procedures vary considerably both in extent and skill of administration. Whilst scores obtained in a single unit may be related to severity of illness, the system is inappropriate for comparison between units.

ACUTE PHYSIOLOGY SCORE (APS)

This comprises the sum of scores relating to 34 variables measured during the first 24 hr of a patient's admission to the ITU (Knaus et al., 1981). The score for each variable increases in proportion to the degree of deviation from normal. In conjunction with a chronic health factor as part of the original APACHE system (see below), the APS has been shown to be reasonably sensitive and specific in determining outcome, but is time consuming. In addition, not all variables are investigated routinely, and missing values are scored usually scored as normal. A simplified acute physiology score (SAPS) has been described consisting of 14 observations. This is as sensitive, but less specific, than APS in determining outcome (Le Gall et al., 1984).

ACUTE PHYSIOLOGY AND CHRONIC HEALTH EVALUATION (APACHE)

The original APACHE system (Knaus et al., 1981) combined the 34-point APS with an estimate of chronic health status. A revised version, APACHE II (Knaus et al., 1985), uses a point score based usually on the worst i.e. most abnormal, value of a simplified physiological score consisting of 12 measurements made during the first 24 hr of admission, together with scores based on age and previous health status in terms of chronic organ dysfunction (Table 71.3). The APACHE II system has been applied prospectively in many thousands of patients in many centres, and has enabled comparison of different methods of treatment (Meakins, 1984). It has also permitted development of a prognostic index. By subdivision of patients according to diagnosis, a relationship may be obtained

Table 71.3 Variables used in calculation of APACHE II score

Acute physiology score

Variable	Maximum score for	
	Low value	High value
Rectal temperature	4	4
Mean arterial pressure	4	4
Heart rate	4	4
Respiratory rate	4	4
Oxygenation		
$(A-a)Do_2$ if $F_{1}O_2 > 0.5$		4
Pao_2 if $F_{1}O_2 < 0.5$	4	
Arterial pH	4	4
Serum sodium	4	4
Serum potassium	4	4
Serum creatinine	2	4
(double score if		
acute renal failure)		
Haemoglobin	4	4
White blood count	4	4
Glasgow coma score (GCS)	Score $= 15 - $ GCS	

Age

Age (yr)	Points
<44	0
45–54	2
55–64	3
65–74	5
>75	6

Chronic health

If history of severe organ system insufficiency or if immunocompromised, then:

1 For non-operative or emergency postoperative patients, 5 points
2 For elective postoperative patients, 2 points

between diagnostic category, severity of illness and outcome. The observations consist of physiological and biochemical measurements undertaken routinely in most ITUs, and thus the frequency of missing values is small. The chronic health and age components add significantly to the sensitivity and specificity of the score.

The APACHE II system has been evaluated in critically ill patients requiring transport (Bion *et al.*, 1985) and to identify the need for total parenteral nutrition (Chang *et al.*, 1986). In a study in which the APACHE II score was evaluated prospectively (Jacobs *et al.*, 1987), there was a highly significant difference between the scores of the non-survivors (mean 25.3) and the survivors (mean 11.0). The sensitivity in predicting death was increased if the scores on the first and third days of admission to ITU were considered; a deteriorating score was associated with poor prognosis. Although the original concept was that of a system which could be used as a database to compare survival, there has been interest in prediction of mortality, and in some countries, these predictions may be used to 'rationalize' admission of patients to ITU (Jacobs *et al.*, 1987).

Monitoring in the intensive therapy unit

Monitoring is essential in the critically ill patient. It assists diagnosis, guides adjustment of therapy and allows early detection of deterioration in the patient's condition. The level of monitoring required for an individual patient is determined by the presenting condition and its predicted course, the existence of concurrent disease, and, in the case of invasive monitoring techniques, the risk : benefit ratio.

In general, instrumental monitoring is indicated if it provides information which is not available from clinical observation, if it is likely to provide early warning of an unpredictable change, or if it helps to quantify a predictable change.

Cardiopulmonary monitoring

Although it is convenient to classify monitoring techniques with respect to physiological systems, haemodynamic and respiratory monitoring should be considered in tandem, as oxygen transport to the cell is dependent on the functions of both the cardiovascular and respiratory systems.

HAEMODYNAMIC MONITORING

Electrocardiography (ECG)

Electrocardiographic monitoring provides information on heart rate and rhythm. Changes in the pattern of the ECG complex may indicate electrolyte disturbances or myocardial ischaemia. Detection of these changes requires regular observation by the nursing and medical staff, although devices are now available which detect changes in ECG pattern and indicate rhythm disturbances or onset of ischaemia.

Arterial pressure

Measurement of arterial pressure is essential. In some patients, intermittent non-invasive measurement is adequate. However, direct pressure monitoring is preferable in any patient whose condition is unstable, as rapid changes in arterial pressure are not detected by intermittent observations. Continuous access to an artery permits also regular measurement of arterial blood gases without the need to perform multiple arterial punctures.

The radial artery is used most commonly for arterial pressure monitoring, although some authorities believe that a larger artery, such as the brachial or femoral artery, is less likely to become occluded because of the higher flow rate of blood around the cannula. Femoral artery cannulation is indicated in the shocked patient, or if difficulty is experienced in inserting a radial artery cannula. Although it has been suggested that the femoral route is more likely to lead to infective complications (Band & Maki, 1979), the overall complication rates for femoral and radial routes are similar (Russell *et al.*, 1983). The incidence of complications resulting from radial artery cannulation may be reduced if a parallel-sided Teflon cannula no larger than 20 gauge in adults, or 22 gauge in children, is used, and if multiple attempts at cannulation are avoided (Russell *et al.*, 1983).

The information provided by an intra-arterial cannula may be inaccurate unless careful attention is paid to the damping of the transducer system. Over-damping may result from a kinked or partially occluded catheter, or the presence of air bubbles in the transducer tubing. An excessive length of tubing may result in underdamping, with overestimation of systolic pressure and underestimation of diastolic pressure. Measurement of arterial pressure by cannulation of the dorsalis pedis artery is subject often to underdamping. The reading from the transducer system should be calibrated regularly by checking the true arterial pressure with a cuff and mercury sphygmomanometer.

There are several potential complications of direct arterial pressure measurement. Disconnection leads to haemorrhage, which may be lethal, especially in children, if it is not noticed and arrested promptly. The risk of haemorrhage is reduced if Luer locks are used at all connections and if the number of connections

is kept to a minimum. Integral tubing systems containing a flushing device, transducer dome and connecting tubing are available which reduce the number of connections, and are cheaper than construction of a system from individual components. The cannula and connecting tubing should always be visible to the nursing staff, and should not be hidden underneath bandages or dressings. Excessive flushing of the cannula at high pressure can produce retrograde flow in the artery, with proximal embolization; this is a particular risk in children.

As with any procedure in which the skin is penetrated, arterial cannulation carries a risk of infection. Septic emboli may result also from an infected arterial cannula. Methods of minimizing the risks of infection are described on p. 1289.

The most feared complication of arterial cannulation is distal ischaemia resulting from arterial occlusion. Occlusion of the radial artery occurs in up to 50% of patients during or after long-term arterial cannulation; patency is re-established usually, but this may take up to 11 weeks (Bedford & Wollman, 1973). Clinical evidence of ischaemia is relatively uncommon (up to 4% during radial artery cannulation), but is not predicted accurately by Allen's test (Allen, 1929) to determine adequacy of the collateral circulation through the ulnar artery. Necrotic damage is rare provided that the cannula is removed promptly when distal ischaemia is recognized.

Central venous pressure

Measurement of central venous or right atrial pressure (CVP, RAP) gives an indication of the preload of the right ventricle. The RAP increases if the right ventricle fails because of overtransfusion, increased pulmonary vascular resistance or increased back pressure from the left ventricle, and decreases in the presence of hypovolaemia with normal ventricular function. Right ventricular failure alone is relatively uncommon in the ITU patient; it is usually secondary to acute pulmonary disease or left ventricular failure. The principal use of RAP measurement in the ITU is therefore assessment of the adequacy of the circulating volume.

The commonest sites for insertion of a central venous catheter are the median cubital vein in the antecubital fossa, the internal jugular vein, the subclavian vein and the femoral vein. The internal jugular route is associated with the highest incidence of correct positioning of the catheter tip in the vena cava or right atrium (over 90%), although insertion into an arm vein has fewest early complications (Rosen *et al.*, 1981). The major complications of the four routes are summarized in Table 71.4.

Two complications are common to all routes of insertion. Infection, which may remain localized or may result in bacteraemia, can be reduced substantially by ensuring that a fully sterile technique is used; this is discussed more fully on p. 1289. The tip of the catheter may not be in the correct position. Extravascular insertion may result in infusion of intravenous fluids into tissues, or more seriously, into the pleural cavity. The catheter tip may remain in a vein, but lie outside the thorax or in an anomalous intrathoracic vessel; this results in inaccurate measurements of pressure, and may cause vascular damage if hypertonic fluids are infused. It is essential to check the position

Table 71.4 Major complications of central venous catheterization

Arm veins
High incidence of incorrect placement (25–30%)
Thrombophlebitis—almost 100% at 48 hr

Subclavian vein
Pneumothorax
Haemothorax
Hydrothorax
Subcutaneous emphysema
Brachial plexus palsy
Phrenic nerve paralysis
Subclavian artery puncture
Innominate vein puncture
Subclavian vein thrombosis
Knotted catheter
Air embolism

Internal jugular vein
Pneumothorax
Haemothorax
Hydrothorax
Carotid artery puncture
Thrombophlebitis
Thoracic duct puncture
Horner's syndrome
Endotracheal tube cuff puncture
Vocal cord paralysis
Air embolism
Superior vena cava thrombosis
Aortic catheterization
Ventricular fibrillation

Fkoral vein
Thrombophlebitis
Femoral and iliac vein thrombosis
Inferior vena cava thrombosis
Serious infection

of the tip after insertion by ensuring that venous blood can be aspirated freely, and by chest radiography; it may be necessary to inject a small volume of radio-opaque dye to highlight relatively radiolucent catheters.

Measurement of RAP or CVP can be undertaken with a water-filled manometer. The true zero reference point is the right atrium; the surface marking is the mid-axillary line opposite the fourth costal cartilage. The normal range of values in the spontaneously breathing patient is 0–6 cmH$_2$O. The manubrio-sternal junction is used often as a more convenient zero reference point, but this is 5–10 cm above the right atrium, depending on body build and the position of the patient, and the CVP value is correspondingly lower.

If drugs are infused through the central venous line, administration ceases during the 30–45 sec during which the CVP measurement is made. It is preferable to use a multi-lumen catheter so that one lumen can be dedicated to measurement of CVP. In many units, CVP measurement is now made continuously using a pressure transducer.

Trends in measurement are more important than the absolute value of RAP. There is considerable interindividual variation in the normal measurement, the zero reference point is not always consistent between patients and the use of positive pressure ventilation increases RAP by an amount which varies with the inspiratory and expiratory pressures and the compliance of the lungs. A downward trend in RAP suggests that the circulating volume is decreasing (e.g. haemorrhage), whilst an upward trend suggests right ventricular failure. In the hypotensive patient with RAP within the normal range, the technique of a 'fluid challenge' is used often to help determine the volaemic status. Factors that influence RAP are summarized in Table 71.5.

Pulmonary artery pressures

A balloon-tipped, flow-guided catheter may be inserted by any of the routes appropriate for central venous catheterization. Because of their larger diameter, pulmonary artery catheters are inserted through a wide-bore cannula following dilatation of the vein with a dilator advanced over a guide wire. When the tip is in a central vein, a pressure transducer is connected to the saline-filled distal lumen and the balloon at the tip is inflated. With careful manipulation, the balloon is encouraged to follow the flow of blood through the

Table 71.5 Factors that influence right atrial (central venous) pressure

Blood volume
Total
Volume of blood on venous side
Rate of transfusion or fluid administration
Left ventricular failure
Cor pulmonale
Venoconstriction
Vasopressor administration
Increased intrathoracic pressure
Mechanical ventilation
Mediastinal emphysema
Pneumothorax
Haemothorax
Postoperative ileus
Pulmonary embolism
Air embolism
Pulmonary arterial hypertension
Superior vena cava obstruction
Pericardial tamponade
Constrictive pericarditis
Artefacts
Blocked catheter
Catheter tip in right ventricle

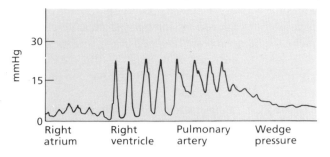

Fig. 71.1 Pressure waveform as a pulmonary artery catheter passes through right atrium, right ventricle and main pulmonary artery to become wedged in a small branch of the pulmonary artery.

right atrium and ventricle and into the main pulmonary artery; its progress is assessed by monitoring the pressure waveform (Fig. 71.1). As the catheter is advanced further, its tip enters a branch of the pulmonary artery with a diameter equal to that of the balloon; at this point, the balloon becomes wedged and the arterial pulsation disappears from the trace. When the balloon is deflated, the pulmonary arterial pressure (PAP) trace returns.

Most pulmonary artery catheters have at least three lumens. The distal lumen is used to record PAP and to obtain samples of mixed venous blood from the pulmonary artery. The proximal lumen, situated approximately 25 cm from the tip, should lie in the right atrium or superior vena cava when the catheter is positioned correctly; it may be used for infusions or for measuring CVP. The third lumen carries air to the balloon at the tip. Additional lumens may be incorporated to carry wires for a thermistor (see below) or for cardiac pacing.

The complications of pulmonary artery catheterization are summarized in Table 71.6. In addition, any of the complications of cannulation at the site of insertion may be encountered. The position of the catheter must be confirmed always by a chest X-ray.

Pulmonary arterial pressure is usually measured continuously, and the waveform displayed on an oscilloscope. When wedging occurs, the PAP trace disappears, and is replaced by a trace similar to that seen in the right atrium, and the pressure declines gradually as blood flows towards the left atrium. The pressure plateaus when pressure in the pulmonary artery branch equilibrates with left atrial pressure (LAP). The pressure measured in this way is not always identical to LAP, and is referred to as pulmonary capillary wedge pressure (PCWP).

Pulmonary capillary wedge pressure should be measured during end-expiration. It is influenced by positive end-expiratory press (PEEP), and on average, PCWP is increased by approximately 40% of the end-expiratory pressure. It should always be less than pulmonary artery diastolic pressure (PADP). Overinflation or eccentric inflation of the balloon, or the presence of mitral regurgitation or complete heart block should be suspected if PCWP exceeds PADP. Pulmonary capillary wedge pressure may reflect LAP inaccurately in severe left ventricular dysfunction, or if it is wedged in the upper zones of the lung where pulmonary capillaries may become occluded during inspiration. The pressure *must* be measured only intermittently, as occlusion of the branch of the

Table 71.6 Complications of pulmonary artery catheterization

Ventricular arrhythmias
Valve erosions
Subacute bacterial endocarditis
Pulmonary emboli
Pulmonary infarction
Pulmonary artery rupture
Arteriovenous fistula
Knot formation in right ventricle
Infection

pulmonary artery for more than 30–45 sec may result in pulmonary infarction; the balloon must be deflated after each measurement has been made, and the return of a PAP waveform confirmed. If the PAP trace assumes a 'wedged' pattern with the balloon deflated, the catheter has probably advanced so that the tip is wedged in a small branch of the artery. Its patency should be checked by aspirating blood, and if the waveform remains unchanged, the catheter should be withdrawn until a pulmonary arterial waveform is obtained.

The indications for pulmonary artery monitoring include clinical or anticipated left ventricular dysfunction, particularly in patients with ischaemic heart disease, and titration of therapy to optimize LAP when dissociation between left and right atrial pressures exists e.g. pulmonary oedema, chronic pulmonary disease and adult respiratory distress syndrome (ARDS). Normal values for PAP and PCWP are shown in 71.7; however, as with RAP, trends are often more useful than absolute values.

The risks of infection and valvular damage associated with pulmonary artery catheters increase with time, and the catheter should be removed after 48 hr unless there are strong clinical indications for its continued use.

Cardiac output

Measurement of cardiac output ($\dot{Q}_T$) may be useful in assessing oxygen delivery, cardiac performance, or the response of the cardiovascular system to treatment. However, all methods of measurement are prone to inaccuracy, and it is important to make other assessments of circulatory adequacy (see below) in conjunction with $\dot{Q}_T$ measurement.

Non-invasive techniques of $\dot{Q}_T$ measurement are available, but, despite manufacturers' claims, they are

Table 71.7 Normal pressures and oxygen saturations in cardiac chambers

	Pressure (mmHg)	Saturation (%)
Right atrium	0–7	77
Right ventricle	14–30/0–7	75
Pulmonary artery	14–30/5–12	75
Left atrium	4–10	97
Pulmonary capillary wedge pressure	4–10	75
Left ventricle	110–135/4–10	97
Aorta	110–135/60–80	96

often inaccurate at measuring absolute values. However, they do reflect changes accurately and may be valuable in following a patient's clinical progress. Impedance cardiography detects voltage changes caused by the ejection of blood from the ventricles. Transcutaneous aortovelography uses ultrasound to detect the velocity of blood flow in the ascending aorta. Stroke volume and cardiac output may be estimated also after injection of technetium-99m-labelled albumin; however, this technique is expensive, and exposes the patient and staff to radioactivity.

Invasive techniques of measuring cardiac output are subject to error also, but at present are more reproducible than any of the non-invasive methods. All are based on the Fick principle. The direct Fick method requires measurements to be made of arterial and mixed venous oxygen contents (Ca_{O_2}, $C\bar{v}_{O_2}$), and oxygen consumption ($\dot{V}_{O_2}$); the latter is calculated by measuring expired minute volume and inspired and mean expired oxygen concentrations. $\dot{Q}_T$ is calculated from the formula:

$$\dot{Q}_T = \frac{\dot{V}_{O_2}}{Ca_{O_2} - C\bar{v}_{O_2}}.$$

However, unless very expensive equipment and microprocessor calculation are used, this technique is time consuming, cumbersome and subject to error particularly in the artificially ventilated patient receiving a high fractional inspired oxygen concentration ($F_{I_{O_2}}$).

Indicator dilution techniques compute $\dot{Q}_T$ by calculating the degree of dilution of a bolus of indicator after mixing with blood. Two indicators are in common use. Indocyanine green may be injected as a bolus into the right atrium or pulmonary artery. Blood is sampled from a peripheral artery, commonly the radial, and the average concentration of dye and its transit time, measured by sampling blood continuously through a densitometer. $\dot{Q}_T$ can be calculated from these data. This method is also rather cumbersome because of the need to draw blood continuously from the peripheral artery using a syringe pump, and because calibration of the densitometer is required for each patient. In addition, indocyanine green accumulates in the circulation and limits the frequency with which measurements can be made.

The thermodilution technique is now the most commonly employed. A known volume of liquid at a known temperature (significantly different from the temperature of the patient) is injected into the right atrium, and the temperature of blood in the pulmonary artery measured using a pulmonary artery catheter with a thermistor at its tip. The 'dilution' of temperature difference is calculated, and cardiac output computed from the mean temperature dilution and the transit time of the temperature drop. The accuracy of the method improves if ice-cold liquid is used, especially in children, small adults or low output states. Errors are introduced by injecting the liquid slowly or irregularly. The mean of three measurements, each of which differs by no more than 10%, is calculated usually in order to minimize the errors of individual measurements. The method is easy to perform; the catheters are precalibrated and thermodilution cardiac output computers are easy to use. There is no problem with a shifting baseline. The major disadvantage is that large volumes of fluid are injected if measurements are made frequently. With both dye and thermodilution techniques, the accuracy depends on the shape of the dilution curve; this should be recorded, and calculations based on unsatisfactory curves should be rejected. Cardiac output varies with respiration. Although reproducibility of cardiac output measurements is improved by injecting the indicator at the same point in the respiratory cycle, the true cardiac output is probably reflected more accurately by averaging values obtained after injection at intervals spread evenly throughout the respiratory cycle (Versprille, 1984).

Derived haemodynamic variables

A number of variables can be calculated after cardiac output and cardiovascular pressures have been measured. Table 71.8 indicates the necessary calculations and normal values of these variables. They are often of value in determining the optimum mode of therapy in the presence of hypotension or cardiac failure. Table 71.9 shows methods of calculating oxygen delivery.

Perfusion

The aim of cardiovascular support in the ITU is usually to obtain satisfactory perfusion of the tissues. This can be assessed clinically by observing the colour and temperature of the skin. However, a more accurate assessment is obtained by monitoring peripheral temperature and urine output. The difference between core temperature and the temperature of the large toe has been related to outcome in critically ill patients

Table 71.8 Derived haemodynamic variables

Variable	Derivation	Normal value (70 kg)
Cardiac output (CO)	SV × heart rate	5 litre/min
Cardiac index (CI)	$\dfrac{CO}{\text{Body surface area}}$	$3.2 \text{ litre} \cdot \text{min}^{-1} \cdot \text{metre}^{-2}$
Stroke volume (SV)	$\dfrac{CO}{HR} \times 1000$	80 ml
Stroke index (SI)	$\dfrac{SV}{\text{Body surface area}}$	50 ml/metre^2
Systemic vascular resistance (SVR)	$\dfrac{\text{Mean arterial pressure} - CVP}{CO} \times 80$	$1000{-}1200 \text{ dyne} \cdot \text{sec}^{-1} \cdot \text{cm}^{-5}$
Pulmonary vascular resistance (PVR)	$\dfrac{\text{Mean pulmonary artery} - \text{left atrial pressure}}{CO} \times 80$	$60{-}120 \text{ dyne} \cdot \text{sec}^{-1} \cdot \text{cm}^{-5}$
Left ventricular stroke work index (LVSWI)	$\dfrac{1.36 \,(\text{Mean arterial} - \text{left atrial pressure})}{100} \times SI$	$50{-}60 \text{ g} \cdot \text{metre} \cdot \text{metre}^{-2}$
Rate pressure produce (RRP)	Systolic arterial pressure × heart rate	
Ejection fraction (EF)	$\dfrac{\text{End-systolic} - \text{end-diastolic volumes}}{\text{End-diastolic volume}}$	> 0.6

Table 71.9 Oxygen delivery

Variable	Derivation	Normal value (70 kg)
Oxygen content (Co_2)	$Hb \times So_2 \times 1.34 + Po_2 \times 0.0225$	18–20 ml/dl
Oxygen delivery ($\dot{D}o_2$)	$CO \times Cao_2 \times 10$	850–1050 ml/min
Oxygen consumption ($\dot{V}o_2$)	$CO \times C(a-\bar{v})o_2$	180–250 ml/min
Oxygen extraction rate	$C(a-\bar{v})o_2/Cao_2$	20–30%

Hb = haemoglobin concentration (g/dl). So_2 = fractional oxygen saturation.
CO = cardiac output (litre/min).   a = arterial.
Po_2 = oxygen tension (kPa). $\bar{v}$ = mixed venous.

(Henning *et al.*, 1979); an increase in this temperature gradient often precedes a change in arterial pressure or cardiac output because vasoconstriction is one of the earliest compensatory mechanisms of the cardiovascular system in response to hypovolaemia or decreased cardiac output. Urine output is also a valuable index of peripheral perfusion, although it may be affected by other factors.

The degree of cardiovascular monitoring, and the frequency with which observations are made, depend on the severity and nature of illness. Indications for invasive monitoring are shown in Table 71.10.

Respiratory monitoring

Ventilatory volume and frequency

Gas volumes are usually measured directly, using one of the devices listed in Table 71.11. Monitoring of tidal or minute volume is relatively easy in the ventilated patient, and many ITU ventilators incorporate either a vane respirometer or pneumotachograph. In the patient who is breathing spontaneously without an endotracheal tube, a closely fitting mask can be applied and connected to a respirometer, but continuous monitoring can be effected with an impedance or inductance plethysmograph. Ideally, tidal or minute volume should be monitored continuously in the patient undergoing mechanical ventilation so that the development of a large leak in the system, or significant changes in volumes from altered pulmonary compliance or resistance, can be detected rapidly. When this is not possible, measurements should be made at regular intervals e.g. every 30–60 min. Respiratory frequency is displayed by a number of types of ventilators, or may be counted by nursing staff; it is important to count also the rate of spontaneous ventilation in patients receiving intermittent mandatory or mandatory ventilation.

Airway pressure

Changes in airway pressure may indicate a change in compliance, as may occur with the development of pulmonary oedema or pneumothorax, or changes in resistance e.g. from bronchospasm. It is difficult to measure airway pressure accurately in the spontaneously breathing patient who is without an endotracheal tube. During artificial ventilation, a short end-inspiratory pause permits monitoring of alveolar pressure, which is related to compliance; the difference between peak and pause pressures is influenced predominantly by airway resistance when constant flow ventilators are used. End-expiratory pressure should be monitored also in patients receiving PEEP or continuous positive airways pressure (CPAP). Airway pressure may be measured mechanically or electronically.

Pressure/flow–volume loops

Using electronic monitoring techniques, pressure–volume or flow–volume loops can be displayed

Table 71.10 Indications for invasive cardiovascular monitoring

High-risk, preoperative patients (e.g. recent MI)
Combined acute cardiac and pulmonary disease
Multiple trauma
Pre-existing cardiorespiratory or renal disease
Multiple organ failure
Septic shock
Pulmonary embolism
Fat embolism

Table 71.11 Methods of measuring gas volumes in the ITU

Respirometer (e.g. Wright's)
Pneumotachograph
Heated wire
Vortex spirometer
Inductance plethysmograph

regularly. Pressure–volume loops are useful in detecting changes in compliance and resistance. The expiratory flow–volume pattern is useful in monitoring the resolution of bronchospasm in asthmatic patients.

Respiratory gas concentrations

The fractional inspired oxygen concentration is an important determinant of alveolar oxygen tension ($P_{A}O_2$). It should be monitored routinely during artificial ventilation so that adjustments can be made accurately as indicated by arterial blood gas analysis, and in order to calculate $P_{A}O_2$ when calculations of alveolar–arterial oxygen tension gradient or intrapulmonary shunt are required. The fractional inspired oxygen concentration is measured usually by a polarographic or fuel cell or using a paramagnetic analyser. These devices have a response time which is too slow to record tidal variations at the airway, and are used only in the inspiratory limb to measure $F_{I}O_2$.

End-tidal carbon dioxide pressure ($P_{ET}CO_2$) is derived from end-tidal carbon dioxide concentration, which is measured most commonly using an infrared spectrometer. These devices have a rapid response time. End-tidal carbon dioxide pressure is related to Pa_{CO_2}, but in patients with pulmonary disease, the gradient between the two may be greater than the normal 0.7 kPa (5.25 mmHg). However, measurement of $P_{ET}CO_2$ is useful in following trends in Pa_{CO_2}, and for calculation of physiological deadspace. Most infrared capnographs show an analogue or digital display of $P_{ET}CO_2$, and many display also the expired carbon dioxide waveform. Computer analysis of this waveform has been used in critically ill patients to analyse pulmonary function (Fletcher et al., 1981).

Mass spectrometry is used in some units to analyse respiratory gases. The mass spectrometer has an extremely fast response time, and can measure simultaneously the concentrations of carbon dioxide, oxygen, nitrogen and anaesthetic gases. Using a tracer gas dilution technique, it is possible also to measure mixed expired concentrations of carbon dioxide and oxygen for calculation of oxygen consumption, carbon dioxide excretion and respiratory quotient.

Blood gas analysis

Arterial oxygen and carbon dioxide tensions and pH are measured usually intermittently from samples of arterial blood drawn from an arterial puncture or indwelling cannula. Modern blood gas analysers contain three electrodes and display P_{O_2}, P_{CO_2} and pH within 1–2 min of inserting a small sample (usually less than 0.25 ml) of heparinized blood. The machines are self-calibrating and may be used by non-technical staff. However, errors may occur unless careful attention is paid to methods of sampling and storage. Excessive heparin in the sampling syringe decreases pH and P_{CO_2}, and results in large errors in calculated bicarbonate and base excess concentrations. When sampling from an indwelling cannula, the heparinized saline in the connecting tube must be aspirated and discarded before the sample is drawn. Bubbles of air in the syringe should be expelled immediately, or the gases dissolved in blood tend to equilibrate with gas in the bubbles. Storage of the sample for more than a few min results in oxygen consumption and carbon dioxide production, particularly by leucocytes; if analysis cannot be carried out immediately, the syringe should be capped and stored in ice-cold water. The syringe should be rotated gently immediately before injection into the analyser in order to ensure complete mixing of blood. The analysing electrodes are maintained at 37 °C, and mathematical corrections are required to all three measurements if the patient's temperature is different.

Frequency of arterial blood gas analysis is determined usually by the clinical condition of the patient. Mixed venous blood gas analysis can be undertaken by sampling from a pulmonary artery catheter when calculation of intrapulmonary shunt is required.

Continuous monitoring of blood gases has been made possible by the development of intravascular catheters with inbuilt electrodes. All of these devices suffer from having a relatively slow response time. Although pH and P_{CO_2} electrodes are available, they are relatively unstable and require frequent calibration. Indwelling oxygen electrodes are more stable, and may be useful in monitoring Pa_{O_2} in the very sick patient. However, pulse oximetry is probably superior in most patients.

Oximetry

Oximeters estimate the oxygenation of haemoglobin by measuring either the reflectance or the transmission of light in the red and infrared ranges. Pulse oximeters (p. 462) are now available readily. Most of these are accurate in all but the severely vasoconstricted patient, and provide a continuous display of oxygen saturation (So_2). As So_2 is almost directly proportional to oxygen content in blood, arterial oxygen saturation (Sao_2) is in many ways a more useful measurement than Pao_2 when arterial oxygenation is impaired. The technique is non-invasive, and its use is likely to increase greatly in the ITU. Continuous measurement of Sao_2 may be of value in the patient in whom it is impossible to maintain a normal Pao_2 (e.g. severe ARDS), and in the spontaneously breathing patient with threatened respiratory failure. It may be useful also during such procedures as physiotherapy or tracheal suction, although there is a relatively slow response time when a finger probe is used.

Continuous measurement of mixed venous oxygen saturation ($S\bar{v}o_2$) can be achieved using a pulmonary artery catheter which incorporates three fibre-optic bundles. Light from light-emitting diodes is transmitted through two of the bundles to the tip of the catheter, and light reflected by pulmonary arterial blood is transmitted up the third bundle to a detector at the proximal end of the catheter. Once calibrated, these systems are accurate in the range of 25–95% saturation. Mixed venous oxygen saturation is influenced by cardiac output in addition to arterial oxygenation, and reflects the average oxygenation of the tissues. The difference between Sao_2 and $S\bar{v}o_2$ indicates oxygen consumption if cardiac output is known. Values of $S\bar{v}o_2$ below 50% in critically ill patients, or failure of $S\bar{v}o_2$ to improve with therapy, are associated with a poor prognosis, whilst values over 65% indicate usually a satisfactory outcome (Kaznitz *et al.*, 1976).

Central nervous system

Clinical examination of the CNS is the single best method of monitoring brain function. However, in the comatose patient, other means may be necessary.

Electroencephalogram

The rhythm, amplitude and waveform pattern of the electroencephalogram (EEG) may be used to monitor patients with suspected CNS dysfunction. However, EEG interpretation requires skilled assistance. In addition, there is considerable variability in the normal EEG, and the relationship between clinical and EEG abnormalities is often poor. Conventional EEG monitoring can be performed only intermittently, and is subject to interference from other apparatus in the ITU.

A variety of methods is available for processing the EEG signal to provide a continuous and more easily interpreted form of monitoring.

Frequency domain analysis. This technique displays the frequency distribution of the EEG. The compressed spectral array (Fig. 71.2) is an example of this form of monitoring. The amplitudes at each frequency are

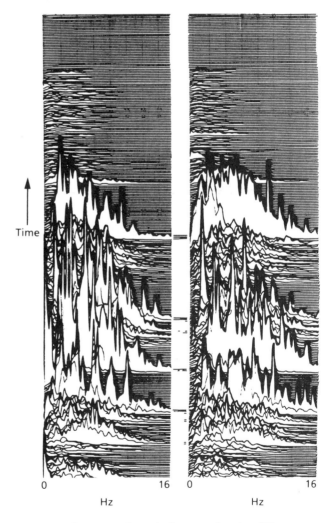

Fig. 71.2 Compressed spectral array, showing fitting followed by electrical silence in a patient with meningoencephalitis. (Reproduced from Willatts, 1985.)

displayed as a series of 'hills' and 'valleys'. Monitoring can be carried out continuously, but interpretation is difficult in the comatose patient unless gross abnormalities are present.

Time domain analysis. The cerebral function monitor (CFM) displays the integrated electrical activity from the cerebral cortex as a trace of amplitude plotted against time (Fig. 71.3). Electrical activity increases in the presence of seizures, and decreases if cerebral ischaemia or hypoxia occur. Sedation with intravenous anaesthetic agents decreases the amplitude of the trace also.

Time and frequency domain analysis. The cerebral function analysing monitor (CFAM) displays the total electrical activity of the brain together with the percentage of that activity which falls into the α-, β-, θ- and δ-frequency bands. Its role in ITU has yet to be established.

Evoked potentials

Auditory- visual- and somatosensory-evoked potentials can be used to assess the integrity of pathways in the brainstem and cerebral cortex. Asymmetrical conduction or absent potentials are poor prognostic signs after cerebral trauma. Delayed conduction may occur in the presence of anaesthetic agents or oedema.

Intracranial pressure

Intracranial pressure (ICP) may increase and cerebral perfusion pressure (CPP) decrease in some categories

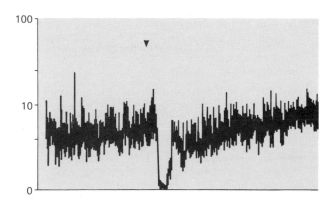

Fig. 71.3 Trace from a cerebral function monitor, showing interruption of the circulation at the arrow causing a transient absence of cerebral activity. (Reproduced from Willatts, 1985.)

of comatose patient e.g. traumatic or metabolic coma. These patients receive often heavy sedation or are paralysed in order to provide artificial ventilation so that adequate oxygenation and a decrease in arterial carbon dioxide tension may be achieved. Consequently, it is virtually impossible to monitor neurological function clinically. The likelihood of permanent cerebral damage increases if ICP exceeds 3.3–4.0 kPa (25–30 mmHg), or if CPP is less than 8 kPa (60 mmHg). Continuous monitoring of ICP permits early therapeutic intervention if ICP starts to increase, and, intuitively, careful control of ICP should help to reduce the probability of secondary cerebral damage occurring. Intracranial pressure is monitored most accurately using a fluid-filled catheter inserted into the lateral ventricle, but this technique is associated with the highest incidence of infective complications. Measurement of pressure in the subarachnoid space can be achieved by insertion of a catheter through a conventional burrhole, or using a 'bolt' threaded into a smaller burrhole in the skull. Despite the anticipated advantages of ICP monitoring, there is little evidence to show that control of ICP improves outcome in patients with severe head trauma. However, computerized analysis of the ICP waveform and automated recognition of patterns of ICP change may be able in future to predict dangerous increases in ICP, and might be useful in improving prognosis.

Infection control

Hospital-acquired (nosocomial) infection complicates the course of at least 40% of patients admitted to ITU. It has been estimated that 150 000 deaths occur each year in the USA alone as a direct result of infections which were not present, and not incubating, in patients at the time of admission to hospital (Farber, 1987). The survivors spend a longer period of time in hospital and require often treatment with the most expensive antibiotics. Intensive therapy unit patients are particularly susceptible to infection for a number of reasons. The body's natural defences are breached by an endotracheal tube, intravascular monitoring cannulae and urinary catheters; the immune system may be depressed by the severity of the patient's illness; infection may be transmitted from other patients after incubation in items of equipment or by staff; and antibiotics prescribed for infection by relatively susceptible micro-organisms may permit superinfection by resistant bacteria.

Pneumonia

Nosocomial lower respiratory tract infections are the third most common type of hospital-acquired infection; only wound and urinary infections are more frequent. However, it has by far the greatest mortality; 30% of patients with nosocomial pulmonary infection die (Farber, 1987). The incidence of nosocomial pneumonia in ITU patients has been estimated at 9–15%. In a more recent European multi-centre study, 33% of patients admitted to ITU with no evidence of pulmonary infection developed pneumonia subsequently (Ruiz-Santana et al., 1987); this higher figure reflects probably the greater number of patients in European ITUs who require tracheal intubation and mechanical ventilation.

CAUSES

A number of factors are known to increase the risk of nosocomial pneumonia (Table 71.12). The most important of these are thoracic or thoraco-abdominal surgery, and artificial ventilation, especially if continued for more than 72 hr. In one study, pneumonia developed in 8.5% of patients intubated for 3 days, and its incidence became progressively greater with time; 45.6% of patients undergoing intubation for longer than 14 days showed evidence of pneumonia (Ruiz-Santana et al., 1987). It is most common in patients who have severe underlying disease, and in those who have received antibiotic treatment for other infections.

The most common causative organisms found in one large study are listed in Table 71.13. Most are

Table 71.12 Factors which increase risk of developing nosocomial pneumonia

Thoraco-abdominal surgery
Mechanical ventilation
Thoracic surgery
Upper abdominal surgery
Smoking
Low serum albumin
Prolonged surgery (> 3 hr)
High ASA classification
Corticosteroids
Prolonged hospital stay (> 40 days)
Other infection
Social class
? Age
? Male gender
? Obesity

Table 71.13 Causative organisms of hospital-acquired pneumonia in decreasing order of frequency. (From Ruiz-Santana et al., 1987)

Pseudomonas aeruginosa
Proteus mirabilis
Escherichia coli
Staphylococcus aureus
Serratia marcescens
Klebsiella pneumoniae
Other Gram-negative aerobes
Enterobacter spp.
Streptococcus pneumoniae
Haemophilus influenzae
Other Pseudomonas spp.
Other Gram-positive aerobes
Other Serratia spp.
Bacteroides fragilis
Bacteroides spp.
Other Gram-negative anaerobes
Fungi

Gram-negative bacilli, although the exact pattern varies in different hospitals and depends in part on the original complaint of the patient. Klebsiella and Staphylococcus aureus infections are more common in obstetric and paediatric patients, and Haemophilus influenzae in ITU patients who have suffered trauma. However, in up to 62% of patients with nosocomial pneumonia, a positive sputum culture is not obtained (Ruiz-Santana et al., 1987), and in almost 50% of patients with bacteraemia and pneumonia, there is no correlation between the organisms isolated from blood and sputum samples. Viruses may be responsible for a proportion of cases of pneumonia in the ITU; these may be transmitted by staff, but are thought more often to be the result of reactivation of latent disease as a result of temporary immunosuppression. Patients with severe immunosuppression may develop infections with uncommon pathogens; this subject is dealt with in a separate section below.

There are three mechanisms by which organisms may infect the lower respiratory tract in the critically ill patient. There may be bloodborne spread. Infected material may be aspirated from the pharynx; this may contain upper respiratory tract flora, or may consist of gastrointestinal contents regurgitated from the stomach. Finally, there may be inhalation of droplets containing bacteria.

Normally, the lung is well protected against entry of foreign material. The laryngeal reflex is usually sufficiently strong to prevent aspiration of pharyngeal contents. The nose and nasopharynx filter out inhaled particles or droplets which exceed 3 μm in diameter, and those larger than 1 μm are deposited on the tracheal or bronchial mucosa, and removed by ciliary transport. The growth of micro-organisms which reach the alveoli is inhibited by surfactant and complement, and removed by phagocytosis, which is stimulated by immunoglobulins and complement products.

These defence mechanisms are altered by disease, and may be influenced by treatment. The gag reflex is depressed in patients with neurological disease involving the cranial nerves, and in those who are semi-conscious or debilitated; 70% of patients with depressed consciousness aspirate during sleep (Huxley et al., 1978). Aspiration is not prevented completely by the presence of a cuffed endotracheal tube. Chronic lung disease and anaesthetic drugs inhibit ciliary movement. Alveolar defences are impaired by nutritional deficiency, pulmonary oedema or ARDS. Tracheal intubation allows droplets of any size to bypass the nasopharynx, and prevents ciliary transport of infected material. High inspired oxygen concentrations inhibit ciliary movement and surfactant production.

The normal bacterial flora of the nasopharynx inhibit the growth of more virulent strains; when antibiotics are administered, staphylococci and coliform bacilli proliferate. Elderly patients who have been hospitalized for some time have colonies of Klebsiella, Escherichia coli or Enterobacter in the oropharynx even if no antibiotics have been administered. The incidence of colonization is highest in those who have been in hospital longest, and those with respiratory infections or severe illness. Gram-negative bacilli may be grown from oropharyngeal cultures in 45% of ITU patients, and nosocomial pneumonia is seven times commoner in these patients than in those whose orophayngeal cultures are negative (Johanson et al., 1972). Thus, aspiration of fluid from the oropharynx appears to be the source of many cases of respiratory infection.

The majority of bacteria which colonize the oropharynx originate in the gut. In patients with ileus, the gastric content is not sterile. Patients treated with antacids or H_2-receptor antagonists have a high gastric pH, and bacteria can be cultured from gastric aspirate. In several studies, the same organism has been cultured from tracheal and gastric aspirates in a large proportion of ITU patients with pneumonia (duMoulin et al., 1982).

Any equipment used to deliver gases may act as a source of infection, particularly if it contains fluids. Nebulizers used during physiotherapy to loosen bronchial secretions, and those used for drug administration, are likely to become colonized with Pseudomonas organisms. Ventilator humidifiers may act as a breeding ground for bacteria unless maintained at an adequate temperature. The expiratory ventilator tubing becomes contaminated with secretions where bacteria multiply; some of this infected material may be re-introduced into the patient's bronchial tree if fluid in the expiratory limb is not collected in traps. The tip of the endotracheal tube becomes contaminated almost always becomes contaminated with infected secretions. The incidence of colonization with Gram-negative organisms is higher if the endotracheal tube is left in place for more than 8 days. During tracheal suctioning, crusts of infected material may be dislodged into the bronchial tree.

PREVENTION

In patients about to undergo major elective surgery, smoking should be discontinued, pre-existing infection treated with appropriate antibiotic therapy and physiotherapy, and any congestive cardiac failure should be controlled. The risk of nosocomial pneumonia in the ITU may be minimized by using only sterile water in humidifiers, and by ensuring that they are maintained at an appropriate temperature. Water in the ventilator tubing becomes infected in both inspiratory and expiratory limbs, and must not be allowed to drain towards the endotracheal tube. Bacteria may migrate along the inspiratory limb towards the humidifier. Because of this, it is normal practice to change humidifier water and ventilator tubing every 24 hr, although there is some evidence that changing ventilator tubing every 48 hr does not increase the risk of contamination. The introduction of infection by droplet spread from the atmosphere may be minimized by placing bacterial filters on the air inlet port of air-entraining ventilators and humidifiers, and filtering gas at the expiratory port reduces contamination of the atmosphere by infected material from the expiratory limb. The use of a filter between the endotracheal tube and the ventilator reduces contamination of the patient's lungs from the inspired gas, of the expiratory limb from the patient's bronchial tree and acts as a condenser humidifier. It has been suggested that this obviates the need for a water humidifier, and so eliminates the risk of humidifier contamination. However, there is some doubt as to whether these filters are efficient enough in the critically ill patient to prevent tracheal secretions from becoming thick and difficult to remove.

Inappropriate use of antibiotics should be avoided, as this may encourage the growth of resistant strains of bacteria in the lungs. Meticulous attention by staff to hand-washing is important in reducing the risk of cross-infection. The use of H_2-receptor antagonists may not be appropriate in patients with a high risk of developing nosocomial pneumonia. Chest physiotherapy is believed to reduce the risk, or at least the severity, of nosocomial pneumonia, although there are few data to confirm this. In the patient who is breathing spontaneously, adequate analgesia must be provided to permit deep breathing and coughing, but excessive sedation must be avoided. After abdominal surgery, there is a decrease in functional residual capacity (FRC), which may decline below closing capacity (CC) (p. 175). Atelectasis is likely to occur in this situation. Positive-pressure breathing produced intermittently by pressure-cycled ventilation applied through a mouthpiece may help to reduce atelectasis. However, the use of CPAP increases FRC, and can be applied comfortably using a mask (Fig. 71.4). Continuous positive airway pressure improves gas exchange and reduces nosocomial infection in patients who have undergone major abdominal or thoracic

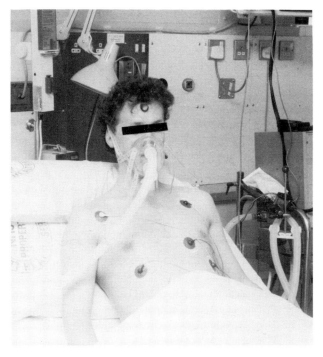

Fig. 71.4 A patient receiving continuous positive airway pressure (CPAP) by mask.

surgery and in those being weaned from intermittent positive-pressure ventilation (IPPV) (Feeley *et al.*, 1975).

Selective decontamination of the gastrointestinal tract in order to reduce the likelihood of aspiration into the lungs of infected gastrointestinal fluid has been investigated recently. Antibiotics used for this purpose should be bactericidal and non-absorbable, and should not be inactivated by food or faecal material. The combination of polymyxin E, tobramycin and amphoterecin B administered through a nasogastric tube and applied also as a paste to the oropharynx reduced the overall infection rate from 81% to 18%, and was particularly effective in reducing the incidence of pneumonia (Stoutenbeek, 1986). Antibiotic resistance did not increase during the study period. Alternative antibiotics which are more palatable and with a broader range of sensitivity have been suggested for this form of treatment, which appears to offer enormous potential for a reduction of nosocomial pneumonia in the ITU patient. A similar form of prophylactic treatment has had promising results in severely immunocompromised patients (see below).

DIAGNOSIS

It is often difficult to make a definite diagnosis of pneumonia in the critically ill patient. Fever may result from infection elsewhere in the body, or from complications of CNS disease. However, a sustained fever with only small fluctuations is caused often by pneumonia from Gram-negative bacilli. Radiological and clinical chest signs may be difficult to distinguish from those of ARDS or pulmonary contusion. Leucocytosis is not specific to pulmonary infection. Impairment of gas exchange is found often, although this may be caused also by ARDS or changes in cardiac output.

Culture of tracheal aspirate is used often as the criterion for diagnosing pneumonia. However, tracheal aspirates often yield positive cultures in patients without pneumonia, and therefore have a low specificity. Specificity is improved to some extent by taking cultures of bronchial secretions through a fibre-optic bronchoscope using a protected specimen brush (Chastre *et al.*, 1984). The most specific method is transthoracic pulmonary aspiration using a fine needle, but this technique is relatively insensitive (i.e. produces false-negatives) and carries a significant risk of pneumothorax. Bronchial lavage may be useful in some conditions e.g. *Pneumocystis carinii* infection. Bacteraemia occurs in only 20% of patients with nosocomial pneumonia, and positive blood cultures are more commonly the result of infection elsewhere.

TREATMENT

Appropriate respiratory and cardiovascular support measures are required often in order to maintain adequate tissue oxygenation. Clearly, the patient's primary illness must be treated if possible. Nutritional support may be required also. Antibiotic therapy should be based ideally on sensitivity studies on bacteria cultured from the patient's lungs. However, this is often impractical, and leads to long delays in starting treatment. A Gram stain of the specimen may give an indication of the pathogenic organism. Most nosocomial lung infections result from Gram-negative bacilli or *Staphylococcus aureus*. The choice of antibiotic therapy should be made in consultation with a microbiologist, and with knowledge of the resistance spectra of similar bacteria isolated recently in the ITU. At present, empirical therapy for Gram-negative bacilli consists often of an aminoglycoside (although serum concentrations at the upper end of the therapeutic range are required because of poor penetration in the lung), or a second- or third-generation cephalosporin; a penicillinase-resistant penicillin should be used for staphylococcal infection.

When sensitivity studies have been undertaken, it may be necessary to change the antibiotic regimen.

PROGNOSIS

Reported mortality from nosocomial pneumonia varies from 20% (Stamm *et al.*, 1977) to 50% (Stevens *et al.*, 1974); the variations reflect probably different patterns of admission, with the lower figures coming from units which tend towards high dependency. In one large study (Ruiz-Santana *et al.*, 1987), mortality from hospital-acquired pneumonia in ITU patients was 47%, but only 17% of patients with pneumonia acquired before admission to hospital died. Mortality is highest in patients with Gram-negative pneumonia. The mortality (and of course the likelihood of developing pneumonia) is related to the severity of the underlying condition. Pneumonia prolongs also the duration of admission in the ITU; in one study (Craig & Connelly, 1984), survivors of nosocomial pneumonia stayed in ITU for an average of 12 days, compared with 4.3 days for a comparable group of patients who did not develop this complication.

Nosocomial bacteraemia

Approximately 5% of all nosocomial infections result in bacteraemia, and 25% of these are related to intravascular cannulae or catheters. The remainder are the result of infection acquired by other routes e.g. secondary to nosocomial pneumonia or abdominal sepsis.

Table 71.14 lists the sites at which infection may be introduced when the integrity of the vascular system is breached by a cannula. The most common site of entry is the area of skin puncture. Contamination from this source is with the patient's own skin flora, such as *Staphylococcus epidermidis*, diphtheroids and some anaerobic organisms. However, the skin of patients who have been hospitalized for some days, and of those who have received antibiotic therapy, is often colonized with more virulent bacteria. Infection may be introduced also by hospital personnel during insertion of the cannula or subsequent dressing of the site. The hands of medical staff and nurses are often contaminated with *Staphylococcus aureus* and Gram-negative bacilli.

Organisms gain access to the circulation by migrating along the cannula, and may then become attached to the fibrin sheath which forms around the intravascular portion of the cannula as a normal reaction to its presence. This sheath may then act as a medium for multiplication of bacteria, whilst also protecting the organisms from antibiotics.

DIAGNOSIS

External signs of infection (erythema, swelling or pus) are present in less than 50% of subsequently proven,

Table 71.14 Sites of introduction of infection to the bloodstream from intravascular devices

Intravenous fluids
Contamination during manufacture
Contamination during insertion of giving set
Contamination introduced with additives
Injection ports
Stopcocks
Transducers
Flush solutions
Connections and Y-junctions
CVP manometers
Catheter insertion site
Skin flora
Contamination of operator's hands
Contaminated or inadequate disinfectants

catheter-related infections, and the diagnosis is made often by process of exclusion when no other source of bacteraemia is found. Catheter-related sepsis should always be considered when appropriate antibiotics are unsuccessful in treating bacteraemia. Positive confirmation is made by culturing the tip of the catheter after its removal. Positive cultures may be obtained from a catheter tip which has been infected secondarily in patients with bacteraemia from another source. However, the number of colonies of bacteria cultured from the catheter tip is lower in these cases. A semi-quantitative culture technique has been described (Maki *et al.*, 1977) which is claimed to identify if the catheter is the source of infection. However, this results in a high false-positive rate. A more recent rapid technique which involves slicing and Gram-staining the catheter tip appears to be more sensitive and specific (Cooper & Hopkins, 1985).

The most common organisms isolated from intravascular cannulae are *Staphylococcus aureus* and *Staphylococcus epidermidis*; although the latter is often thought of as a benign organism, it now appears to be a major pathogen (Ponce de Leon & Wenzel, 1984). *Enterococci*, *Klebsiella* and *E. coli* are also cultured commonly, and occasional reports have been made of infection of intravascular lines with *Candida*.

RELATIONSHIP WITH TYPE OF CATHETER

Peripheral venous catheters are used most commonly throughout the hospital, and most ITU patients have at least one in place. Infection is more common if the cannula is inserted in an emergency, if an aseptic technique is not used, if a surgical cut-down is required, and if left in position for more than 72 hr. Daily dressing changes, the use of semi-permeable dressings and local antibiotic ointment have been recommended, but there is no definite evidence that these reduce the risk of infection. Inline filters reduce the incidence of thrombophlebitis, but have not been proved to reduce infection.

Central venous catheters are often considered to present a higher risk of bacteraemia than peripheral cannulae, but the risk of infection per day of catheterization is lower. The incidence of infection is higher in the presence of distant infection and, in the case of lines inserted in the jugular or subclavian veins, if a tracheostomy is in place. Infection is less common if a strict aseptic technique is used for insertion. Move-

ment of the catheter increases the risk of infection, and it should be anchored well at its site of insertion. Silicone catheters are surrounded by a smaller fibrin sheath than plastic catheters, and are probably associated with a lower risk of infection. There are no strict guidelines regarding the duration of insertion beyond which the infection rate increases substantially. It is also unclear if replacement by insertion of a new catheter over a guide-wire at the same site is associated with a higher incidence of infection than insertion at a new site. Central venous catheters introduced into a peripheral vein should be replaced at least every 72 hr.

Long-term central venous cannulae are used for intravenous nutrition or the administration of chemotherapy. The infection rate is extremely low if insertion is conducted aseptically and the catheter tunnelled subcutaneously so that the exit site in the skin is some distance from the site of venous puncture. The most common site of infection is the exit of the tunnel. Whilst this may be treated by systemic antibiotics, infection throughout the tunnel requires removal of the catheter. Catheters have been left in place successfully for as long as 2.5 yr.

Pulmonary arterial catheters produce all the risks of central venous catheters, but in addition, have a large puncture wound, are handled and manipulated usually to a considerable degree during insertion, are often left in place inside an introducing sheath which is filled with blood and pass through the chambers of the heart resulting in damage to the endocardium. Endocardial lesions occur in over 50% of all patients in whom a pulmonary artery catheter has been inserted (Rowley *et al.*, 1984), and over 10% of these patients are likely to have infective endocarditis. It has been estimated that 3% of pulmonary artery catheters are a source of bacteraemia if left in place for longer than 72 hr.

Arterial cannulae are associated with an increased risk of infection if left in place for more than 4 days. In one study, approximately 14% of arterial cannulae showed signs of local infection, and 4% were responsible for bacteraemia (Band & Maki, 1979). Although bacteraemia is the most serious complication, serious local skin infection may occur also; an abscess containing 30 ml has been reported at the site of a radial artery cannula, with minimal external signs of infection (Lindsay *et al.*, 1987).

(Centers for Disease Control Working Group, 1981)

Insertion

The operator's hands should be washed before insertion of any cannula. Soap and water is appropriate before insertion of a peripheral line, but an antiseptic should be used before insertion of any central line. Sterile gloves should be worn for insertion of any central line, and for insertion of any cannula requiring a cut-down. Veins in the arm or neck are preferable to veins in the leg or groin. The site should be prepared with iodine 1 or 2%, chlorhexidine or 70% alcohol; the solution should be in contact with the skin for at least 30 sec before venepuncture is performed. The cannula should be secured firmly to the skin; if tape is used, it must not cover the puncture site. A topical antiseptic or antibiotic and sterile dressing should be applied. The date and time of insertion should be recorded.

Maintenance

The minimum number of connections between infusion bag and cannula should be made. Injection ports should be swabbed before use. Daily examination of catheter sites should be made, including palpation through the dressing to elicit tenderness. The intravenous administration set sould be changed every 48 hr. The entire administration system should be changed if there is any evidence of sepsis.

Pressure-monitoring systems

Disposable components should be used whenever possible. Those pre-assembled by the manufacturer are preferable. They should not be stored after preparation and flushing. A closed flush system should be used. Glucose solutions should never be used to flush intravascular pressure lines because of the increased risk of infection. Flush solutions should be changed every 24 hr, and the administration and flushing set every 48 hr. If any part of the system is contaminated with blood (except the tubing between catheter and sampling point), it is desirable to replace the contaminated section. Three-way stopcocks should be used only if essential, and covered when not in use. The number of blood samples taken from indewlling lines should be kept to a minimum.

The immunosuppressed patient

The normal immunological defence mechanisms may be impaired by a number of diseases. Immunological depression may occur to some degree in many acute conditions, but specific depression of cellular immunity occurs in patients with Hodgkin's disease, some leukaemias, the acquired immune deficiency syndrome (AIDS), and low levels of immunoglobulins are found in mutliple myeloma. In addition, drug therapy may induce immunological depression. Steroids and chemotherapy for leukaemia, lymphoma and bone-marrow transplantation, depress cellular immunity, and cytotoxic drugs used for some tumours result in impairment of both cellular and humoral immune mechanisms. Patients with a neutrophil count of less than 1×10^9 cell/litre appear to be most at risk. Immunocompromised patients are susceptible to any infection, although specific pathogens which are combatted easily in the normal patient may result also in life-threatening illness. Infections are caused usually by organisms which have colonized the patient before the acute episode; in one study of patients with acute non-lymphocytic leukaemia, almost 50% of these organisms were acquired within hospital (Schmipff *et al.*, 1972).

PREVENTION OF INFECTION IN THE
COMPROMISED PATIENT

Protective isolation

Simple isolation in an isolation room in which all staff wear a gown, mask and gloves, has not been found to reduce the risk of infection in the immunocompromised patient (Nauseef & Maki, 1981). The use of filtered air, which removes virtually all particles greater than 0.3 μm in diameter, has been shown to reduce dramatically the number of airborne micro-organisms. However, neither protective 'bubbles' nor laminar airflow rooms supplied with filtered air have been shown to influence the incidence of infection in immunocompromised patients in most of the randomized trials which have been conducted, although there is some evidence to suggest that the infection rate, and particularly the incidence of pneumonia, is reduced in patients who remain isolated for more than 3 weeks (Yates & Holland, 1974). Patients undergoing bone-marrow grafting for aplastic anaemia or leukaemia have a reduced incidence of graft rejection if isolated in a laminar airflow environment.

REDUCTION OF ENDOGENOUS BACTERIA

The gastrointestinal tract is the major site of colonization with bacteria which may subsequently cause clinically important infection. Hospital food, particularly salads and vegetables, has a high content of pathogens. Immunocompromised patients do not require sterile food, but food with low bacterial counts should be available. Sterilization of the gastrointestinal tract with non-absorbable antibiotics (usually gentamicin, vancomycin and nystatin) is effective in suppressing gut flora, but has not been proved conclusively to influence the incidence of infection; in addition, this regimen causes significant incidences of nausea, vomiting and diarrhoea. Selective suppression of gut flora with trimethoprim and sulphamethoxazole reduces the number of aerobic Gram-negative organisms in the gut, but has little effect on anaerobic bowel flora. This regimen has been shown to reduce the incidence of infections in immunocompromised patients with a variety of types of primary pathology. However, there is an increased risk of fungal infections, and little effect has been seen in the eventual outcome of the patients.

Topical antibiotic or antiseptic regimens have been suggested as a means of reducing skin flora. These involve usually bathing or showering daily in an antiseptic solution, with local antibiotic treatment of mouth and nose. However, it has proved to be virtually impossible to sterilize the skin completely, and the effect on infections remains unclear.

SPECIFIC PROPHYLAXIS

Viral infections are more common in immunocompromised patients. Reactivation of latent herpes simplex virus occurs in up to 40% of patients, but the incidence can be reduced by the administration of acyclovir. The risks of contracting varicella zoster infection in children, and cytomegalovirus infection in all immunocompromised patients, may be reduced by administration of specific immunoglobulins. Trimethoprim/sulphamethoxazole treatment reduces the risk of *Pneumocystis carinii* infection, but is recommended only for patients in areas where infection with this protozoon is common because of fears that resistant strains may develop.

Granulocyte infusions have been shown to reduce the incidence of bacterial sepsis by 60% in patients with leukaemia (Strauss *et al.*, 1981). However, overall infection rates and survival are not altered.

Prevention of spread of infection

There are three mechanisms (Table 71.15) by which infection may spread in the ITU. True airborne transmission in droplets of less than 10 μm in diameter, and transmission in larger droplets (i.e. greater than 10 μm) (which requires relatively close contact), have been implicated in spread of respiratory viral infections such as influenza, para-influenza, varicella, measles, rhinoviruses, rubella, echovirus and adenoviruses. Members of staff, rather than other patients, are usually the source. Paediatric patients are particularly susceptible. *Aspergillus* and other fungi may be present on dust particles in hospital, particularly during rebuilding programmes. *Pseudomonas* and staphylococci may be carried on droplets from infected linen. However, the major source is contaminated respiratory equipment, such as humidifiers and ventilators.

Indirect contact spread may occur if any item of equipment is contaminated by contact with an infected patient or staff member, and used subsequently without being sterilized. Stethoscopes are often contaminated with pathogens, especially *Staphylococcus aureus*, and should be cleaned regularly with 70% alcohol. Endoscopes are contaminated readily, and disinfection is difficult and time consuming. Bacteraemia following gastroduodenal endoscopy occurs in up to 8% of patients, and respiratory infection has been reported after use of contaminated bronchoscopes. Thermometers often harbour pathogenic organisms, despite the use of sheaths; perforation of plastic sheaths is common. Non-disposable items such as endotracheal tubes, suction tubing or drains may also transmit infection, although most units now use only disposable

Table 71.15 Mechanisms of spread of infection and reservoirs in ITU

Contact	Airborne	Ingestion
Mattresses	Ventilators	Food
Bandages	Humidifiers	Enteral feeds
Stethoscopes	Nebulizers	Ice
Endoscopes	Air conditioning	
Bronchoscopes	False ceilings	
Thermometers	Building work	
Suction apparatus	Staff respiratory	
Pressure transducers	infections	
Contaminated		
disinfectants		
Sinks		
Toilets		
Flower vases		

items. Infection may be spread also by contact with the bed, mattress or bed linen.

Indirect spread may result also from contamination of staff. Medical and nursing staff may become contaminated after contact with another patient, or from another source in the unit. Sinks are a common source. *Pseudomonas* has been isolated from up to 59% of hospital sinks, and may contaminate staff either by direct contact or by large droplet spread during hand-washing. Heat traps are effective in reducing contamination of the waste pipe.

Many types of bacteria have been isolated from water in flower vases. Nurses' hands may become contaminated after changing water in vases, or if spillage occurs. In most units, fresh flowers are not permitted for this reason. Contaminated water has been implicated in the transmission of intravascular infection; warm water baths for thawing fresh frozen plasma, and iced water baths for cooling syringes before thermodilution cardiac output measurements, can result in bacteraemia.

Patients with some types of infection present a particular risk both to other patients and to staff. Various degrees of isolation may be required to minimize this risk.

Isolation

Prevention of cross-infection from an infected patient requires that precautions must be taken which are appropriate to the nature of the infective organism, the source (e.g. respiratory tract, body secretions, skin) and the means of transmission. In many cases, adequate isolation may be achieved with the patient in the main area of the ward. However, an isolation room should be available for some categories of patient. This room should have a negative air pressure relative to the main unit, and the room should be vented directly to the outside of the building.

Isolation precautions may be considered as category-specific or disease-specific. Recommendations for category-specific isolation are summarized in Table 71.16, and examples of diseases requiring each category of isolation are shown in Table 71.17.

Antibiotic resistance

Resistance to antibiotics may occur by a number of mechanisms. Bacteria vary in the composition of the cell wall which surrounds the cell membrane; Gram-positive bacteria are relatively permeable to antibiotics,

Table 71.16 Category-specific isolation requirements. (From Garner & Simmons, 1983)

Strict isolation
Private room, door kept closed
Mask, gown and gloves must be worn by all persons entering room
Hands must be washed after touching patient or contaminated articles
Contaminated articles e.g. linen, must be discarded or bagged and labelled before being sent for decontamination

Contact isolation
Private room
Masks should be worn by those in close contact with patient
Gowns should be worn if soiling with infected material likely
Gloves should be worn if touching infected material
Hand-washing and disposal as for strict isolation

Respiratory isolation
Private room
Masks should be worn by those in close contact with patient
Hand-washing and disposal as for strict isolation

Tuberculous isolation
Private room with negative pressure, door closed
Masks should be worn if patient is coughing
Gowns should be worn if gross contamination likely
Hand-washing and disposal as for strict isolation

Enteric precautions
Private room if patient hygiene poor, or if incontinent
Gowns should be worn if soiling likely
Gloves should be worn when touching infected material
Hand-washing and disposal as for strict isolation

Drainage/secretion precautions
Gowns should be worn if soiling likely
Gloves should be worn when touching infected material
Hand-washing and disposal as for strict isolation

Blood/body fluid precautions
Private room if patient hygiene poor, or if incontinent
Gowns should be worn if soiling with blood or body fluids likely
Gloves should be worn if touching blood or body fluids
Hands must be washed immediately if contaminated with blood or body fluids, and always before touching another patient
Needlestick injuries should be avoided
Used needles should be placed immediately in a labelled, puncture-resistant container
Spilt blood should be cleaned immediately with sodium hypochlorite solution
Disposal as for strict isolation

Table 71.17 Category-specific isolation recommendations. (From Garner & Simmons, 1983)

Strict isolation
Varicella
Diphtheria
Viral haemorrhagic fevers (e.g. Lassa fever)
Pneumonic plague

Contact isolation
Multiply resistant, Gram-negative bacilli
Methicillin-resistant *Staphylococcus aureus*
Major wound sepsis
Group A *Streptococcus pneumoniae*
Rubella

Respiratory isolation
Measles
Meningococcal meningitis
Mumps
Pertussis

Tuberculous isolation
Active pulmonary tuberculosis
Laryngeal tuberculosis

Enteric precautions
Cholera
Enteroviral infections
Hepatitis A
Poliomyelitis
Salmonella enteritis

Drainage/secretion precautions
Minor abscess
Conjunctivitis
Minor infected decubitus ulcer
Minor wound infection

Blood/body fluid precautions
Acquired immunodeficiency syndrome
Hepatitis B
Hepatitis non-A, non-B
Malaria

whereas Gram-negative organisms have a more complex wall which is less permeable. Many microorganisms synthesize enzymes which inactivate antibiotics. Beta-lactamases are a group of enzymes which can inactivate the β-lactam ring of a variety of antibiotics including most penicillins and cephalosporins. These enzymes may be excreted into the immediate surroundings of the bacteria, or may exist between the inner and outer cell membranes. They may be a normal constituent of the bacterium, or their production may be induced in the presence of an antibiotic. The capacity to produce the enzymes may be mediated by chromosomes or by plasmids; plasmid-mediated resistance may be transferred to other bacteria of the same, or occasionally of other, species. Some species of Gram-negative bacteria produce β-lactamases which are capable of inactivating the newer β-lactam antibiotics. Aminoglycoside-modifying enzymes are produced by some species of Gram-positive and Gram-negative bacteria, and account for most of the resistance which occurs to these antibiotics. Many of these enzymes are plasmid mediated, and once induced in a hospital strain, resistance spreads rapidly. Chloramphenicol can be inactivated by a specific enzyme produced by some strains of *Haemophilus influenzae* and *Streptococcus pneumoniae*.

Alteration of the cellular target sites is perhaps the most serious method by which resistance can develop. Structural changes may occur in the penicillin-binding proteins, the normal target sites of penicillins of the cytoplasmic membrane. These changes reduce the affinity of the target sites for penicillin molecules, and render these antibiotics useless. This mechanism has been implicated in the development of resistance by enterococci, gonococci, *Haemophilus influenzae* and methicillin-resistant *Staphylococcus aureus*. Similar structural changes account for some types of resistance to other antibiotics, and are plasmid mediated. There is therefore the possibility that this form of resistance could spread rapidly to many bacterial species.

The development of resistant strains of bacteria is related largely to the quantity of antibiotics administered. Almost 30% of hospitalized patients receive one or more antibiotics, and as many as 50% of these may be administered inappropriately. Areas of the hospital with the highest antibiotic usage, such as the ITU, have also the highest incidence of resistant strains (McGowan, 1983). A number of studies have shown that decreased use of an antibiotic to which resistance has developed leads to a decrease in the isolation of resistant strains.

PROBLEM ORGANISMS

Staphylococcus aureus

This organism has produced a succession of phage types resistant to a variety of antibiotics. Previous resistant strains have disappeared without any apparent reason. The current resistant strain is not particularly virulent, but can cause serious postoperative sepsis, especially after vascular surgery. It is extremely resistant to almost all antibiotics, including gentamicin, methicillin and cloxacillin. Vancomycin is one of the few effective agents against this strain.

Staphylococcus epidermidis

The use of intravenous catheters and prosthetic surgery have resulted in this previously commensal organism becoming a serious pathogen. Most strains are resistant to the commonly used antibiotics.

Gram-negative bacteria

Although *Pseudomonas* species and *Klebsiella* are common causes of serious infection in the ITU, more unusual strains have started to emerge in patients treated with broad-spectrum antibiotics. These include *Enterobacter*, *Serratia* and *Acinetobacter*, which are resistant often to most antibiotics.

Infection control policy

Every hospital should have an infection control policy, which defines the criteria for isolation, gives guidance for the use of disinfectants and antiseptics in each department of the hospital, and for the decontamination and disinfection of equipment. It should be revised periodically by an infection control committee, which should be responsible in addition for education of staff, and implementation of the policy. It should give guidance also on local use of antibiotics. Control of antibiotic use varies, but in general, it is best if a hospital confines itself to the use of a single first-line drug in each of the following categories: aminoglycoside, second- or third-generation cephalosporin, broadspectrum penicillin, antistaphylococcal penicillin, tetracycline. Toxicity and cost should be considered when selecting the first-line agents. Antibiotic prophylaxis for surgery should not be given for prolonged periods; in general, there is no advantage in continuing therapy for more than 24 hr. By consultation with the microbiologists, it should be possible in most cases to select an appropriate empirical agent for treatment before culture and sensitivities have been obtained.

Analgesia and sedation

Sedation is required in many patients admitted to the ITU. Patients are exposed to a number of noxious stimuli. They may experience pain after trauma or surgery, distress and discomfort from the presence of an endotracheal tube and mechanical ventilation, and anxiety from appreciation of the severity of their illness. In addition, there are intermittent stimuli during physiotherapy, tracheal suction and nursing procedures such as turning and changing of dressings.

The major complication from sedative and analgesic drugs is respiratory depression. Clearly, this is of little importance in the patient who requires controlled ventilation, but the choice of sedative drug must be made carefully in the patient who is breathing spontaneously, in those treated with intermittent mandatory ventilation and if mechanical ventilation is to be discontinued in the near future.

A number of mechanisms are available for reducing the quantity of pharmacological sedation which patients require. Frequent communication and reassurance from all staff can do much to allay anxiety, and are essential in every patient. Lack of windows in the ITU deprives patients of the normal day–night cycle and of information on seasonal and weather conditions. In one study, the incidence of postoperative delirium was between two and three times higher in patients managed in an ITU without windows than in those nursed in a unit with windows (Wilson, 1972). Intermittent mandatory ventilation reduces the discomfort and distress associated with mechanical ventilation by permitting the patient to take spontaneous breaths on demand. Moderate hypocapnia reduces respiratory drive and improves toleration of mechanical ventilation. Nasotracheal intubation is tolerated better by most patients than an orotracheal tube. One of the major complaints of patients after leaving an ITU is the unpleasant memory of insertion of intravenous and intra-arterial cannulae; these procedures can be made more pleasant by the use of local anaesthesia. Nevertheless, drugs are required to sedate or provide analgesia in most patients, at least in the early days of admission.

Ideal level of sedation

There is no necessity for patients to be rendered totally unconscious during their stay in ITU. If sedation is unnecessarily heavy, recovery times are prolonged. There may be a risk also of immunosuppression and an increased incidence of infection if large doses of intravenous anaesthetic agents (Ward et al., 1985) or opioids (Tubaro et al., 1983) are used. Ramsay et al. (1974) described a six-point sedation score applicable to patients in the ITU (Table 71.18). In most patients,

Table 71.18 Scoring system for assessment of sedation in ITU patients. (From Ramsay *et al.*, 1974)

Level	Response
1	Anxious, and agitated or restless or both
2	Co-operative, orientated and tranquil
3	Responds to commands only
4	Asleep, but brisk response to glabellar tap or loud auditory stimulus
5	Asleep, sluggish response to glabellar tap or loud auditory stimulus
6	No response

adjustment of doses of sedative drugs to maintain a level between points 2 and 3 on their scale is desirable. This ensures that the patient is comfortable, and minimizes the risks of prolonged sedation and respiratory depression when administration is discontinued.

METHOD OF ADMINISTRATION

Most drugs used for sedation are given parenterally. Sedation is achieved most satisfactorily by continuous intravenous infusion, which avoids the peaks and troughs associated with the use of intermittent administration. However, it is often necessary to supplement this basal sedation with small increments of rapidly acting agents (e.g. intravenous anaesthetic, fentanyl or alfentanil) or with an inhalational anaesthetic before painful procedures such as physiotherapy or changing of wound dressings. This is especially true in patients with intracranial hypertension, in whom painful stimulation can cause acute and dangerous rises in intracranial pressure secondary to arterial hypertension, coughing and straining.

Analgesics

Opioids are the most commonly administered drugs for sedation in ITU. In a recent survey, 37% of units used an opioid alone for routine sedation, and a further 60% used an opioid in combination with a benzodiazepine (Bion & Ledingham, 1987). Opioids are appropriate for any patient in whom pain is anticipated, although the dose must be titrated carefully in patients in whom artificial ventilation of the lungs is not anticipated. In the artificially ventilated patient, the antitussive action of the opioids may help toleration of an endotracheal tube. The dose of opioid is dependent in part upon severity of the patient's illness;

less morphine is required to sedate patients with high APACHE II scores (Bion *et al.*, 1986).

Morphine

Morphine is an appropriate drug in many situations in the ITU. Its slow distribution half-life and relative lipid insolubility are disadvantages if a rapid onset of action is required, but in the patient in whom sedation is required for many hr or several days, analgesia may be achieved by a loading dose followed by a continuous infusion. Adjustment of the dose results in a relatively slow change in level of analgesia. A loading dose of 10–15 mg followed by an infusion of 2–3 mg/hr is an acceptable initial regimen in the adult. However, as with all opioid drugs, there is enormous interindividual variation in both pharmacokinetics and pharmacodynamics, and the dose must be adjusted for each patient. Distribution volumes and protein binding may be abnormal in the ITU patient, resulting in an exaggerated or diminished response. However, morphine is less protein bound than other opioids. The clinical effect of alterations in hepatic function on its metabolism is small, although clinical factors which reduce hepatic blood flow, such as shock, would be expected to reduce the elimination of the drug. The main disadvantage of morphine in the ITU patient relates to the elimination of its metabolites, which are excreted normally in the urine. One of the main metabolites, morphine-6-glucuronide (M6G), is an active analgesic, and blood concentrations of M6G may reach high levels after prolonged infusions, particularly in patients with impaired renal function (Osborne *et al.*, 1986). Thus, the infusion rate may have to be decreased after several hours, and there may be a much longer delay between cessation of the infusion and diminution of clinical effect than the elimination half-life of up to 4 hr (Table 71.19) might suggest. If very large doses have been employed, respiratory depression and excessive sedation may last in excess of 24 hr.

Papaveretum

The analgesic effects of this drug, which is the most commonly used opioid in British ITUs (Bion & Ledingham, 1987), result predominantly from the morphine which it contains, but the other alkaloids appear to provide more of a sedative effect than morphine alone. This may be an advantage in many patients, but results in prolonged narcosis if large doses are given, particu-

Table 71.19 Approximate distribution and elimination half-lives of opioid agents in normal patients

Agent	Distribution half-life (min)	Elimination half-life (hr)
Morphine	25	1.5–4
glucuronides	—	3–6
Fentanyl	3	2–5
Sufentanil	1	2–3
Alfentanil	3	1.5–3.5
Phenoperidine	3	1.5–4
Pethidine	7	3–6.5
Nalbuphine	2	3.5–4
Buprenorphine*	3	2–4.5

*The clinical effects of buprenorphine are not related to serum concentration but to receptor binding.

larly to elderly patients or those with hepatic or renal impairment.

Fentanyl

This drug is often thought to be superior to morphine or papaveretum because of its short duration after a single bolus dose. However, this effect is the result of its high lipid-solubility, which permits rapid equilibration between blood and CNS. As the drug is distributed into other tissues also, concentrations in the blood and CNS decay within a few minutes, and its analgesic and respiratory depressant actions wane. However, after repeated administration, or after prolonged infusion, blood and CNS concentrations decrease only as the drug is metabolized, as distribution into other tissues has occured already. The elimination half-life of fentanyl is longer than that of morphine (Table 71.19) after bolus doses; in the elderly, the elimination half-life is extended to 9 hr, and may be as long as 16 hr after prolonged infusion (Shafer et al., 1983). Consequently, fentanyl is *not* a short-acting drug when used for analgesia in the ITU, and offers little advantage over morphine.

Alfentanil

Alfentanil has a small distribution volume and short terminal half-life in most patients. Consequently, it should be a useful drug for administration by infusion, as changes in infusion rate should produce a rapid alteration in clinical effect. However, it is an expensive agent. In some patients, its elimination is delayed and

its duration of action prolonged (Yate et al., 1986). When a prolonged period of analgesia is anticipated, it may be appropriate to use alfentanil to establish analgesia rapidly before transferring to another opioid; its use might be considered also towards the end of the treatment period to reduce the risks of prolonged respiratory depression when the infusion is discontinued.

Pethidine

Pethidine is a useful alternative to morphine, especially in patients prone to bronchospasm. It is rather more lipid soluble than morphine, and its actions are therefore of more rapid onset. However, it depresses myocardial function in high doses, and its major metabolite, norpethidine, has convulsant properties. Blood concentrations of pethidine are increased in the elderly, and its elimination is delayed in patients with hepatic dysfunction.

SIDE-EFFECTS OF OPIOIDS

Respiratory

All pure agonist opioids cause respiratory depression. It is likely that equianalgesic doses of any pure agonist result in equal degrees of respiratory depression. This side-effect is often advantageous during controlled ventilation. However, residual effects of opioids on the respiratory centre may delay weaning from the ventilator. The delay is unpredictable to some extent, even with the shorter-acting agents. The rate of elimination of opioids may vary by a factor of five even in normal individuals, and impaired metabolism and excretion, together with accumulation of active metabolites, may result in a very prolonged duration of action in some patients.

Cardiovascular

All opioids may reduce arterial pressure by causing arterial and venous dilatation. This effect is seen particularly in the hypovolaemic patient. In addition, an initial decrease in arterial pressure may result from the alleviation of pain and anxiety. Fentanyl has less depressant effect on the cardiovascular system than morphine in patients with cardiac disease. Pethidine has vagolytic action which results in an increase in heart rate. The cardiovascular effects can be minimized by ensuring that the circulating volume is adequate, and by providing the initial loading dose as an infusion over 10–15 min rather than as a single bolus dose.

Gastrointestinal

All the opioids delay gastric emptying and decrease intestinal motility. This may impair the ability to absorb enteral feeds, and may increase the risks of regurgitation and aspiration of gastric contents. Spasm of the sphincter of Oddi and an increase in common bile duct pressure may occur, but the clinical significance of this in the ITU patient is not clear.

TOLERANCE AND ADDICTION

Some degree of tolerance to opioids may occur after 3–4 days, and the infusion dose may have to be increased. Tolerance occurs to both the analgesic and respiratory depressant effects. Addiction, reflected by withdrawal symptoms when the drug is discontinued, is extremely uncommon in patients who receive opioids for the treatment of pain, and fear of addiction should not limit dosage adjustments if tolerance develops.

NON-OPIOID ANALGESICS

The combination of opioid and non-opioid analgesics may reduce the dose of opioid drugs required to produce adequate analgesia, and thus reduce the potential for side-effects. *Indomethacin* suppositories reduce the need for morphine after surgery (Reasbeck *et al.*, 1982) and have been used successfully to supplement opioids in patients with blunt chest trauma. However, the incidence of haemorrhagic complications is increased. *Lysine acetyl salicylic acid* can be administered parenterally, and provides good postoperative analgesia (Cashman *et al.*, 1985).

Sedation

Sedative drugs may be used alone, or in combination with opioids, to achieve sleep and anxiolysis in the ITU patient. Provided sufficient analgesia is achieved, not all patients require sedative drugs, particularly after the first 24–48 hr following admission. It is inappropriate to use high doses of opioids to achieve sedation, as the doses required may result in prolonged respiratory depression. Similarly, it is inappropriate to use sedative agents alone for patients who are in pain, as very high doses are required. If patients have no pain, sedatives alone may be administered. In most patients, however, a balanced combination of analgesic and sedative drugs titrated to individual needs results in relief of pain and anxiety, but permits continued communication with staff.

Benzodiazepines

These agents induce sleep, anxiolysis and decrease in muscle tone. Although total sleep-time is increased, there is a reduction in REM (rapid eye movement) sleep.

Diazepam has an elimination half-life of 36 hr, and an active metabolite, *N*-desmethyl diazepam, with an elimination half-life of up to 96 hr. Infusion of diazepam is therefore inappropriate, and it is administered best as a loading dose with maintenance doses every 12–24 hr. Recovery of consciousness may take several days if large doses are administered.

Midazolam has a rapid onset of action, and a shorter duration of action than diazepam. Its elimination half-life in normal individuals is 2–4 hr after a single dose, although this may be prolonged significantly in critically ill patients (Shelly *et al.*, 1987). It has no active metabolites. It is water soluble and may be administered safely into peripheral veins.

Flunitrazepam and *lorazepam* have much longer half-lives (20 and 15 hr respectively). Lorazepam also has a slow onset of action.

Although these agents produce profound amnesia, they often fail to achieve satisfactory sedation. Amnesia *per se* may not prevent subsequent psychological sequelae after traumatic experiences; indeed, memory may be improved by benzodiazepines in anxious individuals (Desai *et al.*, 1983). All the benzodiazepines tend to produce cardiovascular and respiratory depression. However, their major disadvantage relates to the prolonged recovery times after large doses. The benzodiazepine antagonist flumazenil may be useful in reversing the sedative effects of these agents. However, its properties in the critically ill patient have not yet been investigated adequately. It has a short elimination half-life and may need to be given for many hours if the duration of sedation with benzodiazepines has been prolonged. It is very expensive.

Intravenous anaesthetics

BARBITURATES

Thiopentone and pentobarbitone are indicated occasionally in patients with severe head injury, as they help to control intracranial hypertension. However, after prolonged administration, slow elimination results in prolonged coma. In moderate doses (approximately 100 mg/hr) for up to 14 days, recovery of consciousness takes up to 48 hr. In doses high enough to produce an isoelectric electroencephalogram, recovery may take up to 4 days (Stanski et al., 1980). Deep coma induced with thiopentone for treatment of patients with head injury has been associated with an increased incidence of pulmonary infection and ARDS (Ward et al., 1985), possibly as a result of reduced immunological competence. Barbiturates in high doses may result in significant cardiovascular depression.

ETOMIDATE

This relatively recent anaesthetic agent was used widely for sedation in the ITU, although no controlled clinical trials had been undertaken to confirm its safety during prolonged infusion. Careful audit in one unit resulted in the detection of increased mortality associated with infective complications in a group of trauma patients who had received etomidate (Watt & Ledingham, 1984). Further investigations revealed that etomidate induces adrenocortical suppression, even after a single dose (Moore et al., 1985). It is therefore entirely unsuitable as a sedative agent in the critically ill patient.

PROPOFOL

This new agent is insoluble in water, and therefore is formulated in a lipid emulsion. It has a short elimination half-life (less than 1 hr), and recovery of consciousness from anaesthesia after single bolus or short infusion is free of the 'hangover' associated with the use of most other intravenous anaesthetic drugs.

Only limited information is available regarding the safety of propofol for sedation. It has been used successfully for 2.5–18 hr after cardiac surgery (Grounds et al., 1987). The use of propofol was associated with more easily controlled sedation than midazolam, and a shorter requirement for mechanical ventilation. The median time from discontinuation of the infusion to the return of spontaneous respiration was 9.5 min after propofol and 202 min after midazolam.

In a study conducted in five general ITUs (UK Multi-Centre Study), 100 patients were allocated randomly to receive either propofol or midazolam, in combination with a continuous infusion of morphine 2 mg/hr, for up to 24 hr. The level of sedation was adjusted easily during propofol infusion (1–3 mg/hr), and recovery of consciousness was rapid at the end of the study period. Cardiovascular depression did occur with propofol, but appeared to be accompanied by maintenance of peripheral perfusion. It responded to intravenous fluid infusion, and it was not necessary to discontinue propofol administration because of side-effects. There were no biochemical abnormalities attributable to either drug. Although plasma cortisol concentration decreased during the infusion of both drugs, there was no inhibition to the Synacthen test. The lipid solution was not associated with adverse effects.

In a small number of ITU patients who received propofol because of severe agitation, there appeared to be minimal accumulation of the drug over a 4-day period, and recovery times, which were assessed every 24 hr, remained rapid (less than 30 min) (Beller et al., 1988).

However, it must be stressed that experience with this agent is limited. The drug is cleared more slowly in the presence of renal insufficiency. The safety of infusions for longer than 24 hr has not yet been established.

CHLORMETHIAZOLE

This drug is used occasionally to sedate ITU patients. It produces little cardiovascular depression, and may increase heart rate and arterial pressure. However, it is formulated for intravenous use only in a dilute solution, and large volumes are required to provide sedative doses. It is metabolized slowly in patients with hepatic dysfunction, and this may result in prolonged recovery of consciousness.

KETAMINE

This drug has analgesic properties at subanaesthetic doses (0.5 mg/kg). However, its use as a sedative has been disappointing except in patients with severe bronchospasm, where it has been used successfully (Strube & Hallam, 1986).

Inhalational anaesthetic agents

Virtually all the inhalational anaesthetic agents have been used to produce sedation in the ITU. Nitrous oxide is useful in providing intermittent analgesia, for example during physiotherapy or other painful procedures. Concentrations up to 70% have been used, but may be limited by the requirement of the patient for a high inspired oxygen concentration. Prolonged use of nitrous oxide is associated with megaloblastic bone-marrow changes (Amos et al., 1982). Enflurane and isoflurane have been used also, but there have been no adequate investigations of the use of these agents for prolonged periods. Adequate scavenging facilities must be provided if inhalational agents are used.

Neuromuscular blocking drugs

A study published as recently as 1980 (Miller-Jones & Williams, 1980) showed that pancuronium was administered to 'calm' 48 out of 50 ventilated patients, and that it was by far the most commonly used drug for encouraging patients to tolerate artificial ventilation, in some cases without any sedation or analgesia. A subsequent editorial (Editorial, 1981) drew attention to the dangers of such treatment. It is now uncommon for neuromuscular blocking drugs to be used in the ITU; only 16% of units surveyed in 1987 used them, and 71% of these employed them only rarely (Bion & Ledingham, 1987). However, they are still indicated in some circumstances. In patients who are severely hypoxic, oxygenation may be improved if chest-wall compliance is increased by using a neuromuscular blocking drug, particularly if the patient is restless. In patients with intracranial hypertension, improved control of intracranial pressure may be achieved by neuromuscular blocking drugs, probably because of an increase in venous capacitance secondary to a reduction in skeletal muscle tone. It is essential to ensure that the patient is sedated adequately before a neuromuscular blocking drug is given.

Pancuronium achieved popularity in the ITU because of its tendency to increase arterial pressure. However, it induces tachycardia also. Vecuronium and atracurium have little effect on the cardiovascular system. However, vecuronium may accumulate in the critically ill patient (Smith et al., 1987) and atracurium is probably preferable if a neuromuscular blocking drug is indicated.

Regional analgesia

Some patients in ITU may benefit from regional techniques of analgesia, such as the use of extradural local anaesthetic or opioid administration. However, the presence of sepsis or coagulation defects are contra-indications to regional analgesia.

References

Allen E.V. (1929) Thromboangiitis obliterans: methods of diagnosis of chronic occlusive arterial lesions distal to the wrist with illustrative cases. *American Journal of Medical Science* **178**, 237–44.

Amos R.J., Amess J.A.L., Hinds C.J. & Mollin D.L. (1982) Incidence and pathogenesis of acute megaloblastic bone-marrow changes in patients receiving intensive care. *Lancet* **2**, 835–9.

Band J.D. & Maki D.G. (1979) Infections caused by arterial catheters used for hemodynamic monitoring. *American Journal of Medicine* **67**, 735–41.

Bedford R.F. & Wollman H. (1973) Complications of radial-artery cannulation: an objective prospective study in man. *Anesthesiology* **38**, 228–36.

Beller J.P., Pottecher T., Lugnier A., Mangin P. & Otteni J.C. (1988) Prolonged sedation with propofol (Diprivan) in ITU patients: recovery and blood concentration decreases during periodic interruptions of infusion. *British Journal of Anaesthesia* **61** (In press).

Berenson R.A. (1984) *Intensive Care Units (ITUs): Clinical Outcomes, Costs and Decisionmaking (Health Technology Study 28).* Office of Technology Assessment, US Congress, OTA-HCS-28, Washington, D.C.

Bion J.F., Edlin S.A., Ramsay G., McCabe S. & Ledingham I.McA. (1985) Validation of a prognostic score in critically ill patients undergoing transport. *British Medical Journal* **291**, 432–4.

Bion J.F. & Ledingham, I.McA. (1987) Sedation in intensive care—a postal survey. *Intensive Care Medicine* **13**, 215–16.

Bion J.F., Logan B.K., Newman P.M., Brodie M.J., Oliver J.S. & Aitchison T.C. (1986) Sedation in intensive care: morphine and renal function. *Intensive Care Medicine* **12**, 359–65.

Cashman J.N., Jones R.M., Foster J.M. & Adams A.P. (1985) Comparison of infusions of morphine and lysine acetyl salicylate for the relief of pain after surgery. *British Journal of Anaesthesia* **57**, 255–8.

Centers for Disease Control Working Group (1981) Guidelines for prevention of intravascular infections. In *Guidelines for the Prevention and Control of Nosocomial Infections.* VSDHS-PHS.

Chang R.W.S., Jacobs S. & Lee B. (1986) Use of APACHE II severity of disease classification to identify intensive-care-unit patients who would not benefit from total parenteral nutrition. *Lancet* **1**, 1483–7.

Chastre J., Viau F., Brun P., Pierre J., Dauge M.C., Bouchama A., Akesbi A. & Gilbert C. (1984) Prospective evaluation of the protected specimen brush for the diagnosis of pulmonary infections in ventilated patients. *American Review of Respiratory Disease* **130**, 924–9.

Cooper G.L. & Hopkins C.C. (1985) Rapid diagnosis of intravascular catheter-associated infection by direct gram staining of catheter segments. *New England Journal of Medicine* **312**, 1142–7.

Craig C.P. & Connelly S. (1984) Effect of intensive care unit nosocomial pneumonia on duration of stay and mortality.

American Journal of Infection Control 12, 233–8.

Cullen D.J. (1977) Results and costs of intensive care. *Anesthesiology* 47, 203–16.

Deam R., Kimberley A.P.S., Anderson M. & Soni N. (1988) AIDS in ITUs: outcome. *Anaesthesia* 43, 150–1.

Department of Health and Social Security (1970) *Intensive Therapy Unit*. Hospital Building Note (HBN) 27.

Desai N., Taylor-Davies A. & Barnett D.B. (1983) The effects of diazepam and oxprenolol on short term memory in individuals of high and low state anxiety. *British Journal of Clinical Pharmacology* 15, 197–202.

Dudley H.A.F. (1987) Intensive care: a specialty or a branch of anaesthetics? *British Medical Journal* 294, 459–60.

duMoulin G.C., Paterson D.G., Hedley-White J. & Lisbon A. (1982) Aspiration of gastric bacteria in antacid-treated patients: a frequent cause of postoperative colonisation of the airway. *Lancet* 1, 242–5.

Editorial (1981) Paralysed with fear. *Lancet* 1, 427.

Farber B.F. (1987) Nosocomial infections: an introduction. In *Infection Control in Intensive Care* (Clinics in Critical Care Medicine 12) (Ed. Farber B.F.) pp. 1–7. Churchill Livingstone, New York.

Fedullo A.J. & Swinburne A.J. (1983) Relationship of patient age to cost and survival in a medical ITU. *Critical Care Medicine* 11, 155–9.

Feeley T.W., Faumarez R., Klick J.M., McNabb T.G. & Skillman J.J. (1975) Positive end-expiratory pressure in weaning patients from controlled ventilation. A prospective randomized trial. *Lancet* ii, 725–8.

Fletcher R., Jonson B., Cumming G. & Brew J. (1981) The concept of deadspace with special reference to the single breath test for carbon dioxide. *British Journal of Anaesthesia* 53, 77–88.

Garner J.S. & Simmons B.P. (1983) Guideline for isolation precautions in hospitals. *Infection Control* 4, 245–325.

Grounds R.M., Lalor J.M., Lumley J., Royston D. & Morgan M. (1987) Propofol infusion for sedation in the intensive care unit: a preliminary report. *British Medical Journal* 294, 397–400.

Hanson G. (1985) Training doctors for intensive therapy. *Care of the Critically Ill* 1, 4–5.

Henning R.J., Wiener F., Valdes S. & Weil M.H. (1979) Measurement of toe temperature for assessing the severity of acute circulatory failure. *Surgery Gynecology and Obstetrics* 149, 1–7.

Huxley E.J., Viroslav J., Gray W.R. & Pierce A.K. (1978) Pharyngeal aspiration in normal adults and patients with depressed consciousness. *American Journal of Medicine* 64, 564–8.

Intensive Care Society (1984) *Standards for Intensive Care Units*. Biomedica, London.

Jacobs S., Chang R.W.S. & Lee B. (1987) One year's experience with the APACHE II severity of disease classification system in a general intensive care unit. *Anaesthesia* 42, 738–44.

Jennett B. (1984) Inappropriate use of intensive care. *British Medical Journal* 289, 1709–11.

Johanson W.G., Pierce A.K., Sanford J.P. & Thomas G.D. (1972) Nosocomial respiratory infections with gram-negative bacilli. The significance of colonization of the respiratory tract. *Annals of Internal Medicine* 77, 701–6.

Kaznitz P., Druger G.L., Yorra F. & Simmonds D.H. (1976) Mixed venous oxygen tension and hyperlactemia. Survival in severe cardiopulmonary disease. *Journal of the American Medical Association* 236, 570–4.

Keene A.R. & Cullen D.J. (1983) Therapeutic intervention scoring systems: update 1983. *Critical Care Medicine* 11, 1–3.

Kerr J.H., Coates D.P. & Gale L.B. (1985) Use of 'bollards' to improve patient access during intensive care. *Intensive Care Medicine* 11, 33–8.

Knaus W.A., Draper E.A., Wagner D.P. & Zimmerman J.E. (1985) APACHE II: a severity of disease classification system for acutely ill patients. *Critical Care Medicine* 13, 818–29.

Knaus W.A., Zimmerman J.E., Wagner D.P., Draper E.A. & Lawrence D. (1981) APACHE—acute physiology and chronic health evaluation: a physiologically based classification system. *Critical Care Medicine* 9, 591–7.

Ledingham I.McA. (1977) Care of the critically ill. In *Recent Advances in Intensive Therapy* (Ed. Ledingham I.McA.) pp. 1–7. Churchill Livingstone, Edinburgh.

Le Gall J.R., Loirat P., Alperovitch A., Glaser P., Granthil C., Mathieu D., Mercier P., Thomas R. & Villers D. (1984) A simplified acute physiology score for ITU patients. *Critical Care Medicine* 12, 975–7.

Lindsay S.L., Kerridge R. & Collett B.J. (1987) Abscess following cannulation of the radial artery. *Anaesthesia* 42, 654–7.

McGowan J.E. (1983) Antimicrobial resistance in hospital organisms and its relation to antibiotic use. *Reviews of Infectious Diseases* 5, 1033–48.

Maki D.G., Weise C.E. & Sarafin H.W. (1977) A semiquantitative method for identifying intravenous-catheter-related infection. *New England Journal of Medicine* 296, 1305–9.

Meakins J.L. (1984) Surgeons, surgery and pancreatitis. *Gastroenterologie Clinique et Biologique* 8, 531–2.

Miller-Jones C.M.H. & Williams J.H. (1980) Sedation for ventilation. A retrospective study of fifty patients. *Anaesthesia* 35, 1104–7.

Moore R.A., Allen M.C., Wood P.J., Rees L.H. & Sear J.W. (1985) Peri-operative endocrine effects of etomidate. *Anaesthesia* 40, 124–30.

Nauseef W.M. & Maki D.G. (1981) A study of the value of simple protective isolation in patients with granulocytopenia. *New England Journal of Medicine* 304, 448–53.

Osborne R.J., Joel S.P. & Slevin M.L. (1986) Morphine intoxication in renal failure: the role of morphine-6-glucuronide. *British Medical Journal* 292, 1548–9.

Ponce de Leon S. & Wenzel R.E. (1984) Hospital-acquired bloodstream infections with Staphylococcus epidermidis: review of 100 cases. *American Journal of Medicine* 77, 639–44.

Ramsay M.A.E., Savage T.M., Simpson B.R.J. & Goodwin R. (1974) Controlled sedation with alphaxalone/alphadolone. *British Medical Journal* 2, 656–9.

Reasbeck P.G., Rice M.L. & Reasbeck J.C. (1982) Double blind controlled trial of indomethacin as an adjunct to narcotic analgesia after major abdominal surgery. *Lancet* 2, 115–18.

Rosen M., Latto I.P. & Ng W.S. (1981) *Handbook of Percutaneous Central Venous Catheterisation*. W.B. Saunders, London.

Rowley K.M., Clubb S.K., Smith G.J.W. & Cabin H.S. (1984) Right sided infective endocarditis as a consequence of flow-directed pulmonary-artery catheterization. A clinicopathological study of 55 autopsied patients. *New England Journal of Medicine* 311, 1152–6.

Ruiz-Santana S., Jimenez A.G., Esteban A., Guerra L., Alvarez B., Corcia S., Gudin J., Martinez A., Quintana E., Armengol S., Gregori J., Arenzana A., Rosada L. & Sanmartin A. (1987) ITU pneumonias: a multi-institutional study. *Critical Care Medicine* 15, 930–2.

Russell J.A., Joel M., Hudson R.J., Mangano D.T. & Schlobohm R.M. (1983) Prospective evaluation of radial and femoral artery catheterization sites in critically ill adults. *Critical Care Medicine* 11, 936–9.

Schimpff S.C., Young V.M., Greene W.H., Vermeulen G.D., Moody

M.R. & Wiernik P.H. (1972) Origin of infection in acute nonlymphocytic leukemia: significance of hospital acquisition of potential pathogens. *Annals of Internal Medicine* **77**, 707–14.

Shafer A., White P.F., Schuttler J. & Rosenthal M.H. (1983) Use of a fentanyl infusion in the intensive care unit: tolerance to its anesthetic effects? *Anesthesiology* **59**, 245–8.

Shelly M.P., Mendel L. & Park G.R. (1987) Failure of critically ill patients to metabolise midazolam. *Anaesthesia* **42**, 619–26.

Smith C.L., Hunter J.M. & Jones R.S. (1987) Vecuronium infusions in patients with renal failure in an ITU. *Anaesthesia* **42**, 387–93.

Stamm W.E., Martin S.M. & Bennett J.V. (1977) Epidemiology of nosocomial infections due to gram-negative infections; aspects relevant to development and use of vaccines. *Journal of Infectious Diseases* **136**, S151.

Stanski D.R., Mihm F.G., Rosenthal M.H. & Kalman S.M. (1980) Pharmacokinetics of high-dose thiopental used in cerebral resuscitation. *Anesthesiology* **53**, 169–71.

Stevens R.M., Teres D., Skillmann J.J. & Feingold D.S. (1974) Pneumonia in an intensive care unit; a 30-month experience. *Archives of Internal Medicine* **134**, 106–111.

Stoddart J.C. (1986) A career post—with intensive therapy? *Anaesthesia* **41**, 1181–3.

Stoutenbeek C.P., van Saene H.K., Miranda D.R., Zandstra D.F. & Langrehr D. (1986) Nosocomial Gram-negative pneumonia in critically ill patients. A 3-year experience with a novel therapeutic regimen. *Intensive Care Medicine* **12**, 419–23.

Strauss R.G., Connett J.E., Gale R.P., Bloomfield C.D., Herzig G.P., McCullough J., Maguire L.C., Winston D.J., Ho W., Stump D.C., Miller W.V. & Koepke J.A. (1981) A controlled trial of prophyl-actic granulocyte transfusions during initial induction chemo-therapy for acute myelogenous leukemia. *New England Journal of Medicine* **305**, 597–603.

Strube P.J. & Hallam P.L. (1986) Ketamine by continuous infusion in status asthmaticus. *Anaesthesia* **41**, 1017–19.

Tubaro E., Borelli G., Croce C., Cavallo G. & Santiangelif, C. (1983) Effect of morphine on resistance to infection. *Journal of Infectious Diseases* **148**, 656–66.

Versprille A. (1984) Thermodilution in mechanically ventilated patients. *Intensive Care Medicine* **10**, 213–15.

Ward J.D., Becker D.P., Miller J.D., Choi S.C., Marmarou A., Wood C., Newlon P.G. & Keenan R. (1985) Failure of prophylactic barbiturate coma in the treatment of severe head injury. *Journal of Neurosurgery* **62**, 383–8.

Watt I. & Ledingham I.McA. (1984) Mortality amongst multiple trauma patients admitted to an intensive therapy unit. *Anaesthesia* **39**, 973–81.

Willatts S.M. (1985) Physiology of the nervous system. In *Textbook of Anaesthesia* (Eds Smith G. & Aitkenhead A.R.) pp. 72–100. Churchill Livingstone, Edinburgh.

Wilson L.M. (1972) Intensive care delirium. The effect of outside deprivation in a windowless unit. *Archives of Internal Medicine* **130**, 225–6.

Yate P.M., Thomas D., Short S.M., Sebel P.S. & Morton J. (1986) Comparison of infusions of alfentanil or pethidine for sedation of ventilated patients on the ITU. *British Journal of Anaesthesia* **58**, 1091–9.

Yates J.W. & Holland J.F. (1972) A controlled study of isolation and controlled endogenous microbial suppression in acute myelo-cytic leukemia patients. *Cancer* **32**, 1490–8.

72

Drug Intoxication and Poisoning

L. F. PRESCOTT

Self-poisoning is one of the most common causes of acute medical admission to hospital. In the UK, the total number of admissions for self-poisoning approaches 150 000 annually, but the true incidence is considerably higher, as not all patients are admitted or even referred to hospital. In adults and older children, self-poisoning is usually an intentional impulsive act which has been provoked by failure to cope with adverse social circumstances or breakdown in personal relationships. It is fashionable and it no longer carries the stigma of former times. It is indulged in more frequently by females than by males and the peak incidence is in the age range of 18–30 yr. Self-poisoning must always be a game of toxicological roulette to some extent but overall it is very safe. It would certainly not be so popular otherwise. The mortality in hospital patients is approximately 0.5 % (Jacobsen *et al.*, 1984), with most fatalities occurring in the elderly and in patients with serious underlying medical problems. The great majority of deaths from poisoning occur outside hospital and the total number in England and Wales is about 4000 per annum (Osselton *et al.*, 1984).

Epidemiology of acute poisoning

Classification of poisoning

Poisoning may be classified under the following main headings:

INTENTIONAL SELF-POISONING

This is the most common type in adults and older children, and the usual method is the taking of drugs in overdose. The adverse social and personal factors which lead up to the event include broken love affairs, separation, divorce, loneliness, homosexuality, debts, conflict with the law, court appearance, alcoholism, drug abuse, poor housing, unemployment and disordered or inadequate personality. Some patients with intractable social problems, drug or alcohol abuse and inadequate personality poison themselves repeatedly over a period of months or years, despite all efforts at reform. They carry often a mind-boggling burden of psychotropic polypharmacy obtained by repeat prescription. Not only is this unlikely to help them, but potentially depressing drugs such as benzodiazepines and major tranquillizers may actually predispose to self-poisoning (Prescott & Highley, 1985).

Children older than 8–10 yr tend to copy their parents increasingly and take drugs in overdosage when they are unable to cope with pressures at home and at school. In addition, the abuse of drugs and solvents (glue sniffing) has become an increasing problem in school children, especially in boys.

An important minority of patients have serious premeditated and persistent suicidal intent. Some of these suffer from genuine psychiatric illness such as schizophrenia and depression (as distinct from unhappiness, frustration or disappointment), and it is essential that a full psychosocial assessment is carried out in all cases on recovery so that such patients can be identified and treated. It is important also to remember that these patients may make further determined attempts on their life whilst under medical supervision. Other, less severely disturbed patients may require psychiatric follow-up and support also, and official guidance has been issued recently on the psychosocial assessment of self-poisoners (Department of Health and Social Security, 1984). Although described often as a 'suicide attempt' or 'suicide gesture', the intentional taking of drugs and poison is best referred to as 'self-poisonig', as this does not imply any motive. Most patients do not intend to kill themselves and seek only to escape from an intolerable situation.

ACCIDENTAL POISONING

This is common in toddlers and very young children who eat almost anything that they can obtain. An incredible variety of substances and objects may be taken, including the whole range of domestic products together with plants (e.g. berries), nuts and bolts, batteries and fireworks, etc. To these should be added drugs, most of which are now brightly coloured and as irresistible to an inquisitive youngster as Liquorice Allsorts. In 1984, more than 25 000 children were admitted to hospital in England with suspected accidental poisoning, but fortunately serious consequences are rare and the mortality is very low. In a recent survey of 2043 cases in children under 5 yr of age, drugs were involved in 59%, household products in 37% and plants in 3% (Wiseman et al., 1987). Less than 5% of children taking household products suffer serious consequences (Craft et al., 1984).

Accidental poisoning is uncommon in adults and older children, and it occurs usually because of confusion over identity and labelling. All too often poisonous substances (e.g. paraquat concentrate) are decanted into beer or lemonade bottles without warning labels and left carelessly for an unsuspecting victim to drink. Accidental carbon monoxide poisoning may occur with incomplete combustion of carbon-containing fuels (e.g. a gas fire with a blocked flue) and inadequate ventilation. Other forms of accidental poisoning include toxicity caused by stings and bites (e.g. by adders), ingestion of contaminated food and the consumption of poisonous plants and fungi.

NON-ACCIDENTAL POISONING IN CHILDREN

In recent years it has been recognized that parents (usually the mother) may abuse their children by poisoning them with drugs deliberately (Dine & McGovern, 1982). In some cases, the objective may be to quieten the child, in others the circumstances resemble child battering with toxicological rather than physical assault, and in another group, drugs may be used to produce the equivalent of the syndrome of 'Munchausen by proxy'. Subacute and chronic intoxication produced by non-accidental poisoning may lead to extensive and expensive investigation before the true cause is recognized (Rogers et al., 1976).

DRUG ABUSE AND DRUGS 'FOR KICKS'

Drug abuse is a very serious problem, and increasing numbers of young people are referred to hospital with complications (Horn et al., 1987). Overdosage may cause acute behavioural disturbances, coma and cardiorespiratory disasters. The drugs involved include hallucinogens and central stimulants such as lysergic acid diethylamide (LSD), anticholinergics, herbal cigarettes, 'magic mushrooms', cyclizine, sympathomimetics, amphetamines and cocaine, and depressants such as barbiturates, organic solvents (e.g. toluene and trichloroethane) and opioid analgesics. Inexperienced drug takers may become frightened by the effects produced by hallucinogens, whilst others become violent and uncontrollable. Mainlining abusers of 'street' opioids overdose because they are ignorant of the strength and purity of what they inject, and multiple drug abuse is common. Some intravenous opioid abusers intend to kill themselves by overdosage knowing that they are condemned to a miserable and degrading existence from which there seems to be no other escape. Apart from the formidable list of medical complications of intravenous drug abuse, there is now the problem of acquired immunodeficiency syndrome (AIDS), and in some areas a substantial proportion of drug abusers already have positive tests for the HIV antigen (Brettle et al., 1987).

THERAPEUTIC POISONING

This arises usually from the chronic excessive therapeutic use of cumulative drugs such as long-acting benzodiazepines, depot phenothiazines, diphenylhydantoin, phenobarbitone and salicylate. It is particularly likely to occur with drugs which have saturable dose-dependent kinetics within the therapeutic dose range, and diphenylhydantoin and salicylate may be cited as examples. The recognition of therapeutic poisoning is often delayed and the consequences may be serious. Thus, therapeutic salicylate intoxication carries a very high mortality, particularly in the young and the elderly (Anderson et al., 1976).

OCCUPATIONAL POISONING

This form of poisoning is less common with increasing recognition of hazards and legislation to ensure safer working conditions. However, patients may still be exposed inadvertently to toxic substances, and accidents may always occur. Inadequate ventilation may lead to poisoning with agents such as chlorine, oxides of nitrogen, hydrogen sulphide, carbon monoxide and metal fumes from welding. Established safety procedures are not always complied with and protective clothing may not be worn. The latter is particularly important with agents which are absorbed rapidly through the skin e.g. organophosphate insecticides.

HOMICIDAL POISONING

Homicide by poisoning is rare in the UK, but the possibility should always be kept in mind and investigated further if circumstances are in any way suspicious. Traditional poisons such as arsenic and cyanide have given way largely to more subtle agents and paraquat has become fashionable.

Agents used for self-poisoning

Most adults and older children poison themselves on impulse at a time of crisis, and they take usually whatever is immediately at hand. Drugs are taken by the great majority, and the remainder resort mostly to household products such as bleach, detergents and disinfectants. Patients with serious suicidal intent may deliberately choose traditionally dangerous poisons such as phenols ('Lysol'), cyanide, ethylene glycol (antifreeze) and paraquat. They may poison themselves also with carbon monoxide from a car exhaust.

Most self-poisoners have personal problems for which many have consulted their general practitioners during the preceding few weeks. They are often prescribed hypnotics, tranquillizers and antidepressants, and most patients who take overdoses repeatedly are being given these drugs long-term. Not surprisingly, psychotropic drugs are involved in the majority of poisonings (more than 60%), and of these the ubiquitous benzodiazepines lead the field by a substantial margin. Analgesics (usually non-prescription products containing aspirin or paracetamol) are taken by approximately 30% of patients, mostly young women who have not been given prescribed drugs. The remaining patients take a wide range of miscellaneous drugs (Prescott & Highley, 1985). As many as 60% of patients may take more than one drug in overdosage and as prescribing fashions change gradually over time, so too do the drugs used for self-poisoning (Proudfoot & Park, 1978).

Alcohol

Most patients now take ethanol before they poison themselves. This is of considerable toxicological significance, as ethanol potentiates the toxicity of other CNS depressants, and the outcome may be rapidly fatal when it is taken in combination with particularly dangerous drugs such as barbiturates, d-propoxyphene ('Distalgesic') and chlormethiazole (McInnes, 1987). The consumption of ethanol by self-poisoners is related to age and sex. It is taken before an overdose by approximately 75% of males and more than 50% of females aged between 18 and 30 yr.

Diagnosis of poisoning

Contrary to popular belief, many poisons and drugs taken in overdosage do not cause rapid loss of consciousness. However, overdosage must always be considered in the differential diagnosis of coma, and it is by far the most common cause in young to middle aged adults.

The diagnosis of self-poisoning may be made almost always on clinical and circumstantial evidence, and laboratory confirmation is rarely necessary. Personal problems come to light usually with careful questioning of friends and relatives, there are often medicine bottles and containers at the scene and a 'suicide' note may be found. Although the clinical features of poisoning are often non-specific, the diagnosis can be made usually with reasonable certainty on the basis of the clinical state, circumstantial evidence and knowledge of the drugs available to the patient. Certain intoxications produce a characteristic clinical picture (Table 72.1).

Poisons Information Services

The range of toxic substances to which patients might be exposed is enormous, and Poisons Information Services have been established to assist doctors in the management of poisoning. The centres in the UK provide information concerning the composition and toxicity of a wide range of proprietary, domestic, industrial and agricultural products, the toxic principles of plant and animal poisons and the acute toxicity of drugs and medicines. Detailed information is available on the manifestations and management of poisoning. In the case of difficulty, advice should always be sought from the nearest centre. The Scottish Poisons Information Bureau has been converted recently to a computer viewdata system, and the

Table 72.1 Some characteristic clinical manifestations of poisoning

Common clinical manifestations	Drug or poison
Vomiting, deafness, tinnitus, hyperventilation, sweating, vasodilatation, tachycardia, mixed respiratory alkalosis (adults) and metabolic acidosis (young children)	Salicylates
Initial nausea and vomiting, delayed onset of liver tenderness, mild jaundice and biochemical evidence of acute hepatic necrosis. Hepatic and renal failure in severe untreated cases	Paracetamol
Coma, slow respiration, cyanosis, hypotension, pinpoint pupils	Opioid analgesics
Deep peaceful sleep, depressed reflexes, minimal cardiorespiratory depression	Benzodiazepines
Coma, muscle twitching, convulsions, cardiac arrhythmias (tachycardia, absent P-waves, QRS widening), dry mouth, dilated pupils, extensor plantar responses, urinary retention, agitation and delirium on recovery	Tricyclic antidepressants and other anticholinergics
Vomiting, restlessness, delirium, dilated pupils, tremor, hyperreflexia, convulsions, hyperventilation, tachycardia	Theophylline and sympathomimetics
Gross ataxia, dysarthria and nystagmus, stupor, dilated pupils	Diphenylhydantoin
Brief ataxia, muscle twitching, coma, convulsions (usually isolated)	Mefenamic acid
Coma, convulsions, bradycardia, conduction defects, hypotension, severe circulatory failure	β-blockers
Confusion, deafness, tinnitus, cardiac arrhythmias, delayed onset blindness, fixed dilated pupils	Quinine
Vomiting, confusion, coma, hyperventilation (severe metabolic acidosis) circulatory failure, delayed blindness, fixed dilated pupils	Methanol
Vomiting, diarrhoea, colic, sweating, salivation, bronchospasm, pinpoint pupils, bradycardia, hypotension, muscle twitching, paralysis, respiratory failure, confusion, coma, convulsions	Cholinergics (organophosphates)

database is now accessed by users with their own terminals throughout the UK (Proudfoot & Davidson, 1983).

Use of the laboratory

Specific antidotal therapy is available for very few commonly taken poisons. Management is not influenced usually by laboratory identification of drugs or knowledge of their concentrations in biological fluids. On the other hand, clinical biochemical investigation is essential for correct management of the serious complications of poisoning (Table 72.2). Careful monitoring of fluid, acid–base and electrolyte balance is required during forced alkaline diuresis, and laboratory assistance may be required to confirm the diagnosis and monitor treatment in patients with met-haemoglobinaemia and poisoning with carbon monoxide and cholinesterase inhibitors. Laboratory identification is obviously important in medico-legal

cases, and it is helpful usually in the confirmation of non-accidental poisoning in children (Flanagan et al., 1981).

The correct management of some poisonings does depend on emergency measurement of the plasma concentration of the agent in question (Table 72.3). In paracetamol poisoning for example, there are no reliable, early clinical indications of the severity of intoxication. Specific treatment with N-acetylcysteine must be started within 8–10 hr to prevent severe and sometimes fatal liver damage, and only a small minority of patients is at risk. Emergency estimation of the plasma paracetamol concentration is therefore necessary, and treatment is indicated in patients with concentrations above the treatment line shown in Fig. 72.1. Without treatment, 60% of such patients suffer severe liver damage (Prescott, 1983). Ideally, toxic substances should be indentified and quantitated before attempts to enhance their elimination by techniques such as haemodialysis, haemoperfusion or

Table 72.2 Biochemical investigation in acute poisoning

Investigation	Relevant conditions
Arterial blood gas analysis	Respiratory failure, metabolic acidosis (shock, severe poisoning with many agents including methanol, ethylene glycol, metformin, cyanide, salicylate and paracetamol)
Plasma electrolytes	Cardiac arrhythmias, haemolysis, renal failure, rhabdomyolysis, forced diuresis. Poisoning with K^+, saline emetics, salicylate, theophylline, sympathomimetics, digoxin, insulin, etc.
Plasma calcium	Cardiac arrhythmias, ethylene glycol and fluoride poisoning
Plasma urea and creatinine	Renal failure (shock, haemolysis, rhabdomyolysis, poisoning with salicylate, paracetamol, non-steroidal, anti-inflammatory drugs, heavy metals, paraquat, chlorate, ethylene glycol, carbon tetrachloride, etc.)
Liver function tests	Hepatotoxicity—paracetamol, phenylbutazone halogenated hydrocarbons [e.g. carbon tetrachloride, paraquat, metals, Amanita phalloides (the death cap mushroom), etc.]
Prothrombin time ratio	Poisoning with anticoagulants and hepatotoxins, snake bites
Plasma glucose	Poisoning with hypoglycaemics, hepatotoxins, ethanol, salicylate
Plasma creatine phosphokinase and myoglobin	Muscle damage and rhabdomyolysis
Met-haemoglobin	Poisoning with chlorate, nitrites, aromatic amines, phenols, drugs with oxidizing metabolites (sulphonamides, dapsone, phenazopyridine, etc.)
Carboxyhaemoglobin	Carbon monoxide poisoning
Plasma pseudocholinesterase	Organophosphate and carbamate poisoning

Table 72.3 Indications for emergency measurement of plasma concentrations of drugs and poisons

Drug or poison	Indication
Paracetamol	Treatment with N-acetylcysteine
Salicylate	Active removal e.g. forced alkaline diuresis
Iron	Treatment with desferrioxamine
Lithium	Active removal
Phenobarbitone	Active removal
Digoxin	Treatment with antidigoxin Fab fragments
Methanol, ethylene glycol	Treatment with ethanol, active removal
Paraquat	Assessment of prognosis and risk of complications
Other drugs	Removal by haemodialysis or haemoperfusion (Table 72.7)

forced alkaline diuresis, and the efficacy of treatment should be monitored by serial estimation of plasma concentrations. Unfortunately, most hospitals have a very limited repertoire of emergency toxicological analyses, but the position is improving with technical advances and the growth of therapeutic drug monitoring.

Toxicological results should be interpreted with caution, and must be considered always in relation to the clinical state of the patient. Some simple assays necessarily used for emergency work are non-specific and subject to interference by other drugs and inactive metabolites. The relationship between drug concentrations and toxicity is complex. Patients often take multiple drugs in overdosage, ethanol is also often taken, and there is often great individual variation in response. Published lists of 'toxic', 'lethal' or 'potentially lethal' concentrations of drugs and poisons may be useful as a guide (Stead & Moffat, 1983), but they can be very misleading and are often inaccurate.

Drug pharmacokinetics are unpredictably abnormal in severely poisoned patients (Rosenberg et al.,

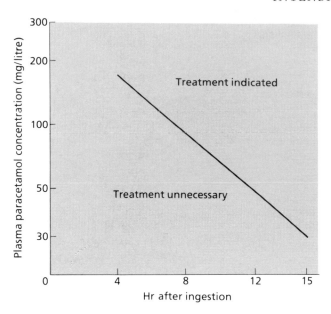

Fig. 72.1 Graph relating plasma paracetamol concentrations to the risk of liver damage after overdosage. Treatment with N-acetylcysteine is indicated in patients with values above the treatment line. Measurements made less than 4 hr after ingestion cannot be interpreted.

1981). Absorption may be slow or delayed, distribution may be restricted because of poor tissue perfusion, plasma protein binding is reduced at high concentrations and elimination is often impaired because of saturation of drug-metabolizing enzymes and reduced hepatic and renal blood flow. Hypothermia may depress drug metabolism also (Koren *et al.*, 1987). The time since ingestion must usually be taken into account in the interpretation of drug concentrations, and serial measurements are much more useful than a single estimation. It is essential to be aware of the units used by the laboratory for drug measurement. Unfortunately, units have not been standardized and although mass units have always been used in clinical toxicology, the recent unofficial introduction of molar units by some laboratories has caused dangerous confusion. To make matters worse, drug concentrations measured in these new units cannot be related to conventional mass units unless the molecular weight is known (Prescott *et al.*, 1987).

Principles of management

Antidotes are available for very few commonly encountered poisons, and treatment is usually non-specific and symptomatic. In such circumstances, management consists of emergency first aid and resuscitation, intensive care and supportive therapy, removal of unabsorbed drug and if appropriate, measures to enhance the elimination of the drug or poison.

Emergency measures and resuscitation

The unconscious patient should be transported and nursed initially in the head-down semi-prone position to minimize the risk of inhalation of gastric contents. The depth of coma is assessed most conveniently according to the Edinburgh coma scale (Table 72.4). The first priority is to establish a clear airway and to ensure that ventilation is adequate. If it is not, the lungs should be ventilated with oxygen and the trachea should be intubated if the conscious level permits. Re-oxygenation often transforms the clinical state of an unconscious, seemingly moribund patient, and can restore rapidly an effective cardiac output and circulation. The adequacy of ventilation should be monitored by arterial blood gas analysis (p. 475). The combination of coma, cyanosis, slow respiration and pinpoint pupils is virtually diagnostic of poisoning with opioid analgesics, and a trial of intravenous naloxone in sufficient dosage (up to 2 mg) is mandatory. Potentially serious abnormalities such as metabolic acidosis, hyperkalaemia and hypoglycaemia may require correction as a matter of urgency.

Hypotension with peripheral circulatory failure is treated first by correction of hypoxia and acidosis, and by elevation of the foot of the bed. If adequate perfusion is not restored by these measures, the circulating volume should be increased by administration of a plasma expander (p. 371). Cardiac arrhythmias are often improved or abolished by correction of hypoxia, acidosis and electrolyte imbalance. The temptation to give antiarrhythmic drugs must be resisted unless control of the rhythm disturbance is absolutely necessary. Many drugs and poisons can cause grand mal convulsions which, if repeated, should be controlled with intravenous diazepam.

The indications for other emergency measures depend on the agent involved and the severity of

Table 72.4 Assessment of depth of coma in poisoned patients (Edinburgh coma scale)

Grade 0	Fully conscious
Grade 1	Drowsy but responding to commands
Grade 2	Ready response to painful stimuli
Grade 3	Minimal response to maximal painful stimuli
Grade 4	No response to any stimulus

intoxication. Oxygen should be given in maximum concentration for carbon monoxide poisoning and transfer for hyperbaric oxygen therapy considered (Norkool & Kirkpatrick, 1985). Specific antidotal therapy may have to be given without delay, and examples include N-acetylcysteine for paracetamol poisoning, glucagon for severe β-blocker intoxication, dicobalt edetate for cyanide poisoning and atropine with pralidoxime for organophosphate intoxication. Once the condition of the patient has been stabilized, decisions can be made about further management.

Removal of unabsorbed drug

Theoretically, unabsorbed drug in the stomach can be removed by gastric aspiration and lavage or by induction of emesis. In practice, neither procedure can be relied upon to empty the stomach, and most drugs and poisons seem to be absorbed surprisingly rapidly. Gastric lavage is performed normally in patients in Grade 3 or 4 coma, and in most other patients who are thought to have taken a potentially toxic dose of drug or poison within the preceding 4 hr. This period is extended to 12 hr with drugs which delay gastric emptying such as opioid analgesics, anticholinergics and salicylates. Gastric lavage is not carried out in unconscious patients unless an effective gag reflex is present or an endotracheal tube is in place, and it is contra-indicated in patients who have ingested corrosives or liquid hydrocarbons. Inhalation of the latter may cause a severe pneumonitis.

The patient is placed head-down on the left side on a trolley and a well-lubricated large bore stomach tube (e.g. Jacques, 30 gauge) is passed. Suction must be available throughout the procedure. After siphoning out as much of the gastric contents as possible, the tube is connected to a large funnel with rubber tubing and successive volumes of 300 ml of warm tap-water poured into the stomach and removed by siphoning. When the return is clear, the tube is removed with its open end occluded.

In most cases, very little drug is removed by gastric lavage, but gratifyingly large amounts can occasionally be recovered. Its routine use has been questioned, and with the changing pattern of drugs taken in overdosage, it is probably unnecessary in at least 50% of patients (Blake et al., 1978). However, used with discrimination, gastric lavage retains an important place in the management of poisoning (Proudfoot, 1984). Complications of gastric lavage include inhalation of gastric contents and, very rarely, rupture of the oesophagus. It may also cause transient hypoxia, tachycardia, arrhythmias and ischaemic ECG changes (Thompson et al., 1987).

Emesis is the preferred method of emptying the stomach in young children, and patients who refuse to submit to gastric lavage. Emetics obviously cannot be used in unconscious patients. Syrup of ipecacuanha is the fashionable emetic currently, and its active principle is emetine. In adults, a dose of 15 ml taken with 200 ml of water usually causes vomiting in 20 min. If there is no response, the dose may be repeated once. Serious complications of ipecac-induced emesis are extremely rare, but Mallory–Weiss oesophageal tears and fatal gastric rupture have been described (Knight & Doucet, 1987). Other emetics should not be used, as they can cause serious toxicity if retained. Saline emetics are prepared often with grossly excessive amounts of salt and can cause fatal hypernatraemia (Goulding & Volans, 1977).

Activated charcoal is a powerful absorbent which is recommended often as a means of reducing the absorption of ingested drugs and poisons. Unfortunately, it has little effect unless given within 1 hr, and most patients arrive in hospital too late for it to be effective. There is no evidence that it limits drug absorption when administered after gastric lavage (Comstock et al., 1982). However, activated charcoal is safe and cheap. It is given as an aqueous suspension and the adult dose is 50–100 g.

Intensive supportive therapy

The primary objective of intensive supportive therapy is to maintain the vital functions to allow time for elimination of the poison and recovery. At the same time, potentially serious complications are anticipated and treated promptly if necessary.

Intensive supportive therapy is based on the principles of conservative intensive care. It includes such measures as the maintenance of respiration with assisted ventilation if necessary, regular removal of bronchial secretions, the use of humidified air or oxygen when the trachea has been intubated, regular chest physiotherapy, cardiovascular support, ECG monitoring, correction of hypo- and hyperthermia, close attention to fluid, acid–base and electrolyte balance, and conventional treatment of complications such as convulsions, pneumonia and renal failure. Central venous pressure monitoring and bladder catheterization may be required, but meddlesome medical interference should be kept to a minimum.

Additional drugs should never be given unless they are necessary. Antibiotics are indicated only for demonstrable infection, and there is rarely, if ever, any need for the use of pressor agents. An exception is dopamine which is often effective in increasing renal blood flow and urine output in hypotensive patients with oliguria. Techniques for enhancing drug elimination should be employed only when justified by the clinical state and when they may be expected to be effective. Skilled nursing care is of great importance. In addition to regular observations and monitoring, this includes regular turning of the patient and removal of secretions, passive movements of the limbs, care of the skin, mouth and eyes and emptying of the bladder by fundal pressure.

Management of the complications of poisoning

Although recovery from self-poisoning is often rapid and uneventful, serious life-threatening toxicity may be caused by many poisons and commonly used drugs taken in large doses. The morbidity and outcome depend on the nature of the toxic agent(s), the dose absorbed, the rates of absorption and elimination, the duration of intoxication and many other factors including age, pre-existing disease, individual susceptibility, associated ingestion of ethanol and environmental temperature. Poisoning can cause serious adverse effects on virtually every organ system (Kulling & Persson, 1986). Coma is the most common complication, but it persists rarely for more than 24–36 hr. It may be prolonged in poisoning with phenobarbitone and baclofen, and with long-acting benzodiazepines such as nitrazepam and flurazepam in the elderly. Intoxication which is severe enough to produce Grade 4 coma is associated with a high incidence of morbidity and mortality (Arieff & Friedman, 1973).

Pulmonary complications

Pulmonary complications are common in unconscious poisoned patients and are important causes of morbidity and mortality (Jay et al., 1975). They include aspiration pneumonia, bronchial obstruction and collapse, infection, hypostatic pneumonia, and adult respiratory distress syndrome (ARDS). These are treated conventionally as described in Chapter 73.

Poisoned patients may develop pulmonary oedema of cardiac or non-cardiac origin. Cardiac pulmonary oedema is caused usually by the administration of excessive fluid, often in attempts to produce a forced diuresis in a severely poisoned patient. In this setting, myocardial and renal function are often impaired (Glauser et al., 1976). In addition, drugs such as salicylate and the non-steroidal, anti-inflammatory drugs cause fluid retention. Cardiac pulmonary oedema should be treated with oxygen, fluid restriction, diuretics and if necessary, removal of excess fluid by haemodialysis.

Non-cardiac pulmonary oedema is a rather uncommon complication of severe poisoning with a variety of agents including opioid analgesics, salicylate, tricyclic antidepressants and quinine. Pulmonary capillary permeability is increased as a result of endothelial injury, and there is leakage of albumin-rich fluid into the interstitial and alveolar spaces. The pulmonary capillary wedge pressure is usually normal or low (Benowitz et al., 1979). A particularly acute form of pulmonary oedema may occur in drug addicts following the intravenous injection of opioid analgesics. More often, there is gradual development of interstitial oedema during the course of the intoxication. Inhalation of irritant gases such as chlorine, sulphur dioxide and oxides of nitrogen produces a chemical pneumonitis with associated pulmonary oedema. The treatment of non-cardiac pulmonary oedema consists of administration of oxygen, and if necessary, ventilation of the lungs with positive end-expiratory pressure (PEEP). Haemorrhagic pulmonary oedema occurs in severe, rapidly fatal paraquat poisoning and in less severe but ultimately fatal poisoning there is delayed onset of progressive proliferation of alveolar cells and pulmonary fibrosis. These changes resemble those of oxygen toxicity and are aggravated by oxygen.

Cerebral oedema

Cerebral oedema may occur in patients who have suffered hypoxic brain damage. It may also follow hypoglycaemia and other forms of metabolic brain damage such as may occur in poisoning with carbon monoxide, cyanide, methanol and salicylate. Cerebral oedema is aggravated by hypercapnia and by overhydration as may occur with misguided attempts at forced diuresis (Mühlendahl et al., 1978). Treatment is directed towards correction of the underlying metabolic disorder and removal of excess fluid. Intracranial pressure may be reduced by administration of osmotic agents such as mannitol and if possible, hypocapnia should be induced by controlled hyperventilation. Dexamethasone is given often but its value in such circumstances is doubtful.

Convulsions and motor disorders

Many poisons and drugs taken in overdosage can cause grand mal convulsions: examples include mefenamic acid, tricyclic antidepressants, d-propoxyphene, theophylline, anticholinergics, antihistamines, monoamine-oxidase inhibitors, organophosphates, baclofen and salicylate. Isolated convulsions such as those produced by mefenamic acid do not require treatment, but repeated convulsions should be controlled with intravenous diazepam. If this fails, it may be necessary to paralyse the patient and ventilate the lungs.

Agents such as strychnine and α-chloralose may also cause extensor muscle spasms and opisthotonus provoked by tactile and auditory stimuli. The patient should be nursed in a dark, quiet room and sedated with diazepam. If the spasms cannot be controlled in this way, the patient should be paralysed.

A malignant neuroleptic hyperthermia syndrome characterized by coma, generalized muscle rigidity, tachycardia, hyperventilation and hyperpyrexia may occur in poisoning with monoamine-oxidase inhibitors and amphetamines, and with combinations of phenothiazines, butyrophenones and lithium. The sustained muscle activity may cause necrosis with myoglobinuria, hyperkalaemia and renal failure. The onset of this syndrome is usually delayed and muscle rigidity and hyperpyrexia can usually be brought under control rapidly with intravenous dantrolene (Harpe & Stoudemire, 1987).

In normal therapeutic doses, the phenothiazines, butyrophenones and metoclopramide may cause bizarre acute dystonic reactions involving primarily the muscles of the head and neck. The onset is delayed usually for 12 hr or more, most cases occur in young adults, and females are affected more often than males. These reactions are probably caused by inhibition of central dopamine receptors and resulting imbalance with the cholinergic system. They can be terminated rapidly with intravenous procyclidine or benztropine.

Hypothermia

Prolonged, deep, drug-induced coma may result in hypothermia, especially in the elderly and when environmental temperatures are low and vasodilators such as ethanol have been taken. Mild hypothermia (down to about 33 °C), is normally reversible rapidly and of little consequence. In more severe hypothermia, there is bradycardia, hypotension and slow respiration, (this is not necessarily harmful, as the metabolic rate is correspondingly depressed). The results of arterial blood gas analysis may appear less worrying if corrected for low temperature, but there is evidence that myocardial function is optimal at an uncorrected blood pH of 7.4 (Matthews et al., 1984). After initial resuscitation, patients with severe hypothermia should be wrapped in a reflective 'space' blanket and nursed in a warm room with extra wool blankets. There is usually a rapid, spontaneous return to normal temperature, and this may be followed by an overshoot to 38 °C or more. Atrial fibrillation with a slow ventricular rate may occur as the temperature rises, but it is usually self-limiting. Active rewarming is potentially dangerous as it causes peripheral vasodilatation with demands for increased cardiac output while the core temperature remains low. It is rarely, if ever, indicated in poisoned patients.

Hypotension

Some degree of hypotension is common in moderate to severe poisoning, and it is almost always present in patients in Grade 3 and 4 coma. It does not require treatment unless there is peripheral circulatory failure with cold extremities or the systolic pressure is less than approximately 10.6 kPa (80 mmHg). Several factors contribute to hypotension, depending on the drugs taken and the severity and stage of intoxication (Benowitz et al., 1979). Many poisons and drugs taken in overdosage cause myocardial depression, and this is aggravated often by factors such as hypoxia and acidosis. In addition, CNS depressants and other drugs impair the autonomic reflex control of vascular tone causing vasodilatation, relative hypovolaemia and a decrease in the venous return to the heart. Hypovolaemia may result also from vascular injury with increased capillary permeability and loss of fluid into the tissues (Shubin & Weil, 1985). Arterial pressure and the circulation can often be improved dramatically by correction of hypoxia and acidosis, and by raising the foot of the bed to increase the venous return. If these measures fail, the blood volume should be increased by infusion of plasma expanders such as albumin solution, preferably with monitoring of the central venous or pulmonary capillary wedge pressure. Pressor agents are not normally recommended because the peripheral resistance may be raised already but dopamine infusion may produce a beneficial increase in cardiac output without decreasing renal blood flow.

Hypertension

Hypertension severe enough to warrant treatment may occasionally complicate overdosage with central stimulants. The administration of labetolol would be logical, and sublingual nifedipine has been used also (Gibson *et al.*, 1987).

Cardiotoxicity and arrhythmias

Many drugs and poisons can cause cardiac arrhythmias and conduction abnormalities. The mechanisms are complex and although the ECG may appear alarming (Fig. 72.2), most rhythm disturbances in poisoned patients are self-limiting. They often respond promptly to correction of hypoxia, acidosis and electrolyte balance. The administration of cardiotoxic antiarrhythmic drugs to a patient with an already poisoned myocardium is fraught with danger. These drugs should only be given, and then with great caution, if the cardiac output is seriously compromised by the abnormal rhythm, or progression to a malignant arrhythmia is considered likely and simpler measures have failed. The chaotic cardiac rhythm in a patient with chloral hydrate intoxication shown in Fig. 72.3 was associated with a good cardiac output, and in this context there was no indication for treatment. However, chloral hydrate sensitizes the myocardium

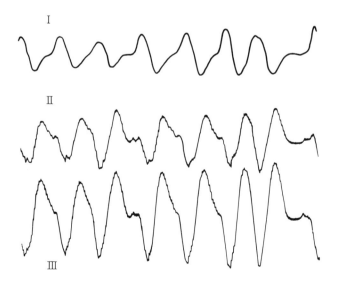

Fig. 72.2 Electrocardiogram (standard leads I, II and III) in a young woman with severe imipramine poisoning. Recovery was uneventful without the use of antiarrhythmic drugs. (Reproduced from Prescott, 1987.)

to catecholamines, and there is a risk of ventricular fibrillation. The multi-focal ventricular ectopic activity was abolished safely with a very small intravenous dose of a β-adrenergic blocker. Pacing may be required occasionally for extreme bradycardia or atrioventricular conduction block.

Solvent abuse may cause chronic cardiotoxicity (McLeod *et al.*, 1987), and heart transplantation has been carried out in a glue sniffer for dilated cardiomyopathy associated with abuse of toluene (Wiseman & Banim, 1987). Myocardial infarction is an uncommon complication of poisoning. It may occur in carbon monoxide poisoning, and it has been described also in glue sniffers (Cunningham *et al.*, 1987) and abusers of cocaine and amphetamine (Carson *et al.*, 1987).

Renal failure

Renal function may be impaired in any poisoned patient with severe hypotension and persistent circulatory failure. In such circumstances it is important to avoid both under- and overhydration, and central venous pressure monitoring with hourly measurement of urine volume is essential for the correct control of fluid balance. Renal blood flow and urine output can be improved usually by infusion of low-dose dopamine (Henderson *et al.*, 1980), and these measures may prevent otherwise irreversible ischaemic renal failure.

Many drugs and poisons (Table 72.2) may cause proximal tubular necrosis and acute renal failure (Kulling & Persson, 1986). Acute drug-induced rhabdomyolysis is another cause of renal failure in poisoned patients (Forwell & Hallworth, 1986). In addition to fluid replacement, correction of acidosis and circulatory support as described above, and the use of antidotes and measures to enhance elimination if appropriate, little can be done to prevent renal failure in such circumstances. There is some evidence that early diuresis may limit nephrotoxic renal damage, but attempts to force a diuresis as renal failure is developing are hazardous and not to be undertaken lightly. Established acute renal failure is treated conventionally as described in Chapter 74.

Liver damage

Acute hepatic necrosis is a common complication of paracetamol overdosage, and it may occur also in poisoning with a number of other agents (Table 72.2). In addition, prolonged hypotension may cause ischaemic liver damage. Acute hepatic necrosis

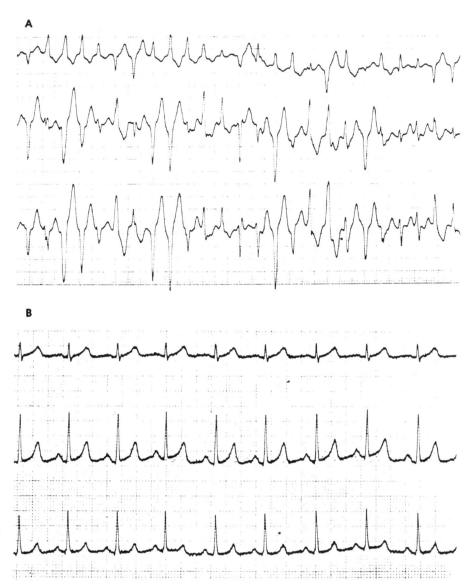

Fig. 72.3 Electrocardiograms in a patient with chloral hydrate intoxication. Gross multi-focal ventricular ectopic activity (**A**) was abolished completely by the intravenous injection of 1 mg of practolol (**B**).

induced by paracetamol can be prevented by the early administration of *N*-acetylcysteine (see below). Otherwise, severe liver damage and hepatic failure are managed as described in Chapter 51.

Skin blisters, peripheral nerve injury and muscle damage

Poisoned patients who remain deeply unconscious and immobile with poor peripheral perfusion for many hours may develop erythema of the skin progressing to bullous blister formation at pressure points. These lesions are caused probably by local ischaemia. Similarly, prolonged pressure may cause ischaemic peripheral nerve injury and muscle necrosis. Injury to

nerves becomes apparent often only on recovery of consciousness, and functional recovery may be delayed for weeks or months. Muscle damage is manifest by swelling, brawny induration, oedema and severe pain on passive movement when consciousness returns. The diagnosis of a compartmental syndrome may be facilitated by direct pressure measurement (Macey, 1987), and fasciotomy may be required to restore the blood supply, relieve pressure on nerves and prevent further muscle necrosis. More generalized muscle damage (rhabdomyolysis) is a less common complication of severe poisoning with a variety of agents including amphetamines, theophylline, opioid analgesics and isopropanol. Myoglobinuria is associated with gross elevation of plasma creatine phosphokinase activity, hyperkalaemia and oliguric renal failure (Forwell & Hallworth, 1986).

Behaviour disturbances

Agitation, restlessness, delirium and hallucinations may be caused by drug abuse and intoxication with a variety of agents, particularly those with a central anticholinergic action. Delirium may persist for several days after consciousness is regained after tricyclic antidepressant overdosage, and phenobarbitone intoxication may cause a prolonged period of disruptive disinhibited behaviour. Sedation may be required to prevent injury in a disturbed patient, but obvious causes of restlessness such as a distended bladder must first be excluded. The safest method, in the author's experience, is oral administration of diazepam in doses of 50–100 mg repeated hourly until the patient is asleep but easily roused. Prevention is always better than cure, but if oral therapy is not practicable, restraint may be necessary and diazepam should be given intravenously in small graded doses. A large total dose may be needed in an acutely disturbed patient and in such circumstances oral or intramuscular chlorpromazine has a potent synergistic effect.

Methods for enhancing drug elimination

The efficacy of regimens for enhancement of drug elimination from the body can be predicted to a large extent if the physico-chemical properties, disposition and pharmacokinetics of the substance are known (Prescott, 1974; De Broe *et al.*, 1986). Nevertheless, these measures have been employed often indiscriminately without clinical or toxicological justification, and in circumstances where only insignificant amounts of drug could be removed. The use of these techniques has been encouraged by numerous anecdotal reports of successful treatment in which survival of the patient is accepted as proof of efficacy. Unfortunately, it is not often possible to obtain proof of clinical benefit with such treatment in controlled clinical trials, but its use can be justified if rapid removal of a toxicologically significant fraction of the total body burden of the active drug can be demonstrated. Invasive and potentially dangerous methods for drug removal should be restricted to seriously poisoned patients who do not improve with conservative management and whose survival would otherwise be in doubt. Ideally, the toxic substance should be identified and its plasma concentrations monitored before, during and after the procedure.

Repeated oral activated charcoal

Repeated oral activated charcoal is effective in accelerating the removal of many drugs and poisons after absorption has occurred (Pond, 1986). It is thought to act by irreversibly binding drug which diffuses from the circulation into the gut lumen under 'sink' conditions and the process has been referred to as gastrointestinal dialysis (Levy, 1982). Compounds which are excreted into the bile during enterohepatic circulation are bound also in the gut and their reabsorption is prevented.

Repeated oral charcoal is most effective with drugs which have a small volume of distribution, a small endogenous clearance and a long half-life (Table 72.5). It is the only means known of enhancing significantly the removal of drugs such as diphenylhydantoin and quinine, and with salicylate and phenobarbitone it is at least as effective as forced alkaline diuresis and haemodialysis (Fig 72.4) (Hillman & Prescott, 1985; Boldy *et al.*, 1986). Efficacy depends on keeping an

Table 72.5 Some drugs which can be removed effectively by repeated oral activated charcoal

Phenobarbitone	Diphenylhydantoin
Carbamazepine	Salicylate
Theophylline	Dapsone
Barbiturate hypnotics	Meprobamate
Digoxin	Digitoxin
Quinine	Cyclosporin

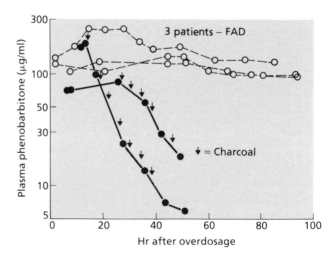

Fig. 72.4 Rapid removal of phenobarbitone by repeated oral activated charcoal in two patients (●—●). The charcoal was administered at the times indicated by the arrows. Plasma phenobarbitone concentrations are shown for comparison in three patients treated by forced alkaline diuresis (FAD) (o – – – o). (Redrawn from Prescott, 1987.)

adequate mass of charcoal moving down the intestine, and on the absorptive capacity of the preparation used. 'Medicoal' is recommended, as it contains non-absorbable polyvinylpyrrolidone which maintains intestinal transit and may cause beneficial diarrhoea. An initial dose of 100 g of charcoal is given as a slurry in 200 ml of water followed by 50 g every 4 hr until recovery. In unconscious patients, the charcoal may be given by nasogastric tube, and the stomach contents should be aspirated before each dose is given. The major disadvantages are unpalatability and difficulty of administration in patients with nausea and vomiting.

Forced diuresis

There are relatively few indications for forced diuresis although it is used frequently. It can only increase the renal clearance of drugs which undergo tubular reabsorption, and it can only enhance usefully the overall elimination of drugs which are excreted unchanged in the urine to the extent of 30 % or more. Diuresis alone has relatively little effect on drug elimination because at best the renal clearance is only proportional to the urine flow rate. In the case of drugs which are weak organic acids and bases with pKa values of 3.0–7.5 and 7.5–10.5 respectively, a much greater effect on clearance can be obtained by manipulation of the urine pH. The lipid-solubility and hence tubular reabsorption of such acidic and basic drugs is decreased in alkaline and acid urine respectively, and their renal clearance is increased correspondingly. This relationship is logarithmic, and theoretically for each change of one unit in urine pH, the renal clearance could change by a factor of 10. Urine pH is therefore much more important than urine flow rate. (Fig 72.5).

In practice, forced alkaline diuresis is restricted largely to poisoning with phenobarbitone and salicylate, although much of the effect in lowering plasma salicylate concentrations results from haemodilution rather than increased urinary excretion (Prescott et al., 1982). Repeated oral activated charcoal is much more effective in removing phenobarbitone (Fig. 72.4), and simple alkalinization of the urine is as effective as forced alkaline diuresis for the removal of salicylate. Alkaline diuresis is effective in the treatment of intoxication with the selective weedkiller 2,4-dichloro-phenoxyacetic acid (Prescott et al., 1979) and it would be effective also in removing chlorpropamide (Neuvonen & Kärkkäinen, 1983). Forced acid diuresis is potentially much more hazardous than alkaline

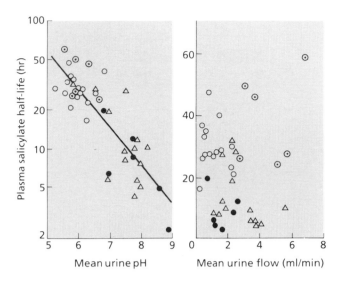

Fig. 72.5 Relationship between plasma salicylate half-life, and urine pH and flow rate in patients with salicylate poisoning treated by forced alkaline diuresis (△), alkali alone (●), forced diuresis alone (■) and in control patients (○). There is a highly significant correlation with urine pH but not with flow rate. (Redrawn from Prescott et al., 1982.)

diuresis, and there are no proven indications for its use.

Before forced diuresis is undertaken, the state of hydration and electrolyte balance should be assessed together with cardiac and renal function. Regular monitoring is necessary during the procedure. A standard 'cocktail' containing sodium bicarbonate and potassium may be used for forced alkaline diuresis in salicylate poisoning (Lawson et al., 1969) and a less aggressive regimen is used to produce alkaline urine at a rate of about 500 ml/hr for phenobarbitone poisoning (Vale & Meredith, 1981). Any form of forced diuresis is potentially dangerous. It is contra-indicated in patients with cardiac and renal impairment, and great caution is needed in the elderly. Complications include water intoxication, disturbances of acid–base and electrolyte balance, left ventricular failure with pulmonary oedema and cerebral oedema. Deaths have occurred as a result of unnecessary and inappropriate forced diuresis (Mühlendahl et al., 1978).

Haemodialysis, peritoneal dialysis and haemoperfusion

These regimens have been used extensively in attempts to enhance the elimination of drugs in poisoned patients. In many cases little clinical benefit could be expected on the basis of the pharmacokinetic characteristics of the drug, and when measured, the amounts removed have often been toxicologically insignificant.

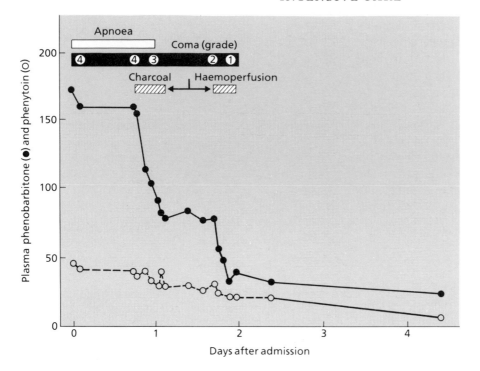

Fig. 72.6 Rapid removal of phenobarbitone by charcoal haemoperfusion in a 29-yr-old woman in Grade 4 coma with prolonged apnoea requiring ventilation following overdosage of phenobarbitone, diphenyl-hydantoin, pentazocine and diazepam. Large doses of naloxone had no effect and she met the criteria for brain death. Adequate spontaneous respiration returned after the first haemoperfusion and consciousness was regained after the second. Note that haemoperfusion had no effect on the plasma concentrations of diphenylhydantoin. Drug concentrations are in mg/litre.

Nevertheless, haemodialysis and haemoperfusion may be very effective in appropriate circumstances (Fig. 72.6) (Pond *et al.*, 1979). The conditions which must be met for the effective removal of toxic substances by haemodialysis and haemoperfusion are summarized in Table 72.6. Apart from the efficacy of removal of the drug from the blood by the device, the most important factors are the volume of drug distribution, the extent of binding to plasma proteins and the ratio of the extracorporeal to endogenous clearance. The maximum extracorporeal clearance cannot exceed the blood flow rate, and an adequate flow may be difficult to obtain in the most seriously poisoned patients. At the end of the day, the most important criteria are the survival of the patient and the amount of active drug removed relative to the total body burden.

Some drugs which can be removed reasonably effectively by haemoperfusion and haemodialysis are listed in Table 72.7. In general, haemoperfusion with coated charcoal or exchange resins is more effective than haemodialysis, although the latter may be preferred for simultaneous correction of acid–base and electrolyte balance (e.g. in salicylate poisoning). Haemodialysis is also the method of choice for removal of methanol, ethylene glycol and lithium. Peritoneal dialysis is much less effective and it is used rarely. It has the advantages that unlike the other methods it can be continued without interruption for long periods and does not require special facilities. The complications of haemodialysis and haemoperfusion include hypotension, haemorrhage, air embolism and removal of white blood cells and platelets. Peritoneal dialysis

Table 72.6 Characteristics necessary for effective removal of drugs by haemodialysis and haemoperfusion

Low molecular size and weight for good dialysance (haemodialysis)
Great affinity for and irreversible binding to adsorbent (haemoperfusion)
Small volume of distribution
Minimal binding to plasma proteins
Rapid transfer from peripheral tissues to the circulation
Extracorporeal clearance similar to or greater than endogenous clearance
Adequate extracorporeal blood flow

Table 72.7 Some drugs which can be removed effectively by haemodialysis and haemoperfusion

Phenobarbitone	Carbamazepine
Other barbiturates	Meprobamate
Salicylate	Theophylline
Dapsone	Most antibiotics
Lithium*	Chloral hydrate*
Methanol*	Ethylene glycol*

* Haemodialysis only.

may be complicated by fluid and electrolyte abnormalities, perforation, peritonitis and adhesions.

Exchange transfusion and plasmapheresis

Drug removal by these regimens is very inefficient, and there is rarely, if ever, any indication for their use in poisoned patients. Even with drugs which have limited tissue distribution such as theophylline, the fraction removed by exchange transfusion is clinically insignificant (Wolff & Dreissen, 1983).

Specific antidotal therapy

Specific antidotes are not available often and they must be given usually without delay for maximum protect-ive action. The mechanisms of reversal of toxicity include pharmacological agonist–antagonist interactions at receptors, inhibition of formation of toxic metabolites, provision of substrates and co-factors to stimulate detoxifying enzyme systems, enzyme regeneration, chelation of metals and the binding of toxins with specific antibodies. Some examples are listed in Table 72.8.

Agonist–antagonist interactions

Toxicity caused by blockade or stimulation of specific receptors may be reversed by administration of pharmacological agonists and antagonists respectively. The overall effect of combinations of competitive

Table 72.8 Specific antidotal therapy

Drug or poison	Specific therapy	Mechanism of protection
Opioid analgesics	Naloxone	Pharmacological antagonism
β-blockers	Isoprenaline Prenalterol Glucagon	Pharmacological antagonism
Sympathomimetics Theopylline	β-blockers	Pharmacological antagonism
Phenothiazines Metoclopramide (acute dystonic reactions)	Anticholinergics (e.g. benztropine)	Pharmacological antagonism
Anticholinergics	Physostigmine	Pharmacological antagonism
Cholinesterase inhibitors	Atropine Pralidoxime	Pharmacological antagonism Enzyme regeneration
Benzodiazepines	Flumazenil (Ro 15-1788)	Pharmacological antagonism
Warfarin	Vitamin K Clotting factors	Pharmacological antagonism Replacement of factors
Ethylene glycol, methanol	Ethanol	Inhibition of metabolic activation
Paracetamol	N-acetylcysteine (methionine)	Stimulation of glutathione synthesis
Digoxin	Antidigoxin Fab	Binding and inactivation of digoxin in tissues
Iron	Desferrioxamine	Chelation
Lead	Calcium sodium edetate, D-penicillamine	Chelation
Other heavy metals	Dimercaprol D-penicillamine	Chelation
Cyanide	Dicobalt edetate Sodium nitrite Sodium thiosulphate	Chelation Met-haemoglobin binds cyanide Provides sulphur for conversion to thiocyanate
Oxidizing agents	Methylene blue	Reversal of met-haemoglobinaemia

agonists and antagonists depends on their relative concentrations, their relative affinities for the receptor, and their intrinsic activities. The dose required to reverse toxicity therefore depends on the drugs involved and the severity of intoxication.

Naloxone has a very high affinity for opioid receptors but is virtually devoid of agonist activity. When given intravenously in adequate dosage it rapidly reverses coma, respiratory depression and hypotension in patients with opioid analgesic intoxication (Evans et al., 1973). The most common mistake is the use of too small a dose, and up to 2 mg may be required initially to obtain a response. Even larger doses are needed to counteract the effects of partial agonist/antagonists such as pentazocine, and the effects of buprenorphine cannot be reversed by naloxone in any reasonable dose. Naloxone has a relatively short duration of action and repeated doses may be necessary in poisoning with long-acting opioids such as methadone. The complete reversal of severe opioid analgesic intoxication with intravenous naloxone results in an abrupt return to full consciousness, with dilatation of the pupils, tremor, pilo-erection, hyperventilation and tachycardia. These latter effects are mediated probably by massive catecholamine release, and this may be relevant to the rare induction of serious ventricular arrhythmias by naloxone (Cuss et al., 1984). It is probably safer to give repeated incremental doses of 0.4 mg to allow a more gradual return to consciousness. The effects of naloxone cannot be regarded as specific, as it can partially reverse coma produced by other CNS depressants such as ethanol, benzodiazepines and clonidine (Kulig et al., 1982; Jeffreys & Volans, 1983).

Other examples of useful receptor interactions include those between adrenergic and cholinergic agonists and antagonists. Poisoning with β-adrenergic blockers can cause severe myocardial depression with virtual electromechanical dissociation. Isoprenaline is the pharmacological antagonist, but very large doses may be required, and safe titration in an emergency is impossible. Although recommended universally, atropine is useless in this situation. Prenalterol may have a wider margin of safety than isoprenaline, and it has been used successfully in β-blocker poisoning (Wallin & Hulting, 1983). However, the preferred treatment for severe poisoning with these drugs is glucagon. It activates cardiac adenyl cyclase by a mechanism independent of that mediated by catecholamines without causing excessive stimulation. In graded intravenous doses up to 10 mg it reverses myocardial depression effectively and restores an effective cardiac output (Illingworth, 1979).

Atropine blocks acetylcholine receptors and antagonizes the toxic effects of cholinergic agonists and cholinesterase inhibitors such as organophosphates. Again, very large doses may be needed. Conversely, anticholinesterases such as physostigmine have been used as antidotes for poisoning with tricyclic antidepressants and other anticholinergics. However, physostigmine is a potent non-specific central stimulant, and it has a very short duration of action which makes it difficult to use. Although it restores consciousness effectively, in mild to moderate poisoning with a variety of drugs, including the tricyclic anti-depressants, it does not reverse the lethal cardiac toxicity produced by the latter. It causes convulsions and asystole has been reported (Pentel & Peterson, 1980). The use of physostigmine may have limited diagnostic value but its therapeutic benefit is minimal (Nilsson, 1982). It is not recommended. The availability of benzodiazepine antagonists such as flumazenil (Ro 15-1788) is of limited relevance to the treatment of overdosage with benzodiazepines as their acute toxicity is rarely serious or life threatening (Johnston, 1985).

Other antidotal therapy is based on receptor-mediated interactions involving parallel or opposing physiological systems. Thus, β-adrenergic blockers such as propranolol antagonize many of the effects attributed to excessive adenyl cyclase activity in theophylline toxicity, atropine may reverse bradycardia in mild β-adrenergic blocker and digoxin poisoning, and other anticholinergics such as benztropine abolish acute dystonic reactions produced by central dopamine antagonists.

Inhibition of metabolic activation

Many agents cause toxicity through the formation of reactive intermediate metabolites by drug-metabolizing enzymes. There are many examples of prevention of this form of toxicity by inhibition of microsomal enzymes in experimental animals. However, the clinical application of this principle is very limited and extends only to the use of ethanol to inhibit the metabolism and reduce the toxicity of other alcohols. Given acutely to maintain a blood concentration of approximately 100 mg/100 ml, ethanol is a potent inhibitor of alcohol dehydrogenase and it reduces the rate of conversion of methanol and ethylene glycol to the highly toxic metabolites formate and glycolate which cause severe acidosis, blindness and encephalo-pathy (Jacobsen & McMartin, 1986).

Stimulation of detoxifying enzyme systems

The capacity of major routes of elimination is an important determinant of toxicity. Drug metabolizing enzymes may become saturated at high toxic concentrations, and the availability of substrates and co-factors may become a limiting factor. Endogenous protective mechanisms such as the conjugation of reactive nucleophilic metabolites with glutathione may fail if substrates for its synthesis become depleted. This is a critical factor in hepatotoxicity following overdosage with paracetamol.

The metabolic activation of paracetamol results in the formation of a minor reactive metabolite (N-acetyl-p-benzoquinoneimine) which is normally inactivated rapidly by conjugation with reduced glutathione. Following overdosage, glutathione is depleted rapidly and the excess metabolite damages liver cells causing necrosis (Mitchell et al., 1974). The availability of cysteine is rate limiting for glutathione synthesis. The administration of precursors such as N-acetylcysteine stimulates glutathione synthesis and it is very effective in preventing liver damage if given intravenously within 8–10 hr. Its protective action declines after this time and it is not effective after 15 hr (Prescott, 1983). Oral methionine has been used also but its absorption and efficacy may be compromised because nausea and vomiting occur in most severely poisoned patients. Only a minority of patients are at risk of severe liver damage and N-acetylcysteine should be given only to those with plasma paracetamol concentrations above the treatment line shown in Fig. 72.1. However, treatment should be started immediately in patients admitted 8–15 hr after the overdose, and it must not be withheld after 8 hr whilst awaiting the laboratory result. N-acetylcysteine may be discontinued if the plasma paracetamol is found subsequently to be below the treatment line.

Glutathione protects against the toxicity of many other agents, including heavy metals and halogenated hydrocarbons such as chloroform. However, the toxicity of carbon tetrachloride is not glutathione dependent, and N-acetylcysteine does not prevent it from causing liver damage in man (Ruprah et al., 1985).

Another example of the enhancement of detoxification is the use of sodium thiosulphate for cyanide poisoning. It provides sulphur which is rate limiting for the inactivation of cyanide through conversion to thiocyanate by the enzyme rhodanase.

Enzyme regeneration

Organophosphate compounds irreversibly phosphory-late the ester site of the cholinesterase receptor and cause severe cholinergic toxicity by inhibiting the hydrolysis of acetylcholine. Spontaneous recovery is very slow as it depends on resynthesis of the enzyme. Pralidoxime binds to the anionic site of the receptor and regenerates the enzyme by forming a stable complex with the organophosphate moiety. Poisoning with organophosphate is treated with large doses of atropine to block the acetylcholine receptors, and pralidoxime is given to regenerate the cholinesterase. Repeated doses may be necessary, and treatment is not effective if it is delayed for more than about 12 hr (Hackett & Buckley, 1983).

Chelation

Chelating agents form inert stable complexes with heavy metals and can reduce their toxicity if administered without delay. Currently available chelating agents include desferrioxamine (for iron), calcium disodium edetate (for lead) and thiols such as dimercaprol and D-penicillamine (for arsenic, antimony, bismuth, gold, mercury, lead and copper). Newer chelating agents such as 2,3-dimercaptosuccinic acid hold promise of greater efficacy and safety (Graziano, 1986). Iron poisoning is relatively common, especially in children, but it does not often cause serious toxicity (Proudfoot et al., 1986). Treatment with desferrioxamine has been recommended in patients with serum iron concentrations above 8–10 mg/litre (145–180 μmol/litre), and vomiting and diarrhoea are useful predictors of severe poisoning with serum iron concentrations above 300 mg/litre (Lacouture et al., 1981). Prompt treatment with desferrioxamine may prevent the acute toxicity of severe iron poisoning but not late complications such as intestinal stricture (Henretig et al., 1983).

Cyanide inactivates cytochrome oxidases and is a very rapidly acting metabolic poison. It has a very high affinity for cobalt, and dicobalt edetate has now replaced sodium nitrite and thiosulphate for the treatment of cyanide poisoning.

Met-haemoglobinaemia

Oxidizing agents cause met-haemoglobinaemia in which the iron of haemoglobin is converted to the ferric form with loss of oxygen carrying capacity (Table 72.2). Met-haemoglobinaemia can be recognized by slatey grey cyanosis which is unrelieved by oxygen and a characteristic chocolate-brown colour of the blood. Severe met-haemoglobinaemia (exceeding 40%) causes symptomatic tissue hypoxia, and it can be reversed with intravenous methylene blue (Hall *et al.*, 1986).

Immunotherapy

The use of antibodies to reverse toxicity is not new but there have been important recent developments, and the treatment of severe digoxin intoxication has been revolutionized by the introduction of digoxin-specific Fab antibody fragments. These fragments are less immunogenic than the complete IgG antibody and they have a much greater affinity for digoxin than binding sites in the myocardium and other tissues. Following their intravenous administration, there is a precipitous decrease in the plasma concentrations of free digoxin, and rapid reversal of life-threatening cardiac arrhythmias and hyperkalaemia (Smith *et al.*, 1982). The inactive complex with digoxin is degraded partially, and excreted eventually in the urine (Schaumann *et al.*, 1986). The dose of Fab fragments is calculated according to the estimated body load of digoxin, but treatment is very expensive and it should be reserved life-threatening intoxication. Digoxin-specific Fab antibody fragments bind other cardiac glycosides also such as digitoxin and lanatoside C. Digoxin toxicity has been treated also by haemoperfusion through columns containing antidigoxin antibodies bound covalently to agarose–polyacrolein microspheres (Savin *et al.*, 1987). Unfortunately, because of the very large distribution volume of digoxin, this ingenious technique could not be expected to remove more than a tiny fraction of the total amount of drug in the body. With recent developments in genetic engineering and DNA biotechnology, the potential exists for effective specific immunotherapy of intoxication with many other lethal poisons.

References

Anderson R.J., Potts D.E., Gabow P.A., Rumack B.H. & Schrier R.W. (1976) Unrecognized adult salicylate intoxication. *Annals of Internal Medicine* 85, 745–8.

Arieff A.I. & Friedman E.A. (1973) Coma following nonnarcotic drug overdosage: management of 208 adult patients. *American Journal of the Medical Sciences* 266, 405–26.

Benowitz N.L., Rosenberg J. & Becker C.E. (1979) Cardiopulmonary catastrophes in drug-overdosed patients. *Medical Clinics of North America* 63, 267–96.

Blake D.R., Bramble M.G. & Grimley Evans J. (1978) Is there excessive use of gastric lavage in the treatment of self-poisoning? *Lancet* II, 1362–4.

Boldy D.A.R., Vale J.A. & Prescott L.F. (1986) Treatment of phenobarbitone poisoning with repeated oral administration of activated charcoal. *Quarterly Journal of Medicine* 235, 997–1002.

Brettle R.P., Bisset K., Burns S., Davidson J., Davidson S.J., Gray J.M.N., Inglis J.M., Lees J.S. & Mok J. (1987) Human immunodeficiency virus and drug misuse: the Edinburgh experience. *British Medical Journal* 295, 421–4.

Carson P., Oldroyd K. & Phadke K. (1987) Myocardial infarction due to amphetamine. *British Medical Journal* 294, 1525–6.

Comstock E.G., Boisaubin E.V., Comstock B.S. & Faulkner T.P. (1982) Assessment of the efficacy of activated charcoal following gastric lavage in acute drug emergencies. *Journal of Toxicology. Clinical Toxicology* 19, 149–65.

Craft A.W., Lawson G.R., Williams H. & Sibert J.R. (1984) Accidental childhood poisoning with household products. *British Medical Journal* 288, 682.

Cunningham S.R., Dalzell G.W.N., McGirr P. & Khan M.H. (1987) Myocardial infarction and primary ventricular fibrillation after glue sniffing. *British Medical Journal* 294, 739–40.

Cuss F.M., Colaço C.B. & Baron J.H. (1984) Cardiac arrest after reversal of effects of opiates with naloxone. *British Medical Journal* 288, 363–4.

De Broe M.E., Bismuth C., De Groot G., Heath A., Okonek S., Ritz D.R., Verpooten G.A., Volans G.N. & Widdop B. (1986) Haemoperfusion: a useful therapy for a severely poisoned patient? *Human Toxicology* 5, 11–14.

Department of Health and Social Security (1984) The management of deliberate self-harm. *Department of Health and Social Security Health Notice* HN(84)25.

Dine M.S. & McGovern M.E. (1982) Intentional poisoning of children —an overlooked category of child abuse: report of seven cases and review of the literature. *Pediatrics* 70, 32–5.

Evans L.E.J., Roscoe P., Swainson C.P. & Prescott L.F. (1973) Treatment of drug overdosage with naloxone, a specific narcotic antagonist. *Lancet* I, 452–5.

Flanagan R.J., Huggett A., Saynor D.A., Raper S.M. & Volans G.N. (1981) Value of toxicological investigation in the diagnosis of acute drug poisoning in children. *Lancet* II, 682–5.

Forwell M.A. & Hallworth M.J. (1986) Nontraumatic rhabdomyolysis and acute renal failure. *Scottish Medical Journal* 31, 246–9.

Gibson R.G., Oliver J.A. & Leak D. (1987) Nifedipine therapy of phenylpropanolamine-induced hypertension. *American Heart Journal* 113.406–7.

Glauser F.L., Smith W.R., Siefkin A. & Morton M.E. (1976) Renal hemodynamics in drug-overdosed patients. *American Journal of the Medical Sciences* 272, 147–52.

Goulding R. & Volans G.N. (1977) Emergency treatment of common poisonings: emptying the stomach. *Proceedings of the Royal Society of Medicine* 70, 766–70.

Graziano J.H. (1986) Role of 2,3-dimercaptosuccinic acid in the treatment of heavy metal poisoning. *Medical Toxicology* 1, 155–62.

Hackett D.R. & Buckley M.P. (1983) Organophosphorous poisoning. *Irish Medical Journal* 76, 146–50.

Hall A.H., Kulig K.W. & Rumack B.H. (1986) Drug- and chemical-induced methaemoglobinaemia: clinical features and management. *Medical Toxicology* 1, 253–60.

Hampel G., Horstkotte H. & Rumpf K.W. (1983) Myoglobinuric renal failure due to drug-induced rhabdomyolysis. *Human Toxicology* 2, 197–203.

Harpe C. & Stoudemire A. (1987) Aetiology and treatment of neuroleptic malignant syndrome. *Medical Toxicology* 2, 166–76.

Henderson I.S., Beattie T.J. & Kennedy A.C. (1980) Dopamine hydrochloride in oliguric states. *Lancet* II, 827–9.

Henretig F.M., Karl S.R. & Weintraub W.H. (1983) Severe iron poisoning treated with enteral and intravenous desferrioxamine. *Annals of Emergency Medicine* 12, 306–9.

Hillman R.J. & Prescott L.F. (1985) Treatment of salicylate poisoning with repeated oral activated charcoal. *British Medical Journal* 291, 1472.

Horn E.H., Henderson H.R. & Forrest J.A.H. (1987) Admissions of drug addicts to a general hospital: a retrospective study in the northern district of Glasgow. *Scottish Medical Journal* 32, 41–5.

Illingworth R.N. (1979) Glucagon for beta-blocker poisoning. *Practitioner* 223, 683–5.

Jacobsen D., Frederichsen P.S., Knutsen K.M., Sorum Y., Talseth T. & Odegaard O.R. (1984) Clinical course in acute self-poisonings: a prospective study of 1125 consecutively hospitalised adults. *Human Toxicology* 3, 107–16.

Jacobsen D. & McMartin K.E. (1986) Methanol and ethylene glycol poisonings: mechanisms of toxicity, clinical course, diagnosis and treatment. *Medical Toxicology* 1, 309–34.

Jay S.J., Johanson W.G. & Pierce A.K. (1975) Respiratory complications of overdose with sedative drugs. *American Review of Respiratory Diease* 112, 591–8.

Jeffreys D.B. & Volans G.N. (1983) An investigation of the role of the specific opioid antagonist naloxone in clinical toxicology. *Human Toxicology* 2, 227–31.

Johnston G.D. (1985) Benzodiazepine overdose: are specific antagonists useful? *British Medical Journal* 290, 805–6.

Knight K.M. & Doucet H.J. (1987) Gastric rupture and death caused by ipecac syrup. *Southern Medical Journal* 80, 786–7.

Koren G., Barker C., Goresky G., Bohn D., Kent G., Klein J., MacLeod S.M. & Biggar W.D. (1987) The influence of hypothermia on the disposition of fentanyl—human and animal studies. *European Journal of Clinical Pharmacology* 32, 373–6.

Kulig K., Duffy J., Rumack B.H. Mauro R. & Gaylord M. (1982) Naloxone for treatment of clonidine overdose. *Journal of the American Medical Association* 247, 1697.

Kulling P. & Persson H. (1986) Role of the intensive care unit in the management of the poisoned patient. *Medical Toxicology* 1, 375–86.

Lacouture P.G., Wason S., Temple A.R., Wallace D.K. & Lovejoy F.H. (1981) Emergency assessment of severity in iron overdose by clinical and laboratory methods. *Journal of Pediatrics* 99, 89–91.

Lawson A.A.H., Proudfoot A.T., Brown S.S., MacDonald R.H., Fraser A.G., Cameron J.C. & Matthew H. (1969) Forced diuresis in the treatment of acute salicylate poisoning in adults. *Quarterly Journal of Medicine* 38, 31–48.

Levy G. (1982) Gastrointestinal clearance of drugs with activated charcoal. *New England Journal of Medicine* 307, 676–8.

Macey A.C. (1987) Compartmental syndromes in unconscious patients: a simple aid to diagnosis. *British Medical Journal* 294, 1472–3.

McInnes G.T. (1987) Chlormethiazole and alcohol: a lethal cocktail. *British Medical Journal* 294, 592.

McLeod A.A., Marjot R., Monaghan M.J., Hugh-Jones P. & Jackson G. (1987) Chronic cardiac toxicity after inhalation of 1,1,1-trichloroethane. *British Medical Journal* 294, 727–9.

Matthews A.J., Stead A.L. & Abbott T.R. (1984) Acid–base control during hypothermia. *Anaesthesia* 39, 649–54.

Mitchell J.R., Thorgiersson S.S., Potter W.Z., Jollow D.J. & Keiser H. (1974) Acetaminophen-induced hepatic injury. Protective role of glutathione in man and rationale for therapy. *Clinical Pharmacology and Therapeutics* 16, 676–84.

Mühlendahl K.E., Krienke E.G. & Bunjes R. (1978) Fatal overtreatment of accidental childhood intoxication. *Journal of Pediatrics* 93, 1003–4.

Neuvonen P.J. & Kärkkäinen S. (1983) Effects of charcoal, sodium bicarbonate, and ammonium chloride on chlorpropamide kinetics. *Clinical Pharmacology and Therapeutics* 33, 386–93.

Nilsson E. (1982) Physostigmine treatment in various drug-induced intoxications. *Annals of Clinical Research* 14, 165–72.

Norkool D.M. & Kirkpatrick J.N. (1985) Treatment of acute carbon monoxide poisoning with hyperbaric oxygen: a review of 155 cases. *Annals of Emergency Medicine* 14, 1169–71.

Osselton M.D., Blackmore R.C., King L.A. & Moffat A.C. (1984) Poisoning-associated deaths for England and Wales between 1973 and 1980. *Human Toxicology* 3, 201–21.

Pentel P. & Peterson C.D. (1980) Asystole complicating physostigmine treatment of tricyclic antidepressant overdose. *Annals of Emergency Medicine* 9, 588–90.

Pond S.M. (1986) Role of repeated oral doses of activated charcoal in clinical toxicology. *Medical Toxicology* 1, 3–11.

Pond S., Rosenberg J., Benowitz N.L. & Takki S. (1979) Pharmacokinetics of haemoperfusion for drug overdose. *Clinical Pharmacokinetics* 4, 329–54.

Prescott L.F. (1974) Limitations of haemodialysis and forced diuresis. In *The Poisoned Patient: the Role of the Laboratory.* pp. 269–82. Ciba Foundation Symposium 26. Associated Scientific Publishers, Amsterdam.

Prescott L.F. (1983) Paracetamol overdoses: pharmacological considerations and clinical management. *Drugs* 25, 290–314.

Prescott L.F. (1987) Drug overdosage and poisoning. In *Drug Treatment* 3rd edn. (Ed. Speight T.M.) pp. 283–302. ADIS Press, Auckland.

Prescott L.F., Balali-Mood M., Critchley J.A.J.H., Johnstone A.F. & Proudfoot A.T. (1982) Diuresis or urinary alkalinisation for salicylate poisoning? *British Medical Journal* 285, 1383–6.

Prescott L.F. & Highley M.S. (1985) Drugs prescribed for self-poisoners. *British Medical Journal* 290, 1633–6.

Prescott L.F., Park J. & Darrien I. (1979) Treatment of severe 2,4-D and mecoprop intoxication with alkaline diuresis. *British Journal of Clinical Pharmacology* 7, 111–16.

Prescott L.F., Proudfoot A.T., Widdop B., Volans G.N., Vale J.A., Whiting B., Griffin J.P. & Wells F.O. (1987) Who needs molar units for drugs? *Lancet* I, 1127–9.

Proudfoot A.T. (1984) Abandon gastric lavage in the accident and emergency department? *Archives of Emergency Medicine* 2, 65–71.

Proudfoot A.T. & Davidson W.S.M (1983) A viewdata system for poisons information. *British Medical Journal* 286, 125–7.

Proudfoot A.T. & Park J. (1978) Changing pattern of drugs used for self-poisoning. *British Medical Journal* 1, 90–3.

Proudfoot A.T., Simpson D. & Dyson E.H. (1986) Management of acute iron poisoning. *Medical Toxicology* 1, 83–100.

Rogers D., Tripp J., Bentovim A., Robinson A., Berry D. & Goulding R. (1976) Non-accidental poisoning: an extended syndrome of child abuse. *British Medical Journal* 1, 793–6.

Rosenberg J., Benowitz N.L. & Pond S. (1981) Pharmacokinetics of drug overdose. *Clinical Pharmacokinetics* 6, 161–92.

Ruprah M., Mant T.G.K. & Flanagan R.J. (1985) Acute carbon

tetrachloride poisoning in 19 patients: implications and treatment. *Lancet* I, 1027–9.

Savin H., Marcus L., Margel S., Ofarim M. & Ravid M. (1987) Treatment of adverse digitalis effects by hemoperfusion through columns with antidigoxin antibodies bound to agarose polyacrolein microsphere beads. *American Heart Journal* 113, 1078–84.

Schaumann W., Kaufmann B., Neubert P. & Smolarz A. (1986) Kinetics of the Fab fragments of dioxin antibodies and of bound digoxin in patients with severe digoxin intoxication. *European Journal of Clinical Pharmacology* 30, 527–33.

Shubin H. & Weil M.H. (1985) The mechanism of shock following suicidal doses of barbiturate, narcotics and tranquillizing drugs, with observations on the effects of treatment. *American Journal of Medicine* 38, 853–63.

Smith T.W., Butler V.P., Haber E., Fozzard H., Marcus F.I., Bremner W.F., Schulman I.C. & Phillips A. (1982) Treatment of life-threatening digitalis intoxication with digoxin-specific Fab antibody fragments. *New England Journal of Medicine* 307, 1357–62.

Stead A.H. & Moffat A.C. (1983) A collection of therapeutic, toxic and fatal blood drug concentrations in man. *Human Toxicology* 2, 437–64.

Thompson A.M., Robins J.B. & Prescott L.F. (1987) Changes in cardiorespiratory function during gastric lavage for drug overdose. *Human Toxicology* 6, 215–18.

Vale J.A. & Meredith T.J. (1981) Forced diuresis, dialysis and haemoperfusion. In *Poisoning Diagnosis and Treatment* (Eds Vale J.A. & Meredith T.J.) pp. 59–68. Update Books, London.

Wallin C-J. & Hulting J. (1983) Massive metoprolol poisoning treated with prenalterol. *Acta Medica Scandinavica* 214, 253–55.

Wiseman M.N. & Banim S. (1987) 'Glue sniffer's' heart? *British Medical Journal* 294, 739.

Wiseman H.M., Guest K., Murray V.S.G. & Volans G.N. (1987) Accidental poisoning in childhood: a multicentre survey. 1. General epidemiology. *Human Toxicology* 6, 293–301.

Wolff E.D. & Dreissen O.M.L. (1983) End kind met theofyllinevergiftiging. *Nederland Tijdschrift voor Geneeskunde* 121, 896–9.

73

Ventilatory Failure

D. ROYSTON

The view that the heart was the furnace where the 'fire of life' kept the blood boiling has long been relegated to antiquity. Current views on cell biology hold that each cell has its own set of furnaces; the mitochondria. These organelles are specialized towards supplying the cell with its energy needs by oxidation of organic substrates. The mitochondrion is equipped with a set of enzymes which degrade sugars to carbon dioxide, extracting hydrogen ions in the process which are, in turn, combined with oxygen to produce water. This fundamental process of energy production by oxidation depends totally on an adequate and continuous supply of oxygen.

The respiratory system is the first part in the complex chain which, by securing effective continuous exchange of oxygen and carbon dioxide between air and blood, enables respiration to proceed at cellular level without interference.

If this exchange between air and blood becomes discontinuous or impaired because of failure of one or more of the normal mechanisms of transfer, respiratory failure occurs.

The purpose of this chapter is to outline the current concepts of the mechanism by which this happens and to discuss the management of this problem. It is worth highlighting that the majority of the modern multidisciplinary intensive therapy units were established on the basis of the ability of anaesthetists to take control efficiently of patients breathing and thereby provide some support for the failing respiratory system. It is important also to underline that the concept of respiratory support units is comparatively new. Whilst major advances have and continue to be made, there are still yawning gaps in our knowledge.

Definition

A primary task is to provide a definition of respiratory failure. Many attempts have been made to provide a universally accepted definition for use by the clinician in all circumstances. As outlined above, the role of the respiratory system is to maintain gas exchange. The definition of failure of the system is based usually on measuring blood gas tensions in the end-organ (arterial blood) and allocating levels of normality. If the tension of carbon dioxide in arterial blood exceeds 6.7 kPa (50 mmHg) or that of oxygen is less than 8.0 kPa (60 mmHg) while the patient is at rest, breathing air at sea level and when there is no primary metabolic alkalosis, this is defined as respiratory failure (Sykes et al., 1976). Whilst this definition is extremely useful in terms of characterizing certain pathophysiological states, it does not necessarily define clinical management strategies. For example, respiratory support with artificial means would probably not be instituted in a patient known previously to have carbon dioxide retention as a consequence of chronic obstruction airway disease at a Pa_{CO_2} of 6.7 kPa (50 mmHg). In contrast, aggressive intervention may be instituted at a lower Pa_{CO_2} in a young asthmatic who fails to respond adequately to medical management of an acute attack.

Nonetheless, the definition of respiratory failure on blood gas tension criteria remains the most accepted and will remain so until other more suitable methds are established.

Failure of respiration

It is axiomatic from the previous section that 'respiratory failure' at a tissue level determines the ability of an organism to survive. The partial failure of the lungs and respiratory system alone may be compensated for by other mechanisms aimed at improving oxygen availability e.g. by improvements in the circulation or the gas transport capacity of the blood. For this reason, failure of the respiratory system alone is not considered in isolation but rather as part of an integrated interactive system. The concept of 'pulmonary failure' may then be discussed in two broad areas.

Failure of ventilation (ventilatory failure)

This may result from problems of mechanics or ventilatory control. In these conditions there is usually an increase in arterial blood carbon dioxide tension in addition to a reduction in oxygen tension.

Failure of tissue oxygenation (hypoxaemic failure)

This type of failure can have both a pulmonary and extrapulmonary aetiology. The majority of such disorders are inflammatory in nature and/or are related to pathology of the pulmonary vasculature with alterations in ventilation and perfusion leading to an increase in shunting of venous blood. Causes unrelated to the lung include reductions in blood flow (found in heart failure) and reductions in oxygen carrying capacity of the blood.

Causes of respiratory failure

As an exhaustive list of causes of respiratory failure would be extremely long, this section deals with the more commonly occurring causes leading to ventilatory and hypoxaemic failure. Although this classification aids description, it is not intended to suggest that the two terms and types of failure cannot be interlinked and the patient may present with hypoxaemic failure and progress rapidly to ventilatory failure.

Ventilatory failure

This is defined by an increase in the arterial carbon dioxide tension. This represents the balance between carbon dioxide production and alveolar ventilation. Ventilatory failure therefore follows if:

1 There is a reduction in alveolar ventilation to an amount which does not allow adequate exchange of carbon dioxide with ambient air.
2 Ventilation cannot increase to compensate for an increased carbon dioxide production.
3 There is inefficient removal from inappropriate matching of pulmonary perfusion and ventilation.

It is usual and convenient to consider the various causes of ventilatory failure by defining the underlying lesion according to its anatomical site.
1 Central nervous system.
2 Neuromuscular.

3 Thoracic cage and pleura.
4 Lungs and airways.

CENTRAL NERVOUS SYSTEM

An increase in total ventilation accompanies emotional surges and is normal prior to energetic physical activity e.g. in athletes immediately prior to a race. However, the vast majority of processes affecting the respiratory neuronal mechanism situated around the fourth ventricle produce depressed respiration.

The main causes of respiratory centre depression are:
1 Drugs.
2 Trauma.
3 Intracranial disease.
4 Hypoxia.
5 Hypercapnia.
The most common cause of respiratory centre depression is the administration of drugs, particularly those used to provide anaesthesia, analgesia and sedation. The mode of action to produce this depression varies between compounds. For example, the opioid analgesics do not affect tidal volume significantly but cause the internal cycling system in the respiratory centre to slow down or stop. The frequency of breathing is thus reduced until apnoea develops. In contrast, the barbiturates and volatile anaesthetics reduce the ventilation by decreasing tidal volume whilst having usually little effect on respiratory frequency.

It is important to remember that in the presence of other causes of CNS depression such as hypoxaemia or trauma the respiratory centre is more sensitive to the effects of sedative and analgesic agents.

Trauma to the brain may produce central depression either as a direct result of trauma itself or secondary to an increased intracranial pressure when there is a reduction in cerebral perfusion pressure and cerebral blood flow. The most extreme example of the effects of trauma and raised intracranial pressure is coning of the medulla leading to apnoea.

Ventilatory depression consequent to raised intracranial pressure from intracranial tumours is usually a preterminal event. However, there are a number of inflammatory diseases of the nervous system which may lead to reductions in ventilation. Encephalitis and bulbar involvement in ascending polyneuritis represent the most commonly seen examples of this type of lesion in the UK. More rarely, patients with poliomyelitis and tetanus may demonstrate also the same derangement in ventilatory control.

Finally, moderate hypoxaemia and hypercapnia act as stimulants to breathing, the former via peripheral chemoreceptors, the latter acting centrally. However, with severe hypoxia the pattern of respiration becomes irregular and of the so-called Cheyne–Stokes pattern; apnoea follows if hypoxaemia is not relieved. Similarly, with elevation of Pa_{CO_2} to values of 11–12 kPa (80–90 mmHg) there is an increasing depression of ventilation with a reduction in conscious level.

NEUROMUSCULAR

In this type of ventilatory failure, there is a normal central respiratory drive but the peripheral neural and muscular responses are abnormal.

There are four main causes of this problem:
1 Drugs and toxins.
2 Spinal cord dysfunction from trauma or infection.
3 Congenital or acquired muscle disease.
4 Myasthenia gravis.

As in the case of the central depression of ventilation, this type of ventilatory failure most commonly follows the administration of drugs, particularly those used to provide neuromuscular blockade. Persistent respiratory inadequacy after their withdrawal is invariably a result of overdosage, especially if these compounds are given in full dosage to patients with myasthenia gravis or Eaton–Lambert syndrome. Other causes of inadequate reversal include disorders of acid–base balance and electrolyte disorders, especially those affecting calcium homeostasis.

Two further causes of myoneuronal blockade now seen rarely are poisoning with organophosphorus insecticides and botulinus toxin. The former acts as an anticholinesterase producing an excess of acetylcholine at the motor end-plate and the latter acts by inducing a failure to release this neurotransmitter. Whilst the final effect of both toxins is to produce a flaccid paralysis, it may be that patients with organophosphorus poisoning have a period of time where there are excitatory phenomena and convulsions.

The most common inflammatory lesion in the UK affecting the spinal cord is acute polyneuritis (Guillain–Barre syndrome) which is usually a self-limiting and reversible condition of the lower motor neurone producing flaccid paralysis. Infections of the anterior horn cell with the poliomyelitis virus are now extremely rare in the UK and USA but are still a considerable cause of morbidity and mortality in the world.

Patients with muscular dystrophies and myositis present occasionally with ventilatory failure. However, ventilatory failure in these conditions more usually follows chest infection, acquired as a complication of treatment rather than to muscle weakness alone.

Patients with myasthenia gravis may present with ventilatory failure either as a consequencee of their disease or as a complication of therapy. In addition, myasthenic patients require often ventilatory support in the perioperative period following thymectomy.

THORACIC CAGE AND PLEURA

This system is the force generator for respiration. Failure of the system leading to hypercapnic respiratory failure results from problems with either the muscles of inspiration or the 'mechanical' connection to provide adequate lung movement.

Inspiratory muscle fatigue (the patient getting 'tired') is probably the most common reason for instituting mechanical ventilatory support. It is also an area in which there is a comparative paucity of well-controlled clinical trials and research.

In addition to the more hereditary muscle diseases such as muscular dystrophy, the respiratory muscles may be compromised in many ways. Increased work of breathing, usually a consequence of an underlying lung problem, mechanical disadvantage, impaired nutritional status, shock, hypoxaemia and electrolyte deficencies (especially potassium, magnesium and inorganic phosphates) are major factors which contribute to respiratory muscle fatigue and failure.

To allow the chest-wall muscles and mechanics to work at their best advantage, the thoracic cage should be both uniform and firm. If the thoracic cage is not uniform (for example in patients with kyphoscoliosis) or has a flail segment (following thoracic trauma), ventilatory failure may develop rapidly. Interestingly, in patients suffering from ankylosing spondylitis with a stiff (or immobile) chest wall but with uniformity of shape, the incidence of ventilatory failure is low.

LUNGS AND AIRWAYS

Ventilatory failure with hypercapnia is a late event in the majority of disease processes affecting the lungs and airways. The majority of patients have hypoxaemia as a primary abnormality.

Large airway disease

The pivotal mechanism by which ventilatory failure is produced in larger airways disease is by airway narrowing. As the flow resistance of an airway is inversely proportional to the fourth power of its radius, small changes in the lumen have profound effects on air flow rates and increase the work of breathing, leading eventually to inspiratory muscle fatigue. By far the most common cause of large airway lumen obstruction is the presence of secretions.

Other less commonly seen but easily treated causes include upper airway obstruction following infection (epiglottitis, laryngotracheitis, 'croup'), trauma (post-intubation) and tumour (either directly or via involvement of the recurrent laryngeal nerve).

Sleep apnoea syndrome

One final cause of ventilatory failure which does not at present fit comfortably into any single classification is the so-called sleep apnoea syndrome. This was described originally as general alveolar hypoventilation (Fishman *et al.*, 1966) and is a syndrome of respiratory and cardiac failure in patients with normal lungs (Strohl *et al.*, 1986). Patients with this condition are usually obese (nearly always 30% greater than their ideal weight, sometimes three times heavier!), although it is not known if this is cause or effect of the disease. During rapid eye movement (REM) sleep, the patients develop complete upper airway obstruction to air flow for periods lasting over 15 sec. The desaturation of arterial blood which follows leads to arousal and relief of the obstruction. Daytime somnolence is a part of the syndrome.

The patients eventually develop crippling pulmonary hypertension with hypoxaemia, hypercapnia and right heart failure. The diagnosis of sleep apnoea syndrome is made by continuously monitoring respiration, oxygen saturation, electroencephalogram (for sleep stages) and electroculography (for eye movement) during sleep. Similar periods of pronounced episodic desaturation related to obstructive hypopnoea and apnoea have been recorded in the first 16 postoperative hours in patients given morphine for analgesia. These episodes are not seen in patients who had analgesia provided by local anaesthetic blockade (Catley *et al.*, 1985).

Lower airway obstruction

Lower airway narrowing is a predominant feature of the respiratory failure associated with a number of diseases, particularly:

1 Asthma.
2 Bronchiolitis.
3 Chronic obstructive lung disease.

The presence of intraluminal secretions has profound effects on airway calibre leading to increasing airway resistance (chronic bronchitis, asthma, bronchiolitis), although airway narrowing by either bronchiolar muscle spasm (asthma) or a lack of appropriate elastic recoil (emphysema) play a part also. Nevertheless, the predominant and primary effect of all these diseases is to produce a mismatching of ventilation and perfusion ($\dot{V}/\dot{Q}$) leading to arterial hypoxaemia; ventilatory failure is usually a late event in these patients.

Hypoxaemic respiratory failure

Hypoxaemia may develop as a consequence of:

1 Low inspired oxygen concentration.
2 Alveolar hypoventilation.
3 Increased $\dot{V}/\dot{Q}$ mismatching.
4 Increase in intrapulmonary shunting.
5 Limitation of diffusion across the alveolar capillary barrier.

The alveolar : arterial oxygen tension difference is normal in the first two causes and elevated in the latter three. Diffusion limitation once held as a major component and cause of hypoxaemia, is currently not believed to contribute to clinical respiratory failure.

The principle underlying lesion in hypoxaemic failure is abnormalities of $\dot{V}/\dot{Q}$ matching in the lung. Table 73.1 shows a number of the disease processes associated causally with the development of hypoxaemic failure from $\dot{V}/\dot{Q}$ mismatch. Although for convenience the diseases have been listed under vascular and alveolar unit causes of this defect, there are certain conditions which overlap these boundaries. For example, patients suffering from the so-called adult respiratory distress syndrome (ARDS) have pulmonary vascular abnormalities in addition to pulmonary oedema and alveolitis.

The predominant effect of most of these diseases is to produce increased stiffness of the lung parenchyma and a reduction in lung compliance necessitating an increased work of breathing to maintain ventilation. Infiltration of the lung parenchyma with inflammatory cells, exudates and oedema fluid is thought to lead to stimulation of the J-receptor in the lung parenchyma. This in turn produces the sensation of shortness of breath which is usually the predominant and primary symptom in patients with such diseases.

Table 73.1 Disease processes associated with the development of hypoxaemia and respiratory failure

Alveolar unit
Pneumonia
Bronchiectasis (cystic fibrosis)
Inhalation
   Firesmoke
   Gastric contents
   Near drowning
Interstitial lung disease
Radiation
Pulmonary haemorrhage and contusion
Opportunist infections in immune-compromised hosts
   Aspergillus and other fungi
   Cytomegalovirus
   Pneumocystis carnii
Respiratory failure with pulmonary oedema following a non-pulmonary disease (ARDS)

Circulation
Cardiac pulmonary oedema
Pulmonary artery embolism
   Fat
   Thromboemboli
   Amniotic fluid
Pulmonary hypertension
   Primary (plexiform lesions)
   Secondary (Eisenmenger's syndrome)

There are two further pathological conditions which lead to impaired tissue oxygenation, although the arterial Po_2 may not be reduced:

1 Limitation of oxygen delivery to the perpheral tissues so that aerobic metabolism cannot be maintained. Examples include severe anaemia, carbon monoxide poisoning and low cardiac output states.
2 Failure to extract oxygen at tissue level to allow its use for aerobic metabolism. The most obvious example of this is poisoning with cyanide. However, there is a recent body of evidence to suggest that in certain disease processes, associated with multi-system failure, improvements in delivery are not matched by increases in peripheral usage.

Principles of management of respiratory failure

These may be classified into two broad categories based on the actiological subgroups.
1 Methods to improve gas transfer to alveoli.
2 Methods to improve tissue oxygenation.

Methods to improve gas transfer

These can be subdivided further into:
1 General methods to improve ventilation.
2 Specific methods based on treating certain known underlying disease processess especially airflow obstruction.

GENERAL MANAGEMENT

Ventilatory failure with a high arterial carbon dioxide tension can be reversed only by altering those factors which affect this gas tension: carbon dioxide production and alveolar ventilation, $\dot{V}_A$.

Carbon dioxide production may be reduced using antipyretics such as aspirin or paracetamol, by surface cooling, using antibiotics in the presence of a proven infection and by the judicious use of sedatives to reduce excessive muscle activity from shivering or agitation.

Alveolar ventilation may be improved by restoring normal control of ventilation, overcoming lung restriction and, most importantly, by reducing airflow obstruction mainly by ensuring clearance of secretions. Tracheal intubation and mechanical support may be necessary if these measures fail.

Retained secretions increase airway resistance and thereby the work of breathing (related to the fourth power of the airway radius).

Clearance of secretions may therefore produce a major reduction in the work of breathing.

Causes of retained secretions include:
1 Mucus hypersecretion as found in asthma or in bronchiectasis (e.g. cystic fibrosis).
2 Impaired ciliary function, most commonly from chronic inhalation of irritants such as tobacco smoke. However, there are many iatrogenic causes of decreased ciliary beat frequency. The most important are increases in inspired oxygen concentration and the administration of anaesthetics, opioids and sedatives.
3 Ineffective or absent cough may occur in patients with neuromuscular disease or following CNS or spinal trauma. Drug overdose either by intent or iatrogenic is a further potent cause of absent cough. Adequacy of cough to expel secretions requires the generation of an explosive expiratory flow. Inability to take a deep breath, weak abdominal muscles or unwillingness to contract them because of pain, and small airways collapse on forced expiration (as occurs in obstructive lung disease) all reduce cough efficiency significantly.
4 Alterations or abnormalities of mucus secretion may be important. The mucus secretions of the large airways are a complex mixture of mucopolysac-

charides which act as a thyxotrope. Purulent sputum has different visco-elastic properties to non-purulent sputum. One factor known to modify the transport velocity of sputum is the degree of hydration. Experimental work has shown that mucus flow may be reduced by 25% in the presence of systemic dehydration.

5 Bronchoconstriction and airway collapse potentiate secretion retention. Airway collapse may lead also to plugging of airways with subsequent atelectasis of the distal segment thereby decreasing lung compliance leading to increased $\dot{V}/\dot{Q}$ inequalities.

THERAPY TO IMPROVE CLEARANCE OF SECRETIONS

From the above outline of causes, a simple management plan to improve clearance should include:

1 Adequate hydration. This is attained by ensuring that humidification of the inspired gas is appropriate using either a nebulizer or hot-water device. Additionally, any systematic dehydration should be corrected. The visco-elastic properties of sputum may also be modified pharmacologically. In particular, N-acetyl cysteine and bromhexene have been suggested as therapies to reduce the 'stickiness' of sputum and aid its removal. Unfortunately, controlled trials have not been in agreement regarding the value of these compounds (Wanner & Rao, 1980).

2 Chest physiotherapy. This is the mainstay of therapy to remove secretions by using techniques such as postural drainage, percussion and vibration when accompanied by cough to clear secretions. If the patient's ability to cough is inadequate, secretions may be expelled with the aid of artificial breaths and suctioning (bagging and sucking). This does not necessarily require tracheal intubation but may be performed using a T-piece and mask following insertion of a nasopharyngeal airway under local anaesthesia.

There are a number of relative contra-indications to chest physiotherapy which include:

(a) Raised intracranial pressure.

(b) Active or recent lung haemorrhage.

(c) Multiple rib fractures when percussion and vibration may lead to pneumothorax.

(d) Lung abscess and empyema unless it is possible to institute powerful endotracheal and endobronchial suction in case of rupture.

(e) Uncontrolled hypoxaemia when postural changes induce haemodynamic disturbances.

(f) Patients with severe shortness of breath, low cardiac output or cardiac arrhythmia should be treated with caution, as the physiotherapy itself is known to produce an increase in $\dot{V}/\dot{Q}$ mismatch during the procedure.

Finally, a number of patients with chronic sputum retention develop acute lobar atelectasis in the perioperative period probably because of mucus plugging. Bronchoscopy and removal of this plug under direct vision is often suggested as the therapy of choice. However, a prospective study of the use of fibre-optic bronchoscopy and physiotherapy in patients with acute lobar atelectasis showed no benefit of bronchoscopy over physiotherapy alone (Marini et al., 1979).

Airflow obstruction may be relieved also by using an *artificial airway* which is used usually for four specific indications:

1 Prevention or reversal of upper airway obstruction e.g. permanent tracheostomy in a patient with sleep apnoea syndrome or laryngeal tumours.

2 Protection against aspiration in patients with impairment of the level of consciousness from drugs or organic CNS disease.

3 Facilitating tracheobronchial toilet. A fine suction catheter via a nasopharyngeal airway passed into the trachea for suctioning at the time of chest physiotherapy is often of great benefit.

4 To allow mechanical ventilation. This is by far the commonest indication for tracheal intubation whether by the oral or nasal route. When choosing the route for tracheal intubation, it is often worth considering the technique proposed to wean the patient from ventilation. There is, for example, little point in passing a 7 mm nasotracheal tube in a patient with chronic obstructive lung disease as the tube itself produces a resistance to air flow some four times higher than that of the patients own airway. In this case it may be that an early tracheostomy with the insertion of a 12 mm tube (which has the same resistance to airflow as the patient) may be more useful.

VENTILATORY SUPPORT

Mechanical support

Mechanical ventilatory support is indicated when there is hypercapnia from CNS depression or neuromuscular disease. In addition, many centres would institute controlled hyperventilation in patients with cerebral trauma in order to produce hypocapnia, to aid the reduction of post-traumatic oedema.

As suggested earlier, the exact timing of institution of ventilatory support based on blood gas criteria is more difficult to define in patients with pulmonary disease. It is based usually on additional clinical criteria such as patient age, chronicity of the underlying disease process and prospects for recovery from the disease.

Probably of equal controversy is the type of ventilation to use and the pattern of ventilation to select. Earlier ventilators were negative-pressure devices of the tank or cuirass type. Until recently, this mode of support has been reserved for patients with normal lungs such as those patients with muscle weakness or neuromuscular dysfunction.

More modern ventilators apply intermittent positive pressure to the airway to promote gas transfer. The simplest such devices provide a near sinusoidal waveform, and only the frequency of breathing and the volume of each breath can be altered independently. Attempts to overcome the many disadvantages and potential deleterious affects of such systems have taxed engineers and clinicians alike. Such systems as assisted mechanical ventilation (AMV) and (synchronized) intermittent mandatory ventilation ((S)IMV) have been developed. It is thought that AMV would spare the patient the energy cost of breathing by providing the inspiratory power from the machine. However, measurements in clinical practice suggest that some patients receiving mechanical assistance with AMV may continue to perform respiratory work at levels which stress the ventilatory reserve and as a consequence work levels during AMV may be comparable to the work of chest inflation during spontaneous ventilation (Marini et al., 1986). Similarly, the use of (S)IMV has failed to show the major benefits ascribed originally to the method (Luce et al., 1981).

High-frequency ventilation (HFV) using high-pressure jets or oscillators has been suggested as an advance in ventilatory support. However, in the presence of airflow limitation, the devices produce a highly predictable increase in resting lung volume with an increased likelihood of barotrauma. In patients with low lung compliance, there is a theoretical benefit for increased respiratory frequency compared to conventional intermittent positive-pressure ventilation (IPPV). However, studies designed to investigate this theory have failed to show any significant benefit of HFV (Brichart et al., 1986). The optimum ventilator and pattern of ventilation which is applicable universally to patients with ventilatory failure remains unclear.

PHARMACOLOGICAL SUPPORT OF VENTILATION

Increased alveolar ventilation may be achieved in certain conditions using pharmacological support. Doxapram stimulates an increase in minute ventilation, and aminophylline and isoprenaline can restore the force of contractility of the diaphragm (Aubier et al., 1981). However, there have been no controlled clinical trials to examine the application and efficiency of such support in acute (and chronic) ventilatory failure.

SPECIFIC THERAPY TO RELIEVE AIRFLOW OBSTRUCTION

There is considerable interest in the definition and concept of airflow limitation and its management. Historically, airflow limitation has been designated according to the response to a set dose of a known bronchodilator. Thus, patients suffered from either reversible disease, perceived as asthma in the young, atopic non-smoker with a family history, or irreversible disease, found in older, tobacco smokers often with bronchitis and emphysema.

The study by Eliasson and de Graff (1985), however, showed that airflow limitation (measured as the forced expiratory volume in 1 sec, $FEV_{1.0}$) would not distinguish between these patients with 'asthma' and those with chronic obstructive airway disease (COAD). These authors questioned the practice of classifying patients with known airflow limitation as either asthmatic or COAD. Studies such as this together with recent reappraisals of the meaning of the term obstructive airway disease (Fletcher & Pride, 1984) imply that the majority of patients with airflow obstruction (except those with fixed upper airway lesions) may benefit from a trial of bronchodilator therapy. Indeed, it has been argued cogently (Luce et al., 1984) that acute ventilatory failure in patients with COAD is manageable nearly always without mechanical ventilation if the patient is alert on admission. This point is amplified by a recent review suggesting that 94 % of patients admitted with respiratory failure and with a history of COAD did not receive ventilatory support and left hospital (Rosen, 1986). In addition, these patients pose a special problem in regard to weaning from ventilatory support and the primary goals of therapy must be to avoid mechanical support.

In cases where ventilatory support is felt to be justified, there is a reported mortality of approximately

25% of patients with COAD requiring more than 24 hr ventilation, compared with a mortality of 80% in patients with multiple organ failure (Gillespie *et al.*, 1986).

Methods to improve tissue oxygenation

Classically, tissue hypoxaemia has been classified into four aetiological subgroups.
1 Hypoxic hypoxia.
2 Anaemic hypoxia.
3 Stagnant hypoxia.
4 Cytotoxic hypoxia.
In patients with respiratory failure, the problem is hypoxic hypoxia where arterial oxygen tension is abnormal as a result of a $\dot{V}/\dot{Q}$ mismatch in the lung. However, in the clinical situation where hypoxaemia is refractory to therapeutic intervention, it may be that therapy to improve oxygen transport (increasing the red cell mass) and availability (improving tissue blood flow) may have profoundly beneficial effects. As other variables can determine tissue oxygenation, the measurement of arterial blood tension of oxygen alone may be misleading. In certain situations, monitoring cardiac output together with oxygen contents of arterial and mixed venous blood may be important.

THERAPY TO IMPROVE ARTERIAL BLOOD
OXYGENATION

Increasing inspired oxygen concentration

Administration of added oxygen is the most obvious first step in reversing or diminishing arterial hypoxaemia. Oxygen is administered often as first-line and potentially life-saving therapy although in theory administration of oxygen to patients with relatively fixed right–left shunting should be ineffective. However, it is important to note that giving added oxygen may not be without dangers. This is true in patients with chronic respiratory failure who present with an acute exacerbation. The hypoxic ventilatory drive diminishes greatly when the Pao_2 increases above 8.7 kPa (65 mmHg). In patients whose breathing is stimulated primarily by hypoxic drive, the administration of added oxygen may produce severe hypoventilation or apnoea.

Additionally high inspired oxygen tensions have other adverse and toxic effects which are discussed more fully in the section on oxygen toxicity. It is therefore important to define the goals of oxygen administration.

The curvilinear relationship between arterial oxygen tension and the saturation of haemoglobin is well known. Because of this relationship, an increase in Pao_2 of, say, 3 kPa (22.5 mmHg) has differing effects depending on the original Pao_2. If this were 6 kPa (45 mmHg), a 3 kPa (22.5 mmHg) increase raises saturation from 75% to 90%, equivalent to oxygen content increasing from 15 ml/dl to 18 ml/dl for a haemoglobin of 15 g/dl. However, a 3 kPa (22.5 mmHg) increase in Pao_2 from 10.7 kPa (80 mmHg) increases haemoglobin saturation by only 3%, a content increase of only about 0.5 ml/dl.

For this reason it is conventional to attempt to maintain Pao_2 at approximately 10 kPa (75 mmHg) in an attempt to balance the beneficial effects of added oxygen against its potentially deleterious effects.

Raising airway pressure

It has been known for some time that by raising end-expiratory pressure [conventionally termed continuous positive airway pressure (CPAP) for spontaneously breathing and positive end-expiratory pressure (PEEP) for patients receiving assisted ventilation] can improve Pao_2. These techniques are used in addition to added inspired oxygen in conditions where there is diffuse, restrictive disease associated with a reduction in functional residual capacity. Classically, these disorders represent the pulmonary complications of anaesthesia, surgery and inadequately treated primary ventilatory failure. Whilst raising the airway pressure has beneficial effects, it can also be deleterious and inappropriate, particularly in patients who already have abnormally high functional residual capacity (FRC) e.g. in obstructive lung disease, raising FRC further may have deleterious effects on gas exchange and simply increase the incidence and severity of barotrauma. Additionally, in patients with large physiological deadspace as a result of vascular occlusions a further increase in this deadspace induced by PEEP/CPAP may result in alveolar hypoventilation and retention of carbon dioxide. The use of PEEP is relatively contra-indicated in the presence of localized and unhomogeneous disease, especially if there is evidence of gas trapping.

Correctly used, PEEP/CPAP can restore an abnormally low FRC towards normal. Nonetheless, there is still lack of agreement concerning the most appropriate means of determining the optimum timing, levels and outcome of the application of PEEP.

Before applying PEEP it is worth asking:
1 Is this manoeuvre likely to benefit the patient?

2 What level of raised airway pressure is optimal for this individual patient?

Therefore the goals of the therapy need to be defined. Application of PEEP in an attempt to allow an adequate Pa_{O_2} at a safe $F_{I_{O_2}}$ should be beneficial in patients with severe hypoxaemia from increased $\dot{V}/\dot{Q}$ mismatch, where the disease is diffuse and where there is a reduction in lung volumes.

Raising lung volumes above normal by raising airway pressure increases both pleural and intra-thoracic pressure throughout both the respiratory and the cardiac cycles. This leads to a reduction in cardiac ouput from decreased venous return to the right atrium. The amount of PEEP necessary to produce this effect is reduced markedly in patients with hypo-volaemia or intrinsic cardiac dysfunction. The increase in venous pressure and reduction in arterial pressure induced by PEEP make this modality of therapy inappropriate also in patients with raised intracranial pressure.

Attempting to minimize shunt from $\dot{V}/\dot{Q}$ mismatch requires usually very high levels of PEEP, an approach which requires intensive and aggressive cardiovascular support. This approach will produce the best Pa_{O_2} for the lowest $F_{I_{O_2}}$ and is appropriate when pulmonary oxygen toxicity may be a significant problem. However, some clinicians aim to maintain relatively low intravascular volumes. It is therefore more appropriate to apply PEEP to a level which has minimal effect on cardiac output whilst hopefully increasing haemoglobin saturation. The concept of optimum PEEP therefore depends on the objective of the therapy.

The application of PEEP and CPAP require usually the presence of an endotracheal tube. However, techniques of applying CPAP by close-fitting mask have been described. This technique may be useful in such conditions as viral pneumonia or following inhalation of toxic smoke and fumes. However, the technique does require that the patient is fully conscious and co-operative and is able to remove the mask if vomiting occurs.

Other deleterious and beneficial effects of PEEP/CPAP are discussed more fully in the later section on adult respiratory distress syndrome (ARDS).

Effects of position

In unilateral lung disease, a change in posture can have profound beneficial effects in returning $\dot{V}/\dot{Q}$ mismatch towards normality. Perfusion is increased to the dependent lung. Ventilation to the upper lung is greatest during controlled ventilation and to the lower lung during spontaneous breathing. In diffuse lung disease postural changes are also of great benefit, mechanical ventilation in the prone position increasing Pa_{O_2} (Douglas *et al.*, 1977).

Hyperbaric oxygenation

Hyperbaric oxygenation may have potential areas of benefit. However, its use in the management of acute respiratory failure has never been justified.

THERAPY TO IMPROVE TISSUE OXYGENATION

This may be classified into:
1 Increasing blood flow.
2 Increasing oxygen transport by haemoglobin or synthetic oxygen carriers.

Measurement of blood flow entails usually the use of a thermodilution cardiac output pulmonary artery catheter. The insertion of such a catheter is not routine in most patients with respiratory failure and their beneficial use in such situations is not known.

Increasing a reduced red cell mass may often have a beneficial effect on tissue oxygen delivery. For example, raising the total oxygen delivery to the tissues from 500 ml/min to 600 ml/min could be achieved by raising the haemoglobin concentration by 1.5 g/dl. This could probably be achieved more easily than raising cardiac output from 5 litre/min to 6 litre/min or the Pa_{O_2} from 8.0 kPa (60 mmHg) to 12 kPa (90 mmHg) to produce the same effect. Notwithstanding the obvious benefits of blood transfusion, there are worries related to the transmission of bloodborne diseases. The quest for synthetic substitutes for haemoglobin has been, and continues to be, the subject of intense research. At present, perflurocarbon preparations (e.g. Fluosol DA) have significant toxic side-effects. However, newer less toxic substances are being prepared and these may lead to significant improvements in the future.

Adult respiratory distress syndrome (ARDS)

Background

The term ARDS is used to designate an episode of acute respiratory failure developing in association with a separate, usually non-pulmonary, medical or surgical illness. Once recognized, the syndrome should be appreciated as simply a statement of an immediate clinical condition, which needs to be defined in terms of the responsible aetiological factors. Although this type of respiratory failure had been described in detail previously (Cameron, 1948), the war in Vietnam emphasized the occurrence of the condition and brought this type of respiratory failure to the notice of a global audience. The paper by Ashbaugh and colleagues in 1967 was the first to describe the problem in civilian practice. They described sudden respiratory distress in 12 adult patients who had no evidence of either prior lung disease or heart failure. The disease was characterized by dyspnoea and reduced lung compliance. In addition, the patients exhibited low arterial oxygen tensions, refractory to increased F_IO_2 and diffuse infiltrates on chest radiography which strongly suggested pulmonary oedema. This condition was termed acute respiratory distress in adults (Ashbaugh et al., 1967).

Later studies by the same group (Petty & Ashbavgh, 1971) centred on the observation that histological damage to the lung and reduced surfactant activity resembled that found in neonates with idiopathic respiratory distress syndrome. They coined the term adult respiratory distress syndrome (ARDS) to describe the clinical syndrome.

Definition, diagnosis and incidence

The obvious first step in understanding and managing a problem is to develop a definition of that problem. Unfortunately, and in common with defining respiratory failure, there is no universally accepted definition of the condition. It is therefore clear that the true incidence of ARDS cannot be known accurately. The Task Force of the National Heart Lung and Blood Institute suggested that 150 000 cases of ARDS occurred each year in the USA alone (Murray, 1977). However, this figure is now thought to be a considerable underestimate. In addition, the likelihood of ARDS developing as a consequence of a specific cause varies also varies with that predisposition. The incidence and mortality for certain 'at-risk' populations is shown in Table 73.2. These data were obtained from prospective studies of ARDS in the USA (Pepe et al., 1982; Fowler et al., 1983). It must be emphasized that the criteria used for the diagnosis of ARDS were extremely strict compared to the original definition (Ashbaugh et al., 1967). The patients had to fulfil the following five criteria for ARDS to be diagnosed.

1 Respiratory failure requiring mechanical ventilation.
2 Alveolar : arterial oxygen tension ratio of less than 0.3.
3 Static respiratory compliance of less than 50 ml/cmH_2O.
4 Bilateral diffuse infiltrates on the chest radiograph.
5 Pulmonary capillary wedge pressure of less than 2.4 kPa (18 mmHg).

Thus, it may be that the incidence of the syndrome was underestimated. It may be also that by using these criteria only the most ill patients fulfilled the authors strict definition of ARDS and this resulted in an increased mortality associated with the condition.

The effect of modifying the definition of ARDS is apparent when the risk factor under investigation is cardiopulmonary bypass.

If the criteria for diagnosing ARDS are more akin to the originally described criteria (Ashbaugh et al., 1967) i.e.
1 Diffuse infiltrates on the chest X-ray,
2 Respiratory failure requiring mechanical ventilation with an F_IO_2 of more than 0.4 (i.e. a greater than 20% shunt),

Predisposition	% patients developing ARDS	% mortality in ARDS patients
Bacteria	30	77.8
Aspiration of gastric contents	36	94
Disseminated intravascular coagulation	22	50
Massive blood transfusion	5	45
Long-bone or pelvic fracture	5	0
Following cardiopulmonary bypass	1.7	50

Table 73.2 The percentage of patients who developed ARDS following a specific predisposing factor. Also included is the mortality in those patients who developed ARDS. (Data from Pepe et al., 1982; Fowler et al., 1983)

3 Absence of heart failure (i.e. low heart filling pressures),

then nearly all patients having open-heart surgery would be diagnosed as having ARDS in the immediate postoperative period. It is true also that simple cardiorespiratory support during the initial period of respiratory distress following open-heart surgery ensures that the mortality from this more loosely defined condition is essentially zero.

Notwithstanding these problems of definition, there is little doubt that acute pulmonary failure as a consequence of a separate non-pulmonary cause is responsible for an increasing proportion of admissions to the intensive therapy unit. Patients with ARDS account for approximately one in 15 patients requiring ventilation in a district general hospital (Searle, 1985) and approximately one in seven non-cardiac surgery patients at the author's institute.

Pathophysiology

The majority of the studies designed to identify and understand the mediators and modulators of this pulmonary injury have been performed in animals. The starting premise for such studies was that there was pulmonary capillary leak of protein-rich oedema fluid into the interstitium and airspaces.

In 1896 Starling defined the relationship between the forces which governed the rate of fluid flux across a capillary membrane. This relationship is stated simply as:

$$Q_{fluid} = K_f \times \Delta P,$$

where Q_{fluid} is the net fluid flow, K_f is the fluid filtration coefficient (or index of the 'leakiness' of the barrier to that fluid) and ΔP is the driving pressure for that fluid across the capillary. The term ΔP comprises the difference between hydrostatic pressure (tending to force fluid out of the circulation) and colloid oncotic pressure (tending to draw fluid into the circulation).

The development of the balloon flotation catheter allowed indirect determination of left heart filling pressures. It soon became obvious that patients with ARDS did not have increased intravascular pressures as the cause of lung failure; the 'cause' must therefore result from changes in K_f, or leakiness of the lung. Further evidence to imply an increased lung leak came from investigations in humans with ARDS who had mean oedema fluid to plasma protein concentration ratios which were statistically greater than those found in patients with cardiac oedema (Sprung et al., 1981).

However, this was not found universally and there was overlap between the results of these protein ratios between the cardiac oedema and ARDS patients.

At the same time as the development of the theory of ARDS based on Starling forces, an animal model was described in which lung lymph was collected from the caudal mediastinal lymph node of the unanaesthetized sheep (Staub et al., 1975). Alteration in the rate of flow of this lymph, together with any changes in the concentration of the constituent proteins, can be ascribed to changes in driving pressure (cardiac oedema) or increased permeability/surface area of the alveolar capillary barrier (non-cardiac permeability oedema).

Increased flows of high-protein lung lymph or frank pulmonary oedema, suggesting increased permeability of the alveolar capillary barrier, have been produced in this model by infusions of bacteria and endotoxin (simulating sepsis), fibrin degradation products (simulating disseminated intravascular coagulopathy, DIC) and microemboli (air or glass beads) (Rinaldo & Rogers, 1982). The ability to produce an ARDS-like syndrome in experimental animals with evidence of increased lung leakiness led to the concept of treatment based on mechanical ventilatory support together with manipulation of Starling forces. However, histological examination of biopsy specimens obtained before and after death from patients with ARDS in the American extracorporeal membrane oxygenator study revealed that the concept of ARDS being purely a capillary-leak syndrome causing non-cardiac, pulmonary oedema was oversimplified. The normal Type I epithelial cells were lost rapidly and replaced with proliferating Type II cells, leading to a greatly thickened alveolar septa. The interstitial space became infiltrated with inflammatory cells and fibroblasts. There was rapid obliteration of alveolae, alveolar ducts and interstitium by fibrous tissue. The pulmonary vasculature became obliterated early in the development of this progressive response (Pratt et al., 1979). These histological features showed clearly that changes which occur over weeks or months in patients not receiving cardiopulmonary support could occur in days in patients receiving such support. With this extremely complex series of events, it is not surprising that mechanical ventilatory support and manipulation of Starling forces has met with little success.

Because of the lack of a beneficial treatment there has been a great deal of effort directed to establishing the mediators and modulators of the acute oedematous lesion. A vast number of humoral and cellular

Table 73.3 Humoral mediators shown to increase macromolecular transport across capillaries. Also shown to indicate potency are molar concentrations of substance producing the effect

Mediator	Effective concentration (M)
Histamine, hydroxytryptamine	10^{-6}
Bradykinin, substance P	10^{-7}
ADP, adenosine, inosine	10^{-5}
Prostaglandins E_1, E_2, F_2	$> 10^{-8}$
Leukotrienes C_4, D_4, E_4, B_4	$> 10^{-9}$
C_3a, C_5a	$> 10^{-9}$
Platelet-activating factor	$> 10^{-9}$
Fibrin-derived products	—
Free-radicals	—
Immune complexes	—

mediators have been implicated. Table 73.3 shows a number of humoral mediators of capillary macromolecule leakage in hamsters (Svensjo & Grega, 1986). Extrapolation of data to pulmonary injury is difficult. For example, histamine but not bradykinin increases lymph flow in sheep (Malik et al., 1985). Similarly, the pulmonary effects of the leukotrienes LTC_4, D_4 and E_4 (slow reacting substance of anaphylaxis, SRSA) depend on the animal studied. Cat and rabbit lungs are relatively immune to the effects of infusions of these leukotrienes. Guinea pig and sheep lungs respond with increased pulmonary vascular pressure and permeability (Malik et al., 1985).

Of the formed elements in the blood, considerable interest has focused on the role of the neutrophil in inducing the lung injury leading to ARDS, specifically the hypothesis that neutrophils are activated, perhaps by complement conversion products. These activated neutrophils sequester in lung where they release cytotoxic substances, which are released normally as part of the body's host defences. Activated neutrophils release reactive oxygen species (ROS). These highly toxic species can degrade DNA and hyaluronic acid, peroxidise membrane lipids, destroy endothelial cells and increase capillary permeability. In addition, they inactivate α1-antiproteinase rapidly, a crucially important defence mechanism against proteolytic enzymes. The neutrophil can also release proteases that destroy collagen, elastin and the adhesive glycoprotein fibronectin. The proteases can also cleave fibrinogen, complement and Hageman factor (Fig. 73.1).

Humans with severe ARDS have evidence of activated neutrophils in the circulation (Zimmerman et al., 1983). There is also evidence in humans for a significant increase in oxidant and proteolytic activity in the lungs of patients with ARDS (Cochrane et al., 1983; Brigham & Meyrick, 1984). However, these mechanisms do not provide a universal explanation.

Complement activation occurs as commonly in ill patients without pulmonary failure as in those with (Weinberg et al., 1984). In addition, ARDS has been reported in patients without evidence of neutrophil involvement (Braude et al., 1985).

The role of platelets in triggering or augmenting the original lung injury of ARDS has not been characterized as thoroughly. In the sheep, infusion of

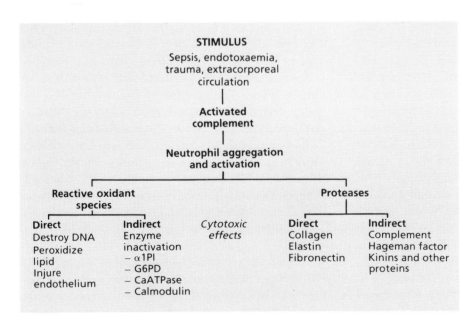

Fig. 73.1 Schematic outline of proposed mechanism of cytotoxic effects of neutrophils leading to ARDS.

study in patients given steroids for neural trauma. They also developed sepsis and multi-system failure more frequently than non-steroid-treated patients (De Maria *et al.*, 1985). Based on this evidence, the use of high-dose steroids to treat patients with ARDS can no longer be recommended routinely.

Considerable interest has been shown in three other areas.

1 Arachidonic acid metabolites and inhibitors of metabolism.
2 Oxidant free-radical scavengers.
3 Fibronectin and antiprotease augmentation.

The vast majority of evidence suggesting efficacy of these approaches has been performed in animal models of lung injury. When human studies have been performed, the results have been less dramatic. In particular, administration of prostaglandin E_1 and the thromboxane synthetase antagonist, dazoxiben, have not been shown to be of benefit (Leeman *et al.*, 1985; Shoemaker & Appel, 1986). Non-steroidal, anti-inflammatory agents have a number of potent toxic side-effects including an increased incidence of gastrointestinal bleeding and renal dysfunction (Patmas *et al.*, 1984).

A number of lung injuries may be reduced by the administration of antioxidants and free-radical scavengers. In particular, the increased lung lymph flow following endotoxin administration in the sheep can be prevented by the prior administration of N-acetyl cysteine (normally used as a source of sulphydryl groups in paracetamol overdose). Unfortunately, this agent increased mortality in other oxidant stress injuries such as the administration of bleomycin (Patterson *et al.*, 1985). Moreover, increasing antioxidant protection to endotoxin-treated sheep by administering superoxide dismutase (SOD) increased the permeability injury (Traber *et al.*, 1985). These data suggest that it would be premature to design clinical trials of antioxidants and free-radical scavengers in ARDS.

Reversal of opsonic deficiencies by administration of cryoprecipitate which is rich in fibronectin has been claimed to be highly beneficial. However, controlled trials have failed to demonstrate clear differences in fibronectin concentrations between survivors and non-survivors in intensive therapy units. The benefit of giving antiproteinase compounds awaits human studies.

Overall, it is obvious that there is currently no specific therapy which reduces the permeability injury of ARDS from any cause.

Increased lymphatic drainage and fluid clearance

Data related to methods of increasing lung fluid clearance are sparse. Essentially nothing is known of the factors which modify active lung lymph flow. There is, however, a body of evidence to suggest active transport plays a major role in lung fluid clearance e.g. infusions of β-agonists increase lung liquid clearance in neonatal lambs. Airway instillation of amiloride (which inhibits sodium transport) slows fluid clearance in adult sheep (Staub, 1983). Obviously, a great deal more needs to be known of such active transport systems before controlled trials and guidelines for therapy can be instituted.

PREVENTION OF COMPLICATIONS

As there is no proven therapy for patients with ARDS, the outcome is dependent on natural healing and prevention of complications, particularly further lung injury manifest clinically as barotrauma or fibrosis. The incidence of barotrauma may be reduced, if not prevented, by measures to minimize airway pressures and lung volumes (Hillman, 1985).

Little is known of the intermediate messages that link the early capillary leak syndrome to the later disordered fibrotic response. As discussed previously, this fibrotic response can occur within 24–48 hr of clinical presentation with the syndrome. Biochemical agents aimed specifically at collagen synthesis have been studied in models of lung injury (Rinaldo & Rogers, 1982). However, there have been no controlled clinical trials of these compounds, and it is clear that some of these agents would have limited use in conditions where collagen turnover is high, for example in healing wounds.

Prevention of infection

Prevention of infection and sepsis is of great importance. In a prospective study of outcome of patients with ARDS, the patients with sepsis had a significantly greater incidence of multiple organ failure and a far greater mortality (Bell *et al.*, 1983). This progression of disease occurred even in those patients who were improving or had recovered from their respiratory failure. As endotoxin is thought to be a major trigger to developing organ failure, there is current interest in developing methods of preventing or reducing the effects of endotoxaemia. Administration of polyclonal antibodies against the core lipid of endotoxin reduced the mortality from sepsis (Ziegler *et al.*, 1982). A human monoclonal antibody has been developed and has been shown to prevent endotoxin-induced lung capillary leak in rats (Feeley *et al.*, 1987). Other methods to increase immunological surveillance are also being developed e.g. the use of muramyl dipeptides (Chedid, 1986).

One further complication may develop and that is the problem of oxygen toxicity which forms the basis of the final section of this chapter.

Oxygen toxicity

Whilst oxygen is necessary for life it is clear also that increased concentrations can be toxic and induce organ dysfunction. There are three major organs at risk of hyperoxic injury.

1 *Central nervous system.* Only affected under hyperbaric conditions.

2 *The lens of the eye in newborns.* High arterial partial pressures of oxygen are associated with neoangiogenesis of the posterior aspect of the lens. These new vessels allow the laying down of fibrous tissue, and this retrolental fibrous dysplasia produces reduced visual acuity and blindness.

3 *The lung.* The effects of hyperoxia in patients who rely on their hypoxic respiratory drive are well known. Similarly, it has been well demonstrated that breathing of 100% oxygen leads to instability of terminal ventilatory units and reversible absorption collapse (Winter & Smith, 1972).

In the next section the mechanisms of oxygen as an agent toxic to lung structure and function will be discussed.

Pathophysiology of pulmonary oxygen toxicity

The inhalation of high partial pressures of oxygen is known to be toxic to the lung of all mammals (Clark & Lambertson, 1971). The improved supportive care of patients with pulmonary failure and especially those with ARDS has resulted in prolonged survival, with a concomitant increase in the length of time the lung is exposed to high concentrations of inspired oxygen. The patient with respiratory failure has an added risk of an increase of the lung injury, as the levels of oxygen partial pressures used in this situation are potentially toxic. A number of questions thus require answers. How does oxygen induce this injury? How does the body normally protect itself from such injury? What are the effects of oxygen therapy on lung injury and repair? Are there means to prevent these deleterious effects?

HOW DOES OXYGEN INDUCE TISSUE INJURY?

In recent years, a biochemical mechanism involving cellular production of partially reduced metabolites of oxygen (sometimes termed oxidant free-radicals) has been proposed as the basis of oxygen toxicity. In brief, the two outer bonding electrons of molecular oxygen have parallel spins (Fig. 73.2). This configuration imparts a dipole to the molecule (which is used in clinical measurement) and it restricts the molecule into accepting further electrons one at a time. This single-step transfer is essential for the controlled electron transport which is necessary for mitochondrial high-energy phosphate production.

Reduction of oxygen may therefore be represented by the equation

$$O_2 + e^- \rightarrow O_2 + e^- \rightarrow O_2^{2-} + 2e^- + 4H^+ \rightarrow 2H_2O.$$

The compound O_2^{2-} is termed superoxide and is a free-radical i.e. a species capable of independent existence which contains an unpaired electron, signified usually by a superscript dot.

The molecular configurations of superoxide and peroxide radicals are shown in Fig. 73.2.

In life, the reaction is more complex as highlighted by the role of co-enzyme Q in electron transport. The

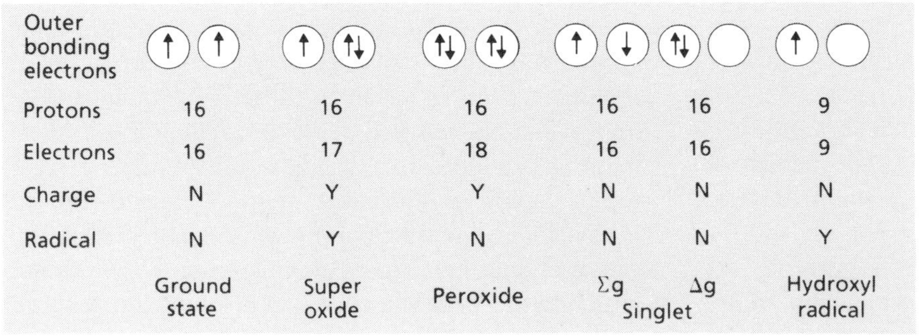

Outer bonding electrons	↑ ↑	↑ ↑↓	↑↓ ↑↓	↑ ↓ ↑↓	↑ ○
Protons	16	16	16	16 16	9
Electrons	16	17	18	16 16	9
Charge	N	Y	Y	N N	N
Radical	N	Y	N	N N	Y
	Ground state	Super oxide	Peroxide	Σg Δg Singlet	Hydroxyl radical

Fig. 73.2 Configurations of oxygen and certain reactive oxidant species to show direction of spin and number of outer bonding electrons, the number of protons and electrons, the presence (Y) or absence (N) of a charge and the definition of the species as a free-radical.

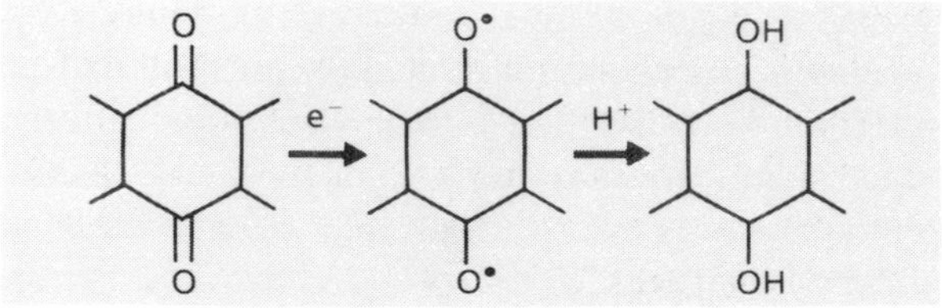

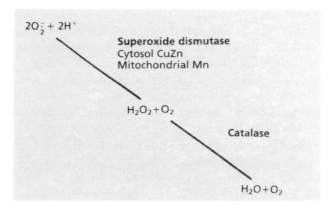

Fig. 73.3 To show the semi-quinone moiety of Co-enzyme Q accepting an electron to produce a free-radical intermediary prior to protonation. This free-radical generation is absolutely essential for the cytochrome chain of ATP production.

Fig. 73.4 Enzymatic conversion of the superoxide radical via hydrogen peroxide to water. Superoxide dismutase is found in humans in the mitochondria (the manganese form) and in the cell cytosol (the copper/zinc form).

active site in CoQ is a semi-quinone (Fig. 73.3) which has two oxygens capable of accepting electrons to produce a semi-quinone free-radical (CoQ^{-}) which is then protonated. In the hyperoxic state the semi-quinone free-radical is thought to react with molecular oxygen to produce superoxide:

$$CoQ + e^- \rightarrow CoQ^- + O_2 \rightarrow CoQ + O_2^-.$$

Although superoxide and peroxide radicals are oxidizing agents, they are relatively unreactive. The danger lies in their ability to react or combine to form other species of considerable potency and reactive capability, in particular hydroxyl radical (OH·) and singlet oxygen ($^1O_2$). Molecular configerations of these moities are shown in Fig. 73.2.

Four cell and tissue components are at greatest risk from oxidant attack:

1 Sulphydryl-containing enzymes and proteins. Most importantly α1-antiproteinase is inactivated rapidly. Glucose-6-phosphate dehydrogenase and enzymes of the citric acid cycle are also at risk.

2 Nucleic acids are damaged irreversibly by oxidants; a useful mode of action of a number of antitumour agents such as bleomycin. Cell death follows as intracellular components are not regenerated.

3 Collagen and glycoproteoglycan oxidation is thought to play a major part in the development of emphysema.

4 Peroxidation of polyunsaturated cell membrane lipids by oxidants leads to an increase in membrane permeability associated with a decreased fluidity.

PROTECTION FROM FREE-RADICAL TISSUE INJURY

It is obvious that with such a potential destructive ability the body has developed a system of antioxidant defences. These defences are based on two systems: an enzymatic system for aiding removal of superoxide and hydrogen peroxide (Fig. 73.4) and a system directed towards minimizing the effects of oxidant tissue injury

by removing the secondary free-radicals, usually lipids (designed ROO·) produced by the initial radical injury. Reduced glutathione can provide a source of protons from sulphydryl groups to protonated lipid radicals. The reduced glutathione is itself oxidized and the oxidized glutathione regenerated using energy dependent processes (Fig. 73.5). Other compounds, α-tocopherol ascorbate, caeruloplasmin, etc., act to reduce oxidant injury usually by accepting the free electron of the free-radical species (Halliwell & Gutteridge, 1985).

These antioxidant defences are found in high concentrations in metabolically active organs such as the liver and kidney. The lung is relatively poorly supplied with these defences and may therefore be at greater risk of hyperoxic injury.

WHAT ARE THE EFFECTS OF HYPEROXIA ON
THE LUNG AND ON LUNG INJURY?

Breathing 100% oxygen produces profound effects on the lung over a short time-period; within hours there

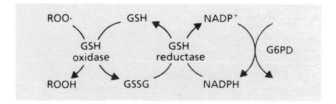

Fig. 73.5 Antioxidant protection using the tripeptide glutathione (GSH). Glutathione is oxidized during protonation of the lipid free-radical (ROO·) to produce the non-reactive lipid hydroperoxide and oxidized glutathione (GSSG). The reduced glutathione is regenerated using energy from the pentose phosphate pathway.

is severe substernal pain, associated with cessation of mucociliary transport. Inflammation of the airways follows within 18 hr. The vital capacity decreases after approximately 24 hr followed by abnormalities of carbon dioxide-diffusing capacity and a widening of the alveolar:arterial oxygen tension difference. Confirmation of lung toxicity in ventilated patients comes from a study in 10 patients who were diagnosed as brain-dead. Five patients ventilated with oxygen had oedematous, heavy lungs associated with increased alveolar:arterial oxygen tension differences, reduced compliance and increased deadspace:tidal volume ratios (Barber *et al.*, 1970). However, the patients in the study had received steroid therapy which may have affected the outcome.

The majority of studies determining the effects of added oxygen on injured lung have been performed in animals or *in vitro*. Oxygen promoted increased fibrosis in injured mouse lungs. Exposure of normal mouse lung to 70% oxygen for 24 hr or 50% for 6 days produced no effects. However, the same dose × time regimens given to animals whose lungs where injured previously with butylated hydroxytoluene produced extensive interstitial fibrosis (Witsch *et al.*, 1981).

Potentiation of oxygen toxicity is induced by a number of pharmacological and physical interventions (Table 73.4). The role of steroids in augmenting or reducing oxygen toxicity to the lung depends on their time of administration. Pretreatment with dexamethasone augmented lung injury, associated with decline in lung antioxidant defences. However, when dexame-

Table 73.4 Agents known to augment pulmonary oxygen toxicity in animals. (References may be found in Clark & Lambertson, 1971)

Agents which increase tissue metabolism
Thyroxine (or hyperthyroidism)
Adrenaline
Amphetamines
Hyperpyrexia

Exogenous agents
Paraquat
Nitrofurantoin
Disulphfiram (Antabuse)
Ionizing radiation

Dietary deficiency
Selenium
Copper
Vitamin C
Vitamin E
Sulphcontaining amino acids

thasone was administered at the end of exposure to oxygen, the effect was protective (Koizumi *et al.*, 1985).

It is not known if there is toxic interaction between oxygen administration and any of the mass of antibacterial, vasoactive or inotropic agents used in critically ill patients.

It has been argued cogently (Rinaldo & Rogers, 1982) that oxygen may increase or affect lung injury in a variety of different ways. Oxidants deactivate the lung antiprotease defences and induce alveolar macrophages to release neutrophil chemotaxins. Oxygen reduces the lung host defences by causing cessation of cilial action, by reducing alveolar macrophage migration and by increasing the adherence of Gram-negative organisms to lower respiratory tract epithelium.

In the light of this array of potential damaging effects, it is not surprising that the 'toxic threshold' for oxygen to the injured lung is unknown.

PREVENTION OF OXYGEN TOXICITY

Augmenting the lung antioxidant defences has been studied as a means of reducing toxicity.

Administration of excess vitamin C or E has no effect. However, liposome-encapsulated enzymes superoxide dismutase and catalase had beneficial effects (Brigham, 1986). Unfortunately, giving liposomes is associated with a depression of bacterial clearance and killing (McDonald *et al.*, 1985).

Stimulation of production of enzymatic protective mechanisms may be achieved by increasing the concentration of inspired oxygen slowly, although this method has limited clinical usefulness.

A further approach is the administration of endotoxin. Paradoxically, this manoeuvre leads to protection from hyperoxic pulmonary injury in the rat. Originally, this protective effect was thought to be via increasing enzymatic antioxidants. More recent studies have failed to demonstrate increases in enzyme levels despite protection by endotoxin (Spence *et al.*, 1986)

There is great interest currently in attempting to modify the endotoxin molecule to produce protective substances which have no inherent toxic action, so-called endotoxoids.

Finally, there is evidence that instillation of erythrocytes into the lung will protect animals from oxygen toxicity, possibly by increasing lung glutathione content (Brigham, 1986).

We are left with the conclusion that oxygen is known to be a potent damaging agent to the lung.

However, the significance of this to human disease is still far from clear.

Conclusion

Imminent and actual failure of respiration is still the most common reason for admission of patients to a critical care facility. Over the years the emphasis has changed from providing support for the patient with a single disease and relatively normal lungs to the complexities of managing severe lung injuries in the context of multiple organ failure.

The fundamental principles of management of the patient with failing respiration, however, have not altered radically i.e. having adequate ventilation whilst maintaining tissue oxygenation using methods with absent or minimal deleterious effects. The optimum and universally applicable methods of achieving these goals are, however, still not well defined.

References

Ashbaugh D.G., Bigelow D.B., Petty T.L. & Levine B.E. (1967) Acute respiratory distress in adults. *Lancet* ii, 319–23

Aubier M., De Troyer A. & Sampson M. (1981) Aminophylline improves diaphragmatic contractility in man. *New England Journal of Medicine* **305**, 249.

Barber R.E., Lee J. & Hamilton W.K. (1970) Oxygen toxicity in man; a prospective study in patients with irreversible brain damage. *New England Journal of Medicine* **283**, 1478–84.

Bell R.C., Coalson J.J. & Smith J.D. (1983) Multiple organ failure and infection in adult respiratory distress syndrome. *Annals of Internal Medicine* **99**, 293–8.

Braude S., Apperley J., Krausz T., Goldman J.M. & Royston D. (1985) Adult respiratory distress syndrome after allogenic bone marrow transplantation; evidence for a neutrophil independant mechanism. *Lancet* i, 1239–42.

Brichart J.F., Rouby J.J. & Viars P. (1986) Intermittent positive pressure ventilation with either positive end-expiratory pressure or high frequency jet ventilation (HFJV), or HFJV alone in human acute respiratory failure. *Anesthesia and Analgesia* **65**, 1135–42.

Brigham K.L. (1986) Role of free radicals in lung injury. *Chest* **89**, 859–63

Brigham K.L. & Meyrick B.O. (1984) Interactions of granulocytes with the lungs. *Circulation Research* **54**, 623–35.

Cameron G.R. (1948) Pulmonary oedema. *British Medical Journal* 965–72.

Catley D.M., Thornton C., Jordan C., Lehane J.R., Royston D. & Jones J.G. (1985) Pronounced episodic oxygen desaturation in the postoperative period; its association with ventilatory pattern and analgesic regimen. *Anesthesiology* **63**, 20–8.

Clark J.M. & Lambertson C.J. (1971) Pulmonary oxygen toxicity; a review. *Pharmacological Reviews* **23**, 37–134.

Cochrane C.G., Spragg R. & Revak S.D. (1983) Pathogenesis of the adult respiratory distress syndrome; evidence of oxidant activity in bronchoalveolar lavage fluid. *Journal of Clinical Investigation* **71**, 754–61.

Chedid L. (1986) Synthetic muramyl peptides; their origin, present status and future prospects. *Federation Proceedings* **45**, 2531–44.

De Maria E.J., Reidman W., Kenney P.R., Armitage J.M. & Gann D.S (1985) Septic complications of corticosteroid administration after central nervous system trauma. *Annals of Surgery* **202**, 248–52.

Douglas W.W., Rehder K., Beynen F.M., Sesslet A.D. & Marsh M.H. (1977) Improved oxygenation in patients with acute respiratory failure; the prone position. *American Review of Respiratory Disease* **115**, 559–65.

Dreyfuss D., Basset G., Soler P. & Saumon G. (1985) Intermittent positive-pressure hyperventilation with high inflation pressures produces pulmonary microvascular injury in rats. *American Review of Respiratory Disease* **132**, 880–4.

Eliasson O. & de Graff A.C. (1985) The use of criteria for reversibility and obstruction to define patient groups for bronchodilator trials. *American Review of Respiratory Disease* **132**, 858–64.

Feeley T.W., Minty B.D., Scudder C.M., Jones J.G., Royston D. & Teng N.H.H. (1987) The effect of human antiendotoxin monoclonal antibodies on endotoxin induced lung injury in the rat. *American Review of Respiratory Disease* **135**, 665–70.

Fishman A.P., Goldring R.M. & Turino G.M. (1966) General alveolar hypoventilation: a syndrome of respiratory and cardiac failure in patients with normal lungs. *Quarterly Journal of Medicine* **35**, 261–75.

Fletcher C.M. & Pride N.B. (1984) Definition of emphysema, chronic bronchitis, asthma and airflow obstruction; 35 years from the CIBA symposium. *Thorax* **39**, 81–5.

Fowler A.A., Hausmann R.F., Good J.T., Benson K.H., Baird M., Eherle D.G., Petty T.L. & Hyers T.M. (1983) Adult respiratory distress syndrome; risk with common predispositions. *Annals of Internal Medicine* **98**, 593–7.

Gillespie D.J., Marsh H.M.M., Divertie M. & Meadows J.A. (1986) Clinical outcome of respiratory failure in patients requiring prolonged (> 24 hours) mechanical ventilation. *Chest* **90**, 364–9.

Grega G.J. (1986) Role of the endothelial cell in regulation of microvascular permeability to molecules. *Federation Proceedings* **45**, 75–95.

Halliwell B. & Gutteridge J.M.C. (1985) *Free radicals in Biology and Medicine* p.67. Clarendon Press, Oxford.

Hillman K. (1985) Pulmonary barotrauma. *Clinics in Anesthesiology* **3**, 877–98.

Koizumi M., Frank L. & Massaro D. (1985) Oxygen toxicity in rats. Varied effects of dexamethasone treatment depending on duration of hyperoxia. *American Review of Respiratory Disease* **131**, 907–11.

Leeman M., Boeynaems J.M., Degante J.P., Vincent J.L & Kahn R.J. (1985) Administration of Dazoxiben, a selective thromboxane synthetase inhibitor in the adult respiratory distress syn-drome. *Chest* **87**, 727–30.

Luce J.M., Pierson D.J. & Hudson D. (1981) Intermittent mandatory ventilation; a critical review. *Chest* **79**, 678–85.

Luce J.M., Tyler M.C. & Pierson D.J. (1984) *Intensive Respiratory Care* p.195. W.B. Saunders, Philadelphia.

McDonald R.J., Berger E.M., White C.V., Freeman B.A. & Repine J.E. (1985) Effect of superoxide dismutase encapsulated in liposomes or conjugated with polyethylene glycol on neutrophil bactericidal activity *in vitro* and bacterial clearance *in vivo*. *American Review of Respiratory Disease* **131**, 633–7.

Malik A.B., Selig W.M. & Burhop K.E. (1985) Cellular and hormonal mediators of pulmonary edema. *Lung* **163**, 193–219.

Marini J.J., Pierson D.J. & Hudson L.D. (1979) Acute lobar atelectasis; a prospective comparison of fibreoptic bronchoscopy and respiratory therapy. *American Review of Respiratory Disease* 119, 971–8.

Malik A.B., Selig W.M. & Burhop K.E. (1985) Cellular and hormonal mediators of pulmonary edema. *Lung* 163, 193–219.

Marini J.J., Rodriguez J. & Lamb V. (1986) The inspiratory workload of patient initiated mechanical ventilation. *American Review of Respiratory Disease* 134, 902–9.

Murray J.F. (1977) Mechanisms of acute respiratory failure. *American Reviews of Respiratory Disease* 115, 1071–8.

Nolop K.P., Braude S., Taylor K.M. & Royston D. (1987) Epithelial and endothelial solute flux after bypass in dogs: effect of positive end expiratory pressure. *Journal of Applied Physiology* 62, 1244–9.

Patmas M.A., Wilborn S.L. & Shankel S.W. (1984) Acute multi-system toxicity associated with the use of the non-steroid anti-inflammatory drugs. *Archives of Internal Medicine* 144, 519–21.

Patterson C.E., Butler J.A., Byrne F.D. & Rhodes M.E. (1985) Oxidant lung injury; intervention with sulfhydryl reagents. *Lung* 163, 23–32.

Pepe P.E., Hudson L.D. & Carrico C.J. (1984) Early application of positive end expiratory pressure in patients at risk from the adult respiratory distress syndrome. *New England Journal of Medicine* 311, 281–6.

Pepe P.E., Potkin R.T., Rens D.N. (1982) Clinical predictors of the adult respiratory distress syndrome. *American Journal of Surgery* 144, 124–30.

Pesenti A.A., Pelizzola D., Muscheroni L., Uzriel E., Pirovano U., Fox L., Galtinoni L. & Kolobow T. (1981) Low frequency positive pressure ventilation with extracorporeal CO_2 removal (LFPPV-$ECCO_2R$) in acute respiratory failure (ARF): technique. *Transactions—American Society for Artificial Internal Organs* 27, 263–6.

Petty T.L. & Ashbaugh D.G. (1971) The adult respiratory distress syndrome clinical features, factors influencing prognosis and principles of management. *Chest* 70, 223–9.

Pratt P.C., Vollmen R.T., Shelburne J.D. & Crape J.D. (1979) Pulmonary morphology in a multihospital collaborative extracorporeal membrane oxygenation project. *American Journal of Pathology* 95, 191–214.

Renken E.M. (1985) Capillary transport of macromolecular pores and other endothelial pathways. *Journal of Applied Physiology* 58, 315–25.

Rinaldo J.E. & Rogers R.M. (1982) Adult respiratory distress syndrome; changing concepts of lung injury and repair. *New England Journal of Medicine* 306, 900–9.

Robin E.D., Carey L.C., Grenvik A., Glansen F. & Gandio R. (1972) Capillary leak syndrome with pulmonary oedema. *Archives of Internal Medicine* 130, 66–71.

Rosen R.L. (1986) Acute respiratory failure and chronic obstructive lung disease. *Medical Clinics of North America* 70, 895–907.

Royston D., Braude S. & Nolop K.B. (1987) Clearance of aerosolised 99mTcDTPA does not predict outcome in patients with adult respiratory distress syndrome. *Thorax* 42, 494–9.

Searle J.F. (1985) The outcome of mechanical ventilation; report of a five year study. *Annals of the Royal College of Surgeons* 67, 187–9.

Shoemaker W.C. & Appel P.C. (1986) Effects of prostaglandin E, in adult respiratory distress syndrome. *Surgery* 99, 275–82.

Shoemaker W.C., Bland R.D. & Appel P.L. (1985) Therapy of critically ill postoperative patients based on outcome prediction and prospective trials. *Surgical Clinics of North America* 65, 811–33.

Sibbald W.J., Anderson R.R., Reid B., Hollidy R.C. & Diriedger A.A. (1981) Alveolar capillary permeability in human septic ARDS; effect of high dose corticosteroid therapy. *Chest* 79, 133–42.

Slavin G., Nunn J.F., Crow J. & Dore C.J. (1982) Bronchiolectasis —a complication of artificial ventilation. *British Medical Journal* 285, 931–4.

Spence T.H., Jenkinson S.G., Johnson K.H., Collins J.F. & Lawrence R.A. (1986) Effects of bacterial endotoxin on protecting copper-deficient rats from hyperoxin. *Journal of Applied Physiol-ogy* 61, 982–7.

Sprung C.L., Rackow E.C., Fein A., Jacob A.L. & Isikoff S.K. (1981) The spectrum of pulmonary edema; differentiation of cardiogenic, intermediate and non cardiogenic forms of pulmonary edema. *American Review of Respiratory Disease* 124, 718–22.

Staub N.C. (1983) Alveolar flooding and clearance. *American Review of Respiratory Disease* 1, 544–51.

Staub N.C., Bland R.D., Brigham K.L. & Woolverton C. (1975) Perforation of chronic lung lymph fistulas on sheep. *Journal of Surgical Research* 19, 315–21.

Strohl K.P., Cherniak N.S. & Gotle B. (1986) The physiological basis of therapy for sleep apnoea. *American Review of Respiratory Disease* 134, 791–802.

Svensjo E. & Gregor G.J. (1986) Evidence for endothelial cell mediated regulation of macromolecular permeability by post capillary venules. *Federation Proceedings* 45, 89–95.

Sykes M.K., McNicol R. & Campbell E.J.M. (1976) Introduction. In *Respiratory Failure* 2nd edn., p. xi. Blackwell Scientific publications, Oxford.

Traber D.L., Adams T., Sziebert L., Stein M. & Traber L. (1985) Potentiation of lung vascular responses to endotoxin by superoxide dismutase. *Journal of Applied Physiology* 58, 1005–9.

Wanner A. & Rao A. (1980) Clinical indications for and effects of bland, mucolytic and antimicrobial aerosols. *American Review of Respiratory Disease* 122 (suppl.), 79–87.

Webb H.H. & Tierney D.F. (1974) Experimental pulmonary edema due to intermittent positive pressure ventilation with high inflation pressures; protection by positive end expiratory pressure. *American Review of Respiratory Disease* 120, 556–65.

Weigelt J.A., Norcross J.F., Bormon K.R. & Snyder U.K. (1985) Early steroid therapy for respiratory failure. *Archives of Surgery* 120, 536–40.

Weinberg P.F., Matthay M.A., Welsten R.O., Roskos K.V., Goldstein T.M. & Murray J.F. (1984) Biologically active products of complement and acute lung injury in patients with the sepsis syndrome. *American Review of Respiratory Disease* 130, 791–6.

Winter P.M. & Smith G. (1972) The toxicity of oxygen. *Anesthesiology* 37, 210–41.

Witsch H.R., Haschek W.M., Klein M., Szanto A.J.P. & Hakkinen P.J. (1981) Potentiation of diffuse lung damage by oxygen; determining variables. *American Review of Respiratory Disease* 123, 98–103.

Zapol W. & Snider M. (1977) Pulmonary hypertension in severe acute respiratory failure. *New England Journal of Medicine* 296, 476–80.

Ziegler E.G., McCutchan J.A., Fierer J., Glansen M.P., Sadoff J.C., Douglas H. & Braude A.I. (1982) Treatment of Gram negative bacteremia and shock with human antiserum to a mutant *Escherichia Coli*. *New England Journal of Medicine* 307, 1225–30.

Zimmerman G.A., Renzetti A.D. & Nill H.R. (1983) Functional and metabolic activity of granulocytes from patients with adult resiratory distress syndrome: evidence for activated neutrophils in the pulmonary circulation. *American Review of Respiratory Disease* 127, 290–300.

74

Renal Failure

A. INNES AND G.R.D. CATTO

Acute renal failure, which may occur following trauma, infection and surgery, continues to carry a high mortality of approximately 50%. Its prevention and treatment present considerable challenges if mortality and morbidity are to be reduced. As patients with chronic renal failure now have a considerably longer life expectancy than 20 yr ago, anaesthetists care for such patients in an increasing number of surgical procedures which may or may not be related to their initial renal disease. Renal transplantation has become an accepted form of treatment for patients with end-stage renal disease, enabling successful recipients to have a relatively normal quality of life. However, these patients present anaesthetists with particular problems because of their necessary non-specific immunosuppressive therapy and consequent increased risk of opportunistic infections. All of these aspects of the management of patients with renal failure necessitate a combined approach to their care by surgeon, anaesthetist and nephrologist.

Chronic renal failure

Although the definition is arbitrary, with the onset of symptoms often related poorly to the degree of renal impairment, chronic renal failure is considered usually to be present when the glomerular filtration rate (GFR) is less than 12–15 ml/min.

The incidence of chronic renal failure is higher in the elderly. In all age groups it shows a marked racial difference (188 per million per year in the black population and 44 per million per year in Caucasians). The overall incidence has been estimated as approximately 90 per million of the population (Easterling, 1977). Chronic renal failure may result from any underlying renal disease but the most frequent causes are glomerulonephritis, hypertension, diabetes mellitus, interstitial nephropathy and polycystic disease.

Pathophysiology

Once renal function starts to decline, the effects of progressive nephron loss are compensated by glomerular hyperfiltration in the remaining intact nephrons. This is achieved by increasing the glomerular capillary plasma flow and glomerular transcapillary hydrostatic pressure. Such adaptation allows patients to remain relatively asymptomatic until approximately 80% of nephrons are destroyed. These vascular protective changes are, however, deleterious and the resulting hyperfiltration may damage the remaining nephrons and cause glomerulosclerosis—indeed this may be one mechanism by which renal function continues to deteriorate even after the initial damaging stimulus is no longer detectable as in many cases of chronic glomerulonephritis (Olsen et al., 1982). When serum creatinine concentration is greater than 200–400 μmol/litre, the GFR almost invariably declines gradually or until end-stage renal failure results.

NITROGEN BALANCE

Nitrogenous waste products of protein metabolism accumulate in chronic renal failure and cause increases in serum urea, creatinine and urate concentrations. These substances are important only because they are relatively simple to measure and not because they are particularly toxic; they may be regarded as representative of a large number of poorly characterized substances excreted normally by glomerular filtration. However, it is known that the factors responsible for the toxicity of uraemia have a molecular weight in the range 500–5000—intermediate in size between small substances removed by dialysis such as urea and large non-dialysable proteins; they have been termed 'middle molecules' but have not been characterized further (Contreras *et al.*, 1982).

Serum urea

As the GFR decreases, serum urea concentration does not increase proportionately—it increases above the upper limit of normal only when the filtration rate is reduced to less than 50% of its normal value. Thus, an individual with mild renal disease may have a GFR as measured by creatinine or ^{51}Cr-EDTA clearance of 80 ml/min and a normal serum urea concentration; with progression of the renal disease, the GFR may decline to 10 ml/min and serum urea increase to 30 mmol/litre.

Serum urea concentrations are influenced not only by changes in GFR but also by: (1) the protein content of the diet; (2) hypercatabolic states such as severe infection, yrauma and surgery; and (3) urinary flow rates—urea is a relatively small molecule which tends to diffuse out of the tubules back into the circulation during states of reduced urine flow. For all these reasons, urea provides a less satisfactory measure of GFR than serum creatinine concentrations.

Serum creatinine

In patients not gaining or losing muscle rapidly, creatinine is produced at a constant rate in proportion to the muscle mass, and is excreted largely by glomerular filtration; only a small proportion is excreted by tubular secretion. Serum creatinine concentration thus provides a useful method of assessing GFR. Because individuals vary widely in muscle mass, single measurements of serum creatinine concentration must be evaluated with care—a concentration of 125 μmol/litre may indicate a normal GFR in a healthy young man but suggests a marked decrease in GFR in a frail elderly woman. When in doubt, GFR should be measured by ^{51}Cr-EDTA or creatinine clearance techniques (Shemesh *et al.*, 1985).

Serum urea and creatinine concentrations

When serum concentrations of both urea and creatinine are measured, additional diagnostic information may be available.

1 Serum urea and creatinine concentrations are elevated equally in established renal failure, both acute and chronic.

2 Serum creatinine may be raised out of proportion to urea because of:

(a) Rhabdomyolysis, associated with elevation of muscle enzymes,

(b) Long-term dialysis treatment as urea molecules are smaller and more readily dialysable than creatinine.

Occasionally, drugs such as aspirin or cotrimoxazole cause a similar but more minor effect by blocking the tubular secretion of creatinine.

3 Serum urea may be raised out of proportion to creatinine because of:

(a) Salt and water depletion or diuretic therapy.

(b) Dietary protein or gastrointestinal haemorrhage.

(c) Hypercatabolic states resulting from surgery, trauma and infection or drugs such as corticosteroids and tetracyclines (except doxycycline) which have an antianabolic effect.

4 Serum urea concentration may be decreased out of proportion to creatinine in liver failure, low-protein diet, high fluid intake and pregnancy.

SODIUM AND WATER BALANCE

As the GFR decreases, there is a compensatory increase in the fractional excretion of both sodium and water from each nephron. It is postulated that the decline in GFR leads to sodium retention and expansion of blood volume, stimulating volume receptors which decrease sodium reabsorption from the renal tubules.

Recently, atrionatriuretic peptides have been discovered. These factors, which are stimulated by atrial distention and cause a marked natriuresis, may be responsible for the increased fractional excretion of sodium observed in chronic renal failure (Ballermann & Brenner, 1985).

In chronic renal failure, the kidney is less efficient in varying urinary sodium excretion. Eventually, nephrons lose their ability to dilute or concentrate urine and cannot excrete more than 200 mmol of sodium per day. As a result of the osmotic gradient created by excess sodium in body fluid, water is generally retained together with salt and the serum sodium concentration remains normal. When sodium intake exceeds output, extracellular volume increases, hypertension develops, body weight tends to increase and features of cardiac failure may become apparent. As a result of the adaptive increase in fractional sodium excretion, clinical problems of oliguria, severe fluid overload and oedema are uncommon until chronic renal failure is advanced—although minor degrees of sodium retention contribute undoubtedly to the hypertension which affects 75 % of patients with renal failure (Bricker, 1982).

Conversely, as such patients are unable to reduce urinary sodium excretion rapidly when intake is diminished, they are at risk of volume depletion, especially after surgery or during intercurrent infection e.g. gastroenteritis. Clinically, they present with polyuria, anorexia, nausea and hypotension. Obligatory urinary sodium losses may cause a decrease in extracellular fluid volume and a further reduction in GFR perhaps producing 'acute-on-chronic' renal failure. In this situation, an intravenous infusion of saline is essential to restore extracellular fluid volume, renal perfusion and renal function.

POTASSIUM BALANCE

Potassium is filtered normally by the glomerulus and then reabsorbed almost completely in the proximal tubule and loop of Henle. As renal function declines, potassium homeostasis is maintained by increasing secretion at the distal tubule and decreasing fractional reabsorption. Faecal loss of potassium increases three- or four-fold as a further adaptive mechanism in chronic renal failure. However, animal studies have shown that despite these homeostatic changes, an acute potassium load is not tolerated well in uraemia (Linas et al., 1979).

These adaptive mechanisms help to maintain potassium balance until an advanced stage of renal failure—despite the reduction in GFR and the shift of potassium from intracellular to extracellular fluid which accompanies the development of acidosis. Moderate hyperkalaemia is noted usually when the GFR decreases to below 15 ml/min; as renal function deteriorates further, severe hyperkalaemia may occur —particularly if the patient becomes oliguric.

ACID-BASE BALANCE

A mild metabolic acidosis develops when the GFR declines to 25 % of normal and is therefore present at a relatively early stage of the disease. The compensatory mechanisms involved in acid-base balance are less efficient than those governing sodium, potassium and water homeostasis. These mechanisms include:
1 Respiratory hyperventilation and loss of carbon dioxide;

$$HCO_3^- + H^+ \rightarrow H_2O + CO_2.$$

2 Buffering by the alkaline skeletal calcium salts; calcium is leached from bone with increased urinary calcium excretion as hydrogen ions are buffered.
3 Secondary hyperparathyroidism—increases the buffering capacity of an acute acid load by increasing the excretion of titratable acid and mobilizing extra-renal buffers.
4 Renal responses—increasing ammonia production $(NH_3 + H^+ \rightarrow NH_4^+)$, enhanced reabsorption of bicarbonate, increased titratable acid excretion and increased distal tubular delivery of sodium, and potassium for hydrogen ions.

In spite of these measures, there is a reduction in serum bicarbonate concentration, a decrease in P_{CO_2} and a decrease in arterial pH. Initially, the anion gap is normal, but as renal function deteriorates, the gap increases by retention of sulphate and phosphate. The anion gap is calculated by subtracting the sum of the serum bicarbonate and chloride concentrations from the serum sodium concentration; normally the result obtained is within the range 10–16 mmol/litre.

The acidosis is exacerbated further by decreased ammonia secretion leading to decreased hydrogen ion excretion, although the urinary pH may remain low. Proximal tubular reabsorption of bicarbonate is impaired also. Clinically, acidosis is exacerbated if diarrhoea (bicarbonate loss), hypotension or a hypercatabolic state are present.

HAEMOPOIETIC AND IMMUNE SYSTEMS

When the creatinine concentration increases to over $300 \mu mol/litre$, anaemia invariably develops. Thereafter, there is only a poor correlation between the degree of anaemia and the reduction in GFR. The aetiology of the anaemia is multi-factorial. There is decreased production of erythropoietin, decreased bone-marrow activity and increased red cell fragility leading to decreased red cell half-life and micro-angiopathic haemolysis (the latter being an acquired abnormality of the red cell pentose phosphate pathway) (Fisher, 1980).

The haemoglobin concentration decreases to below 5 g/dl rarely. Compensatory mechanisms are again important; a shift in the oxyhaemoglobin dissociation curve to the right (from acidosis and the red cell 2, 3-diphosphoglycerate concentration), releases more oxygen to the tissues and there is also an increase in cardiac output.

Thrombocytopenia is uncommon, but platelet function is abnormal with decreased adhesiveness. Bleeding time is prolonged and prothrombin consumption increased (Carvalho, 1983).

Increased susceptibility to infection with impairment of both cellular and humoral immunity may be noted also. Neutrophil chemotaxis and antibody responses are reduced, and there is a decrease in the number of circulating lymphocytes.

Symptoms

GASTROINTESTINAL SYSTEM

Early morning nausea and vomiting with progressive anorexia are common features of chronic renal failure. Hiccups may be troublesome and the stomach-emptying time prolonged (often doubled in patients on dialysis)—of particular relevance in anaesthetic practice.

NEUROLOGICAL SYSTEM

Neurological complications of uraemia can vary from minor mental changes to grand mal seizures, drowsiness and coma. Uraemic twitching, cramps and restless legs may occur also. The peripheral neuropathy of chronic renal failure is sensory in type initially, but may progress to a mixed sensory and motor pattern. It is almost invariably present electromyographically when the GFR is less than 10 ml/min. Myopathy and autonomic dysfunction may occur also, particularly in patients with end-stage disease. The cerebrospinal fluid (CSF) in uraemia often has an increased protein content but there are no changes in pressure, cell count or glucose concentration.

RESPIRATORY SYSTEM

The anaemia and acidosis of uraemia contribute to the dyspnoea of chronic renal failure. The so-called 'uraemic lung' is probably largely the result of pulmonary oedema due to fluid overload and improves generally when the patient is dialysed adequately. There are, however, peculiar abnormalities associated with uraemia. Transfer factor and vital capacity are both reduced. Fibrosis can occur and calcification has been noted in alveolar septa. Pleural effusions present in 20% of patients may be either exudates or transudates—serous, serosanguinous, or even haemorrhagic in type.

CARDIOVASCULAR SYSTEM

Fluid overload, hypertension and anaemia all contribute to the congestive cardiac failure which is common in chronic renal failure. Expansion of the extracellular fluid compartment causes hypertension in 90–95% of patients. Hypertension is a result also of increased activity of the renin–angiotensin system and over-activity of the autonomic nervous system. Approximately 30% of patients have hyperreninaemia, and although bilateral nephrectomy used to be advocated, it produced no improvement in 20% of cases, and, by further reducing erythropoietin, inevitably exacerbated the anaemia. Plasma catecholamine concentrations are elevated also. Autonomic neuropathy may occur particularly in dialysis patients and is often evidenced by marked hypotension, particularly postural, despite volume expansion.

Pericarditis, a frequent late complication of uraemia, is present in 60% of untreated patients. Tamponade occurs in only 20% of patients with pericarditis and constrictive pericarditis in 12% of individuals on chronic dialysis. Two types of pericarditis are found. 'True' uraemic pericarditis occurs in late untreated disease or in inadequately dialysed patients. This form, found rarely in patients treated by peritoneal dialysis, causes few symptoms and seldom causes tamponade; any pericardial effusion consists of serous fluid. The aetiology is unclear although viral infection may be implicated in addition to the uraemia and a satisfactory response to increased dialysis is usual. The second form, dialysis-related pericarditis, occurs early after commencing dialysis and is more likely to produce pain, fever and a leukocytosis. The condition does not respond to intensive dialysis. Tamponade is not uncommon and the risk is increased by the heparin therapy required during haemodialysis; the fluid is often haemorrhagic. Echocardiography is useful in establishing the diagnosis and in assessing the severity of the condition. When tamponade is present, a pericardial drainage catheter should be inserted immediately and some form of more permanent solution such as pericardiectomy considered for the long term. Thoracic surgery of this type is a major undertaking for these seriously ill uraemic patients (Renfrew et al., 1980).

Other cardiac manifestations include uraemic cardiomyopathy—although its existence as a distinct entity is disputed. Peripheral vascular disease is present frequently as a result of the increased incidence of hypertension and atherosclerosis in uraemic patients. Calcification of blood vessels is noted often on X-ray and complicates vascular surgical procedures frequently.

CALCIUM AND PHOSPHATE HOMEOSTASIS

In conservatively treated chronic renal failure, a falling

GFR leads to an increase in serum phosphate and a decrease in serum calcium concentrations. The ionized fraction of the serum calcium concentration is, however, protected by the systemic acidosis and hence tetany is rare. However, these patients should not be given bicarbonate routinely in order to control the acidosis or Kussmaul's respiration, as this may precipitate tetany and generalized convulsions.

Deficiency of the active form of vitamin D (1,25-dihydroxyvitamin D_3) produced normally by the renal tubular cells, leads to defective mineralization of bone and reduced calcium absorption from the gut. As serum calcium concentrations decrease, secretion of parathyroid hormone (PTH) is stimulated. The increased PTH tends to raise serum calcium and reduce serum phosphate concentrations, initially through its effects on the kidney but later at the expense of increased bone resorption; when this happens, serum phosphate concentrations may increase considerably, as both calcium and phosphate are released from bone into the blood and the excess phosphate cannot be excreted in the urine because of the renal impairment. Eventually, the solubility product of calcium phosphate is exceeded and soft tissue calcification may develop. Although particularly noted in blood vessels and around joints (especially when the calcium ;ts phosphate product exceeds 4 mmol/litre), it may occur at any site including lungs, myocardium and the bundle of His. With the continued stimulation of hypocalcaemia, the mass of the parathyroid glands becomes very large and a degree of autonomous (tertiary) hyperparathyroidism with hypercalcaemia may develop.

Renal bone disease is manifest by osteomalacia, osteosclerosis and osteoporosis. Osteitis fibrosa cystica and subperiosteal erosions of the phalanges, usually with an increase in serum alkaline phosphatase activity, are thought to be pathognomic of parathyroid overactivity. Clinically, patients may complain of bone pain but fractures are unusual. Indeed, radiological changes themselves are now uncommon as most patients are treated before these become manifest (Eastwood et al., 1973).

OTHER ENDOCRINE EFFECTS

Chronic renal failure reduces the production of certain hormones and increases the effect of others by reducing their degradation and elimination. Erythropoietin and 1,25-dihydroxyvitamin D, as discussed previously, are reduced. The concentrations of many peptides are elevated—insulin (giving glucose intolerance), somatostatin, calcitonin, glucagon, vasopressin, growth hormone and gastrointestinal peptides. Peripheral insulin resistance may occur in non-diabetic patients. Moreover, as the kidney is an important site for insulin metabolism, insulin dosage may have to be decreased substantially in diabetic patients developing end-stage renal failure (DeFronzo & Alvestrand, 1980).

The clinical symptoms and signs of uraemia relate to the pathophysiological processes in chronic renal failure. These features are summarized in Table 74.1.

Conservative treatment of chronic renal failure

In this section, the treatment of chronic renal failure at the stage before the need for renal replacement

Table 74.1 Clinical features of chronic renal failure

Dermatological
Pallor
Pruritus
Purpura

Cardiovascular
Hypertension
Congestive cardiac failure
Pericarditis
Cardiomyopathy

Respiratory
Infection
'Uraemic lung'
Acidotic respiration

Haemopoietic
Anaemia
Platelet dysfunction
Bleeding tendency

Nervous system
Tremor
Convulsions
Lethargy
Malaise
Peripheral neuropathy
Autonomic neuropathy

Gastrointestinal
Anorexia
Nausea, vomiting
Hiccups
Ulceration
Parotitis
Mouth ulcers

Endocrine and metabolic
Renal bone disease
Hyperuricaemia
Carbohydrate intolerance

therapy is discussed. When possible, any underlying cause should be treated. However, in practice this is confined usually to urinary obstruction, hypertension and drug-induced causes. Treatment is otherwise directed towards ameliorating the biochemical and toxic consequences of uraemia.

DIETARY MEASURES

Protein

Dietary protein restriction has long been used in the symptomatic management of patients with chronic renal failure. There have been recent claims that such treatment may slow or halt the progression of renal disease. In animal studies, the survival rate of animals with chronic renal failure given a low protein diet is increased. At present, the case for such diets in man has not been established firmly, and although symptoms may be relieved, nutritional problems may ensue.

Restriction of protein to 20 g/day is possible with a Giordano–Giovanotti diet, nitrogen balance being maintained by supplements of essential amino acids. However, this regimen is very monotonous, leads to weight loss and is unacceptable to most patients. A 40 g protein diet is reasonably palatable and does not lead to nitrogen imbalance. At present, it seems reasonable to restrict protein intake to 40–50 g/day when serum creatinine concentration exceeds 200 μmol/litre, at least until more objective evidence of any long-term benefits becomes available. Dietary advice of this type will help also to reduce the systemic acidosis but must provide a high calorific content, to prevent catabolism of skeletal muscle. All protein-restricted diets have a low calcium content and below 30 g/day deficiencies of iron and zinc may occur also. The use of essential amino acids or ketoacid analogues as supplements to low-protein diets remains controversial. Most studies involving the use of essential amino acids have been short term and not long enough to assess any changes in GFR. There are no data which demonstrate an advantage of ketoacid analogue supplements and some evidence that severe muscle wasting can occur. When the facilities exist, it is preferable to commence patients on some form of renal replacement therapy (dialysis or transplantation) rather than persevere with such difficult conservative measures which in any event carry a poorer prognosis.

One problem in assessing the effects of low-protein diets lies in monitoring the nutritional status of patients with chronic renal failure. Weight is a poor indicator of nutritional status in advanced uraemia. Significant muscle loss has been observed without any change in serum albumin or transferrin concentrations. Urinary 3-methylhistidine has been used to determine breakdown of skeletal muscle protein but is affected by both renal failure and dietary protein intake (El Nahas & Coles, 1986; Giovannetti, 1986).

Potassium

Restriction of potassium is usually necessary only in the late stages of the disease. The patient should be advised on a reduced potassium diet (40 mmol/day) and told which foods contain high concentrations of potassium.

Sodium

Sodium restriction is indicated for most patients with chronic renal failure who have evidence of salt and water retention and hypertension. The average Western diet contains approximately 100 mmol of sodium per day. Diets containing less than 20 mmol/day are unpalatable but an intake of 60 mmol/day can be achieved by avoiding salted foods such as salted crisps.

Thus, in patients with advanced chronic renal failure, a commonly prescribed diet would contain 40 g protein, 40 mmol potassium and 40 mmol sodium.

RENAL OSTEODYSTROPHY

Treatment consists of maintaining serum phosphate concentrations within normal limits by dietary means or by giving oral phosphate-binding agents if necessary (Maschio *et al.*, 1980). Aluminium hydroxide, the most effective of these drugs, is now known to cause aluminium toxicity—a severe form of fracturing bone disease and a type of progressive dementia. Oral calcium carbonate binds phosphate, buffers the acidosis and provides calcium supplements. It is given usually in a dose of 2 g/day together with calcitriol (1,25-dihydroxyvitamin D_3), 0.25 μg/day, or alfacalcidol (1α-hydroxyvitamin D_3), 0.25-0.5 μg/day, to patients with normo- or hypocalcaemia (Muirhead *et al.*, 1982). Hypercalcaemic patients cannot be treated in this way and are subjected usually to parathyroidectomy and then given vitamin D replacement therapy. Fragments of excised parathyroid gland may be embedded in forearm muscles; this allows the patient to re-establish normal calcium homeostasis in the event of a future renal transplant or to have the gland excised easily should hyperparathyroidism develop again. Whilst these aspects of therapy are described well in dialysis patients, their value in patients treated conservatively is still debated (Neilsen et al., 1980).

ACIDOSIS

The metabolic acidosis of chronic renal failure is normally tolerated reasonably well by patients. However, it may contribute to other problems with potassium homeostasis and to dyspnoea and lethargy. If symptoms resulting from the acidosis become severe, this is usually an indication that dialysis is required. Before this, oral sodium bicarbonate therapy may be considered but its use is limited by the high sodium content which may lead to oedema and worsening of arterial pressure control, and the increased risk of tetany as discussed earlier.

ANAEMIA

Because of the shift in the oxygen dissociation curve, anaemia is tolerated well also. A change from the characteristic normochromic, normocytic pattern should be investigated and any concomitant vitamin, folate or iron deficiency treated. The symptomatic improvement produced by blood transfusion is short-lived and may suppress erythropoiesis further; transfusions are given currently to patients with chronic renal failure for the improvement in subsequent graft survival rates they produce.

HYPERTENSION, SALT AND WATER BALANCE

The salt and water overload that occurs in chronic renal failure responds usually to loop diuretics. There is a dose relationship with the falling GFR. Frusemide is the drug of choice in doses of 250–500 mg/day given in a single dose. Potassium-sparing diuretics should be avoided because of the risk of producing hyperkalaemia. Dietary sodium restriction should be instituted if there is evidence of salt and water excess—despite the potential danger of volume depletion leading to a decrease in renal perfusion. In practice, it is often useful to allow a small amount of peripheral oedema to remain towards the end of the day as a safeguard against excessive volume depletion.

Beta-blockers are used widely to control arterial pressure, although they tend to reduce both renal blood flow and GFR. Atenolol and nadolol are excreted unchanged by the kidney and doses should be reduced in renal failure; metoprolol which is metabolized by the liver, may prove more useful in practice.

Methyldopa increases the GFR even in chronic renal failure but still requires dosage modification; unfortunately, its numerous side-effects limit its acceptability to patients. Captopril has led to further deterioration in renal function in patients with renal artery stenosis and pre-existing renal impairment and is not to be recommended in renal failure. Calcium antagonists appear to be safe drugs, although they have been shown to interact with cyclosporin A in transplant recipients.

ADDITIONAL THERAPY

Pruritus is a common and extremely distressing symptom of uraemia. It can be difficult to control adequately, and scratching may provoke secondary infection. Occasionally, the itch results from deposition of phosphate salts in the skin. This may respond to correction of serum calcium and phosphate concentrations as discussed previously. Chlorpheniramine may give some symptomatic relief.

Persistent nausea and vomiting is usually an indication that dialysis is necessary. Metoclopramide may give some temporary benefit.

The onset of peripheral neuropathy is a further indication for dialysis which usually produces an improvement. Continuous ambulatory peritoneal dialysis (CAPD) appears to be more effective in this regard. Should dialysis not result in an improvement, other causes of neuropathy must be sought; alcohol and nitrofurantoin are common aetiological factors often overlooked in uraemic patients.

Factors of particular relevance to anaesthesia

The complications of chronic renal failure pose special problems for anaesthetic practice. Antihypertensive therapy should be continued up to and including the day of anaesthesia and surgery. Cannulae should not be inserted into forearm veins, as these may be required later as vascular access for haemodialysis.

The compensatory mechanisms in uraemic anaemia generally permit adequate oxygenation of the tissues. However, preoxygenation for 5 min is recommended to improve the removal of nitrogen. Anaemia decreases the blood : gas partition coefficients of halothane and methoxyflurane and thus assists rapid induction when these agents are used. Rapid recovery from anaesthesia occurs also.

Intraoperative fluid and electrolyte balance should be monitored carefully. In chronic renal disease, adequate hydration and the administration of isotonic saline preoperatively may prevent the further deterioration in renal function often associated with major surgery. Serum potassium concentration should be measured and ECG monitoring is essential; ECG abnormalities associated with potassium excess are tall peaked T-waves, loss of P-waves and widening of the QRS complex. Catabolic states, infection or increasing acidosis may all produce dangerous elevation of the serum potassium concentration. The metabolic acidosis is usually mild but, when severe, it has been suggested that hyperventilation be maintained during anaesthesia.

After thiopentone and a neuromuscular blocking agent are given, tracheal intubation should be performed with cricoid pressure applied. The problem of delayed stomach emptying has been discussed previously.

Reversal of muscle paralysis may be achieved with neostigmine, although its half-life is prolonged in renal failure. Pyridostigmine has been preferred because of the possibility of recurarization. If there is weak hand grip or poor head lift, ventilation may be required until full reversal is obtained. Postoperatively, supplemental oxygen should be continued for at least 4–6 hr (Deutsch, 1969).

ANAESTHETIC AGENTS

Barbiturates

In uraemia, the induction dose of thiopentone may be reduced by up to 75%. The sleeping time after a single dose is increased in proportion to the degree of renal impairment. High levels of the unbound drug are noted and caused by reduced serum albumin concentrations or displacement from albumin by nitrogenous toxins and acidosis. It has been suggested also that the blood–brain barrier is altered in uraemia, increasing the effects of lipid-soluble agents (Dundee & Richards, 1954).

Inhalation agents

These are useful agents in anaesthetizing patients with chronic renal failure. They are eliminated rapidly from the body, independent of renal function, and reduce also the total requirement of neuromuscular blocking drugs needed. However, there is an adverse effect on cardiac contractility with reductions in renal blood flow and GFR.

Methoxyflurane and enflurane may lead to increased levels of inorganic fluoride with its associated nephrotoxicity. This is noted particularly in patients on long-term treatment with barbiturates or tolbutamide. Enflurane is metabolized to a lesser extent than methoxyflurane, and only appears to increase inorganic fluoride concentrations in the presence of renal insufficiency. Halothane and isoflurane are safe if cardiovascular stability can be maintained.

Opioid drugs

Although most opioids undergo hepatic metabolism, renal function may influence their duration of action and lead to prolonged respiratory depression. Thus, in advanced renal disease, the dose of opioids should be reduced. Fentanyl appears to be the opioid of choice in chronic renal failure, as it causes the least haemodynamic effect.

Succinylcholine

This is useful in a rapid-sequence induction in chronic renal failure because of the delay in gastric emptying. Given intravenously in a dose of 1 mg/kg body weight, it causes potassium release from skeletal muscle during the process of depolarization and increases the serum potassium by 0.5–0.7 mmol/litre, even in normal individuals. It is considered safe to use succinylcholine only when the serum potassium is less than 5.5 mmol/litre. If advanced uraemic neuropathy has led to immobilization, succinylcholine should be avoided, as an exaggerated hyperkalaemic response can occur. Prolonged apnoea is seldom a problem (Miller et al., 1972).

Non-depolarizing, neuromuscular blocking drugs

A decreased total dose of these agents is required because of the reduction in muscle mass in some patients with chronic renal failure. Potentiation of these agents may occur in the presence of acidosis, hypokalaemia, hypocalcaemia, hypermagnesaemia, aminoglycoside antibiotics, frusemide and mannitol. Hence, the lowest dosage required should be given and neuromuscular activity monitored with a peripheral nerve stimulator.

D-tubocurarine is a drug of choice in this group, as there is no increased sensitivity in renal disease. The disadvantages are ganglionic blockade and peripheral vasodilatation producing hypotension.

Pancuronium is more dependent on renal excretion, but there is some hepatic transformation to inactive or less active metabolites. Prolonged paralysis has been reported but it causes less cardiovascular instability than d-tubocurarine.

Vercuronium, a monoquaternary derivative of pancuronium, produces few cardiovascular problems and its excretion is predominantly biliary. Atracurium has a short duration of action and may be useful in chronic renal failure. Metocurine and gallamine should be avoided in renal failure, as they undergo renal excretion.

Atropine and hyoscine

Atropine is excreted almost entirely in the urine. As only 1% is excreted by the kidney, hyoscine would appear to be the drug of choice.

Droperidol

In combination with fentanyl, droperidol causes a small decrease in GFR, effective plasma flow and urine output. Neuroleptanalgesia has been recommended as a safe procedure in renal failure.

Regional anaesthesia

This technique avoids the problems of anaesthetic agents and intubation of the trachea in patients with chronic renal failure. Nerve blocks or plexus anaesthesia are useful for the insertion of shunts or arteriovenous fistulas. The bleeding tendency of chronic renal failure has been postulated as a problem with spinal or extradural anaesthesia but seldom causes practical difficulties in adequately treated patients. Sympathetic blockade which may occur with extradural or spinal anaesthesia causes hypotension and a fall in the GFR. Regional anaesthesia is contra-indicated generally in patients with uraemic neuropathy and the concomitant use of adrenaline with local agents may lead to cardiac arrhythmias in an acidotic, hyperkalaemic individual. Acidosis decreases also the threshold for toxic effects of local anaesthetic agents and dose reduction is required in this situation (Bromage & Gertel, 1972).

Acute renal failure

Acute renal failure has been defined as a sudden decrease in GFR sufficient to cause uraemia. Oliguria (less than 15 ml/hr) is a usual feature, but non-oliguric acute renal failure may occur. In contrast to chronic renal failure, acute renal failure develops over days or weeks, rather than months or years, and some forms are reversible or potentially reversible. Often, however, the distinction between the two conditions is difficult and an acute deterioration in a patient with chronic renal impairment (acute-on-chronic) may occur.

The classification of acute renal failure into post-renal, prerenal and intrinsic renal failure is probably satisfactory for most purposes. The three groups and their specific management will be discussed separately. The treatment of the general sequelae of acute renal failure will be considered under intrinsic renal failure category.

Table 74.2 Causes of acute renal failure

Postrenal
Calculi
Papillary necrosis
Tumour
Retroperitoneal fibrosis
Bladder dysfunction
Renal vein thrombosis
Prerenal
Haemorrhage
Cardiogenic shock
Cardiac surgery
Cardiac failure
Sepsis
Gastrointestinal loss
Burns
Urinary loss
Muscle damage
Hypercalcaemia
Hepatorenal syndrome
Intrinsic renal
Postischaemic acute tubular necrosis (ATN)
Nephrotoxins
Antibiotics
Analgesics
Heavy metals
Myeloma protein
Acute glomerulonephritis
Acute interstitial nephritis
Polyarteritis nodosa
Acute pyelonephritis
Postpartum renal failure
Haemolytic uraemic syndrome
Acute cortical necrosis
Thrombotic thrombocytopenic purpura

The major causes of acute failure in each category are listed in Table 74.2.

Postrenal renal failure

The possibility of obstruction should always be considered as it is a potentially treatable condition. An obstructive lesion is suggested by a history of total anuria, haematuria, urinary infection or loin pain. Occasionally, partial obstruction may result in paradoxical polyuria as the back-pressure of urine may impair the concentrating ability of the collecting ducts. A history of previous urological problems, such as urinary calculi, should be sought.

Rectal or pelvic examination may reveal a palpable bladder caused by outlet obstruction. Calculi or blood clots, if bilateral or occurring on the side of a solitary functioning kidney, may cause acute renal failure. Analgesic abuse may produce papillary necrosis leading to ureteric obstruction. Intermittent oliguria is a common feature of retroperitoneal fibrosis and, perhaps surprisingly, pain is often absent.

The possibility of an obstructive aetiology is supported by the absence of proteinuria or urinary casts. Real-time ultrasound may be used to confirm or exclude obstruction (more accurately, dilatation of the urinary tract) and has the advantages of being non-invasive and portable. Isotope renography and infusion pyelography (particularly with tomography) may be useful in establishing the diagnosis. Retrograde pyelography is now seldom indicated—the site of obstruction is defined usually by antegrade pyelography performed under local anaesthesia with ultrasound control.

Removal of the obstruction is the aim of treatment. Normal renal function may not return immediately, particularly if prerenal elements (e.g. dehydration or sepsis) are present, and supportive therapy including dialysis may be necessary.

Prerenal acute renal failure

Reduction in renal perfusion leads to the development of acute renal failure; common causes are listed in Table 74.2. Clinically, the signs of incipient shock may be found; reduced skin tissue turgor, oliguria, hypotension and tachycardia. These features may be obscured in patients undergoing artificial ventilation, the elderly and obese. Septicaemia may cause profound hypotension and marked vasodilatation mediated by bacterial toxins. In complex situations, central venous or pulmonary wedge pressures should be monitored to allow circulating plasma volume to be restored to normal by adequate but not excessive fluid replacement. Failure to restore plasma volume will result in the development of intrinsic renal failure, and at that stage renal function will not return to normal with fluid replacement. The renal response to hypoperfusion is to produce a small volume of concentrated urine. Urinary sodium concentration is less than 20 mmol/litre, and urinary osmolality increased; the ratio of the osmolality in urine and plasma (U:P ratio) is greater than 1:1. The ratio of urinary urea:serum urea concentrations is greater than 10:1. Whilst these measurements may be useful clinically, they can be unreliable in the presence of sodium depletion, diuretic therapy and in patients with acute-on-chronic renal failure. The conditions of prerenal uraemia and established renal failure are two ends of a clinical spectrum and intermediate grades of disease may give confusing results.

If the conditions producing renal hypoperfusion are not corrected, one type of intrinsic renal failure, acute tubular necrosis, may develop. In this situation, fluid replacement above the restoration of normal circulating volume results in fluid overload and pulmonary oedema.

Intrinsic renal failure

The major causes of acute renal failure from intrinsic renal lesions are given in Table 74.2. If untreated, prerenal uraemia progresses to produce a potentially reversible form of intrinsic renal failure, known as acute tubular necrosis (ATN). This form of renal lesion is both common and, because of its good prognosis, important clinically. It can be caused not only by ischaemia but also by nephrotoxins e.g. following excessive doses of gentamicin, paracetamol or heavy metals. The kidneys become swollen, the cortex pale and the medulla dark and congested. Histologically, the glomeruli appear intact but tubular damage predominates. This may be patchy in postischaemic renal failure but it is widespread and confluent following nephrotoxic damage. In both situations, the proximal tubules are affected predominantly.

PATHOPHYSIOLOGY

A number of pathophysiological mechanisms (Table 74.3) have been proposed. It should be noted that these are not mutually exclusive.

Table 74.3 Proposed pathophysiological mechanisms in acute renal failure

Tubular obstruction
Vascular alterations
Tubular fluid back-leak
Altered glomerular permeability
Tubuloglomerular feedback

Tubular obstruction

Abnormally high intratubular pressures are present early in acute renal failure; there is impaired sodium reabsorption and an inability to concentrate urine. Obstruction of the tubules by debris and swollen tubular cells may be a major factor, and it is possible that the high back-pressure within the tubules prevents glomerular filtration.

Vascular alterations

Renal blood flow has been shown to be reduced both in man and in animal models of acute renal failure. This may decrease glomerular capillary pressure to a level at which filtration ceases and causes ischaemia of the tubular cells.

Tubular fluid back-leak

The tubular epithelium loses its integrity and it has been proposed that glomerular filtrate may leak back through the damaged epithelium. Following open-heart surgery, a back-leak of inulin of between 5 and 50% has been noted.

Altered glomerular permeability

This has been proposed and indeed a diminished ultrafiltration coefficient has been observed in acute renal failure. The presence, however, of intact glomerular histology makes this a less likely mechanism in the pathogenesis of acute renal failure.

Tubuloglomerular feedback

Reduced sodium and/or chloride reabsorption results in increased salt within the distal tubule. This is detected by the cells of the macula densa which forms one side of the triangle containing the juxtaglomerular apparatus (the other sides being the afferent and efferent glomerular arterioles). The local renin–angio-tensin system is activated, and angiotensin II causes constriction of the afferent arteriole and a reduction in the GFR.

DIAGNOSIS OF INTRINSIC RENAL ACUTE RENAL FAILURE

A thorough history is essential. Previous episodes or a history of the nephrotic syndrome may suggest acute glomerulonephritis. Documented or possible exposure to occupational, environmental or iatrogenic nephro-toxins may be important.

On urinalysis, red-cell casts suggest strongly a diagnosis of acute glomerulonephritis. In acute pyelo-nephritis a positive urinary culture may be obtained. Evidence of a multi-system disorder or vasculitis may be apparent clinically.

Autoantibodies, antistreptolysin-O titres and complement levels may aid the investigation of intrinsic disease also. An eosinophilia may indicate an acute interstitial nephritis—induced generally by analgesic or antibiotic therapy.

Abdominal ultrasound is valuable in determining renal size (and thus helping to identify the small shrunken kidneys of chronic renal failure) and in detecting the dilatation of the renal tract associated with obstructive nephropathy. Renal biopsy may be required to confirm a diagnosis although in seriously ill patients, severe hypertension or a coagulopathy may preclude such an invasive technique. It is useful to determine if glomerular disease is present—important if cases of crescentic nephritis presenting as acute or rapidly progressive renal failure are to be treated adequately; it is also of value in elucidating the histological features and hence the prognosis in those patients who were thought to have a form of ATN but whose renal function has failed to return after several weeks. Routine renal biopsy is not indicated in most cases of ATN (Wilson et al., 1976).

COMPLICATIONS OF ACUTE RENAL FAILURE

When oliguria persists despite correction of prerenal factors and there is no evidence of obstructive uropathy, intrinsic acute renal failure has almost certainly developed. Non-oliguric renal failure is seen increasingly and is encountered most often in patients with ATN secondary to burns or nephrotoxins. The prognosis is better and the hospital stay shorter than for the oliguric form.

Fluid balance

Prerenal uraemia may remain undiagnosed occasionally and therefore untreated in severely debilitated or unconscious patients. More commonly, however, fluid overload is present due either to injudicious fluid replacement or to the inappropriate use of large quantities of sodium bicarbonate in an attempt to correct the acidosis. Fluid overload can lead to hypertension, peripheral, pulmonary and cerebral oedema.

Sodium balance

Hyponatraemia, is common in acute renal failure, and this may be dilutional due to fluid overload or may indicate true sodium loss (e.g. caused by vomiting or diarrhoea). Hypernatraemia is noted less frequently but may occur in situations of volume depletion when more water than salt is lost, or, rarely, after excessive sodium infusion.

Potassium balance

Hyperkalaemia when not caused by foods, drinks, drugs and infusion containing potassium, results most frequently results from leak of intracellular potassium and is associated often with hypercatabolic states such as severe infection or trauma. Acidosis also exacerbates the hyperkalaemia by aiding the shift of potassium from the intracellular compartment. Electrocardiogram changes are common once the serum potassium increases above 6.5 mmol/litre and can lead ultimately to ventricular arrhythmias, cardiac arrest and death.

Acid–base balance

A metabolic acidosis is usual in acute renal failure and may exacerbate already existing hypotension and hyperkalaemia. Rarely, alkalosis can occur when gastrointestinal fluid losses are substantial. Respiratory acidosis may be present also if pulmonary infection, trauma or oedema are present.

Anaemia

Bleeding, haemodilution or haemoconcentration may all obscure the initial stages of acute renal failure. Subsequently, a normochromic normocytic anaemia develops as in patients with chronic renal failure. A rapidly falling haemoglobin concentration may result from bleeding or disseminated intravascular coagulopathy.

Uraemia

The accumulation of uraemic toxins is noted particularly in hypercatabolic states, and the serum urea concentration may increase rapidly. An acute fibrinous pericarditis may occur with the danger of tamponade. Hiccups and gastrointestinal bleeding are common. If untreated, the patient's mental condition deteriorates rapidly from apathy and confusion to coma, convulsions and death.

Calcium balance

Hypocalcaemia is usual and accompanies the increase in serum phosphate concentrations caused by the decreased GFR. Plasma concentrations of 1,25-dihydroxyvitamin D_3 are reduced, and it is believed that the elevated phosphate concentrations cause precipitation of insoluble calcium phosphate complexes in soft tissues and exacerbate the tendency to hypocalcaemia. The precise mechanisms are understood only poorly. The systematic acidosis protects against tetany.

Infection

In addition to being a cause of acute renal failure, infection may occur as a complication of the disease itself. Chest, urinary and oral infections predominate and should be sought and treated actively.

TREATMENT OF INTRINSIC RENAL FAILURE

If practicable, treatment should be directed towards removal of the underlying cause or withdrawal of an offending nephrotoxin. When, as is usual, primary treatment of this type is not possible, the principal aim of management is to prevent death from uraemia or any other cause while the kidneys are recovering from ATN. When the acute renal failure results from a non-reversible renal lesion, the patient should receive the appropriate treatment and rehabilitation necessary to prepare for some form of renal replacement therapy—dialysis or transplantation.

MANAGEMENT OF THE CONSEQUENCES OF
ACUTE RENAL FAILURE

Conservative therapy may be all that is required for patients with mild disease who are not hypercatabolic or oliguric. Conversely, patients who are severely ill following trauma, sepsis or major surgery often require continuing supportive measures and dialysis.

Fluid balance must be monitored stringently by daily weighing of the patient, accurate fluid balance charts and central venous pressure (CVP) measurements when appropriate. Evidence of infection should be sought actively and treated with a non-nephrotoxic antibiotic. Blood and urine cultures should be obtained from all patients presenting with acute renal failure. Physiotherapy is essential for patients undergoing artificial ventilation and those with severe chest infections. Prophylactic systemic antibiotics are not recommended as they may produce superinfection of the mouth and gastrointestinal tract.

If a prerenal element is suspected, a fluid challenge with a test infusion of saline (1 litre in 1 hr) may be helpful. If within 1–2 hr the urine flow doubles, the infusion should be continued—provided the CVP remains below 8–10 cmH$_2$O. If a saline infusion proves ineffective and after ensuring that the patient is volume replete, treatment with frusemide may increase urinary output as it improves renal blood flow and induces a salt diuresis. Although it does not reduce the number of dialyses required, the overall mortality or the period of renal insufficiency, it may, in doses of 1–3 g/day, convert oliguric to non-oliguric renal failure.

Mannitol has been advocated in renal failure because of its effects of increasing renal perfusion and urine flow by inducing an osmotic diuresis. Intravenous mannitol will, however, cause a considerable increase in extracellular fluid volume by attracting water from the intracellular fluid. There is little evidence that it is effective in preventing the development of intrinsic acute renal failure and because of the risks of pulmonary oedema, cerebral dehydration and haemolysis should seldom be used.

When cardiac failure has caused renal hypoperfusion, CVP monitoring may be inadequate, as right-sided cardiac filling pressure may not reflect left-sided pressure. In this situation, a catheter should be inserted into the pulmonary artery so that the pulmonary capillary wedge pressure, and thus, indirectly, the left-sided filling pressure, may be monitored.

Fluid replacement may not abolish hypotension even though the circulating volume returns to normal. In this situation, dopamine and/or dobutamine are useful pressor agents. Both have renal vasodilator effects at low dosage in addition to acting as cardiac inotropes at higher dosage. Unfortunately, as the dose of each increases, the renal vasodilator effect becomes a pressor effect and may well result in a further impairment of renal perfusion. It is probably best to commence with dopamine at a dose of $2\,\mu g \cdot kg^{-1} \cdot min^{-1}$, increasing to a maximum of $10\,\mu g \cdot kg^{-1} \cdot min^{-1}$. If a generalized pressor effect is still required because of persistent hypotension, the addition of dobutamine at a dose of $2.5\,\mu g \cdot kg^{-1} \cdot min^{-1}$ may provide an adequate pressor effect while maintaining or improving renal perfusion (Henderson et al., 1980).

Hyperkalaemia, if mild, may be controlled by diet and by avoiding potassium supplements and potassium-sparing diuretics. If this is insufficient, ion-binding resins (e.g. calcium resonium 15 g 6-hourly) given either orally or rectally are effective in 24–48 hr. In situations of severe life-threatening hyperkalaemia, a combination of soluble insulin (10 units) and dextrose (50 g) given intravenously drives potassium into the intracellular compartment. Its effect is short-lived and may have to be repeated. Calcium gluconate does not lower the serum potassium level, but appears to protect the myocardium from the deleterious effects of hyperkalaemia. The treatment of hyperkalaemia is summarized in Table 74.4.

It is important when investigating patients with acute renal failure to consider first those conditions

Table 74.4 Treatment of severe hyperkalaemia

Calcium gluconate (10%) 10–30 ml i.v. Sodium bicarbonate 50–150 mmol i.v.	Immediate therapy to stabilize cell membrane and shift potassium into cells
Glucose 50 g i.v. Soluble insulin 10 units i.v.	Effective within 15–30 min in shifting potassium into cells
Cation exchange resins (Na or Ca) 30–60 g rectally or 30 g orally	Acts within 1–2 hr and removes potassium from the body
Haemodialysis and peritoneal dialysis	Used only in renal failure and begins to remove potassium from the body within 15–30 min of starting treatment

which, if treated specifically, may be reversible. This applies to postrenal and prerenal factors in particular. Many patients may be so ill on admission that treatment, often including dialysis, must precede all but the most basic investigations. The incidence of gastrointestinal haemorrhage, which is a common problem in such acutely ill patients, has been decreased by the prophylactic use of H_2-antagonists (Priebe et al., 1980).

When immediate life-threatening problems have been tackled, the difficulties of maintaining adequate hydration whilst limiting excessive protein or potassium intake remain. Fluid balance is clearly critically important. Overhydration overloads the cardiovascular system and predisposes to pulmonary oedema; underhydration with a reduction in the extracellular fluid volume delays the return of renal function. For most afebrile patients in temperate climates it is sufficient generally to supply 500 ml fluid daily in addition to the volume of urine excreted.

Dietary protein intake may have to be decreased but it is very important that a high-energy diet (at least 12 000 kJ or 3000 cal) be provided to prevent catabolism of endogenous proteins. When the facilities are available, it is preferable to begin dialysis early and encourage adequate nutrition, if necessary by total parenteral nutrition, than to persist in prolonged conservative measures.

Dialysis is therefore normally required in acute renal failure to control hyperkalaemia, acidosis and fluid overload, and to relieve the symptoms and signs of uraemia. The current trend is to introduce dialysis early, as uraemic complications are reduced if the serum urea is maintained below 33 mmol/litre (Rainford, 1977).

Peritoneal dialysis, which requires no specialized facilities, may be sufficient in non-catabolic patients and is useful in small children, the elderly and those with bleeding problems. It is less efficient than haemodialysis in removing large amounts of fluid and cannot be used after abdominal surgery. Protein depletion and peritonitis can occur and respiration may be compromised in debilitated patients.

Haemodialysis is discussed in greater detail subsequently. It is more satisfactory for fluid removal (using ultrafiltration or haemofiltration) and more useful in correcting biochemical abnormalities rapidly. It requires specialized facilities and vascular access. It is more efficient in correcting serum biochemical abnormalities than peritoneal dialysis in hypercatabolic patients. Such patients may also need total parenteral nutrition—the large amounts of fluid which can be removed by ultrafiltration (or haemofiltration) may enable adequate nutrition to be provided.

RECOVERY FROM ACUTE TUBULAR NECROSIS

The prognosis in acute renal failure depends on the aetiology (Table 74.2). For some conditions, the prognosis is poor and patients may require long-term renal replacement therapy. Conversely, patients with ATN generally recover and the principal aim of management is to support the patient until recovery of some function occurs—usually within 6 weeks (Moran & Myers, 1985). Recovery is marked by a diuretic phase during which urinary output generally increases; rarely, a patient may pass 10 litre/day of dilute urine. This polyuria, which may require considerable fluid and potassium replacement, occurs partly as a result of the osmotic diuresis induced by the retained urea, creatinine, etc. and partly because the medullary hypotonicity, and hence renal concentrating ability, has been lost (Swann & Merrill, 1953).

Recovery of renal function as measured by a reduction in serum urea and creatinine concentration lags usually a few days behind the diuresis. Even when adequate renal function has returned, some impairment of GFR or tubular defects in urinary concentration or acidification may remain.

The overall mortality of acute renal failure from ATN has not changed in the last 30 yr and remains approximately 50%. However, there has been an improvement in mortality from traumatic and obstetric causes. In medical conditions an increase in the average age of the patients treated and the more serious primary conditions precipitating acute renal failure have offset the considerable improvement in patient management and dialysis techniques developed during the last 25 yr (Kennedy et al., 1973).

Factors of particular relevance to anaesthesia

Overall, trauma and surgery predispose to over 50% of cases of acute renal failure. Anaesthetists caring for seriously ill and postsurgical patients in intensive therapy units are responsible for considerable numbers of patients with renal failure. Prerenal uraemia is the most common form usually, but this may progress to established acute renal failure, especially if appropriate treatment is not given rapidly. Close monitoring of urinary output, fluid intake, weight and CVP is necessary. Early correction of hypovolaemia and sepsis increases urinary output and decreases blood urea.

The prognosis is dependent primarily on the factors which precipitated acute renal failure initially and the prognosis of the underlying disease. The prognosis is worse in patients with oliguric acute renal failure compared with the non-oliguric form. Mortality from obstetric causes is very low and, indeed, the incidence of acute renal failure from such causes has fallen markedly in recent years.

In contrast, the mortality in patients with burns, trauma and sepsis remains very high (approximately 50%) and has not changed significantly in the past 20 yr. Death is a result usually of gastrointestinal haemorrhage or sepsis. Jaundice at presentation indicates a poor prognosis. The unchanging prognosis in severely ill patients probably reflects the underlying condition and the degree to which acute renal failure can be prevented in less ill patients. Patients with both adult respiratory distress syndrome (ARDS) and acute renal failure have a particularly poor prognosis (Sweet et al., 1981).

Renal replacement therapy

End-stage renal disease (ESRD) has been defined as the situation in which, despite conservative therapy, the patient with chronic renal failure dies without renal replacement therapy. It may be defined in terms of clinical and biochemical criteria. Renal replacement therapy includes both haemodialysis and CAPD, and transplantation.

The overall incidence of ESRD is unknown, and the incidence of new patients requiring treatment for ESRD is difficult to obtain. In the USA, a figure of 100 patients per million of the population per year is given. In the UK (in the age group 15–60 yr) a figure of approximately 40 patients per million is claimed. Many European countries are now treating 50–60 patients per million population per year (European Dialysis and Transplant Association Registry, 1986). The reasons for these marked differences in national data depend partly on the great variation in the provision of facilities for treating patients with ESRD and partly on such medico-political considerations as a statutory right to treatment which pertains in some countries. Ideally, the need for treatment should be determined solely on medical criteria and all patients with ESRD should be assessed by a nephrologist. The indications for dialysis are listed in Table 74.5.

Table 74.5 Indications for dialysis in ESRD

Uraemic symptoms
Peripheral neuropathy
Pericarditis
Acidosis
Hyperkalaemia

Haemodialysis

Both haemodialysis and peritoneal dialysis are based on the ability of crystalloids but not colloids to diffuse down a concentration gradient through a semi-permeable membrane separating two solutions—blood and an ideal dialysis fluid, the dialysate. For haemodialysis, the membrane is made usually of cellulose derivatives whilst in peritoneal dialysis the peritoneum itself serves as the membrane.

Haemodialysis requires the circulation of blood through an artificial kidney at 200 ml/min and therefore repeated access to the circulation is necessary. For short-term use, particularly in acute renal failure, percutaneous catheterization of central veins is the method of choice. This is achieved by cannulation of either the femoral or the subclavian vein. Subclavian cannulation may be used for longer-term dialysis (for several months) by tunnelling the cannula through a subcutaneous track to reduce the risk of infection.

An arteriovenous (Scribner) shunt was the first method of obtaining repeated access to the circulation (Quinton et al., 1960). A shunt is a moulded silastic tube: one limb is inserted into an artery, the other into a vein to provide blood flow from and to the patient. When not being used for dialysis, blood simply flows through the loop formed by joining arterial and venous limbs. If possible, the shunt should be inserted in the leg to preserve arm vessels for subsequent fistula construction if the patient should require long-term dialysis. The lifetime of a shunt is limited by clotting or infection. With great care, the arterial limb can last up to 5 yr, but the venous limb rarely exceeds 12–18 months.

These problems have led to the use of arteriovenous (Cimino) fistulas (Brescia et al., 1966). The formation of a fistula, however, must be regarded as an elective procedure as the arterialized venous drainage may not produce the distended veins suitable for repeated vascular access for several weeks. The forearm is the most suitable site. Once mature, the fistula can be used for dialysis either by inserting needles at two sites on the fistula for inflow and outflow, or by using a double-lumen cannula. Using specialized equipment, single-needle dialysis is possible also.

The use of an extracorporeal circulation requires anticoagulation. In patients on long-term dialysis, this is provided by a loading dose of heparin (3000–5000 IU) followed by a constant infusion of 1000–1500 IU/hr. In ill patients, particularly those with clotting problems, minimal or regional heparinization should be used to prevent bleeding problems. Minimal heparin therapy involves a loading dose of 1500 IU or less, and additional doses of 500 IU as necessary to maintain the clotting time in the range 15–20 min. Regional heparinization requires an infusion of heparin into the blood leaving the patient, and protamine sulphate into the blood returning to the patient. The aim, difficult to achieve in practice, is to maintain a clotting time in the extracorporeal circuit of 15–20 min with normal values in the patient.

Modern haemodialysis machines provide equipment to generate dialysate from a concentrate and integrate blood and anticoagulant pumps with a system of alarms and monitors. They require a flow of suitably purified water of approximately 500 ml/min. Dialysers are available in a variety of models with different ultrafiltration and clearance capabilities. These have a surface area of semi-permeable membrane of 1.0–1.2 metre², although smaller areas are available for children and larger areas may be useful when increased efficiency is required.

Fluid removal is achieved by ultrafiltration. This involves transfer of water from the blood compartment to the dialysate by varying the suction pressure applied across the dialysis membrane.

Although haemodialysis removes fluid and toxins and corrects the biochemical abnormalities of uraemia, it does so intermittently and therefore, between dialyses, considerable dietary restrictions remain necessary. In adequately nourished patients, an intake of 0.75–1.0 g/kg body weight of protein with a calorie intake of approximately 2000 kcal is recommended. Both sodium and potassium intake has to be restricted, whilst any fluid restriction depends upon urine output and clinical status of the patient.

COMPLICATIONS OF HAEMODIALYSIS

Failure to adhere to salt and water restrictions or a change in the ideal body weight causes fluid overload with weight gain, hypertension, peripheral and pulmonary oedema. Hypertension is usually salt and water dependent and responds to ultrafiltration. This may, however, not be tolerated well, and antihypertensive therapy may remain necessary. Hypotension and cramps are common complications of haemodialysis. Hypotension may develop within minutes of starting dialysis and is related usually to myocardial insufficiency, inadequate response of peripheral blood vessels and poor filling of the vascular bed from the interstitial space. Other reasons invoked have been the use of acetate dialysis, autonomic neuropathy and hypoxaemia. The problem may be alleviated by using either bicarbonate in place of the conventional acetate buffer or sequential ultrafiltration and haemodialysis. Bicarbonate haemodialysis has been advocated for severely ill patients with acute renal failure, hypotension and impaired myocardial contractility.

Anaemia is almost invariable in dialysis patients; the exceptions are patients with polycystic kidneys who may have haemoglobin values in the normal range. In addition to the causes discussed earlier, there is a small amount of blood lost at each dialysis (3–5 ml) although larger quantities can be lost occasionally as a result of membrane rupture, clotting of blood within the dialyser or haemorrhage from a fistula or shunt. It is necessary, therefore, to provide iron supplements to compensate for this loss and most units also give folic acid, although in adequately nourished patients this may be unnecessary.

Hyperlipidaemia, a common finding, may require further dietary restrictions. Renal osteodystrophy is a frequent feature in patients with ESRD and has been discussed previously. Treatment is based on the use of oral phosphate-binding agents and vitamin D analogues (alfacalcidol) or active vitamin D (calcitriol). Vitamin D therapy may lead to hypercalcaemia and the serum calcium should be monitored frequently.

In common with other trace materials, aluminium is not eliminated in renal failure, and toxicity can result from the use of aluminium-containing phosphate-binding agents and aluminium-rich dialysis water. Aluminium is deposited in the bones causing an osteodystrophy (Parkinson et al., 1979). Multiple fractures are common, particularly of the ribs. Histologically, the lesion resembles osteomalacia but serum alkaline phosphatase concentrations (and PTH) are normal. A characteristic encephalopathy may occur also. Water supplies should be treated by reverse osmosis to reduce the aluminium content of the dialysate. Desferrioxamine has been used to chelate aluminium from the tissues with subsequent removal by dialysis and has produced some clinical improvement in the encephalopathy and osteodystrophy. Other phosphate-binding agents which do not contain an aluminium salt can be used. Magnesium-containing antacids (though having a weaker binding effect) have been investigated. Hypermagnesaemia is prevented by using dialysate low in magnesium.

Acquired cystic disease of the kidneys has been described in dialysis patients who did not have any form of renal cystic disease as a cause of their renal failure (Rudge, 1986).

Hepatitis B, once a scourge of dialysis centres, is now an uncommon problem in the UK since screening of blood donations and stringent aseptic techniques have been adopted widely. Within the UK, all staff and patients are screened regularly for HBsAg and positive patients are treated in a separate dialysis unit. Acquired immunodeficiency syndrome (AIDS) is at present a relatively uncommon condition in long-term dialysis patients, but is likely to increase in the near future (Goldman et al., 1986). It is clearly a major problem in young drug addicts, many of whom may present with acute renal failure secondary to septicaemia.

Peritoneal dialysis

Peritoneal dialysis makes use of the peritoneum as the semi-permeable membrane separating blood from the ideal fluid solution, the dialysate. Until recently, difficulty in obtaining repeated access to the peritoneal cavity and problems of malnutrition and peritonitis restricted this simple but relatively inefficient technique to the treatment of patients with non-hypercatabolic acute renal failure. The development, almost 20 yr ago, of the permanent indwelling Tenckhoff catheter, made of flexible silastic and anchored to the anterior abdominal wall by dacron cuffs, allowed peritoneal dialysis to be used for the long-term treatment of patients with chronic renal failure.

Intermittent peritoneal dialysis, performed generally by an automated peritoneal dialysis machine, was used by some renal units but costs and technical problems limited its usefulness. It has now been replaced largely by CAPD, developed a decade ago. A combination of the two therapies, so-called continuous cycling peritoneal dialysis (CCPD), is used by some units to ease the burden of frequent exchange with CAPD. Continuous ambulatory peritoneal dialysis is now used widely in the UK where 50% of children and 30% of adults are treated in this way. It has enabled units to increase the numbers of patients treated for ESRD (Nicholls et al., 1984). Despite this growth in its use, its future is uncertain. With high failure rates, these large numbers of patients treated with CAPD need adequate back-up facilities for haemodialysis. Of patients with CAPD, 80% have required haemodialysis at some time.

Nevertheless, once the catheter system is inserted, the technique for dialysis is simple and rapidly learned by patients (Fig. 74.1). Training is achieved in 7–10 days, it can be performed at home, no complicated equipment is necessary and no costly adaptations to the home are required.

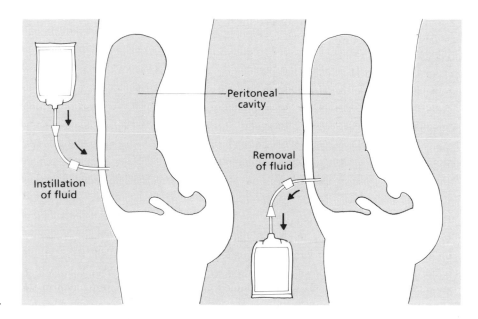

Fig. 74.1 The technique of CAPD.

Contra-indications are usually relative. Intraperitoneal adhesions or abdominal stomas may both cause problems. Hernias should be repaired before CAPD is commenced. Inflammatory bowel disease and diverticular disease may be associated with the spread of bowel organisms. Difficulties either due to visual handicap, comprehension or arthritis may interfere with the aseptic technique. The advantages of CAPD to patients are several. There is better removal of middle molecular weight solutes, patients often feel better on CAPD and an improvement in peripheral neuropathy may be noted.

Haemoglobin concentrations are higher than in patients on haemodialysis, making patients more active physically and increasing their feeling of well-being. Fluid and dietary restrictions are less severe than with haemodialysis and an increased protein intake is required to counteract protein loss into the peritoneal cavity.

No vascular access is required, making this form of treatment useful in children (with a low vascular volume), diabetics and arteriopaths with poor peripheral vasculature. The haemodynamic fluctuations and their associated symptoms, noted on haemodialysis, are avoided. Growth rates in children may be better and control of osteodystrophy is equal to that achieved on haemodialysis. Blood glucose control in insulin-dependent diabetics is easily achieved generally, although insulin requirements are increased. Insulin may be added to the CAPD bags and is thus given intraperitoneally rather than subcutaneously.

Conversely, the technique has considerable disadvantages. There is a high technical failure and drop-out rate. Only 72% of those beginning CAPD in 1981 were still using the technique 10–12 months later. A recent study found only 40% of patients remained on CAPD 2 yr later. Hyperglycaemia and hyperlipidaemia result from the use of necessarily hypertonic solutions with a high glucose content. This may pose problems in existing diabetics leading to poor control and increased insulin requirements and may worsen the hyperlipidaemia which occurs in many renal patients.

Some data suggest that there is long-term damage to the peritoneal membrane. There is a gradual reduction in the efficiency of dialysis with time, and by 2 yr, 30% of patients have lost a substantial proportion of their ultrafiltration capacity (Slingeneyer et al., 1983). This is often the result of recurrent bacterial infections. The use of dialysis solutions containing acetate has been implicated also, although it has been reported as well when lactate-containing solutions are used. Occasionally 'resting' the membrane by using haemodialysis for a period allows recovery of function to take place.

Psychological and psychosocial problems may occur in patients and their relatives who feel unable to cope with the presence of the catheter, bag and tubing.

Peritonitis is a frequent complication of CAPD treatment. The incidence varies but is probably around one episode per 4–12 patient months. It arises usually from contamination of the dialysate when the bags are changed; less frequently, it may pass through the anterior abdominal wall down the catheter track or arise from the bowel. Peritonitis presents as a cloudy CAPD bag (caused by polymorphonuclear leukocytes in the peritoneal effluent) with or without abdominal pain and fever. Approximately 50% of infective episodes are caused by Gram-positive cocci, usually Staphylococcus epidermidis and 20% by Gram-negative bacteria. A sterile peritonitis is usually a result of inadequate bacteriology or previous antibiotic therapy. Fungal peritonitis may occur, often following treatment of bacterial infection. Antifungal therapy is seldom effective, and catheter removal may be essential. For bacterial infection, intraperitoneal antibiotics given with the dialysate are usually satisfactory. As Gram-positive cocci are almost always sensitive to vancomycin and Gram-negative bacteria to netilmycin, treatment with a combination of these antibiotics may be commenced while bacterial sensitivities are awaited. Drug concentrations should be monitored. Infections of the catheter exit site and track may occur. Antibiotic therapy is often ineffective and removal of the catheter may be required.

Subacute sclerosing peritonitis is a rare complication of CAPD. The small bowel becomes encapsulated in thickened fibrosed peritoneum. This causes loss of ultrafiltration and a subacute small bowel obstruction. The cause is uncertain, although certain antiseptic solutions (Chlorhexidine) and acetate have been implicated. Surgical relief may be unsuccessful and mortality is high (Gandhi et al., 1980).

There appears to be little difference in terms of cost between CAPD and haemodialysis when hospitalization, peritonitis, antibiotic therapy and loss of earnings are taken into consideration. Differences in survival rates between the two techniques are difficult to assess. A Canadian study found survival rates at 2 yr to be the same for patients on CAPD and haemodialysis (Posen et al., 1984). A European report also noted no survival differences at one year but thereafter there was an increase in mortality for those patients on CAPD (Kramer *et al.*, 1984). Most studies comparing survival rates had noted, however, that those on CAPD have a higher prevalence of cardiovascular disease and diabetes.

Continuous ambulatory peritoneal dialysis, therefore, appears to be an acceptable form of treatment for certain groups of patients. Individuals with severe cardiovascular disease, children, diabetics, the elderly and those who fear machines may all benefit from this form of therapy. In the absence of a successful transplant, haemodialysis continues to be the treatment of choice for most other categories of patient.

Transplantation

Renal transplantation is now the treatment of choice for most patients with ESRD. Initially successful only between identical twins, kidneys from unrelated cadaver donors and from living-related donors are now transplanted with increasing chances of success. This continuing improvement (with grafts from living-related donors having a graft survival rate at 1 yr of 95% and from cadavers of 75–80%) is a result largely of advances in immunosuppressive therapy; patient survival at 1 yr is now approximately 95%.

When a living-related transplant is performed, anaesthesia is required for both donor and recipient. In some countries, when cadaver donors are used, the anaesthetist may be called upon to supervise ventilation and maintain cardiovascular stability.

Suitable cadaver donors are patients under 70 yr of age, in whom a diagnosis of brain death has been made. Potential donors are excluded if sepsis or malignancy (apart from primary cerebral tumours) is present. Significant hypertension or a history of renal disease are also exclusions.

Transplantation must be based on the principles of ABO compatability. Matching for HLA A, B and DR specificities has been shown to improve graft survival. In living-related donor transplantation, a single haplotype mismatch is suitable if a complete two haplotype match is not available. A complete match for DR and B specificities is considered currently to give the best results in a cadaver donor transplantation (Van Rood *et al.*, 1985).

For many years, blood transfusion of potential graft recipients was avoided to prevent sensitization of patients to Class I antigens (HLA A, B and C). More recently it has been observed that transplant recipients who had received pretransplant blood transfusions from third-party donors had improved graft survival (Terasaki *et al.*, 1983). The reasons for this improvement or enhancement of graft survival are still not understood fully. It is also not known how many blood transfusions are required nor their optimum timing. A beneficial effect of pretransplant blood transfusions is documented less easily in patients treated with the relatively new immunosuppressive agent, cyclosporin A.

Hyperacute rejection with rapid graft destruction within hours of transplantation was a not uncommon occurrence. It was caused by preformed cytotoxic antibodies present in recipient serum and directed to the graft and has fortunately become much less frequent following the introduction of the 'cross-match test'. Donor lymphocytes from spleen or lymph node are incubated with recipient serum in the presence of complement. A positive test in which the serum kills the donor cells indicates the presence of cytotoxic antibodies to donor tissue and precludes transplantation.

The surgical techniques are beyond the scope of this chapter. The anaesthetist is, however, responsible for patients with ESRD; these patients may be considered in terms of two subgroups. The recipient of a living-related donor transplant will be prepared adequately, hydrated optimally and dialysed recently. By contrast, the recipient of a cadaver transplant will have been notified at short notice and may require haemodialysis and preparation before theatre. Patients should not be volume depleted before surgery, and fluid losses during the transplant operation need to be replaced cautiously and potassium balance monitored in case the transplanted kidney does not function immediately.

IMMUNOSUPPRESSION

Within the graft, donor cells possess surface antigens differing from those of the recipient. The more important of these are encoded by the genes of the HLA gene complex, the human major histocompatibility complex, located on the short arm of the sixth chromosome. Recognition of these antigens by the recipient initiates cellular and humoral responses leading to acute rejection. Current immunosuppressive regimens which vary considerably are used to prevent rejection occurring or are given as additional therapy to reverse acute rejection. The most commonly used regimen at present depends on cyclosporin A, either alone or with low-dose prednisolone. Cyclosporin A, which inhibits lymphocyte proliferation mediated by interleukins I and II, results in a reversible impairment of T-cell-dependent immunity. Its use has resulted in graft survival figures for cadaver donor transplants now approaching those achieved in living-related transplants. It has led to a decrease in steroid dosage and the related serious effects. Unfortunately, however, cyclosporin A therapy has significant but different side-effects, notably hepatic and renal toxicity—the latter is often difficult to distinguish from rejection (Bennett & Pulliam, 1983).

Since 1962, prednisolone has been used as an immunosuppressive agent in combination with azathioprine. Steroids are now given in relatively low doses of 20–30 mg prednisolone in daily or alternate day regimens (Morris et al., 1982). To treat episodes of acute rejection, higher doses of steroids (oral prednisolone 200 mg daily or intravenous methylprednisolone 0.25–1 g daily) are used. Such treatment reverses episodes of acute rejection in 90% of cases but in 50% this reversal is only temporary; repeated immunological attack may prove unresponsive to further steroid therapy.

Antilymphocytic globulin, used in 1966 initially, is obtained by immunizing animals with human lymphoid cells. It has led to 15–20% improvement in graft survival but is associated with fever, thrombocytopenia, leukopenia and, rarely, anaphylactoid reactions. In the future, monoclonal antibodies more specifically directed to recipient cytotoxic T-lymphocytes may prove therapeutically useful. Irradiation of the graft, cyclophosphamide, plasmapheresis and depletion of lymphocytes by thoracic duct drainage have all been advocated as immunosuppressive regimens but are seldom used today.

COMPLICATIONS OF RENAL TRANSPLANTATION

Early complications of renal transplantation are related usually to failure of the graft to function. Delayed function may result from a degree of ATN in the graft whereas decreasing function may result from acute rejection, cyclosporin A nephrotoxicity or mechanical problems with the transplanted ureter. A later decline in renal function may result from chronic rejection, further ureteric problems, stenosis of the arterial anastomosis, urinary infection or recurrence of the original pathology (e.g. glomerulonephritis). A chronic rejection process is usually unresponsive to antirejection therapy.

Other long-term complications relate to the need for persisting immunosuppressive therapy. Infection is a major cause of morbidity and mortality after transplantation (Mackowiak, 1978). Bacterial chest infections are produced by common pathogens generally, such as pneumococci or Haemophilus influenzae. Tuberculosis may, however, be reactivated in immunosuppressed patients. 'Opportunistic infections' with fungae and protozoa are encountered frequently. Oral candidiasis usually responds readily to topical nystatin. Pulmonary infections may be caused by Aspergillus, Histoplasma and Cryptococcus which may produce a meningitis also. Pneumocystis carinii is the most common protozoal infection encountered and presents usually as an undiagnosed pulmonary infiltrate in a febrile dyspnoeic patient. Diagnosis depends on lung biopsy and cotrimoxazole is the treatment of choice.

Cytomegalovirus is a common problem in some centres and presents usually with fever and leukopenia. Herpes simplex and varicella zoster infection can occur but respond to therapy with the antiviral agent, acyclovir.

Despite the problems associated with transplantation, cadaver graft survival figures of over 80% have been obtained. Successful transplantation offers the patient with ESRD the best opportunity of achieving a normal lifestyle.

Haemofiltration

Haemofiltration differs from conventional haemodialysis in that no dialysate is used. It is used most frequently in the treatment of acute renal failure, but in some countries it is used also for long-term dialysis despite the expense involved. In haemofiltration, a 'high flux' membrane very permeable to water and solutes is used. Fluid and molecules of molecular weight 6000–12000 in size are removed by convection. Twenty-five to 30 litre of ultrafiltrate can be removed at one 4-hr session—the equivalent of a GFR of 17–20 ml/min for that day. The advantages over haemodialysis are less hypotension and hypoxia during treatment, better control of hypertension, improved control of plasma lipids, peripheral and autonomic neuropathy. One disadvantage is that to maintain volume homeostasis large quantities of crystalloid solution have to be re-infused such that the net removal of fluid may only be 2 litres per session. It may, however, be useful in patients with a tendency to hypotension on dialysis who have not benefited from a change to bicarbonate haemodialysis.

Continuous prolonged haemofiltration can be used in acute renal failure to remove fluid overload and will also permit parenteral feeding to be achieved without fluid restriction or overload.

Drugs and the kidney

Many drugs are excreted at least partially by the kidney, and dosage schedules require modification frequently in patients with chronic renal failure. Drugs which are excreted by non-renal routes may require dosage modification also as the volume of distribution, protein binding of the drug and response of the target organ may all be altered in renal failure. In patients undergoing renal replacement therapy, either haemodialysis or peritoneal dialysis may complicate dosage regimens further as some drugs are removed by these routes. The particular problems of agents used in anaesthetic practice have been dealt with in a previous section. In this part of the chapter, the general principles of drug modification in renal failure are discussed.

In uraemia, some drugs which are excreted normally by the kidney, may be metabolized or excreted by other organs, notably the liver and gastrointestinal tract. Conversely, drug accumulation may occur when normal hepatic pathways such as oxidation, conjugation and acetylation are affected adversely by the biochemical effects of uraemia. Chronic renal failure affects also the protein binding of certain drugs. Drugs which are anionic, including warfarin, frusemide, phenytoin, sulphonamides and salicylates are less protein bound in uraemic patients. Non-ionic drugs, such as propranolol, morphine and diazepam are not affected in this manner by renal failure. In nephrotic patients, the reduction in plasma albumin concentration will alter also the binding of acidic drugs.

If more than 50% of a drug or its active metabolite undergoes renal excretion, the dosage usually requires to be modified when the GFR is less than 40–50 ml/min or the serum creatinine is greater than 200–250 μmol/litre. The loading dose of a particular drug should not be changed but thereafter the dosage can be modified by prolonging the interval between doses or by reducing subsequent doses. Recommended doses for patients with chronic renal failure are given in the British National Formulary.

References

Ballerman B.J. & Brenner B.M. (1985) Biologically active atrial peptides. *Journal of Clinical Investigation* 76, 2041–8.

Bennett W.M. & Pulliam J.P. (1983) Cyclosporin nephrotoxicity. *Annals of Internal Medicine* 99, 851–4.

Brescia M.J., Cimino J.E., Appel K. & Hurwich B.J. (1966) Chronic haemodialysis using venipuncture and a surgically created arteriovenous fistula. *New England Journal of Medicine* 275, 1089–92.

Bricker N.S. (1982) Sodium homeostatis in chronic renal disease. *Kidney International* 21, 886–97.

Bromage P.R. & Gertel M. (1972) Brachial plexus anaesthesia in chronic renal failure. *Anesthesiology* 36, 488–93.

Carvalho A.C.A. (1983) Bleeding in uremia—a clinical challenge. *New England Journal of Medicine* 308, 38–9.

Contreras P., Later R., Navarro J., Touraine J.L., Freyria A.M. & Traeger J. (1982) Molecules in the middle molecular weight range. *Nephron* 32, 193–201.

DeFronzo R.A. & Alvestrand A. (1980) Glucose intolerance in uremia: site and mechanism. *American Journal of Clinical Nutrition* 33, 1438–45.

Deutsch S., Bastron R.D., Pierce G.C. & Vandam L.D. (1969) The effects of anaesthesia with thiopentone, nitrous oxide, narcotics and neuromuscular blocking on renal function in normal man. *British Journal of Anaesthesia* 41, 807–14.

Dundee J.W. & Richards R.K. (1954) Effect of azotemia upon the action of intravenous barbiturate anesthesia. *Anesthesiology* 15, 333–46.

Easterling R.E. (1977) Racial factors in the incidence and causation of end-stage renal disease. *Transactions of the American Society of Artificial Internal Organs* 23, 28–33.

Eastwood J.B., Bordier P.J. & De Wardener H.E. (1973) Some biochemical, histological, radiological and clinical features of renal osteodystrophy. *Kidney International* 4, 128–40.

El Nahas A.M. & Coles G.A. (1986) Dietary treatment of chronic renal failure: ten unanswered questions. *Lancet* i, 597–600.

European Dialysis and Transplant Association Registry (1986) *Demography of Dialysis and Transplantation in Europe 1984.* pp. 1–8.

Fisher J.W. (1980) Mechanism of the anaemia of chronic renal failure. *Nephron* 25, 106–111.

Gandhi V.C., Humayun H.M., Ing T.S., Daugirdas J.T., Jablokow V.R., Iwatsuki S., Geis P. & Hano J. (1980) Sclerotic thickening of the peritoneal membrane in maintenance peritoneal dialysis patients. *Archives of Internal Medicine* 140, 120–3.

Giovannetti S. (1986) Answers to ten questions on the dietary treatment of chronic renal failure. *Lancet* ii, 1140–2.

Goldman M., Vanherweghem J.L., Liesnard C., Dolle N., Sprecher S., Thiry L. & Toussaint C. (1986) Markers of AIDS-associated virus in a haemodialysis unit. *Nephrology, Dialysis, Transplantation* 1, 130.

Henderson I.S., Beattie T.J. & Kennedy A.C. (1980) Dopamine hydrochloride in oliguric states. *Lancet* ii, 827–8.

Kennedy A.C., Burton J.A., Luke R.G., Briggs J.D., Lindsay R.M., Allison M.E.M., Edward N. & Dargie H.J. (1973) Factors affecting the prognosis in acute renal failure. *Quarterly Journal of Medicine* 42, 73–86.

Kramer P., Broyer M., Brunner F.P., Brynger H., Challah D., Oules R., Rizzoni G., Selwood N.H., Wing A.J. & Balas E.A. (1984) Combined report on regular dialysis and transplantation in Europe XIV 1983. *Proceedings of the European Dialysis and Transplantation Association* 21, 2–68.

Linas S.L., Peterson L.N., Anderson R.J., Aisenbrey G.A., Simon F.R.

& Berl T. (1979) Mechanisms of renal potassium conservation in the rat. *Kidney International* **15**, 601–11.

Mackowiak P.A. (1978) Microbial synergism in human infections. *New England Journal of Medicine* **298**, 21–6, 83–7.

Maschio G., Tessitore N., D'Angelo A., Bonucci E., Lupo A., Valvo E., Loschiavo C., Fabris A., Morachiello P., Previato G. & Fiaschi E. (1980) Early dietary phosphorus restriction and calcium supplementation in the prevention of renal osteodystrophy. *American Journal of Clinical Nutrition* **33**, 1546–54.

Miller R.D., Way W.L., Hamilton W.K. & Layzer R.B. (1972) Succinylcholine-induced hyperkalemia in patients with renal failure. *Anesthesiology* **36**, 138–41.

Moran S.M. & Myers B.D. (1985) Pathophysiology of protracted acute renal failure in man. *Journal of Clinical Investigation* **76**, 1440–8.

Morris P.J., Chan L., French M.E. & Ting A. (1982) Low dose oral prednisolone in renal transplantation. *Lancet* **i**, 525–7.

Muirhead N., Adami S., Sandler L.M., Fraser R.A., Catto G.R.D., Edward N. & O'Riordan J.L.H. (1982) Long-term effects of 1,25-dihydroxyvitamin D_3 and 24, 25-dihydroxyvitamin D_3 in renal osteodystrophy. *Quarterly Journal of Medicine* **51**, 427–44.

Neilsen H.E., Romer F.K., Melsen F., Christensen M.S. & Hanson H.E. (1980) 1-alpha hydroxyvitamin D_3 treatment of non-dialysed patients with chronic renal failure. Effects of bone metabolism and kidney function. *Clinical Nephrology* **13**, 103–8.

Nicholls A.J., Waldek S., Platts M.M., Moorhead P.J. & Brown C.B. (1984) Impact of continuous ambulatory dialysis on treatment of renal failure in patients aged over 60. *British Medical Journal* **288**, 18–19.

Olsen J.L., Hostetter T.H., Rennke H.G., Brenner B.M. & Venkatachlam M.A. (1982) Altered glomerular permselectivity and progressive sclerosis following extreme ablation of renal mass. *Kidney International* **22**, 112–26.

Parkinson I.S., Ward M.K., Feest T.G., Fawcett R.W.P. & Kerr D.N.S. (1979) Fracturing dialysis osteodystrophy and dialysis encephalopathy. *Lancet* **i**, 406–9.

Posen G., Lam E. & Rappaport A. (1984) CAPD in Canada in 1982. *Peritoneal Dialysis Bulletin* **4**, 72–4.

Priebe H.J., Skillman J.J., Bushnell L.S., Long P.C. & Silen W. (1980) Antacid versus cimetidine in preventing acute gastrointestinal bleeding. *New England Journal of Medicine* **302**, 426–30.

Quinton E., Dillard D. & Scribner B.H. (1960) Cannulation of blood vessels for prolonged haemodialysis. *Transactions of the American Society of Artificial Internal Organs* **6**, 104–13.

Rainford D.J. (1977) The immediate care of acute renal failure. *Anaesthesia* **32**, 277–81.

Renfrew R., Buselmeier T.J. & Kjellstrand C.M. (1980) Pericarditis and renal failure. *Annual Review of Medicine* **31**, 345–60.

Rudge C.J. (1986) Acquired cystic disease of the kidney: serious or irrelevent. *British Medical Journal* **293**, 1186–7.

Shemesh O., Golbetz H., Kriss J.P. & Myers B.D. (1985) Limitations of creatinine as a filtration marker in glomerulopathic patients. *Kidney International* **28**, 830–8.

Slingeneyer A., Canaud B. & Mion C. (1983) Permanent loss of ultrafiltration capacity of the peritoneum in long term peritoneal dialysis: an epidemiological study. *Nephron* **33**, 133–8.

Swann R.C. & Merrill J.P. (1953) The clinical course of acute renal failure. *Medicine* **32**, 215–92.

Sweet S.J., Glenney C.U., Fitzgibbons J.P., Friedmann P. & Teres D. (1981) Synergistic effect of acute renal failure and respiratory failure in the surgical Intensive care unit. *American Journal of Surgery* **141**, 492–6.

Terasaki P.I., Perdue S.T., Sasaki N., Mickey M.R. & Whitby L. (1983) Improving success rates of kidney transplantation. *Journal of the American Medical Association* **250**, 1065–8.

Van Rood J.J., Hendriks G.F.J., D'Amaro J., Gratama J.W., Jager M., van Es A. & Persijn G.G. (1985) HLA matching, patient survival and immune response genes in renal transplantation. *Transplantation Proceedings* **XVII**, 681–5.

Wilson D.M., Turner D.R., Cameron J.S., Ogg C.S., Brown C.B. & Chantler C. (1976) Value of renal biopsy in acute intrinsic renal failure. *British Medical Journal* **2**, 459–61.

75

Cardiovascular Failure

I. WRIGHT AND I. McA. LEDINGHAM

Cardiovascular failure may be defined as a pathological state in which the tissues are perfused insufficiently in relation to their metabolic needs. In the context of the intensive therapy unit (ITU), this condition may have a variety of causes and often demands prompt and aggressive intervention.

In order to understand and treat cardiovascular failure in the ITU, it is necessary to possess a good working knowledge of the relevant cardiovascular physiology, to understand the underlying physiological derangement caused by specific disease processes, to know the indications for, and the limitations and possible hazards of, available monitoring techniques, to be aware of the spectrum of treatment options and their rationale and to be able to set treatment goals which correlate with increased survival.

Applied physiology

Regulation of cardiac output (see also Chapter 8)

STROKE VOLUME

Cardiac output is determined by the product of stroke volume and heart rate. Stroke volume is determined by the preload, contractility and afterload (Table 75.1).

Preload

Starling's law of the heart states that the force of contraction is a function of the length of the myocardial fibres prior to contraction; an increase in length (preload) produces a more forceful contraction. In the intact heart, preload is taken to be the volume of blood in the ventricle at the end of diastole: the end-diastolic volume (EDV). For any given EDV, the end-diastolic pressure (EDP) depends on the compliance of the ventricle; the less compliant (i.e. stiffer) the ventricle, the higher the EDP for any EDV. It is possible to measure EDV using radionuclide imaging, and modern techniques using short half-life tracers such as ^{195}Au allow repeated estimations of EDV (Mathay & Berger, 1983). There are technical problems of separation of counts from the different chambers of the heart, and the technique is expensive, and not available widely. For these reasons, it is usual to measure EDP as an index of preload, although this involves certain assumptions which if unrecognized may be misleading.

The pressure–volume relationship is alinear (Fig. 75.1) such that at higher volumes, a further small increase in EDV causes a disproportionate increase in EDP. Compliance of the ventricle is not only determined by the elasticity of the myocardium but also by the geometry and wall thickness of the ventricle and ultimately, by the constricting effect of the intact pericardium (Alderman & Glantz, 1976). A single curve cannot describe ventricular compliance, and a family of parallel curves provides a more accurate illustration of changes in compliance. For example, a decrease in compliance associated with ischaemia or the use of some inotropic drugs shifts the curve upwards and to the left, and conversely an increase in compliance shifts the curve downwards and to the right (Fig. 75.1).

It can be seen, therefore, that a high EDP need not reflect a high EDV. However, although compliance may be altered acutely either by disease or treatment, it is still valid to investigate the relationship between EDP and EDV, and this can be achieved best by noting the response to a fluid challenge (see below). A rapid increase in EDP (or some other pressure taken as an indication of preload) in response to a bolus of fluid,

Table 75.1 Determinants of stroke volume

Factors affecting preload

Increase	Decrease
Transfusion*	Hypovolaemia
Venoconstriction	Venodilatation
Posture	Raised intrathoracic pressure
Muscle pump	Raised intrapericardial pressure
	Decreased ventricular compliance
	Loss of atrial transport

Factors affecting contractility

Increase	Decrease
Sympathetic stimulation	Ischaemia
Endogenous catecholamines	Hypoxia
Inotropes*	Metabolic derangement
Improved myo-cardial oxygenation	Negatively inotropic drugs*
Tachycardia	

Factors affecting afterload

Increase	Decrease
High aortic impedance	Low aortic impedance
Arteriolar constriction	Arteriolar dilatation
Increased ventricular radius	Decreased ventricular radius
	Intra-aortic balloon pump*

* Iatrogenic influence.

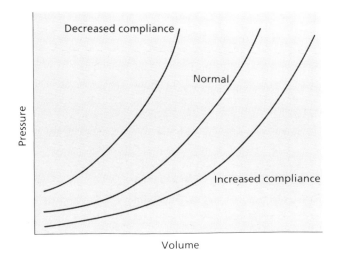

Fig. 75.1 Ventricular compliance curves (see text for details).

indicates that the ventricular pressure–volume relationship lies on the steeply ascending portion of the compliance curve, and that further volume expansion should be considered carefully.

Many factors affect preload in the intact patient. The venous return to the atrium is determined by the balance between circulating volume and venous capacitance, and the presence or absence of the skeletal 'muscle pump' and is reduced by a high intrathoracic or intrapericardial pressure [as a consequence of, for example, intermittent positive pressure ventilation (IPPV) with or without positive end-expiratory pressure (PEEP), pericardial fibrosis or tamponade]. The loss of atrial transport during arrhythmias or ventricular pacing may reduce preload crucially, especially in a non-compliant ventricle, as may also atrioventricular valve dysfunction (Ganong, 1983). The preload is altered also by changes in myocardial contractility and afterload (see below).

Contractility

It is a useful concept to plot a graph with preload on the abscissa and some parameter of ventricular performance on the ordinate, such as stroke volume (end-diastolic volume – end-systolic volume) or more usually stroke work (mean arterial pressure × stroke volume) or even in the clinical setting, cardiac output. Such a graph is described as a ventricular function curve (VFC) (Fig. 75.2) and allows contractility to be deduced. If the afterload (see below) is held constant, increasing contractility produces a greater degree of work for any given preload. This is seen clinically with sympathetic nerve stimulation, release of catecholamines or exogenously administered inotropes. The VFC moves upward and to the left. The converse applies with negatively inotropic influences such as hypoxia, ischaemia, metabolic and acid–base derangements and certain drugs (see below) (Braunwald *et al.*, 1977). The concept of the VFC is useful clinically, as exemplified by the technique of 'fluid challenge'. A bolus of colloid (of the order of 50–200 ml depending on the size and condition of the patient) is given over a short period of time, and this may be repeated. Variables reflecting preload and myocardial performance are measured [e.g. pulmonary capillary wedge pressure (PCWP) and cardiac output], and when further fluid challenges do not result in improvements in myocardial performance, the circulating volume should not be expanded further. The end-point of a series of fluid challenges is indicated usually by a rapid

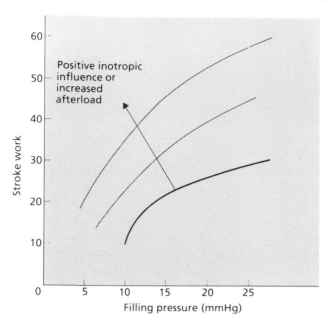

Fig. 75.2 Ventricular function curves (see text for details).

increase in filling pressures in response to a bolus of fluid. This increase reflects the position of the ventricle on the steeply ascending part of the compliance curve (Fig. 75.1) and implies that further volume challenge produces only an increase in venous pressures with the attendant risk of systemic or pulmonary oedema.

Afterload

The tension in the ventricular wall during systole is taken to be the afterload on the ventricle, and is determined partly by the resistance against which the ventricle ejects blood, and partly by the physical characteristics of the ventricle (Braunwald *et al.*, 1977).

The outflow resistance is determined by the aortic impedance (rate of change of pressure divided by instantaneous aortic flow i.e. a reflection of aortic compliance) and arteriolar run off. For any given stroke volume, if the aorta and major vessels are non-compliant (e.g. atherosclerotic) or the patient vaso-constricted, the pressure generated, and thus the afterload, are increased.

Ventricular wall tension is related to ventricular radius and intracavitary pressure by Laplace's law: $P = 2T/R$ (P = intracavitary pressure, T = wall tension, R = ventricular radius) i.e. for any given pressure, as the radius increases, so does the wall tension.

The clinical importance of afterload is that for any given preload and contractility, if the afterload increases, either the ventricular stroke work (and oxygen consumption) has to increase, or cardiac output decreases.

HEART RATE

The denervated sinoatrial node depolarizes spontaneously at a rate of approximately 120 beat/min, and the predominant vagal tone acting on the heart slows this rate to 55–100 beat/min in the normal resting heart.

As the heart rate slows, diastole lengthens, which leads to increased ventricular filling, increased end-diastolic volume, and cardiac output is therefore maintained. At very low rates e.g. less than 40 beat/min, it is not possible for the normal heart to increase stroke volume sufficiently to compensate, and the diseased heart copes even less well. This is especially so if the slow rate is nodal or ventricular in origin.

As the heart rate increases, diastole shortens, and diastolic stress relaxation produces a reduction in compliance (Covell & Ross, 1973). Diastolic filling is therefore compromised, and stroke volume and cardiac output tend to decrease. This effect is overcome at rates up to 180 beat/min by the intrinsic increase in contractility caused by an increased heart rate (the 'treppe' effect; Braunwald *et al.*, 1977) and the positive inotropic effect of sympathetic stimulation (which is usually the cause of the tachycardia) which leads to a relative shortening of systole. At very high rates (180 beat/min or greater), diastolic filling is so compromised that this compensation is ineffective, especially if atrial transport is lost as in many supraventricular arrhythmias, or if ventricular function is compromised by ventricular arrhythmias or myocardial depression (Ganong, 1983).

Determinants of myocardial metabolism
(Table 75.2)

The haemodynamic alterations in disease and ITU treatment have profound implications for myocardial metabolism. Direct measurement of adequacy of perfusion and oxygenation of the myocardium is difficult. Coronary sinus lactate or cardiac enzyme levels may indicate inadequate myocardial perfusion, but provide only retrospective evidence of poor perfusion and/or myocardial damage and may not reveal significant regional ischaemia. Acute changes in the ECG may reflect ischaemia, but the commonly used, continuous,

Table 75.2 Determinants of myocardial oxygen metabolism

Oxygen supply
Arterial oxygen content
Coronary vessel calibre (the concentration of myocardial metabolic products and the P_{CO_2})
Coronary perfusion pressure (diastolic — LVEDP)
Coronary perfusion time (1/heart rate)

Oxygen demand
External work (mean arterial pressure × stroke volume)
   Preload
   Contractility
   Aortic compliance and arteriolar run-off
Internal work (during isovolumic contraction)
   Pressure generated
   Ventricular radius
Heart rate

single-lead display monitors only one region of the heart and serious hypoperfusion can be concealed. A knowledge of the determinants of myocardial oxygen supply and demand allows prediction of the effects of alteration of haemodynamic parameters.

MYOCARDIAL OXYGEN SUPPLY

This is determined by arterial oxygen content (proportional to haemoglobin concentration × oxygen saturation) and coronary blood flow, which depends on coronary vessel calibre, perfusion pressure [diastolic pressure − left ventricular end-diastolic pressure (LVEDP)] and perfusion time (i.e. duration of diastole).

Inotropes, pressor agents, vasodilators and P_{CO_2} may affect coronary vessel calibre directly (except in rigid, atherosclerotic vessels). However, the predominant determinant of calibre is accumulation of local metabolites (in response to increased myocardial work) which causes vasodilatation and overrides the direct effects of vasoactive drugs.

The pressure in the left ventricle during systole is slightly greater than in the aorta, and subendocardial vessels are compressed by the increased wall tension during systole, so perfusion of the left ventricular muscle occurs predominantly during diastole (although the atria and right ventricle are perfused throughout the cardiac cycle). Perfusion pressure depends, therefore, on the differences between aortic diastolic pressure and LVEDP. As heart rate increases, diastole shortens, and perfusion time is therefore inversely proportional to heart rate.

Coronary blood flow is affected also by viscosity of blood, and may be decreased locally by atherosclerotic lesions.

MYOCARDIAL OXYGEN DEMAND

Oxygen demand is proportional to the amount of work performed by the ventricle. Stroke work is calculated as the product of mean arterial pressure and stroke volume (although it should be noted that this is only an estimate of external work performed by the ventricle, and takes no account of internal work performed when the inflow valve is closed and the outflow valve has not yet opened). Factors which increase myocardial oxygen consumption are therefore increased ventricular wall tension, increased contractility, increased stroke volume and increased heart rate. 'Pressure' work raises oxygen consumption much more than 'volume' work, reflecting the internal work performed in increasing wall tension before the ejection phase (Sonnenblick & Skelton, 1971) and this demonstrates the importance of afterload as a prime determinant of myocardial oxygen consumption.

MAINTENANCE OF INTRAVASCULAR VOLUME

There is a complex series of inter-relating mechanisms to maintain circulating volume and vascular capacity within the normal range, which in the short term are protective but may cause further problems eventually and indeed lead to the breakdown of cellular integrity. These mechanisms may be considered under the headings of neurohumoral and passive responses.

Neurohumoral response (Fig. 75.3)

Reduction in blood volume stimulates vascular mechanoreceptors in the great vessels of the chest leading to release of antidiuretic hormone (ADH). Baroreceptor stimulation increases heart rate and causes peripheral vasoconstriction, and activation of the renin–angiotensin–aldosterone axis leads to salt and water retention. Afferent stimuli integrated in the hypothalamus cause release of stress hormones from the arterior pituitary, chiefly adrenocorticotrophic hormone (ACTH) but also growth hormone and prolactin, and lead also to a massive outpouring of catecholamines from the adrenal medulla, in addition to direct sympathetic stimulation. Benedict and Grahame-Smith (1978) observed that adrenaline concentrations exceeded noradrenaline concentrations in hypovolaemic shock whilst the reverse applies

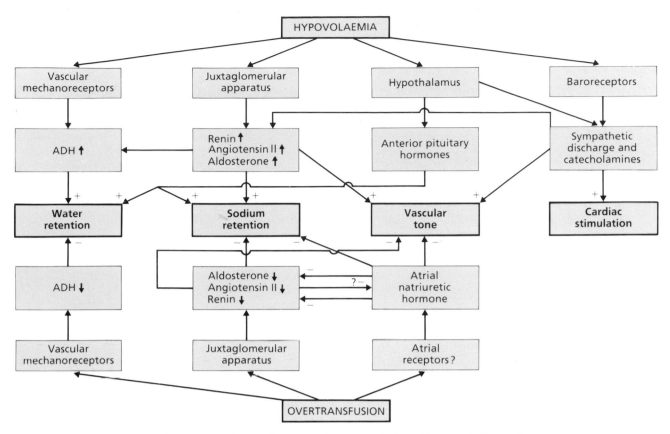

Fig. 75.3 The neurohumoral response to hypovolaemia and overtransfusion. ADH = antidiuretic hormone.

in septic shock (Griffiths, 1972). The net result of these responses is to reduce vascular capacity by sympathetic nervous system and catecholamine-induced vasoconstriction, to increase circulating volume by causing salt and water retention and incidentally to mobilize energy reserves directly and as a result of insulin antagonism. Release of β-endorphin from the anterior pituitary and met-enkephalin from the adrenal medulla caused by these same stimuli tends to antagonize the actions of catecholamines (Watson *et al.*, 1984).

An increased blood volume partially reverses the response noted above and causes vasodilatation and diuresis, chiefly via reduced plasma ADH and renin concentrations. Recently, atrial natriuretic hormone has been identified. Granules in the atrial wall contain a substance (now synthesized) which causes a natriuresis by increasing glomerular filtration rate, exerting an antirenin and antiangiotensin action, and directly relaxing vascular smooth muscle. The stimulus for release of this hormone is at present unknown, although atrial distension may be an important factor (Laragh, 1985).

Passive response

The transfer of fluid between the intravascular and interstitial fluid compartments is governed by Starling's hypothesis that a net outward hydrostatic force is balanced by a slightly smaller inward oncotic force. Thus, there is a net outflow of fluid from the intravascular compartment into the interstitial compartment under normal circumstances, and this returns to the circulation via the lymphatics.

The balance of these forces is altered in cardiovascular failure. In the early stages of shock, the effects of sympathetic stimulation result in constriction of the resistance vessels on both sides of the capillary bed. Precapillary resistance is increased (by arteriolar constriction) to a greater extent than postcapillary (venular) resistance. This reduces the intravascular pressure so that there is net transfer of fluid from the interstitial space to the intravascular space. Both the gel and the free fluid phases of the interstitium are involved (Haljamäe, 1984), and because the interstitial compartment contains approximately four times the volume of fluid compared with the intravascular compartment, there is considerable scope for auto-transfusion to occur. However, as the shock process continues and in the absence of effective resuscitation, there is a marked change in vascular reactivity. The arteriolar constriction 'fades' much more rapidly than venular constriction, and the accumulation of local metabolites such as lactate has a greater vasodilatory effect on arterioles than venules. The result is an increased mean capillary pressure which causes net transfer of fluid initially into the interstitium and later into the cells. This process is exacerbated by the increase in capillary permeability from vasoactive mediators such as histamine and kinins released early in septic shock but eventually in all types of shock.

METABOLIC RESPONSE TO CARDIOVASCULAR FAILURE

Hormonal and substrate variations (Table 75.3)

The initial metabolic response to injury is uniform, whatever the mechanism of the injury. Hypergly-caemia occurs early, and increased uptake of precursor substrates such as lactate, pyruvate and gluconeogenic amino acids cause increased hepatic glucose production (Wilmore *et al.*, 1980). The hormones adrenaline and cortisol, released as part of the systemic response to injury, and glucagon, released by adrenaline, have a synergistic hyperglycaemic action (Heath, 1980). Plasma adrenaline concentrations increase rapidly, causing extensive muscle glycolysis, and the lactate produced is converted to glucose in the liver. Glucagon

Table 75.3 Metabolic response to injury

Hormonal response	Substrate response
Increased adrenaline	*Carbohydrate*
Increased glucagon	Increased glycogenolysis
Increased cortisol	Increased peripheral glycolysis
	Increased hepatic gluconeo-genesis
	Increased lactate and pyruvate
	Increased glucose (late fall in sepsis)
	Lipid
	Increased lipolysis
	Increased free fatty acids (down in severe injury)
	Protein
	Increased visceral protein turnover
	Negative nitrogen balance

increases later, reaching a peak within 2 hr, and stimulates hepatic glycogenolysis, gluconeogenesis and amino acid uptake. Cortisol, released rapidly and in proportion to the severity of the insult (Stoner *et al.*, 1979), increases and prolongs the action of adrenaline and glucagon, and stimulates peripheral release of amino acids. Relative insensitivity to insulin occurs 2–7 days after injury; this is termed insulin resistance and potentiates the hyperglycaemia.

Catecholamine-induced lipolysis leads to an increase in plasma free-fatty acid concentration initially, in concert with increasing severity of injury, but this correlation no longer holds in severe injury because of poor perfusion of fat depots, and re-esterification stimulated by increasing lactate concentrations (Stoner *et al.*, 1979).

Injury causes an increase in whole-body protein turnover, breakdown increasing more than synthesis (especially in severe injury or sepsis) resulting in a net negative nitrogen balance. Rennie and Harrison (1984) suggest that visceral protein turnover predominates over muscle protein turnover and that this is independent of nutritional manipulation.

These metabolic changes are exaggerated in sepsis (Wardle, 1979); lipolysis is prominent and there may be a marked lipaemia. Intracellular glucose oxidation and ketone body utilization are decreased in muscle, and there is therefore increased utilization of branched-chain amino acids. Hyperglycaemia with insulin resistance is superseded by hypoglycaemia, produced by depletion of glycogen stores, depressed gluconeogenesis (Wilmore *et al.*, 1980) and increased tissue utilization of glucose, and hypoinsulinaemia from depressed pancreatic secretion associated with high plasma catecholamine concentrations.

Plasma lactate concentrations correlates with severity of injury as shown by the Injury Severity Score (Stoner *et al.* 1979). This may reflect direct hypoperfusion as a result of hypotension, but in severe cardiovascular failure, especially that associated with sepsis, there is evidence that blood may traverse arteriovenous anastamoses or preferred route capillaries rather than nutrient vessels (Silver, 1977).

Cellular dysfunction

Failure of perfusion of the respiring tissues deprives the cells of oxygen and substrate, and causes inability to remove products of cellular metabolism. This damages the cell in three ways: altered cell volume regulation, altered energy metabolism and intracellular release of lysosomal enzymes. Anaerobic metabolism leads to a reduction in cellular adenosine triphosphate (ATP) content. This essential energy source for the ionic pump of the plasma membrane is broken down normally to adenosine diphosphate (ADP) and phosphate in the presence of ATPase. The absence of high-energy phosphate bonds leads to depression of pump function and cell swelling, the cells tending to approach Gibbs–Donnan equilibrium with an increase of intracellular sodium, calcium and water content and a loss of potassium and magnesium.

When oxygen tension decreases to below 0.1 kPa (0.75 mmHg) in the mitochondria (Nunn, 1977) electron transport stops immediately. Oxidative phosphorylation is uncoupled and ATP production ceases, and eventually structural changes appear in the outer and inner mitochondrial membranes. These mark the 'point of no return' (Trump *et al.*, 1976) beyond which the mitochondria and therefore the cells are damaged irreparably.

Adenosine triphosphate deficiency and intracellular lactic acidosis alter calcium flow within the cell, and the excess intracellular calcium has been postulated as a major cause of irreversibility of damage in ischaemia (Jennings, 1976). The reduced intracellular pH causes alteration in lysosomal structure and function leading to release of hydrolases from the lysosomes. This seems to be a late effect however, and not a causative event in the sequence of cellular derangement (Trump *et al.*, 1976).

Aetiology of shock

The three classical clinical subdivisions of shock (Table 75.4) are discussed in this section. Their causes, the resulting primary physiological insults and compensatory reactions are described. The clinical pictures, and the effects on myocardial metabolism and tissue perfusion follow logically from these descriptions, although the complexity of septic shock makes interpretation difficult.

Hypovolaemia

The effects of hypovolaemia vary with its nature, severity and duration, the patient's age and general health, and with the speed and adequacy of resuscitation. The causes of hypovolaemia are well known, have been reviewed recently (Ledingham & Ramsay, 1986) and are therefore not considered further. Whatever the cause, the primary physiological insult is a reduction in venous return which causes reduction

Table 75.4 Aetiology of shock

Hypovolaemic shock
Haemorrhage
Burns
Salt and water deficits e.g.
   Addison's disease
   Gastrointestinal fistulae
   Diabetes insipidus

Cardiogenic shock
Primary myocardial failure e.g.
   Ischaemia
   Arrhythmias
   Valvular damage
   Cardiomyopathy
Secondary myocardial failure e.g.
   Drugs
   Hypoxia
   Acute rise in afterload

Distributive shock
Sepsis
Anaphylaxis
Late stages of hypovolaemic shock

in cardiac output and a reduction in major organ perfusion. In early and uncomplicated hypovolaemia, the intravascular space is replenished at the expense of the interstitial space. The neurohumoral response to hypovolaemia causes salt and water retention, sympathetic stimulation of the heart and peripheral vasoconstriction which tends to redistribute blood centrally, notably improving perfusion of the heart and the brain at the expense of skin, muscle and splanchnic circulation.

The cumulative effect of the primary insult and the compensatory mechanisms leads to the development of the typical clinical picture: clouding of consciousness, tachypnoea, pallor, hypotension, tachycardia, poor peripheral perfusion and oliguria.

Prompt and effective resuscitation reverses this picture. However, if the shock is prolonged or especially severe, secondary complications may arise as a consequence of reduced perfusion of the heart and other organs.

The effect of hypoperfusion on the heart is to reduce coronary perfusion pressure, and the compensatory tachycardia reduces the duration of coronary perfusion. In addition, arterial oxygen content is often reduced as a result of anaemia and hypoxia. Sympathetic stimulation increases heart rate and contractility, and peripheral vasoconstriction increases afterload. The net effect of these changes is to reduce myocardial oxygen supply and increase myocardial oxygen demand, which may cause myocardial failure, especially in elderly patients with pre-existing cardiac disease.

Prolonged ischaemia causes irreversible cellular dysfunction as noted above, but the susceptibility of different cells is variable. Astrocytes cease to function after seconds, whilst skeletal muscle functions anaerobically for 30 min, and hepatocytes for several hr. The effects of hypovolaemia may be complicated by, for example, the release of myocardial depressant factor (MDF) from hypoxic pancreatic cells (Lefer, 1978) or absorbtion of endotoxin from underperfused bowel (Haglund & Lundgren, 1978; Wardle, 1978). Ultimately therefore, a patient with hypovolaemic shock may manifest signs also of cardiogenic or septic shock as a preterminal event.

Cardiogenic shock

Cardiogenic shock results from pump failure, a mechanical dysfunction which is caused usually by myocardial infarction involving more than 40% of the ventricle. It may be especially severe where rupture of a papillary muscle or a ventricular septal defect interferes with normal forward flow of blood.

In the past, attention has focused on left ventricular dysfunction, but the important role of acute right ventricular dysfunction is increasingly recognized (Ducas & Prewitt, 1988). Right ventricular infarction is relatively rare as an isolated entity. Much more common is right ventricular dysfunction result-ing from increase in right ventricular afterload, the right ventricle being unable to generate high intra-cavitary pressures (Mathay & Berger, 1983; Sibbald et al., 1986). Failure of the right ventricle causes distension of the systemic venous system which therefore sequesters a proportion of the intravascular volume, left ventricular preload decreases, and thus, cardiac output diminishes (Furey et al., 1984). Right ventricular dilatation may occur also in an attempt to maintain right ventricular output. The interventricular septum bulges into the left ventricle causing an acute decrease in left ventricular compliance and consequently in cardiac output (Sibbald & Driedger, 1983).

Even if right or left ventricular failure is the primary cause of the cardiogenic shock, failure is exacerbated by brady- or tachyarrhythmias.

The initial physiological derangement is therefore reduced cardiac output, with acutely decreased ventricular compliance resulting in high ventricular end-diastolic pressures in the face of normal or slightly increased end-diastolic volumes. Increased pulmonary and sytemic venous pressures result in net outflow of fluid from the intravascular to the interstitial space, whilst the neurohumoral response tends to cause salt and water retention, peripheral vasoconstriction and increased sympathetic stimulation of the heart. There is usually a tachycardia but contractility may be little enhanced because of intrinsic myocardial dysfunction.

The clinical picture is similar to hypovolaemia with clouding of consciousness, tachypnoea and orthopnoea, hypotension, tachycardia, poor peripheral perfusion, an elevated jugular venous pressure and oliguria.

Pulmonary oedema may cause hypoxia, coronary perfusion pressure and time is reduced, and coronary vessel lesions decrease myocardial oxygen supply further. Tachycardia and peripheral vasoconstriction increase myocardial oxygen demand, and the worsening myocardial oxygen supply : demand ratio may lead to further deterioration of myocardial function and increase in the size of myocardial infarction, resulting in a downward spiral of clinical deterioration.

Hypoperfusion results in cellular dysfunction (see above) and the effects are liable to be worsened by critical stenotic lesions in major vessels (e.g. the carotid and renal arteries), such that ischaemia occurs at a higher mean pressure than would otherwise be the case. As major organ dysfunction supervenes the metabolic derangement and hypoxia worsens, endotoxaemia may occur from gut hypoperfusion, and secondary myocardial depression exacerbates the physiological derangement.

Distributive shock

In distributive shock, cardiac output may be increased, but altered distribution of blood flow causes hypoperfusion of respiring tissues. The prime example of this type of shock is septic shock.

Sepsis may be defined as the systemic response to micro-organisms of all types. In the past it was thought that the response to sepsis depended on the organism involved but more recent work has shown that the response is host determined and is not peculiar to a specific pathogenic micro-organism (Wiles et al., 1980). A proportion of septic patients proceed to frank septic shock, displaying either unexplained systemic hypotension [exceeding 10.6 kPa (80 mmHg) systolic] or reduced systemic vascular resistance (exceeding 800 dyne· sec · cm^{-5}) or unexplained metabolic acidosis. Such patients comprise 1% of the hospital population, or 100 000–300 000 cases per year in the USA, with a mortality rate approaching 60% (Wardle, 1979).

Cellular and humoral mechanisms underlie the septic response. These mechanisms and their inter-relations are summarized and simplified in Fig. 75.4.

It is difficult to predict the effect of these often opposing influences, and indeed it is often impossible to know if the release of such substances represents the cause or effect of the septic response. However, the physiological dysfunction in sepsis has been well characterized and reflects the combined actions of the above mediators on vascular tone, patency and permeability. In the past, hyperdynamic and hypodynamic responses to sepsis have been described (MacLean et al., 1967,

Kwaan & Weil, 1969) and both forms of clinical presentation are common. However, it is increasingly accepted that the hypodynamic, low cardiac output, high systemic vascular resistance picture is a result of either inadequate volume resuscitation and/or intrinsic myocardial disease (Wiles et al., 1980). It is thought that the primary response to sepsis is a profound reduction in systemic vascular resistance which is maintained until the moment of death in the majority of non-survivors, presumably as a result of locally released mediators, and that this reduction is often refractory to exogenous vasopressors, even in large doses (Parker et al., 1984a). An apparent increase in capillary permeability leads to a net outflow of fluid from the intravascular to the interstitial space (Fleck et al., 1985), and this, in addition to the peripheral

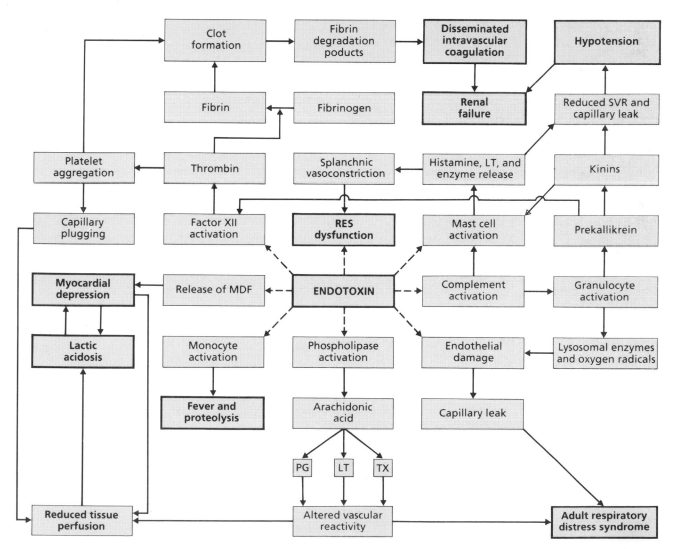

Fig. 75.4 The cellular and humoral effects of endotoxin. SVR = systemic vascular resistance; RES = reticuloendothelial system; MDF = myocardial depressant factor; PG = prostaglandins; LT = leukotrienes; TX = thromboxanes.

vasodilatation, causes a relative hypovolaemia. Pulmonary vascular resistance is increased, and the combination of raised pulmonary arterial pressure and leaking capillaries causes interstitial and often intra-alveolar oedema formation.

The compensatory response to the septic insult is one of salt and water retention and increased cardiac output. However, myocardial function is depressed by a number of factors, including myocardial oedema, hypoxia and metabolic derangement, right heart failure (consequent upon acute increases in pulmonary vascular resistance), coronary hypoperfusion and possibly circulating substances such as MDF (see above). Providing there is adequate volume replacement, cardiac output is increased to supranormal levels as a result of increased preload associated with dilatation of the heart (Parker *et al.*, 1984b). Despite this compensation, the reduction in systemic vascular resistance is so profound that the patient often remains hypotensive.

The clinical picture in volume-repleted septic shock is one of variable confusion, tachypnoea associated with a characteristic 'white-out' pattern on the chest X-ray consistent with pulmonary oedema, warm, dilated extremities with tachycardia and bounding pulse, hypotension and oliguria.

The effect on the myocardial oxygen supply: demand ratio is marked. Supply decreases as a result of decreased arterial oxygen content and decreased coronary perfusion pressure and duration. The increase in heart rate produces an increased demand, and the tendency for afterload to decline as a result of peripheral vasodilatation is counter-balanced by an increase as ventricular radius enlarges.

Cellular dysfunction results from a number of factors in sepsis. In addition to hypotension, microvascular thrombi, direct endothelial damage, increased interstitial fluid and diversion of blood through arterio-venous anastamoses and preferred-route capillaries result in failure of oxygenation of the respiring tissues. Serum lactate concentrations increase markedly and oxygen consumption declines, reducing the arterio-venous oxygen content difference (Shoemaker, 1971).

Pathogenesis of cardiovascular failure
(Table 75.5)

The preceding section dealt with three types of shock and made clear distinctions between them. In fact, the situation is rarely so clear: hypovolaemia may be complicated by the manifestations of sepsis in pro-

Table 75.5 Pathogenesis of cardiovascular failure

Primary myocardial failure

Secondary myocardial failure

Peripheral circulatory failure
{ Hypovolaemia
  Regional redistribution of flow
  Microvascular changes
    Thrombosis
    Interstitial space expansion
    Opening of arteriovenous fistulae
    Opening of preferred route capillaries

longed shock, sepsis may be complicated by absolute or relative hypovolaemia, and hypotension may precipitate myocardial infarction leading to cardiogenic shock. It is more useful for immediate therapeutic purposes to assess the underlying mechanism of the cardiovascular failure in terms of physiological dysfunction. A short summary of myocardial failure is followed by a more complete account of peripheral circulatory failure, although it should be noted that the two often coexist.

Myocardial failure

Myocardial failure may precipitate or complicate an admission to the ITU, and may result either from primary myocardial dysfunction or secondary to other disease processes or treatment (Fig. 75.5).

PRIMARY MYOCARDIAL DYSFUNCTION

The incidence of coronary artery disease increases with increasing age, and cardiac ischaemia with or without frank infarction is a common finding in patients in the ITU, either causing the admission, or as a result of adverse effects on the myocardial demand: supply ratio as detailed above, complicating other disease processes. Tachy- and bradyarrhythmias are often a cause of myocardial failure and may be difficult to treat. Rarer causes include cardiomyopathies, pericardial tamponade, acute or chronic valvular dysfunction as a result of ischaemic, traumatic or infective damage, and blunt or penetrating myocardial trauma. Some of these causes are not obvious immediately in the context of a complex ITU patient, but they should be borne in mind and excluded if necessary.

SECONDARY MYOCARDIAL DYSFUNCTION

This is probably more common in the general ITU than primary dysfunction. There may be global myocardial

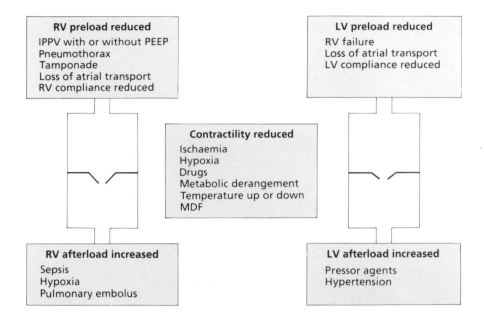

Fig. 75.5 The causes of secondary myocardial failure. RV = right ventricular; LV = left ventricular; MDF = myocardial depressant factor.

dysfunction or one or the other ventricle may be primarily affected.

Global dysfunction is seen in hypoxia (especially in patients with pre-existing coronary disease; Coetzee *et al.*, 1984), electrolyte imbalance (especially hypokalaemia) and metabolic derangement (especially acidosis). Negatively inotropic drugs such as sedative agents or β-blockers may be given therapeutically or taken in overdose, and hyper- or hypothermia may cause myocardial dysfunction also. In sepsis, or the late stages of other forms of shock, MDF may be released.

Specific ventricular dysfunction is seen with acute changes in the preload or afterload occurring in either ventricle. For example, right ventricular preload may be reduced by a tension pneumothorax, or IPPV with or without PEEP (Fig. 75.6). Acute changes in right ventricular afterload have been discussed above, as has the inter-relationship between increased right ventricular afterload and left ventricular preload and compliance. Left ventricular afterload may be altered acutely by vasodilators or pressor agents, the effect on cardiac output depending on the balance between direct effects and changes secondary to altered myocardial perfusion.

Peripheral circulatory failure

Tissue perfusion may be inadequate as a result of disturbances in the peripheral circulation. These may result from an absolutely or relatively inadequate circulating volume, regional redistribution of blood flow, or microvascular changes including diversion of blood away from respiring tissues, intravascular thrombi and interstitial compartment expansion as a result of increases in vascular permeability.

Hypovolaemia is the most common cause of shock in a general hospital population (Ledingham *et al.*, 1974). There may be absolute hypovolaemia, as in loss of fluid from the body, transfer of fluid from the intravascular compartment to the interstitial or intracellular compartments, or to closed body cavities (e.g. pleural effusion, ascites), or relative hypovolaemia produced by dilatation of blood vessels, often venous capacitance vessels.

During shock, there is autoregulation of blood flow to the brain and heart, and to a lesser extent the kidneys, mediated partly by an intrinsic property of the vascular smooth muscle and partly by accumulation of metabolites such as adenosine. However, if cardiac output reduces whilst blood flow to these organs is maintained, it implies that there is regional redistribution of blood flow such that muscle, skin and the splanchnic circulation are relatively deprived. Gilmour *et al.* (1980) showed that a 10% reduction in blood volume produced negligible alterations in arterial pressure and heart rate, but a 30% reduction in colon blood flow and oxygen availability, and Kram *et al.* (1986) showed that 30 ml/kg blood loss in a dog was associated with a linear reduction in intestinal oxygen saturation whilst renal oxygen saturation was maintained at significantly higher levels.

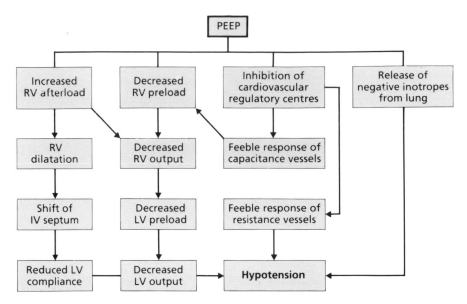

Fig. 75.6 The haemodynamic effects of PEEP. RV = right ventricular; IV = interventricular; LV = left ventricular.

The most important effect of this redistribution of blood flow is a reduction in gut perfusion, which produces also a reduction in hepatic perfusion (because 80% of hepatic perfusion is via the portal vein). The gut wall becomes permeable and allows release of gut organism-derived endotoxin into the circulation (Wardle, 1978). Hepatocellular and reticuloendothelial function is reduced, and since 85% of the fixed macrophages are in the liver, clearance of particulate debris, bacteria and endotoxin is greatly impaired (Prytz *et al.*, 1976).

Microcirculatory disturbances are difficult to quantify and treat, but become increasingly important in the late stages of cardiovascular failure, especially in sepsis. Vasoconstriction occurs partly as a response to circulating catecholamines and angiotensin II, and partly as a response to locally released mediators such as the prostaglandins, leukotrienes and thromboxanes.

Such alterations in vascular tone and increased capillary permeability cause fluid shifts which tend to expand the interstitial compartment, impairing delivery of oxygen and substrates to the respiring cells and removal of products of metabolism. Complement-mediated aggregation of white cells, aggregation of platelets and activation of the clotting cascade leads to intravascular thrombi formation in the microcirculation, impairing perfusion further. The reduced arteriovenous oxygen content difference in complicated shock (Shoemaker, 1971) may be explained either by diversion of blood away from normally respiring tissue, or by direct metabolic disturbances inhibiting cellular respiration (which occurs typically in septic shock).

Oxygen consumption is normally independent of oxygen delivery (Fig. 75.7). As oxygen delivery declines, capillary recruitment occurs, thereby reducing the mean distance between the respiring cells and the capillaries; oxygen extraction ratio is consequently increased. Below a critical level of total oxygen delivery, no further recruitment takes place and therefore consumption becomes supply dependent, with an increase in lactate. In sepsis, oxygen extraction appears to be defective as a result of many reasons, including microvascular occlusion. As a result, oxygen consumption is supply dependent over a much greater range, induced by reduced capillary reserve (Cain, 1986).

The above observations indicate why mixed venous oxygen measurement may be of limited value in the

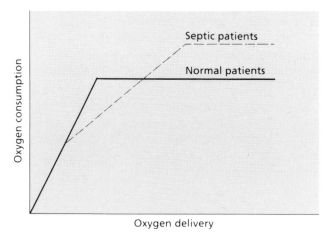

Fig. 75.7 Oxygen delivery–consumption relationships in normal patients and those with septic shock.

diagnosis and treatment of some complex forms of cardiovascular failure.

Monitoring

It is important to examine the critically ill patient regularly from top to toe. This has the dual function of stimulating a fresh assessment of each system on at least a daily basis, allowing early identification of new problems or deterioration of the existing complaint, and ensures also that the patient is treated as a whole.

A vast array of complex, invasive and expensive investigations and monitoring procedures has developed in the last 10–15 yr, but the temptation to monitor comprehensively every patient should be resisted. There is a risk : benefit ratio for every procedure, and in these days of increasing medical expenditure, costs cannot be ignored. Monitoring of cardiovascular failure may include invasive and non-invasive monitoring of haemodynamic parameters, and monitoring of the biochemical consequences of hypoperfusion.

Non-invasive haemodynamic measurement

These techniques are used most commonly in the general wards, but have a limited role in the ITU. The most commonly recorded parameters are pulse and arterial pressure measurement, and although these may alter markedly in cardiovascular failure, they are not diagnostically or prognostically useful (Shoemaker et al., 1973). Core/peripheral temperature gradient is a useful index of the adequacy of peripheral perfusion and may follow closely changes in cardiac output (Joly & Weil, 1969); it is not, however, synonymous with systemic vascular resistance (Woods et al., 1987). Similarly, hourly measurements of urine output reflect renal perfusion and intrarenal distribution of blood flow.

Transcutaneous measurement of oxygen tension has been evaluated, and correlates well with arterial oxygen tension providing the subject is haemodynamically stable (Fink et al., 1984). However, artefacts are introduced by the necessity to heat the skin to arterialize the circulation, and haemodynamic stability cannot be assumed in ITU patients. At best therefore, this device provides an early warning system: if transcutaneous oxygen tension declines, either arterial oxygen tension or tissue perfusion has decreased and further diagnostic steps are necessary. Transconjunctival oxygen tension may be measured also, using an unheated electrode which therefore avoids heating artefacts. Fink et al. (1984) and Shoemaker et al. (1984) have shown that transconjunctival oxygen tension ($Tcjo_2$) correlates well with arterial oxygen tension when cardiac output is stable, and with cardiac output if arterial oxygen tension is stable. During hypovolaemia, the $Tcjo_2$ reflected oxygen delivery, and the conjunctival temperature (as measured by the electrode) decreased to below $33\,°C$ when hypovolaemia became significant. On an experimental model, $Tcjo_2$ was shown to be a substantially more effective measurement of the adequacy of resuscitation than mean arterial pressure (Abraham & Fink, 1986).

Pulse oximetry is a new technique in which the oxygen saturation is determined by the absorption of light in a finger tip or ear lobe, intermittent (i.e. arterial) absorption being electronically distinguished from constant (i.e. capillary and venous) absorption. It reflects accurately the arterial oxygen tension, but errors occur in low flow states, hypothermic and jaundiced patients. It is important also to appreciate that because of the alinearity of the oxygen dissociation curve above approximately 90% saturation, small changes in saturation reflect large changes in oxygen tension. Its main use is probably to identify acute hypoxic episodes associated with physiotherapy, suctioning and similar patient care manoeuvres (Taylor & Whitwam, 1986). Continuous monitoring of the ECG is useful, enabling changes in rhythm to be identified early, and frequent chest X-rays may record the causes or effects of myocardial and peripheral circulatory failure.

Two-dimensional echocardiography and radio-nuclide ventriculography both enable the physician to quantitate ventricular function accurately. One needs to perform only one or the other of these two tests if an estimate of ventricular function is required. Which test is selected depends on a number of local factors such as which test is more rapidly, easily and accurately performed, their relative costs and the particular information sought. In general, echocardiography is a useful diagnostic tool and provides qualitative information on myocardial function; radio-nuclide studies quantitate cardiac volumes and ejection fraction.

Invasive haemodynamic measurement

Invasive monitoring is ubiquitous in the ITU, and often provides continuous measurement of physiological variables. Diagnosis becomes more exact, treatment is regulated more rigorously, and prognostic information may be derived (Shoemaker *et al.*, 1973). These benefits should be balanced by a recognition of the risks involved, the problems of interpretation of the data and the often large costs incurred.

Continuous intra-arterial pressure monitoring is employed frequently, and provides beat-to-beat display of changes in arterial pressure, in addition to allowing repeated blood sampling for blood gas and other estimations. There is a small incidence of thrombosis, and local infection can occur which may act as a focus for systemic spread (Band & Maki, 1979). The same drawbacks apply as with indirect measurement, in that the information is not useful diagnostically or prognostically, but the technique is accurate and is used as the standard against which other methods of arterial pressure measurement are judged (Johnson & Kerr, 1985).

Preload is determined most accurately by measurement of end-diastolic volume, but for practical reasons, pressure monitoring is employed generally. The ideal would be to measure end-diastolic pressure directly, but again for practical reasons, 'upstream' pressures are used.

Insertion of a central venous catheter (via a central vein or threaded up the brachial vein) allows saline manometry of the right atrial pressure. This measurement is taken as an indirect index of left ventricular preload and by measuring a variable which reflects left ventricular function, commonly arterial pressure, a ventricular function curve may be constructed using the concept of a fluid challenge (Fig. 75.2). Although this technique is useful in a patient without previous cardiorespiratory disease and an uncomplicated clinical course in the ITU, it is inappropriate in patients with more complex problems. An understanding of the underlying physiological concepts, complications and data interpretation problems may allow rational selection of the optimum monitoring technique.

Using right atrial pressure as an indirect index of left ventricular end-diastolic pressure depends on normal physiology and a patent anatomical pathway between the two cardiac chambers i.e. normal tricuspid valve, pulmonary vasculature, mitral valve and left ventricular compliance. If there is marked abnormality in any of these sites, left-sided pressures have to be monitored. Examples of indications for a pulmonary artery catheter therefore include conditions in which a marked disparity of ventricular function is expected, as after a large myocardial infarction, conditions where low-pressure or non-cardiogenic pulmonary oedema is likely, and conditions such as sepsis where more detailed physiological measurements are needed for diagnostic, therapeutic and prognostic purposes. A balloon-tipped, flow-directed pulmonary artery catheter may be inserted and this measures pulmonary artery pressures and also PCWP (Fig. 75.8). The pulmonary artery catheter may have a thermistor attached to the distal end, and this enables derivation of cardiac output by thermodilution. Mixed venous blood samples may be obtained also. The composite information may be used to construct a physiological profile, consisting of pulmonary and systemic vascular resistances, right and left ventricular stroke work, oxygen delivery and oxygen consumption. Pulmonary artery catheters provide a wealth of data, but their use has not always been selective (Robin, 1985). In addition to the normal risks of central venous cannulation (chiefly haemopneumothorax, bleeding and infection), insertion of a pulmonary artery catheter may cause arrhythmias (Patel *et al.*, 1986), thrombosis (Hoar *et al.*, 1981), damage to or endocarditis of the pulmonary valve or even pulmonary artery rupture.

The PCWP is a valid reflection of LVEDP only if the tip of the catheter is in Zone III of the lung, the dependent part of the lung in which vascular pressures are always higher than the airway or alveolar pressure (West *et al.*, 1964). In fact, this zone correlates with that part of the lung below the level of the left atrium (Tooker *et al.*, 1978), which accounts for 54% of total lung volume in the supine position (Friedman *et al.*, 1986).

In a non-compliant ventricle, the LVEDP is raised at a normal LVEDV and is therefore less useful in assessing preload, especially as small changes in LVEDV cause large changes in LVEDP.

The transmural PCWP is equal to the measured value minus pleural pressure. In normal, spontaneously breathing subjects, pleural pressure approximates to zero and transmural pressures are the same as measured values. This does not apply in conditions where there may be large variations in pleural pressure such as in asthma or in association with IPPV especially if PEEP is applied. These effects may be lessened by using a graphical representation of the pressure tracing and reading only end-expiratory values (Stevens *et al.*, 1985) (a digital readout averages readings over several sec and gives a falsely high measurement), and by reducing PEEP to the lowest level compatible with good oxygenation. In patients with stiff lungs, low-level PEEP does not affect the measured value greatly (Zapol & Snider, 1977).

Having assessed preload, contractility may be

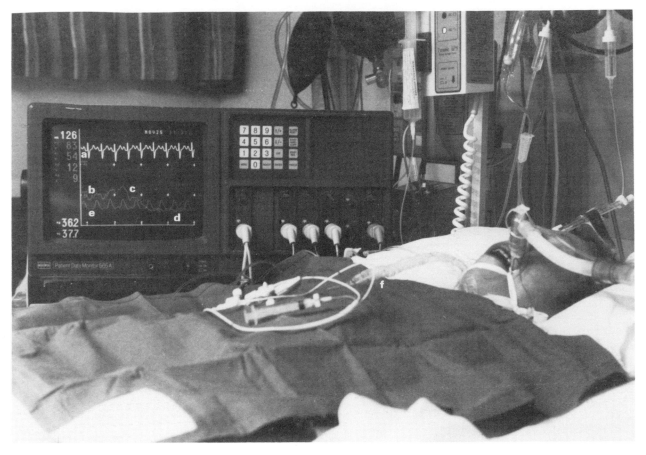

Fig. 75.8 Continuously monitored ECG, pulmonary arterial, and radial arterial traces. (**a**) ECG trace; (**b**) pulmonary arterial trace; (**c**) balloon inflated; (**d**) wedge pressure trace; (**e**) systemic arterial trace; (**f**) pulmonary artery flotation catheter.

inferred from construction of a ventricular function curve as described previously. Afterload is assessed indirectly by calculating systemic vascular resistance which takes into account aortic impedance and arteriolar run-off.

The above comments apply to the systemic circulation, but in acute right heart failure, either primary or secondary to changes in the pulmonary circulation, the appropriate right-sided parameters should be obtained. Right atrial pressure assesses preload, contractility is assessed as before and pulmonary vascular resistance is an index of afterload (Ducas & Prewitt, 1987).

Pulmonary vascular resistance is a summation of the pre- and postcapillary resistances. The precapillary resistance provides the bulk of the resistance normally, in which case the pulmonary capillary pressure is equal to the PCWP. If, however, the postcapillary resistance is increased disproportionately as in histamine release or endotoxaemia for example (D'Orio *et al.*, 1986), pulmonary capillary pressure exceeds

PCWP and pulmonary oedema may occur at normal or low PCWP (Editorial, 1986). The pulmonary capillary pressure may be determined from the point of inflection (Fig. 75.9) between the fast and slow components of the decreasing pressure profile after pulmonary artery occlusion (Cope *et al.*, 1986) and should be determined in conditions such as sepsis so that left-sided preload may be optimized whilst keeping pulmonary capillary pressure as low as possible, thus minimizing extravasation of fluid into the pulmonary interstitium.

A pulmonary artery catheter enables mixed venous blood samples to be taken from the pulmonary artery, and the oxygen saturation may be determined either intermittently or continuously using fibre-optic filaments. The mixed venous oxygen saturation varies directly with arterial oxygen saturation and cardiac output and inversely with oxygen consumption. However, because all these variables may change separately or together, knowledge of this parameter is of little diagnostic or prognostic value; Boutros and Lee

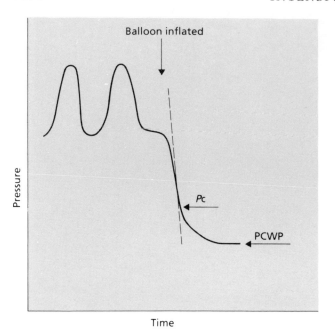

Fig. 75.9 Pressure tracing following inflation of pulmonary artery flotation catheter balloon: the point of inflection between the fast and slow components of the diminishing pressure profile indicates the pulmonary capillary pressure. Pc = pulmonary capillary pressure; PCWP = pulmonary capillary wedge pressure.

(1986) were unable to document any incident in which awareness of the mixed venous oxygen saturation would have resulted in a different and more appropriate line of management. On the other hand, continuous measurement of arterial and mixed venous oxyhaemoglobin saturation using combined pulse and pulmonary artery oximetry has been shown to provide a more rapid assessment of acute cardiorespiratory changes than existing techniques, and on-line display of ventilation/perfusion index (a parameter derived from the two values of saturation) is a valuable indicator of gas exchange (Downs & Rasanen, 1987).

Calculation of oxygen delivery (cardiac output × arterial oxygen content) and oxygen consumption (cardiac output × arteriovenous oxygen content difference) is a useful exercise, and Shoemaker has repeatedly (1971, 1973, 1983) emphasized the diagnostic and prognostic importance of these parameters.

Biochemical monitoring

The function of the cardiovascular system is to provide sufficient perfusion such that the cells are provided adequately with oxygen and substrates and metabolic products are removed. Haemodynamic monitoring provides diagnostic information but does not usually reflect tissue perfusion directly, and this function is performed better using biochemical monitoring which measures substrate supplied to and metabolites derived from the respiring tissues.

Blood gas analysis is the most common form of biochemical monitoring. The arterial oxygen tension may fall as a result of cardiovascular failure (e.g. as a result of pulmonary oedema) or may reveal the cause of secondary myocardial depression. Acid–base analysis (from pH, standard bicarbonate and base deficit values given by most blood gas machines) may likewise show an acidosis as the result of poor tissue perfusion leading to anaerobic metabolism, or may reveal the cause of secondary myocardial depression. The hormonal and substrate changes in shock as detailed in a previous section have been characterized but unfortunately are of limited clinical value. For example, measurement of serum lactate, a product of anaerobic metabolism, has shown good correlation with outcome in traumatic and simple hypovolaemic shock, but the correlation is less valid in septic shock (Vitek & Cowley, 1971; Cowan et al., 1984). Serial lactate measurements were better than a single estimation, but haemodynamic variables showed a significantly better correlation with survival (Cowan et al., 1984). Haupt et al. (1985) identified a group of septic patients with high initial lactate values who increased oxygen consumption in response to an increased oxygen delivery, but similarly, no difference in 24-hr or ultimate survival was noted.

Attempts to construct more complex biochemical 'profiles' have proved to be of value as a research tool but so far are not used routinely in clinical practice.

Knaus et al. (1985) have derived a scoring system (APACHE II) which ascribes a weighted value to derangements of haemodynamic and metabolic parameters from normal. When measured as a single value on admission to the ITU, a close correlation with outcome has been demonstrated. The difficulty is that overlap between different score bands makes it impossible to apply to the individual patient, although it is valuable as a research and audit tool. In addition, although the general relationship that increasing APACHE II score is associated with increasing mortality is true, the precise correlation varies with different categories of disease. Patients with haematological malignancy, for example, have a higher mortality for any particular APACHE II score than the average (Lloyd-Thomas et al., 1986).

Treatment

In considering treatment of cardiovascular failure in the ITU, indirect influences which contribute to myocardial dysfunction and peripheral circulatory failure should be identified and minimized.

Hypoxaemia should be regarded as a major priority and treated initially by increasing inspired oxygen concentration. Ultimately, IPPV with or without PEEP may be required, accepting that the latter may have deleterious effects on myocardial performance. There are occasions when intractable hypoxaemia dictates the use of IPPV with PEEP despite cardiovascular instability. A balance has to be struck between high levels of PEEP producing good oxygenation but less than optimal tissue perfusion, and low levels of PEEP producing good tissue perfusion but less than adequate oxygenation. In these circumstances, PEEP may be optimized by maximizing oxygen delivery (cardiac output × arterial oxygen content), or by adjusting the level of PEEP until pulmonary compliance is maximal, so-called 'best PEEP' (Suter *et al.*, 1975). Rarely, oxygen consumption may need to be reduced. This can be achieved by increasing sedation and analgesia, with or without the use of relaxant drugs, although it should be borne in mind that such agents are often both negative inotropes and peripheral vasodilators.

Metabolic parameters should be restored to as near normal as possible. Electrolyte derangements (especially hypokalaemia) and acid–base abnormalities (especially acidosis) are both arrhythmogenic and negatively inotropic, and may impair the action of inotropic agents.

Drugs taken in overdose or given therapeutically often have adverse effects on myocardial performance, the intracardiac conducting system and peripheral vascular tone. Unfortunately, a drug that is vital for treatment may have unwelcome side-effects e.g. the arrhythmogenicity of many inotropic agents, but each drug given should be scrutinized carefully and its risk : benefit ratio assessed. The adverse effects of many drugs are not recognized easily. For example, etomidate was used by infusion as a sedative agent in the ITU before it was noted that it increased mortality (Ledingham & Watt, 1983).

Having dealt with indirect influences, treatment of cardiovascular failure *per se* is now considered (Fig. 75.10). In order to perfuse the respiring tissues, an adequate cardiac output is required, and this goal is achieved by ensuring optimal preload, heart rate, contractility and afterload. Cardiac output should be

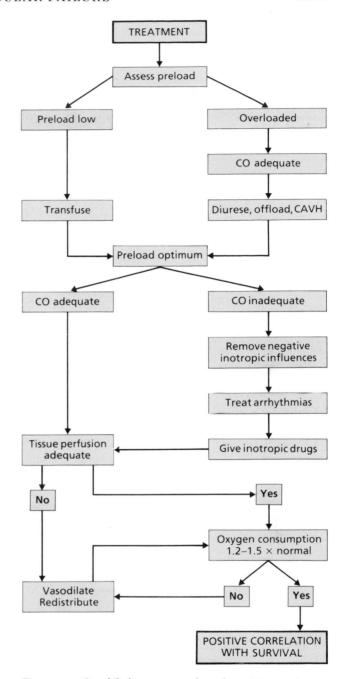

Fig. 75.10 Simplified treatment algorithm. CO = cardiac output; CAVH = continuous arteriovenous haemofiltration.

distributed appropriately between and within vital organs. Treatment is best considered, therefore, under these headings.

Optimization of preload

The effective circulating volume should be increased or decreased to optimize preload.

In increasing the circulating volume, two questions must be considered: what fluid to administer and how much? A controversy has raged for years between the proponents of crystalloids (such as normal saline or Hartmann's solution) and colloids, substances which remain in the intravascular space when transfused e.g. modified gelatin solutions, hydroxyethyl starch (Macintyre *et al.*, 1985) or plasma protein derivatives.

Proponents of crystalloids state that because of passive fluid shifts (see above) the whole of the extracellular space (intravascular plus interstitial space) is depleted in hypovolaemia, and because crystalloids are distributed to both spaces (in a 3 : 1 interstitial : intravascular ratio), crystalloids are more appropriate (Shires *et al.*, 1960; Virgilio *et al.*, 1979). There is less likely to be a rapid increase in preload because 75% of the fluid is distributed to the interstitial space (Virgilio *et al.*, 1979), and crystalloids are free from the risk of infection or anaphylaxis seen occasionally with colloids (Messmer, 1984). Crystalloids are also considerably cheaper.

Proponents of colloid state that it is more logical to replenish circulating volume with a substance that not only remains in the intravascular space, but by increasing plasma oncotic pressure may increase circulating volume further by aiding passive transfer of fluid from the interstitium: as a smaller volume is infused, resuscitation is more rapid (Shoemaker *et al.*, 1981; Twigley & Hillman, 1985). In addition, crystalloids expand the interstitial space, and even small volumes may increase closing volume and decrease pulmonary compliance (Collins *et al.*, 1973), eventually leading to overt hypoxaemia (Rackow *et al.*, 1983).

As in most such long-standing controversies, a choice, based on personal experience, is made. Where circulating volume needs to be replenished rapidly to restore tissue perfusion or where the interstitial space is already overloaded, colloid may be used with advantage. Because preload, which measures the adequacy of intravascular volume replacement, is measured readily, fine control of repletion with colloid is achieved easily. Maintenance fluid requirements are estimated according to less rigorous and exact parameters such as clinical judgement, plasma electrolyte concentrations and measured losses, and crystalloids or water (as dextrose 5%) are more appropriate, especially if deficits of the interstitial space are expected, as, for example, in losses from gastrointestinal fistulae.

More crucial than the particular choice of fluid used is the volume required for restoration of adequate perfusion. A balance has to be struck between an insufficient transfusion causing inadequate tissue perfusion and overloading causing cardiorespiratory embarrassment. In all critically ill patients a ventricular function curve should be constructed as described previously using the technique of fluid challenge. The sicker the patient, the more invasive the measurements tend to be: for example, a young, healthy trauma victim who is obviously hypovolaemic, may reasonably have central venous pressure used as an index of preload and arterial pressure as an index of cardiac performance, whilst the elderly septic patient may require more frequently a pulmonary artery catheter and PCWP plotted against cardiac output. The principle remains the same, however, that repeated fluid challenges should be given until the preload increases and there is no further improvement in cardiac performance. Of course, contractility and afterload may vary during treatment, prompting continual reassessment of the optimum preload. Studies have been carried out to determine optimum filling pressures e.g. Packman and Rackow (1983) suggested that the PCWP should not exceed 1.6 kPa (12 mmHg) in septic and hypovolaemic patients. However, they (and others in similar studies) arrived at this figure by a process of fluid challenge as outlined above, and it is preferable to treat each patient as an individual.

Some patients may become relatively fluid overloaded as a result of overenthusiastic replacement, renal failure or myocardial failure, and such patients need a reduction in their effective circulating volume. This is accomplished most simply by the use of appropriate diuretic therapy, given as a bolus or by infusion, which reduces intravascular and interstitial fluid volumes, and exerts direct effects on cardiovascular haemodynamics (Brater & Chennavasin, 1984). Unfortunately, many patients in the ITU have impoverished renal function which, although not precluding this approach, makes it less feasible, especially if rapid reductions in circulating volume are necessary. In these circumstances, the use of vasodilators, especially venodilators such as isosorbide dinitrate or nitroglycerin (Williams *et al.*, 1975) may be used to reduce filling pressures rapidly whilst slower methods of fluid removal are instituted.

In the past, removal of fluid from a patient with renal impairment involved haemodialysis and ultrafiltration, a technique which often causes hypotension and is, by definition, intermittent. It is expensive and requires specially trained personnel, and in the UK at least is only available at a restricted number of centres. A recently introduced technique is that of continuous arteriovenous haemofiltration (CAVH) in which blood passes from a patient's artery over a dialysis membrane and is returned to a vein. Under the influence of the patient's own hydrostatic pressure, an ultrafiltrate of plasma is formed and extracellular fluid is therefore removed. Small volumes may be removed to allow, for example, intravenous feeding and drug administration, or up to 20 litre/day may be removed, and partially replaced by crystalloid fluids. By manipulation of the fluid intake and output in this way, a net loss of fluid can occur. This technique is inexpensive, does not require specially trained personnel and is tolerated very well haemodynamically. Coraim et al. (1986) demonstrated its efficacy in shocked patients [mean arterial pressure 6.6 kPa (50 mmHg)] and showed that cardiac index, oxygen consumption and Pao_2 increased, and levels of MDF diminished during CAVH.

Recently, venovenous haemofiltration with pump assistance has been introduced; its attractions include greater safety and efficiency.

Optimization of heart rate

The effect of brady- and tachyarrhythmias has been discussed above; both may cause acute reductions in cardiac output. Arrhythmias in patients in the ITU are often secondary to hypoxia and/or metabolic disturbance, and are tolerated poorly by patients whose cardiovascular system is compromised from underlying illness. Hypotension, poor tissue perfusion and disturbances of gas exchange occur rapidly (Edwards & Kishen, 1986).

Most antiarrhythmic drugs are negative inotropes and vasodilators, and are often ineffective in critically ill patients. The first line of treatment is to correct as far as possible underlying physiological disorders. For example, in six carefully documented patients whose atrial fibrillation proved refractory to digoxin and DC cardioversion, correction of hypovolaemia was associated with prompt improvement in cardiac output and reversion to sinus rhythm (Edwards & Wilkins, 1987). Further treatment should be directed initially to optimizing heart rate rapidly. Bradyarrhythmias may require atropine, a chronotropic drug such as isoprenaline, or transvenous pacing. Supraventricular tachyarrhythmias may respond to verapamil given by infusion and titrated against heart rate (Edwards & Kishen, 1986). It should be noted that sinus tachycardia is often necessary to maintain adequate cardiac output, and attempts to slow such a rate with β-blockers, for example, may prove disastrous.

If the pragmatic approach outlined above is ineffective, a selection of conventional agents to meet individual requirements has been described (Rae & Hutton, 1986; Fig. 75.11).

Increasing contractility

Correction of preload or heart rate disturbances often leads to restoration of adequate tissue perfusion but occasional recourse has to be made to augmentation of cardiac contractility.

Calcium salts are potent short-acting inotropes, and may be given as a bolus dose in an emergency to maintain tissue perfusion whilst other agents are diluted and administered. Calcium may be of value also in overcoming the negative inotropic effects of calcium antagonists such as verapamil.

The most common inotropic agents are the adrenergic agonists, which bind to specific receptors and exert their action via the second messenger, cyclic AMP. They are given usually by infusion via a central vein, and are used to improve myocardial performance for any given pre- and afterload, thus shifting the VFC upwards and to the left. They have also other direct and indirect actions which alter heart rate, afterload and myocardial oxygen supply and demand, and rational selection of a particular inotrope should take these actions into account.

Dopamine

In low doses ($0-5\ \mu g \cdot kg^{-1} \cdot min^{-1}$) dopamine (DA) has a specific action on DA_1-receptors in the renal and mesenteric vascular beds. In doses of $5-20\ \mu g \cdot kg^{-1} \cdot min^{-1}$, its β_1 actions predominate, increasing the force of contraction and heart rate, and thus cardiac output (Fig. 75.12). In doses exceeding $20\ \mu g \cdot kg^{-1} \cdot min^{-1}$, α_1 actions are most obvious, and although arterial pressure is maintained by vasoconstriction, it may be at the expense of tissue perfusion. In higher doses, it may cause an increase in PCWP, pulmonary vascular congestion and arterial desaturation (Loeb et al., 1977), tachycardia and an increased incidence of ventricular ectopics (Leier et al., 1978).

With increasing dose, the increased contractility, heart rate and afterload increase myocardial oxygen demand, although supply is maintained by locally mediated coronary vasodilatation and high diastolic pressures. Stemple et al. (1976), using epicardial ST-mapping and coronary sinus lactate estimation, showed that dopamine worsened myocardial ischaemia after coronary occlusion.

In septic shock, there is no close relationship

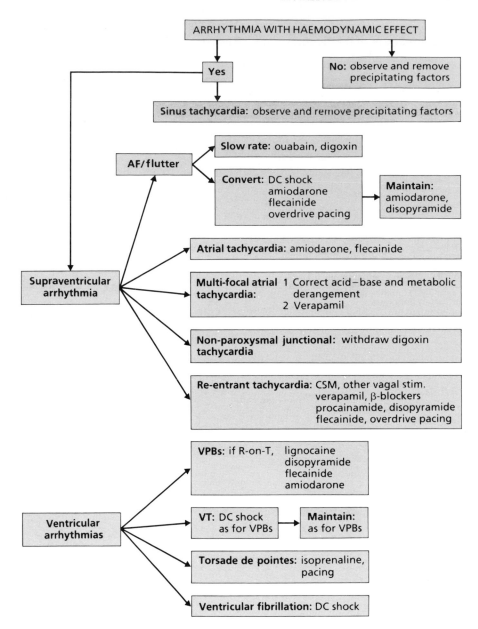

Fig. 75.11 Algorithm for the treatment of cardiac arrhythmias. VPBs = ventricular premature beats. CSM = carotid sinus massage. (Redrawn from Rae & Hutton, 1986.)

between dose of dopamine and haemodynamic effects; optimal response to dopamine administration should be assessed, therefore, by detailed and frequent haemodynamic measurement in individual patients (Edwards & Tweedle, 1986).

Dobutamine

Dobutamine is given in a dose range of 0–40 $\mu g \cdot kg^{-1} \cdot min^{-1}$, and has both β_1 and β_2 actions. The β_1 actions increase the heart rate and force of contraction. Its β_2 actions tend to cause vasodilatation in skeletal muscle, which reduces afterload. It has only weak α activity and no effect on DA-receptors. In

contrast to dopamine, PCWP often decreases with dobutamine infusions (Leier *et al.*, 1978).

The net effect of these actions is that dobutamine increases cardiac output, whilst reducing right and left ventricular afterload, and the myocardial oxygen supply:demand ratio may be unchanged (Vatner *et al.*, 1974a). Gillespie *et al.* (1975) could demonstrate no increase in cardiac enzymes in patients with evolving myocardial infarctions treated with dobutamine. It is therefore of special value in the treatment of myocardial failure; Shoemaker *et al.* (1986) demonstrated significant increases in oxygen delivery and oxygen consumption in critically ill surgical patients. A recent study in elderly patients with septic shock

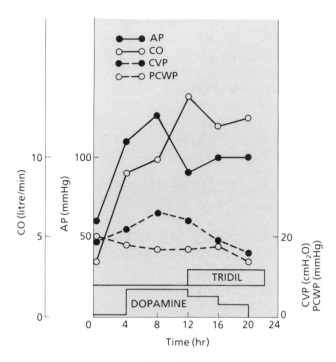

Fig. 75.12 An inotropic dose of dopamine increased arterial pressure (systolic) and cardiac output to adequate levels, but at the expense of unacceptably high filling pressures. The addition of a small dose of tridil (nitroglycerin) reduced the filling pressures, and although arterial pressure decreased, cardiac output increased.

suggests that dobutamine may be a useful adjunct to treatment with dopamine (Tell *et al.*, 1987).

Adrenaline

Adrenaline is given in a dose range of 0.1–0.2 μg · kg^{-1} · min^{-1}, and has α, β_1 and β_2 actions. It is a potent and effective inotrope but in higher doses its α actions predominate and may reduce major organ blood flow critically (Stephenson, 1976). Its effect on contractility and afterload worsens the myocardial oxygen supply:demand ratio as would be expected. Having noted that, some patients with severe cardiovascular failure may need such a potent and effective inotrope, and the invariable increase in cardiac output may increase peripheral perfusion paradoxically despite the direct α effects.

Noradrenaline

Noradrenaline in doses of 0.01–0.1 μg · kg^{-1} · min^{-1} is a pressor agent rather than an inotrope, with principally α-agonist actions. The vasoconstriction in the renal, mesenteric and peripheral vascular beds increases afterload vastly, often causing a reflex bradycardia, and although arterial pressure is increased, cardiac output often decreases. The vast increase in afterload worsens the oxygen supply : demand ratio usually, and vital organ perfusion is reduced (Vatner *et al.*, 1974b). It is used mainly in an effort to overcome the profound reduction in systemic vascular resistance caused by sepsis, but in addition to the drawbacks noted above, may be unable to overcome such locally mediated vasoconstriction (Parker *et al.*, 1984a); even when beneficial haemodynamic effects occur, changes in oxygen delivery and consumption are inconsistent (Meadows *et al.*, 1988).

Isoprenaline

Isoprenaline acts on β_1- and β_2-receptors causing an increase in force of contraction, heart rate and peripheral and pulmonary vasodilatation. Cardiac output increases significantly, but at the expense of a greatly increased myocardial oxygen demand consequent upon the tachycardia, and a reduced supply consequent upon reduced diastolic pressures (Gunnar & Loeb, 1972) and its role in myocardial failure is therefore questionable.

Glucagon

The pancreatic polypeptide, glucagon, causes an increase in contractility and heart rate by stimulating adenyl cyclase which increases intracellular cyclic AMP concentrations. Nausea and vomiting, a dose-dependent side-effect, limits its use, but it may be useful in β-blocker overdose, since its action does not depend on drug receptor interaction (Gunnar & Loeb, 1972).

All the above inotropes have an adverse effect on myocardial oxygen supply:demand ratio to a greater (noradrenaline) or lesser (dobutamine) extent. Combining an inotrope with a vasodilator (Fig. 75.12) to minimize this effect is useful (Foex, 1983) and efforts have been made to synthesize agents which combine the attributes of both.

The most notable example so far has been amrinone which showed early promise; later assessment has shown that its predominant action was vasodilatory and toxicity limited its use (Editorial, 1985). A newer agent, dopexamine, has inotropic and dopaminergic properties, but it awaits formal evaluation.

Whatever the theoretical risks in terms of myocardial perfusion, in practice inotropes are often necessary to ensure adequate peripheral perfusion. Attempts should be made to keep the dose as low as possible, and low-dose dopamine is often combined with potent inotropes in an effort to maintan renal perfusion (Richard et al., 1983). Inotropes should be discontinued as soon as possible by a slow weaning process, and in many instances volume loading is necessary as the inotrope is reduced, relating preload to myocardial performance as usual.

Afterload manipulation

LEFT SIDED

Vasodilators act on the systemic circulation and may reduce afterload predominantly by arteriolar dilatation (e.g. hydralazine) or may reduce pre- and afterload by arteriolar and venular dilatation (e.g. sodium nitroprusside). The result of this therapy is to increase cardiac index, stroke volume index and stroke work index whilst decreasing left ventricular filling pressures (Chatterjee et al., 1976).

Hydralazine acts directly on arteriolar smooth muscle causing vasodilatation and a reduction in afterload. Arteriolar pressure may decrease but the myocardial oxygen supply : demand ratio improves, and cardiac output increases despite lower filling pressures as a result of the improvement in myocardial energetics (Mehta et al., 1978).

Sodium nitroprusside acts on both the arterial and venous sides of the circulation, and therefore lowers both preload and afterload by a direct action on vascular smooth muscle. Its dose should be titrated against effect, although the total dose should not exceed 1.5 mg/kg to avoid the risk of cyanide toxicity.

Its principal action is to reduce afterload, thus increasing cardiac output (Chatterjee et al., 1976), and, providing diastolic pressure is not reduced too far, exerting a beneficial effect on the myocardial oxygen : supply ratio. Preload is reduced also, and if that decreases markedly, cardiac output decreases, although this effect may be offset by volume replacement with colloid (Miller et al., 1977).

Vasodilators tend to reduce preload, afterload and myocardial oxygen demand, but vital organ perfusion may decline as a result of systemic hypotension. Inotropes increase cardiac output and arterial pressure, but may increase preload and afterload, and increase myocardial oxygen demand. The two are often combined e.g. dopamine is used as an inotrope and isosorbide dinitrate is used to reduce preload (Stephens et al., 1978), or sodium nitroprusside is used to reduce myocardial oxygen consumption (Miller et al., 1977).

The intra-aortic balloon pump (IABP) is a mechanical method of reducing left-sided afterload. A balloon is inserted via the femoral artery into the descending aorta; in synchrony with the pressure waveform or the ECG, the balloon is inflated during diastole, thus increasing coronary perfusion, and deflated during systole, reducing afterload. Myocardial oxygen supply is increased and demand reduced, this combination being especially useful in primary myocardial failure (Scheidt et al., 1973).

RIGHT SIDED

As described previously, acute increases in right ventricular afterload reduce left ventricular preload (Furey et al., 1984). The right ventricle dilates in an attempt to maintain output by the Starling mechanism, the interventricular septum bulges into the left venticle and reduces left ventricular compliance, and cardiac output decreases (Sibbald & Driedger, 1983). In these circumstances, further volume challenge merely increases right ventricular dilatation, leading to a greater reduction in cardiac output. Therapy should be directed therefore towards lowering pulmonary vascular resistance: isoprenaline, hydralazine and sodium nitroprusside are effective pulmonary vasodilators, and provided coronary perfusion pressure is maintained (if necessary with pressor agents to avoid systemic hypotension) cardiac output increases (Prewitt & Ghignone, 1983). Matthay and Berger (1983) reviewed the use of vasodilators and β_2-agonists in patients with high pulmonary artery pressures and described the salutory effects of aminophylline, terbutaline and nifedipine.

Redistribution of blood flow

Manipulation of cardiac output is usually straightforward using the methods outlined above. There is no guarantee, however, that vital organs are perfused, or if they are, that blood is distributed to the respiring tissues rather than bypassing them via arteriovenous anastomoses or preferred route capillaries (Silver, 1977). Attempts have therefore been made to manipulate the circulation at this level.

The use of low-dose dopamine to improve renal perfusion, and the combination of inotropes and vasodilators to improve vital organ perfusion has been described already. The problems of this approach are exemplified by septic shock, where hypotension, a low systemic vascular resistance and increasing acidosis reflect poor tissue perfusion despite a greatly increased cardiac output which is maintained, in some instances, until cardiac arrest occurs, despite attempts at manipulation with inotropes and pressor agents (Parker et al., 1984a,b).

The role of centrally and peripherally released endogenous opioid peptides in shock has become clearer recently. Consequently, naloxone and partial opioid agonists (such as meptazinol and nalbuphine), have been evaluated in several types of shock. Results of clinical trials have been equivocal and their routine use is not recommended currently (Hinds & Donaldson, 1988).

It is postulated that the microcirculatory disturbances of shock are mediated via locally released substances of which there are a large (and increasing) number. The microcirculatory changes are reversed readily if the cause of shock is eliminated promptly, and several pharmacological agents are known to attenuate or even reverse some of the adverse effects, for example ATP–MgCl$_2$ (Chaudry et al., 1983), glucose–insulin–potassium (Bronsveld et al., 1984), calcium-channel blockers (Hackel et al., 1981) and steroids (Goldfarb & Glenn, 1983). None of these agents is of proven clinical value.

A number of inhibitors of eicosanoid synthesis have been evaluated in animal models with some success, but it has proved difficult to extrapolate these experimental findings to the clinical situation. It remains a promising area for future research, in which the precise role of eicosanoids in shock may be elucidated (Ball et al., 1986).

Chernow and Roth (1986) reviewed the pharmacological manipulation of the peripheral vasculature in shock, emphasizing its unresponsiveness to exogenous catecholamines, probably because of release of local mediators and down-regulation of α-receptors. Future areas of investigation will probably concentrate on methods of bypassing the adrenergic receptors e.g. increasing intracellular calcium using calcium-channel agonists.

Specific treatment

Although treatment is directed initially towards correcting physiological derangements, specific prob-

lems may require specific treatment. It may be impossible to treat the patient without first combatting the initiating insult e.g. in major haemorrhage, the source of bleeding should be identified and secured as a priority before or at the same time as resuscitation is proceeding. On the other hand, in septic shock where a septic focus must be drained, the surgical procedure is tolerated better following initial resuscitation in the ITU.

The choice of fluid for restoration of circulating volume in hypovolaemia has been covered previously, but controversy still surrounds the optimum haematocrit necessary to maximize oxygen delivery to the tissues. The greater oxygen carrying capacity as the haematocrit increases is counter-balanced by increased viscosity which reduces flow through smaller vessels. In the normal subject, a compromise is reached at a haemoglobin value of approximately 9–9.5 g/litre, but this may not hold for the severely ill and septic patient.

A recent development in the treatment of myocardial infarction has been the administration of fibrinolytic agents. These were administered directly into a coronary artery, but cost and lack of availability of specialized staff and equipment led to the adoption of the intravenous route for administration (Marder & Francis, 1984).

The mainstay of the treatment of sepsis remains efficient surgical drainage (Meakins et al., 1980), and laparotomies may have to be repeated if sepsis is to be eradicated effectively. Broad-spectrum antibiotics (guided where possible by positive bacteriology) have a lesser role to play. Episodes of infection in patients in the ITU are acquired often from endogenous sources such as the gut or oropharynx. The gut flora may be modified by non-absorbable antibiotics given enterally, such that Gram-negative aerobes are reduced in number while anaerobes remain to prevent overgrowth with resistant organisms. Recent studies (Ledingham et al., 1988) have shown a reduced infection rate and mortality with such a regimen of selective decontamination of the digestive tract.

Conclusion

Throughout this chapter, emphasis has been placed on the physiology of the cardiovascular system; how it alters in disease, how to assess the physiological derangement and how to manipulate the cardiovascular system in the light of such knowledge.

A sound understanding of the relevant cardio-vascular physiology is essential, as it is imperative to diagnose, monitor and treat the underlying physio-logical derangement before it worsens (Shoemaker *et al.*, 1973).

Before using invasive monitoring procedures, a risk : benefit assessment should be considered. This entails objective evaluation of the severity of the illness using a measure such as the APACHE II score, and using clinical experience to identify those patients at risk of further deterioration. Having assessed the disordered physiology, rational treatment may then be applied. The question remains as to what end-point should be sought when deciding on treatment. The ultimate goal is obviously survival of the patient but there is surprisingly little information on interim treatment goals. Shoemaker and his co-workers have repeatedly (1971, 1973, 1979, 1982, 1983; Abraham *et al.*, 1984) stressed that those parameters measured most commonly, such as arterial pressure, pulse rate, and filling pressures, are of no predictive value, and returning them to within a range of normal values does not increase survival; these authors identify oxygen consumption as the single most useful variable which correlates strongly with survival or non-survival. Of greater practical value, they suggest a spectrum of parameters (Shoemaker *et al.*, 1973) on the basis of empirical studies which, when achieved, lead to an increased chance of survival. A later study calculated a predictive index of survival on a similar basis with a 94% sensitivity and 90% specificity (Shoemaker *et al.*, 1983). It is salutary to note that many of the parameters represent increases of the values into the supraphysiological range. These observations would be consistent with the recently acquired understanding of the relationship between oxygen supply and demand at the microcirculatory level (Haupt *et al.*, 1985; Cain, 1986). In the case of septic shock, the flow-dependent oxygen consumption is pathological and a higher than normal oxygen supply may be required to achieve optimal oxygen consumption and elimination of lactic acidosis (Astiz *et al.*, 1987).

Cardiovascular failure remains a condition in which mortality is high and the improvement in intensive care over the last 20 yr has not improved survival greatly in the individual case. Advances in future must include enhanced understanding of the disordered physiology, realistic treatment goals and the ability to manipulate the circulation at the microvascular level.

References

Abraham E., Bland R.D., Cobo J.C. & Shoemaker W.C. (1984) Sequential cardiorespiratory patterns associated with outcome in septic shock. *Chest* **85**, 75–80.

Abraham E. & Fink S. (1986) Cardiorespiratory and conjunctival oxygen tension monitoring during resuscitation from haemorrhage. *Critical Care Medicine* **14**, 1004–9.

Alderman E.L. & Glantz S.A. (1976) Acute haemodynamic interventions shift the diastolic pressure–volume curve in man. *Circulation* **54**, 662–71.

Astiz M.E., Rackow E.C., Falk J.L., Kaufman B.S. & Weil M.H. (1987) Oxygen delivery in patients with hyperdynamic septic shock. *Critical Care Medicine* **15**, 26–8.

Ball H.A., Cook J.A., Wise W.C. & Halushka P.V. (1986) Role of thromboxane, prostaglandins, and leukotrienes in endotoxic and septic shock. *Intensive Care Medicine* **12**, 116–26.

Band J.D. & Maki D.G. (1979) Infections caused by arterial catheters used for haemodynamic monitoring. *American Journal of Medicine* **67**, 735–41.

Benedict C.R. & Grahame-Smith D.G. (1978) Plasma noradrenaline and adrenaline concentrations and dopamine-B-hydroxylase activity in patients with shock due to septicaemia, trauma and haemorrhage. *Quarterly Journal of Medicine* **47**, 1–20.

Boutros A.R. & Lee C. (1986) Value of continuous monitoring of mixed venous blood oxygen saturation in the management of critically ill patients. *Critical Care Medicine* **14**, 132–4.

Brater D.C. & Chennavasin P. (1984) Prolonged haemodynamic effect of furosemide in congestive heart failure. *American Heart Journal* **108**, 1031–2.

Braunwald E., Ross J. & Sonnenblick E.H. (1977) Mechanisms of contraction of the normal and failing heart. *New England Journal of Medicine* **277**, 910–20.

Bronsveld W., van Lambalgen A.A., van den Bos G.C., Thijs L.G. & Koopmans P.A.R. (1984) Effects of glucose–insulin–potassium (GIK) on myocardial blood flow and metabolism in canine endotoxic shock. *Circulatory Shock* **13**, 325.

Cain S.M. (1986) Assessment of tissue oxygenation. *Critical Care Clinics* **2**, 537–50.

Chatterjee K., Swan H.J.C., Kaushik V.S., Jobin G., Magnusson P. & Forrester J.S. (1976) Effects of vasodilator therapy for severe pump failure in acute myocardial infarction on short-term and late prognosis. *Circulation* **53**, 797–802.

Chaudry I.H., Ohkawa M., Clemens M.G. & Baue A.E. (1983) Alterations in electron transport and cellular metabolism with shock and trauma. In *Molecular and Cellular Aspects of Shock and Trauma* (Eds Lefer A.M. & Schumer W.) pp. 67–88. Liss, New York.

Chernow B. & Roth B.L. (1986) Pharmacologic manipulation of the peripheral vasculature in shock: clinical and experimental approaches. *Circulatory Shock* **18**, 141–55.

Coetzee A., Foex P., Holland D., Ryder A. & Jones L. (1984) Effect of hypoxia on the normal and ischaemic myocardium. *Critical Care Medicine* **14**, 1027–31.

Collins J.V., Cochrane G.M., Davis J., Benatar S.R. & Clark J.H. (1973) Some aspects of pulmonary function after rapid saline infusion in healthy subjects. *Clinical Science* **45**, 407–10.

Cope D.K., Allison R.C., Parmentier J.L., Miller J.N. & Taylor A.E. (1986) Measurement of effective pulmonary capillary pressure using the pressure profile after pulmonary artery occlusion. *Critical Care Medicine* **14**, 16–22.

Coraim F.J., Coraim H.P., Ebermann R. & Stellwag F.M. (1986) Acute respiratory failure after cardiac surgery: clinical experience of continuous arteriovenous haemofiltration. *Critical Care Medicine* **14**, 714–18.

Covell J.W. & Ross J. (1973) Nature and significance of alterations in myocardial compliance. *American Journal of Cardiology* **32**, 449–55.

Cowan B.N., Burns H.J.G., Boyle P. & Ledingham I.McA. (1984) The relative prognostic value of lactate and haemodynamic measurements in early shock. *Anaesthesia* **39**, 750–5.

D'Orio V., Halleux J., Rodriguez L.M., Wahlen C. & Marcelle R. (1986) Effects of *E. Coli* endotoxin on pulmonary vascular resistance in intact dogs. *Critical Care Medicine* **14**, 802–6.

Downs J.B. & Rasanen J. (1987) Dual oximetry in assessment of cardiopulmonary function. In *Update in Intensive Care and Emergency Medicine* (Ed. Vincent J-L.) pp. 342–8. Springer Verlag, Berlin.

Ducas J. & Prewitt R.M. (1988) Right ventricular dysfunction, detection and treatment. In *Recent Advances in Critical Care Medicine*, number 3 (Ed. Ledingham I.McA.) pp. 109–18. Churchill Livingstone, Edinburgh.

Editorial (1985) Intravenous amrinone: an advance or a wrong step? *Annals of Internal Medicine* **102**, 399–400.

Editorial (1986) Pulmonary capillary pressure? *Critical Care Medicine* **14**, 76–7.

Edwards J.D. & Kishen R. (1986) Significance and management of intractable supraventricular arrhythmias in critically illpatients. *Critical Care Medicine* **14**, 280–2.

Edwards J.D. & Tweedle D.E. (1986) Haemodynamic response to dopamine in severe human septic shock. *British Journal of Surgery* **73**, 503.

Edwards J.D. & Wilkins R.G. (1987) Atrial fibrillation precipated by acute hypovolaemia. *British Medical Journal* **294**, 283–4.

Fink S., Ray W., McCartney S., Ehrlich H. & Shoemaker W.C. (1984) Oxygen transport and utilization in hyperoxia and hypoxia: relation of conjunctival and transcutaneous oxygen tensions to haemodynamic and oxygen transport variables. *Critical Care Medicine* **12**, 943–8.

Fleck A., Hawker F., Wallace P.G.M., Raines G., Trotter J., Ledingham I. McA. & Calman K.C. (1985) Increased vascular permeability. A major cause of hypoalbuminaemia in disease and injury. *Lancet* **1**, 781–4.

Foex P. (1983) Inotropic and vasodilator agents. In *Recent Advances in Critical Care Medicine*, number 2 (Eds Ledingham I.McA. & Hanning C.D.) pp. 45–66. Churchill Livingstone, Edinburgh.

Friedman P.J., Peters R.M., Botkin M.C., Brimm J.E. & Meltvedt R.C. (1986) Estimation of the volume of the lung below the left atrium using computed tomography. *Critical Care Medicine* **14**, 182–7.

Furey S.A., Zieske H.A. & Levy M.N. (1984) The essential function of the right ventricle. *American Heart Journal* **107**, 404–10.

Ganong W.F. (1983) *Review of Medical Physiology* 11th edn., pp. 414–506. LMP, California.

Gillespie T.A., Roberts R., Ambos H.D. & Sobel B.E. (1975) Salutory effects of dobutamine on haemodynamics without exacerbation of arrhythmia or myocardial injury. *Circulation* **52** (Suppl. II), 76.

Gilmour D.G., Aitkenhead A.R., Hothersall A.P. & Ledingham I.McA. (1980) The effect of hypovolaemia on colon blood flow in the dog. *British Journal of Surgery* **67**, 82–4.

Goldfarb R.D. & Glenn T.M. (1983) Regulation of lysosomal membrane stabilisation via cyclic nucleotides and prostaglandins: the effects of steriods and indomethacin. In *Molecular and Cellular Aspects of Shock and Trauma* (Eds Lefer A.M. & Schumer W.) pp. 147–66. Liss, New York.

Griffiths J. (1972) The sequential assay of plasma catecholamines and whole blood histamine in early septic shock. In *Conference on 'Shock'* (Eds Ledingham I.McA. & McAllister T.A.) pp. 76–83. Kimpton, London.

Gunnar R.M. & Loeb H.S. (1972) Use of drugs in cardiogenic shock due to acute myocardial infarction. *Circulation* **45**, 1111–24.

Hackel D.B., Mikat E.M., Reimer K. & Whalen G. (1981) Effect of verapamil on heart and circulation in haemorrhagic shock in dogs. *American Journal of Physiology* **241**, H12–17.

Haglund U. & Lundgren O. (1978) Intestinal ischaemia and shock factors. *Federation Proceedings* **37**, 2729–33.

Haljamäe H. (1984) Interstitial fluid response. In *Clinical Surgery International*, vol. 9. Shock and Related Problems (Ed. Shires G.T.) pp. 44–60. Churchill Livingstone, New York.

Haupt M.T., Gilbert E.M. & Carbon R.W. (1985) Fluid loading increases oxygen consumption in septic patients with lactic acidosis. *American Review of Respiratory Disease* 912–16.

Heath D.F. (1980) Carbohydrate metabolism after injury. The development and maintenance of hyperglycaemia. In *Advances in Physiological Science*, vol. 26. Homeostastis in Injury and Shock. (Eds Biro Z.S., Kovách A.G.B., Spitzer J.J. & Stoner H.B.) pp. 63–70. Pergamon, Oxford.

Hinds C.J. & Donaldson M.J.S. (1988) Endogenous opioid peptides. In *Recent Advances in Critical Care Medicine* number 3 (Ed. Ledingham I.McA.) Churchill Livingstone, Edinburgh.

Hoar P.F., Wilson R.M., Mangano D.T., Avery G.J., Szarnicki R.J. & Hill J.D. (1981) Heparin bonding reduces thrombogenicity of pulmonary artery catheters. *New England Journal of Medicine* **305**, 993–5.

Jennings R.B. (1976) Relationship of acute ischaemia to functional defects and irreversibility. *Circulation* **52** (Suppl. 1), 26–9.

Johnson C.J.H. & Kerr J.H. (1985) Automatic blood pressure monitors. A clinical evaluation of five models in adults. *Anaesthesia* **40**, 471–8.

Joly H.R. & Weil M.H. (1969) Temperature of the great toe as an indication of the severity of shock. *Circulation* **39**, 131–8.

Knaus W.A., Draper E.A., Wagner D.P. & Zimmerman J.E. (1985) APACHE II: a severity of disease classification system. *Critical Care Medicine* **13**, 818–29.

Kram H.B., Appel P.L., Fleming A.W. & Shoemaker W.C. (1986) Assessment of intestinal and renal perfusion using surface oximetry. *Critical Care Medicine* **14**, 707–13.

Kwaan H.M. & Weil M.H. (1969) Differences in the mechanism of shock caused by bacterial infections. *Surgery, Gynecology and Obstetrics* **128**, 37–45.

Laragh J.H. (1985) Atrial natriuretic hormone, the renin–aldosterone axis, and blood pressure–electrolyte homeostastis. *New England Journal of Medicine* **313**, 1330–40.

Ledingham I.McA., Alcock S.R., Eastaway A.T., McDonald I.C., McKay I.C. & Ramsay G. (1987) Triple regimen of selective decontamination of the digestive tract, systemic cefotaxime, and microbiological surveillance for prevention of acquired infection in intensive care. *Lancet* **1**, 785–90 (1987).

Ledingham I.McA., McArdle C.S., Fisher W.D. & Maddern M. (1974) The incidence of shock syndrome in a general hospital. *Postgraduate Medical Journal* **50**, 420–4.

Ledingham I.McA. & Ramsay G. (1986) Hypovolaemic shock. *British Journal of Anaesthesia* **58**, 169–89.

Ledingham I.McA. & Watt I. (1983) Influence of sedation on mortality in critically ill multiple trauma patients. *Lancet* **1**, 1270.

Lefer A.M. (1978) Properties of cardioinhibitory factors in shock. *Federation Proceedings* **37**, 2734–40.

Leier C.V., Heban P.T., Huss P., Bush C.A. & Lewis R.P. (1978) Comparative systemic and regional haemodynamic effects of dopamine and dobutamine in patients with cardiomyopathic heart failure. *Circulation* **58**, 466–75.

Lloyd-Thomas A.R., Wright I.H. & Hinds C.J. (1986) Intensive therapy for life-threatening medical complications of malignancy. *Intensive Care Medicine* **12** (Suppl.), 249.

Loeb H.S., Bredakis J. & Gunnar R.M. (1977) Superiority of dobutamine over dopamine for augmentation of cardiac output in patients with chronic low output cardiac failure. *Circulation* **55**, 375–81.

Macintyre E., Mackic I.J., Ho D., Tinker J., Bullen C. & Machin S.J. (1985) The haemostatic effect of hydroxyethyl starch (HES) used as a volume expander. *Intensive Care Medicine* **11**, 300–3.

MacLean L.D., Mulligan W.G., McLean A.P.H. & Duff J.H. (1967) Patterns of septic shock in man—a detailed study of 56 patients. *Annals of Surgery* **166**, 543–62.

Marder V.J. & Francis C.W. (1984) Thrombolytic therapy for acute transmural myocardial infarction. Intracoronary versus intravenous. *American Journal of Medicine* **77**, 921–8.

Matthay R.A. & Berger H.J. (1983) Noninvasive assessment of right and left ventricular function in acute and chronic respiratory failure. *Critical Care Medicine* **11**, 329–38.

Meadows D., Edwards J.D., Wilkins R.G. & Nightingale P. (1988) Reversal of intractable septic shock with norepinephrine therapy. *Critical Care Medicine* **16**, 663–6.

Meakins J.L., Wicklund B., Forse R.A. & McLean A.P.H. (1980) The surgical intensive care unit: current concepts in infection. *Surgical Clinics of North America* **60**, 117–32.

Mehta J., Pepine C.J. & Conti C.R. (1978) Haemodynamic effects of hydralazine and glyceryl trinitrate paste in heart failure. *British Heart Journal* **40**, 845–50.

Messmer K. (1984) Blood substitutes in shock therapy. In *Clinical Surgery International*, vol. 9. Shock and related Problems (Ed. Shires G.T. III) pp. 192–205. Churchill Livingstone, Edinburgh.

Miller R.R., Awan N.A., Joye J.J., Maxwell K.S., DeMaria A.N., Amsterdam E.A. & Mason D.T. (1977) Combined dopamine and nitroprusside therapy in congestive heart failure. Greater augmentation of cardiac performance by addition of inotropic stimulation to afterload reduction. *Circulation* **55**, 881–4.

Nunn J.F. (1977) *Applied Respiratory Physiology* 2nd edn., p. 378. Butterworths, London.

Packman M.I. & Rackow E.C. (1983) Optimum left heart filling pressure during fluid resuscitation of patients with hypovolaemic and septic shock. *Critical Care Medicine* **11**, 165–19.

Parker M.M., Shelhamer J.H., Bacharach S.L., Green M.V., Natanson C., Frederick T.M., Damske B.A. & Parillo J.E. (1984a) Profound but reversible myocardial depression in patients with septic shock. *Annals of Internal Medicine* **100**, 483–90.

Parker M.M., Shelhamer J.H., Natanson C., Masur H. & Parillo J.E. (1984b) Serial haemodynamic patterns in survivors and non-survivors of septic shock in humans. *Critical Care Medicine* **12**, 311.

Patel C., Laboy V., Venus B., Mathru M. & Wier D. (1986) Acute complications of pulmonary artery catheter insertion in critically ill patients. *Critical Care Medicine* **14**, 195–7.

Prewitt R.M. & Ghignone M. (1983) Treatment of right ventricular dysfunction in acute respiratory failure. *Critical Care Medicine* **11**, 346–52.

Prytz H., Holst-Christensen B., Korner B. & Liehr H. (1976) Portal venous and systemic endotoxaemia in patients without liver disease and systemic endotoxaemia in patients with cirrhosis. *Scandinavian Journal of Gastroenterology* **11**, 857–63.

Rackow E.C., Falk J.L., Fein E.I., Siegel J.S., Packman M.I., Haupt M., Kaufman B.S. & Putnam D. (1983) Fluid resuscitation in circulatory shock: a comparison of the cardiorespiratory effects of albumin, hetastarch, and saline solutions in patients with hypovolaemic and septic shock. *Critical Care Medicine* **11**, 839–50.

Rae A.P. & Hutton I. (1986) Cardiogenic shock and the haemodynamic effects of arrhythmias. *British Journal of Anaesthesia* **58**, 151–68.

Rennie M.J. & Harrison R. (1984) Effects of injury, disease, and malnutrition on protein metabolism in man. *Lancet* **1**, 323–5.

Richard C., Ricome J.L., Bottineau G. & Auzepy P. (1983) Combined haemodynamic effects of dopamine and dobutamine in cardiogenic shock. *Circulation* **67**, 620–6.

Robin E.D. (1985) The cult of the Swan–Ganz catheter. Overuse and abuse of pulmonary flow catheters. *Annals of Internal Medicine* **103**, 445–9.

Scheidt S., Wilner G., Mueller H., Summers D., Lesch M., Wolff G., Krakauer J., Rubenfire M., Fleming P., Noon G., Oldham N., Killip T. & Kantrowitz A. (1973) Intra-aortic balloon counter pulsation in cardiogenic shock. *New England Journal of Medicine* **288**, 979–84.

Shires G.T., Braun F.T., Canizaro P.C. & Somerville N. (1960) Distributional changes in extracellular fluid during haemorrhagic shock. *Surgery Forum* **11**, 115–17.

Shoemaker W.C. (1971) Cardiorespiratory patterns in complicated and uncomplicated septic shock. *Annals of Surgery* **174**, 119–25.

Shoemaker W.C., Appel P. & Bland R. (1983) Use of physiologic monitoring to predict outcome and to assist in clinical decisions in critically ill postoperative patients. *American Journal of Surgery* **146**, 43–50.

Shoemaker W.C. Appel P. & Kram H.B. (1986) Haemodynamic and oxygen transport effects of dobutamine in critically ill general surgical patients. *Critical Care Medicine* **14**, 1032–7.

Shoemaker W.C., Appel P., Schwartz S., Hopkins J. & Chang P. (1982) Clinical trials of an algorithm for outcome prediction in acute circulatory failure. *Critical Care Medicine* **10**, 390–7.

Shoemaker W.C., Chang P. & Bland R. (1979) Cardiorespiratory monitoring in postoperative patients: II. Quantitative therapeutic indices as guides to therapy. *Critical Care Medicine* **7**, 243–9.

Shoemaker W.C., Fink S., Ray W. & McCartney S. (1984) Effect of haemorrhagic shock on conjunctival and transcutaneous oxygen tensions in relation to haemodynamic and oxygen transport changes. *Critical Care Medicine* **12**, 949–52.

Shoemaker W.C., Montgomery E.S., Kaplan E. & Elwyn D.H. (1973) Physiologic patterns in surviving and non-surviving shock patients. *Archives of Surgery* **106**, 630–6.

Shoemaker W.C., Schluchter M., Hopkins J.A., Appel P.L., Schwartz S. & Chang P. (1981) Fluid therapy in emergency resuscitation: clinical evaluation of colloid and crystalloid regimens. *Critical Care Medicine* **9**, 367–8.

Sibbald W.J. & Driedger A.A. (1983) Right ventricular function in acute disease states: physiologic considerations. *Critical Care Medicine* **11**, 339–45.

Sibbald W.J., Driedger A.A., Cunningham D.G. & Cheung H. (1986) Right and left ventricular performance in acute hypoxemic respiratory failure. *Critical Care Medicine* **14**, 852–7.

Silver I.A. (1977) Local factors in tissue oxygenation. *Journal of Clinical Pathology* **30** (Suppl. II), 7.

Sonnenblick E.H. & Skelton C.L. (1971) Myocardial energetics: basic principles and clinical implications. *New England Journal of Medicine* **285**, 688–75.

Stemple D., Griffin J.C., Kernoff R.S. & Harrison D.C. (1976) Metabolic and electrophysiologic effects of nitroprusside and dopamine in experimental acute myocardial infarction. *Clinical Research* **24**, 141A.

Stephens J., Dymond D. & Spurrell R. (1978) Enhancement by isosorbide dinitrate of haemodynamic effects of dopamine in chronic congestive cardiac failure. *British Heart Journal* **40**, 838–44.

Stephenson L.W. Blackstone E.H. & Kouchoukos N.T. (1976) Dopamine vs. epinephrine in patients following cardiac surgery. *Surgery Forum* **27**, 272–5.

Stevens J.H., Raffin T.A., Milum F.G., Rosenthal M.H. & Stetz C.W. (1985) Thermodilution cardiac output measurement. Effects of the respiratory cycle on its reproducibility. *Journal of the American Medical Association* **243**, 2240–2.

Stoner J.D., Bolen J.L. & Harrison D.C. (1977) Comparison of dobutamine and dopamine in treatment of severe heart failure. *British Heart Journal* **39**, 536–9.

Stoner H.B., Frayn K.M., Barton R.N., Threlfall C.J. & Little R.A. (1979) The relationship between plasma substrates and hormones and the severity of injury in 277 recently injured patients. *Clinical Science* **56**, 563–73.

Suter P.M., Fairley H.B. & Isenberg M.D. (1975) Optimum end-expiratory airway pressure in patients with acute pulmonary failure. *New England Journal of Medicine* **292**, 284–9.

Taylor M.B. & Whitwam J.G. (1986) The current status of pulse oximetry: clinical value of continuous noninvasive oxygen saturation. *Anaesthesia* **41**, 943–9.

Tell B., Majerus T.C. & Flanebaum L. (1987) Dobutamine in elderly septic shock patients refractory to dopamine. *Intensive Care Medicine* **13**, 14–18.

Tooker J., Huseby J. & Butler J. (1978) The effect of Swan–Ganz catheter height on the wedge pressure–left atrial pressure relationship in edema during positive-pressure ventilation. *American Review of Respiratory Disease* **117**, 721–5.

Trump B.F., Mergner W.J., Kahng M.W. & Saladino A.J. (1976) Studies on the subcellular pathophysiology of ischaemia. *Circulation* **53** (Suppl. 1): 17–25.

Twigley A.J. & Hillman K.M. (1985) The end of the crystalloid era? *Anaesthesia* **40**, 860–71.

Vatner S.F., Higgins C.B. & Braunwald E. (1974b) Effects of norepinephrine on coronary circulation and left ventricular dynamics in the conscious dog. *Circulation Research* **34**, 812–23.

Vatner S.F., McRitchie R.J. & Braunwald E. (1974a) Effects of dobutamine on left ventricular performance, coronary dynamics, and distribution of cardiac output in conscious dogs. *Journal of Clinical Investigation* **53**, 1265–73.

Virgilio R.W., Rice C.L., Smith D.E., James D.R., Zarins C.K., Hobelmann C.F. & Peters R.M. (1979) Crystalloid vs. colloid resuscitation: is one better? *Surgery* **85**, 129–39.

Virgilio R.W., Smith D.E. & Zarins C.K. (1979) Balanced electrolyte solutions: experimental and clinical studies. *Critical Care Medicine* **7**, 98–106.

Vitek V. & Cowley R.A. (1971) Blood lactate in the prognosis of various forms of shock. *Annals of Surgery* **173**, 308–13.

Wardle E.N. (1978) A review of endotoxin and its absorption from the gut. In *Antigen Absorption by the Gut* (Ed. Hemmings W.A.) pp. 183–8. MTP, Lancaster.

Wardle E.N. (1979) Bacteraemic and endotoxic shock. *British Journal of Hospital Medicine* **21**, 223–8.

Watson J.D., Varley J.G., Hinds C.J., Bouloux P., Tomlin S. & Rees L.H. (1984) Adrenal vein and systemic levels of catecholamines and metenkephalin like immunoreactivity in canine endotoxic shock; effects of naloxone administration. *Circulatory Shock* **13**, 47.

West J.B., Dollery C.T. & Naimark A. (1964) The distribution of blood flow in isolated dog lung: relation to vascular and alveolar pressures. *Journal of Applied Physiology* **19**, 713–22.

Wiles J.B., Cerra F.B., Siegel J.H. & Border J.R. (1980) The systemic septic response: does the organism matter? *Critical Care Medicine* **8**, 55–60.

Williams D.O., Amsterdam E.A. & Mason D.T. (1975) Haemodynamic effects of nitroglycerin in acute myocardial infarction: decrease in ventricular preload at the expense of cardiac output. *Circulation* **51**, 421–7.

Wilmore D.W., Goodwin C.W., Aulick L.H., Powanda M.C., Mason A.D. & Pruitt B.A. (1980) Effect of injury and infection on visceral metabolism and circulation. *Annals of Surgery* **192**, 491–500.

Woods I., Wilkins R.G., Edwards J.D., Martin P.D. & Faragher E.B. (1987) The danger of using peripheral/core temperature gradient as a guide to therapy in shock. *Critical Care Medicine* **15**, 850–2.

Zapol W.M. & Snider M.T. (1977) Pulmonary hypertension in severe acute respiratory failure. *New England Journal of Medicine* **296**, 476–80.

76

Nutrition

S. M. WILLATTS

Nutritional disturbances are extremely common in patients requiring intensive care, and such disturbances have far-reaching consequences. The critically ill develop a marked stress response to trauma with disturbances of carbohydrate, fat and protein metabolism. Oxygen consumption is increased, fluid overload common and susceptibility to sepsis is high.

The effects of malnutrition are legion. This topic is discussed by Cahill (1970), although Studley (1936) first noticed the adverse effect of a reduction in body weight. Acute weight loss in excess of 20% is associated with a postoperative mortality of 33%, compared with 3.5% in those who have lost less weight. Marton et al. (1981) found that approximately 30% of patients who had physical disease causing loss of body weight died within 2 yr. This does not concur with the findings of Ryan and Taft (1980), who found no increase in intraoperative risk in patients who had lost weight. However, malnutrition is held generally to lead to progressive weakness (and other well-known effects, listed in Table 76.1), although the efficacy of perioperative parenteral nutrition in reducing mortality and morbidity has been questioned by Biebuyck (1981). The ability to respond to infection is attribut-

able in part to a group of proteins, leucocyte endogenous mediators, which are reduced in malnutrition and restored by increasing protein intake.

In a group of patients with severe complications after abdominal surgery, Lawson (1965) showed that those who lost more than 30% of their original weight died. It has been estimated that 40–50% of medical and surgical patients exhibit protein energy malnutrition at some time during their hospital stay (Bistrian et al., 1974). Unfortunately, we do not have a simple nutritional index of sufficient predictive power to define that group of patients who need feeding (Baker et al., 1982). Whilst malnutrition is clearly widespread in hospitalized patients and many of its effects are evident and at least partially preventable, associated disturbances in drug disposition (Pantuck et al., 1984; Vessell & Biebuyck, 1984) neurotransmitter release (Pardridge, 1983) and conscious level (Glaeser et al., 1983) are more difficult to manage.

The volume of nutritional support is often limited by salt and water retention produced by increased aldosterone and antidiuretic hormone (ADH) secretion whilst complications of overzealous nutritional replacement can be severe, ranging from respiratory failure to hyperosmolar states. An understanding of basic metabolism and energy requirements is therefore very important. It is illogical to infuse nutritional substances without knowledge of energy requirements and metabolic measurement of the consequences (Biebuyck, 1983).

The energy substrates

Carbohydrate

Under normal circumstances of adequate nutrition, carbohydrate is ingested almost always in excess of requirements but blood glucose concentration is kept

Table 76.1 Effects of malnutrition. (From Irvin, 1978)

Progressive weakness
Reduced vital capacity, respiratory rate, minute volume
Increased risk of respiratory infection
Difficulty in weaning from ventilatory support
Reduced cardiac output, myocardial contractility and compliance
Reduced tensile strength of skin, increased wound dehiscence
Breakdown of anastomoses
Reduced plasma proteins, susceptibility to salt and water overload
Reduced host resistance

between 4 and 8 mmol/litre. Carbohydrate is absorbed from the gut as hexoses (glucose, fructose, galactose) and reaches the liver in the portal circulation where the major uptake occurs. Some glucose bypasses the liver and is metabolized in other tissues, especially muscle where it is used to replenish glycogen stores. The arrival of glucose at the liver has two major effects.

1 Inhibition of endogenous glucose production.

2 Phosphorylation of the glucose to glucose-6-phosphate, which is converted into glycogen or metabolized first to pyruvate via the Embden–Myerhof pathway and thence to acetyl co-enzyme A (CoA) and fatty acids.

There are several mechanisms whereby ingested carbohydrate is stored, either as carbohydrate or lipid, for use during fasting. However, the human body has only limited reserves of energy substrates, and hepatic glycogen is depleted rapidly in starvation (Table 76.2). In the normal human body, the CNS is dependent entirely on glucose except in the starved state. Red blood cells and the adrenal medulla are entirely glucose dependent. Glucose is the main substrate, therefore, for oxidative metabolism, and the only one for anaerobic metabolism. Oxidative metabolism continues *in vivo* with a small mitochondrial P_{O_2} 0.067 kPa (0.5 mmHg), producing 38 mole of adenosine triphosphate (ATP) from 1 mole of glucose. Whilst adequate ingested carbohydrate is essential to maintain a normal blood glucose, there are dangers of hyperglycaemia which, if persistent, gives rise to increased polyol accumulation in tissues, hyperlactataemia, hormone imbalance and glycosylation of tissue proteins including haemoglobin. In this respect, an increase in the proportion or absolute amount of starchy foods may be of benefit to both carbohydrate and fat metabolism because of its reduced hyperglycaemic response.

REGULATION OF CARBOHYDRATE METABOLISM

Mechanisms of regulation of carbohydrate metabolism are summarized in Table 76.3.

Table 76.3 Mechanisms of regulation of carbohydrate metabolis

Endocrine	Non-hormonal
Anabolic Insulin	*Glucose infusion* Inhibits hepatic glucose output
Catabolic Glucogen Cortisol Catecholamines Growth hormone	*Glucose–FA–KB cycle* Increased circulating FAs and KBs inhibit glucose oxidation in heart and muscle

In the fed state, insulin secretion increases in response to carbohydrate and protein feeding. The effect of insulin is to increase phosphorylation of glucose, to activate glycogen synthetase and allow rapid disposal of glucose into glycogen stores. Insulin also increases glycolysis and pyruvate dehydrogenase activity with an increase in acetyl CoA carboxylase which therefore directs glucose towards fatty acid (FA), (implying non-esterified fatty acid) synthesis (Table 76.4).

The net effect of insulin secretion (Table 76.4), therefore, is to increase glucose transport into muscle and fat, to inhibit lipolysis and proteolysis and thus to reduce gluconeogenic precursors. In starvation, plasma insulin concentrations are low and act mainly to inhibit catabolism.

CATABOLIC HORMONES

Most of the hormonal effects on glucose metabolism are mediated by endocrine receptors found in all cells. Hormones may affect the action of each other by altering the affinity or the number of receptors for the other hormones. Both cortisol and growth hormone alter insulin receptors, and insulin can 'down-regulate' its own receptors which is of importance in insulin resistance of stress states.

Carbohydrate metabolism, therefore, depends on the balance between circulating insulin and catabolic

	kg	Duration	kcal
Carbohydrate (mainly liver glycogen)	0.2	6–12 hr	800
Fat	12–15	20–25 days	109 000–136 000
Protein (mainly muscle)	4–6	10–12 days	16 000–24 000

Table 76.2 Nutritional reserves of a 70 kg man

Table 76.4 Effects of insulin

Stimulates
Glucose phosphorylation
Glycogen synthetase
Pyruvate dehydrogenase
Acetyl CoA carboxylase, directing glucose towards fat synthesis

Inhibits
Glycogenolysis
Gluconeogenesis
Lipolysis
Proteolysis

Table 76.5 Catabolic hormones

Glucagon
Maximal effects between feeding
Stimulates glycogenolysis (short term)
Stimulates hepatic uptake of amino acid

Cortisol
Enhances peripheral proteolysis
Increases FA release for gluconeogenesis

Catecholamines
Glycogenolysis
Increase lactate output

Growth hormone (GH)
Short-term increase in glucose transport to muscle
Longer-term impairs glucose uptake, increasing use of alternative substrates

Catecholamines inhibit GH and insulin via β-stimulation and stimulate GH and glucogen via α-receptors. Glucagon stimulates secretion of insulin, GH and cortisol (via adrenocorticotrophic hormone; ACTH), and in pharmacological amounts increases catecholamine secretion. Growth hormone may also increase insulin secretion and cortisol increase secretion of insulin and glucagon.

hormones (Table 76.5). In the fed situation, insulin predominates; if the subject is fasted, there is a predominance of catabolic hormones. In circumstances where the stress response is activated, despite the fed state, a surge of catabolic hormones occurs.

Fat

Lipids make a large contribution to energy stores and they may be stored as compact water-insoluble droplets in adipose tissue. Triacylglycerol (TAG) is the current term for the combination of three FAs with glycerol, termed previously neutral fat or triglyceride. Triacylglycerol has a very high calorie content (9.3 kcal/g). Ketone bodies (KBs) are produced from lipids especially during starvation when they may reduce the requirements for glucose, and minimize gluconeogenesis from amino acids.

After 4 days of fasting, triacylglycerol, non-esterified FA and KB constitute approximately 85% of the potential energy available in plasma (Table 76.6). Fat exists in the body in a great variety of forms: the main ones are summarized in Table 76.7.

METABOLISM OF LIPIDS AND KETONE BODIES

Ingested lipid is hydrolysed in the duodenum to glycerol and FAs. These latter are absorbed by epithelial cells and resynthesized into TAG which is incorporated into chylomicrons (CMs) and apoproteins A and B, and pass eventually into the thoracic duct and then the circulation. Some TAG is taken up by the liver where essential FAs are possibly removed. Some is taken up by heart and muscle but most goes to adipose tissue. Non-esterified FAs are very important fuels of respiration with half-lives in the circulation of 2–3 min.

The liver converts FAs into TAG and very low-density lipoproteins (VLDLs) or oxidizes FAs to KBs. Adipose tissue stores TAG and controls its

Table 76.6 Fuels in circulation

Substrate	Overnight fast		Four-day fast	
	Concentration (μmol/ml)	Available energy (%)	Concentration (μmol/ml)	Available energy (%)
FAs	0.42	9	1.15	20
TAG	1.0	65	1.0	54
Glucose	4.7	25	3.6	16
Lactate	0.5	<1	0.5	<1
KBs	0.03	<1	2.9	9

Table 76.7 Fats in the body

TAG	8–100 nm, soluble in aqueous media, carried in plasma as micelles with lipoproteins, found in liver and intestine
CMs	100–1000 nm, produced by intestine and liver from dietary fat, removed rapidly from plasma
Lipoproteins	Structure aids carriage and delivery, TAG to target tissues
VLDLs	30–80 nm, produced from TAG in liver, secreted into plasma, an important energy source
Low-density lipoproteins	25–30 nm, cholesterol enriched, correlation with atherosclerosis
High-density lipoproteins	8–20 nm, esterify cholesterol, mediate exchange of apoproteins, inverse correlation with atherosclerosis
Apoproteins	synthesized in liver and intestine, used in assembly of VLDLs and CMs, activate enzymes, interact with specific cell-wall receptors, mark residual fat particles for removal by reticuloendothelial system
FAs	Non-esterified FAs transported in plasma bound to albumin, at pH 7.4 carboxyl group almost completely dissociated
KBs	β-hydroxybutyrate and acetoacetate are lipid derived and relatively polar

release as FAs. Lipoproteins are confined to the intravascular space. Metabolism of CMs depends on hydrolysis in the circulation to FAs and glycerol. Glucose cannot be synthesized directly from FAs but glycerol is a gluconeogenic precursor and FAs can be converted into ketone bodies. Hydrolysis of TAG is catalysed by lipoprotein lipase which is found on the luminal surface of capillaries in adipose tissue, heart and skeletal muscle. Fatty acids can then cross capillary membranes where they can be used by most tissues except the CNS for oxidation and TAG synthesis as a local energy reserve. In heart muscle, FAs are preferred to glucose and when both are present, glucose uptake and oxidation are reduced greatly. Synthesis of TAG requires glucose as the precursor of glycerol-3-phosphate. During starvation, insulin secretion is reduced thereby reducing glucose uptake and TAG synthesis. Lack of glucose favours lipolysis and release of FAs. Lipolysis is stimulated by catecholamines, cortisol and thyroxine.

The concentration of KBs is increased during starvation, diabetes, uraemia, a high fat diet, exercise, infancy and the perinatal period. All tissues except the liver have the ability to oxidize KBs. The plasma concentration depends on the balance between hepatic synthesis and peripheral utilization. Oxidation of KBs reduces the demand for glucose, the necessity for gluconeogenesis and the degradation of protein, and in starvation the concentration of insulin, an antili-

polytic hormone, decreases. Infants and children have more active KBs transport systems and a greater capacity to extract KBs from blood. This mechanism may be important particularly in children who can become hypoglycaemic (and hyperketonaemic) after a very short fast.

The influence of hormones on fat metabolism is summarized in Table 76.8.

Brown fat is found in cervical, interscapular, axillary, intrathoracic and perirenal depots and is responsible for buffering changes in food intake. Catecholamine stimulation of brown fat increases the supply of FAs for mitochrondrial oxidation. The calorigenic effect of catecholamines may result from

Table 76.8 The influence of hormones on fat metabolism

Insulin
Promotes esterification of FAs
Inhibits lipolysis
Stimulates glucose entry into fat cells
(glycerol-3-phosphate)
Stimulates intracellular lipase
Reduced supply of FAs to liver inhibits KB formation

Glucagon
Stimulates lipolysis, possibly only when insulin level is low
Stimulates gluconeogenesis
Inhibits glycolysis and FA synthesis

Cortisol, GH, catecholamines, thyroid hormones together and separately mobilize FAs from adipose tissue. All reversed by insulin.

their effect of mobilizing free FAs. Heat is dissipated by uncoupling of mitochondria and heat production proceeds at maximal level. Central control mechanisms for this activity lie in the hypothalamus (Himms-Hagen, 1984).

The grossly obese patients have apparently defective thermogenesis in the mitochondria of brown fat. Exposure of anaesthetized, paralysed patients to a cold environment induces non-shivering thermogenesis, which is greater in lean subjects, with accompanying increased oxygen consumption. Obese patients have higher basal metabolic rates than lean ones and higher energy expenditure during normal life. Self-recorded energy intakes tend to be underestimated in the obese (Prentice et al., 1986).

Fasting

During fasting, glucose must be produced at 180 g every 24 hr. This is effected by glycogenolysis and gluconeogenesis. These two processes occur in the liver where phosphorylase is activated to produce glucose-6-phosphate from which free glucose is liberated. The substrates for gluconeogenesis are lactate, pyruvate, glycerol and the glucogenic amino acids (AAs); alanine, glutamine and glycine. Lactate provides approximately 50% of the precursor pool. Under normal circumstances, the liver can remove up to 400 g of lactate daily from the circulation, but if hypoxia intervenes, liver blood flow and function are impaired. Glycerol provides 5–10% of the gluconeogenic precursor pool. The liver metabolizes normally 80–90% of available glycerol which in the fasting state is converted to glucose. The remainder of new glucose is derived from amino acids, especially alanine which is formed by transamination of pyruvate in peripheral tissues.

As glycogen reserves are limited, most glucose is derived from gluconeogenesis, and protein breakdown occurs to provide the AAs. This process is limited by keto-adaptation. The CNS may use KBs as oxidative fuels in conditions of starvation, such that the total glucose requirement of the CNS decreases by 50% after approximately 5 weeks of starvation. During starvation, overall energy needs of the body are reduced, energy expenditure diminishes by up to 35%, ketoacids are substituted for glucose as brain fuel and the pool of free FAs increases.

Short-term starvation consumes glycogen stores, and proteolysis and lipolysis begin. As proteolysis proceeds, there is a reduction in muscle mass and muscle weakness and respiratory complications develop with an increased incidence of infection resulting occasionally in death. The greatest losses of nitrogen after trauma occur in well-fed young men. After long-term starvation, nitrogen losses in the urine are low because of protein-sparing mechanisms which come into play. These include enhanced KB production and their utilization by the CNS. In total starvation, the basal metabolic rate (BMR) declines by 20% after 3 weeks and 40% by 6 months. However, when the stress response is activated postoperatively, insulin concentrations increase, lipolysis is inhibited and metabolism is more dependent on glucose again. In the fasting state, the heart can metabolize FAs as a primary energy substrate. In the presence of a high concentration of glucose and insulin, myocardial stores of glycogen can be increased, which is valuable (should the heart suddenly become hypoxic) to provide substrate for anaerobic metabolism.

PROTEIN TURNOVER

Protein synthesis and degradation are under independent control. Muscle plays a key role in uptake of AAs after a meal and in release of AAs during fasting. Protein synthesis decreases by 50% during starvation. During periods of rapid growth, protein synthesis increases but this is associated also with increased protein degradation.

In animals, starvation leads to loss of pulmonary surfactant and reduced acetyl CoA carboxylase activity and FA synthesis.

Loss of weight in the first few days after surgery is likely to result from water loss, but after 10–14 days is produced by loss of protein and fat. Kinney and Hessov (1981) calculate that the protein contribution to this weight loss could amount to 10–14% over a 3-week period. In a very ill catabolic patient with sepsis, up to 22% of the resting energy expenditure (REE) is derived from protein.

Stress response to trauma

Surgery or trauma activates a typical metabolic and hormonal response which may be mediated by pain or some other neural mechanism (Fig. 76.1) and may be accompanied by immunosuppression (Bardosi & Tekeres, 1985). Cuthbertson and Tilstone (1969) described an 'ebb' and a 'flow' phase. Loss of nitrogen (N_2), potassium (K) and sodium (Na) from the body are greatest during the flow phase and changes recede if the patient recovers and anabolism begins.

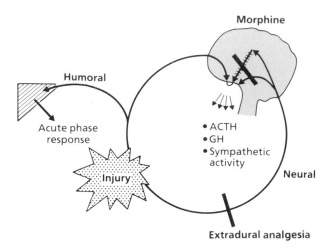

Fig. 76.1 Neuroendocrine response to stress. (Reproduced from Elliott & Alberti, 1983)

In rats, division of afferent fibres from the site of injury suppresses development of the neuroendocrine response. Extensive extradural analgesia (Engquist *et al.*, 1977) to block both somatic and sympathetic afferent activity, centrally acting morphine, fentanyl, alfentanil and high spinal-cord lesions also suppress the response which can be modified by pre-existing fear and anxiety. There is some evidence for a humoral pathway, which would not be modified by the above measures. Prostaglandins, bacterial endotoxin and other pyrogens have been postulated as 'wound hormones'. Interleukin-1 is the most investigated wound hormone which increases lysosomal protein degradation, an action which is mediated by prostaglandin E_2 (Baracos *et al.*, 1983) although other peptides are involved also.

ENDOCRINE CHANGES

The hypothalamus acts as a final common pathway for the neuroendocrine response which involves secretion of pituitary hormones and sympathetic activity (Table 76.9). Most hormones increase in proportion to the severity of the surgery although ACTH is a poor index of the severity of injury and the GH response may vary with age.

Insulin secretion is depressed during surgery (Allison *et al.*, 1969), presumably by increased concentrations of noradrenaline (Nakao & Miyata, 1977). Insulin concentrations can be increased by α-blockade, but suppression is short-lived in uncomplicated surgery (Aarimaa *et al.*, 1978), returning to normal in about 7 days. Plasma glucose concentration and β-adrenergic activity increase. There is evidence also of tissue

Table 76.9 Hormones involved in the endocrine response to surgery

Neuroendocrine response	Systemic response
ACTH	Insulin
Vasopressin	Cortisol
GH	Glucagon
TSH	Thyroxine, triiodothyronine
Adrenaline	Aldosterone
Noradrenaline	Angiotensin

resistance to insulin (Thomas *et al.*, 1979). Early hyperglycaemia (6–18 hr) is probably the result of adrenal medullary output rather than sympathetic nervous discharge.

The increase in plasma cortisol concentration is rapid, occurring within a few hours and is in proportion to the severity of surgery (Stoner *et al.*, 1979). Cortisol is termed the permissive hormone as it has little effect on glucose production, but by stimulating peripheral release of AAs which act as substrates increases gluconeogenesis. The increase in glucagon is related also to the severity of injury and reaches a peak 18–48 hr after injury. Increased glucagon is thought to be caused by increased catecholamines (Porte & Robertson, 1975). Gluconeogenesis, glycogenolysis and AA uptake are stimulated in the liver (Woolfe *et al.*, 1979).

Changes in thyroid hormones are variable (Goode *et al.*, 1981) but extradural analgesia which suppresses cortisol has no effect on the thyroid hormones (Brandt *et al.*, 1976). Changes may be secondary to increased oxygen consumption after surgery. Growth hormone has only a minor effect, a normal metabolic response to trauma occurring in hypophysectomized patients receiving steroid replacements.

These hormonal effects stimulate mostly glucose production and catabolic processes, the so-called 'catabolic drive'.

There is an increased demand for glucose after surgery to provide energy for wound repair. Whilst glycogenolysis continues, stimulated by catecholamines and glucagon, there is also an increase in lactate and pyruvate release from muscle. Pyruvate is taken up by the liver as a gluconeogenetic substrate.

In severe injury, whole-body protein turnover increases but breakdown increases more than synthesis (Birkhahn *et al.*, 1980). There is very little evidence for the assumption that the nitrogen loss in injury is produced by muscle breakdown (Rennie & Harrison, 1984), although new isotope techniques may resolve this. Measurement of whole-body protein breakdown and 3-methyl histidine excretion in fasting shows a reduction in 3-methyl histidine excretion by total parenteral nutrition (TPN). However, increased non-muscle tissue breakdown is probably common in depleted patients (Lowry *et al.*, 1985). There is a complex interaction between nutritional state and the degree of injury in severe trauma, burns and sepsis, and protein breakdown is relatively resistant to nutritional modification. Catecholamine infusions used in these circumstances further increase glyco-genolysis and hepatic gluconeogenesis and worsen insulin resistance.

Fat breakdown increases the release of glycerol and FAs which may be taken up by muscles and used directly as an energy source or by the liver for conversion into KBs. Adrenaline and glucocorticoids stimulate adipose tissue lipolysis whilst glucagon speeds intrahepatic conversion of FAs to KBs.

One of the most prominent features of the stress response is therefore hyperglycaemia; both glucose oxidation and turnover are increased and the primary disturbance is one of increased hepatic output of glucose (Wilmore *et al.*, 1980).

Severe metabolic derangements occur in the septic state with increased glucose utilization (Ryan, 1976) and often inappropriately low insulin concentrations, which correlates with cardiovascular decompensation, reduced cortisol (Sibbald *et al.*, 1977) and reduced GH both of which are associated with a high mortality. Recovery is associated with return of a normal reciprocal relationship between insulin and glucagon.

Total-body oxygen consumption is increased. This may result from the hypermetabolism of infection (Gump *et al.*, 1970a), catecholamine induced after injury or following administration of excess glucose during TPN (Askanazi *et al.*, 1980). This is discussed further below.

EFFECT OF ANAESTHETIC AGENTS

Some aspects of the stress response to trauma may be modified by anaesthetic agents with the potential to improve postoperative nitrogen balance. In dogs receiving phentolamine and propranolol during a standard operation, urinary nitrogen losses, glutamine flux and the muscle glutamine were not reduced by hormonal block but hindquarter nitrogen flux was diminished. Thus, hormonal block inhibits *net* skeletal muscle catabolism without altering whole-body nitrogen loss (Hulton *et al.*, 1985).

Intrathecal diamorphine delays the hypergly-caemic response to colonic surgery and reduces cortisol compared with intravenous opioids. Extradural anal-gesia with local analgesic drugs and, to a lesser extent, opioids can improve nitrogen balance in the first 5 postoperative days and suppress plasma glucose and FA concentrations. Although midazolam obtunds catecholamine secretion during stress in animals through a central GABA (γ-aminobutyric acid) interaction, there is no blunting of the glycaemic response to surgery in man (Dawson & Sear, 1986). Most anaes-thetic techniques modify the response to surgery only for the duration of their intervention and pain relief *per se* may have little effect (Hjortso *et al.*, 1985).

Malnutrition

The effects of malnutrition

A reduction in protein and calorie intake reduces protein turnover, synthesis and breakdown (Reeds & James, 1983). During repletion there are both in-creased synthesis and increased breakdown, but the former predominates with net accumulation of protein. Starvation occurring in the previously well-nourished patient increases plasma concentrations of branched-chain amino acids (BCAAs) and glycine and reduces plasma alanine. Specific plasma amino acid patterns are found in sepsis and hepatic failure, but these do not reflect necessarily the AA concentration of the muscle or the total pool of free AAs.

Nutritional assessment

Most patients requiring intensive therapy show some evidence of malnutrition (Boles *et al.*, 1984), although the aim in general is identification of patients with marginal malnutrition who might benefit from nutri-tional intervention to reduce postoperative mortality and morbidity. A great variety of clinical and labora-tory parameters have been recommended in the past for evaluation of malnutrition (Table 76.10) but few are specific enough to be of much help. In screening for protein energy malnutrition, a plastic strip band to indicate malnourished, borderline and normal has proved helpful in children (Shakir & Morley, 1974). Mid-upper arm circumference was found to be as effective as other nutritional indices in predicting death in malnourished children in Bangladesh (Briend *et al.*, 1986).

Table 76.10 Clinical and laboratory values and malnutrition

Parameter and standard	Degree of malnutrition		
	Mild	Moderate	Severe
Weight loss (of usual)	<10%	10–20%	>20%
Weight (of ideal)	80–90%	70–79%	<70%
Anthropometric measurements			
Triceps skin fold (of standard)	80–90%	60–79%	<60%
Arm muscle circumference (of standard)	80–90%	60–79%	<40%
Creatinine—height index (of standard)	60–80%	40–59%	<40%
Biochemical measurements			
Serum albumin (3.5–5.0 g/dl)	3.0–3.4	2.9–2.1	<2.1
Serum transferrin (175–300 mg/dl)	150–175	100–150	<100
Thyroxin-binding prealbumin (28–35 mg/dl)	25.2–28	23–25.2	<23
Retinol-binding protein (3–6 mg/dl)	2.7–3	2.4–2.7	<2.4
Immune competence			
Total lymphocytes (1500–5000/mm³)	1200–1500	800–1200	<800
Delayed cutaneous hypersensitivity	Reactive	Relative energy	Non-reactive

These may be supplemented by dynamometry, measurement of 3-methylhistidine, creatinine excretion index and tests for muscle fatigue.

Clinical and laboratory values and malnutrition

It is difficult to obtain an ideal body weight in very ill patients and loss of body components is the final stage of malnutrition. Most other methods of assessment have their limitations, and plasma concentrations of visceral proteins are affected by conditions other than malnutrition such as hydration and sepsis (Jeejeebuoy et al., 1982). Three-methylhistidine was thought originally to be a valuable indication of muscle breakdown, but there is doubt regarding its specificity (Rennie & Millward, 1983). It is, therefore, still difficult to identify at-risk patients. Daly et al. (1979) use two of the following three parameters:
1 Unintentional weight loss greater than 10%.
2 Albumin less than 35 g/litre.
3 A negative reaction to five skin antigens.

However, plasma proteins vary with liver disease, septicaemia and other protein-losing states, so albumin is a non-specific measure of malnutrition. Of equal value may be a history and clinical examination in conjunction with the haemoglobin concentration and acute visceral proteins.

Pettigrew and Hill (1986) found that anthropometric measurements did not identify patients who subsequently had complications after operation but that decreased plasma proteins did, probably because they were reduced by preoperative sepsis rather than nutritional status. Even hand grip (an index of muscle function) is effected by factors other than nutrition (e.g. 35% reduction in acute sepsis, 50% after administration of sedative drugs) (Elia et al., 1984).

An interesting new approach to assessing the benefit of TPN is that of Chang et al., (1986) who attempted to identify those patients admitted to ITU who would not benefit from TPN by using APACHE II scoring (Knaus et al., 1985). One problem with such an approach is the possibility of withholding TPN inappropriately thereby ensuring mortality.

The effect of malnutrition on immune function

Malnutrition modifies immune function (Table 76.11). Cell-mediated immunity may be assessed by response to recall skin antigens. A marked reduction in response has been found to correlate with severe sepsis and poor outcome. Although such testing has been advocated as a useful indication of malnutrition, it is non-specific, and routine use of delayed hypersensitivity skin testing was not considered justified by Brown et al. (1982), as they found no significant increase in the incidence of sepsis nor a higher mortality in anergic patients compared with controls with normal delayed hypersensitivity reactions. In Kwashiorkor, however, impaired cellular immunity is improved after nutritional therapy. Fibronectin levels are reduced in malnutrition with resultant impaired macrophage activity.

Table 76.11 Effects of severe malnutrition on immune functions. (From Shizgal, 1981)

Phagocytic activity
Polymorphonuclear leucocytes are normal in number
Chemotaxis, opsonic function and phagocytic function are usually normal
Intracellular killing decreases

Lymphoid organs
Thymus, spleen, lymph nodes and Peyer's patches markedly atrophic

Lymphocyte functions
Lymphocytes normal in number
T-cells reduced
B-cells normal or increased
Null cells increase
Gamma-globulins usually normal (low in severe undernutrition)
Immunoglobulins usually normal (IgM, IgA and IgE may be increased)
Antibody response: primary usually depressed, secondary less affected
Cell-mediated immunity impaired (as perhaps is delayed cutaneous hypersensitivity)
Complement decreases (except C4)

Reliability of assessment

Forse and Shizgal (1980) evaluated the reliability of nutritional assessment by comparing the various parameters with simultaneous body composition measurements. Correlations were poor, the best being weight:height ratio. Many of the parameters are useful for epidemiological studies but not for individual nutritional assessment. Nutritional indices have poor discriminant value for individual prediction of survival (Apelgren et al. (1982).

Klidjian et al. (1980) found hand-grip dynamometry to be a useful screening test for detecting malnutrition. Loss of muscle power does predict those patients likely to show serious postoperative morbidity. Measurements of muscle fatigue are being investigated by Jeejeebuoy (1985), who obtains a force frequency curve for adductor pollicis which correlates with that obtained from the diaphragm. Development of fatigue is a consistent finding in malnutrition and one which is not abnormal in non-specific situations such as sepsis, administration of steroids, anaesthesia or moderate trauma.

The abnormalities of muscle contraction reported in malnourished patients are reviewed by Newham (1986). They include:

1 Excessively high force generation at low versus high stimulating frequencies.

2 Slow relaxation.

3 Increased fatiguability.

Moreover, measurements of fatigue are reversible with refeeding at a time when other indices of body composition remain abnormal (Russel et al., 1983). Brough et al. (1986) found that the ratio of force of contraction of the adductor pollicis at 10 Hz and 20 Hz gave the best combination of sensitivity (87%) and specificity (82%). After TPN, abnormal muscle function tests returned to normal before changes were detectable in anthropometric variables or plasma albumin concentration. However, these abnormal tests have been improved significantly by a regimen of glucose–potassium loading in preoperative malnourished patients (Chan et al., 1986).

However nutritional depletion is assessed, and loss of muscle power is at present the best guide, all patients require adequate nutrition administered ideally by the enteral route, but if this is not possible then parenterally. Early enteral feeding is thought to reduce secretion of catabolic hormones and return immune responsiveness more rapidly.

Feeding

Some attempt should be made to evaluate the degree of existing malnutrition (see above). The American Society of Anesthesiologists (ASA) classification may be helpful (Table 76.12). Alternatively, three patient categories may be defined: normal, depleted and hypercatabolic.

Many authors stress the deficiencies in current methods used to define malnutrition (Baker et al., 1982) and that whilst a definitive single test of malnutrition is not available, clinical evaluation may be sufficient. It may be argued that all tests for malnutrition return to normal with resolution of the disease process regardless of the adequacy of nutritional therapy, but some continuous assessment of nutritional status should be made.

The diet should be as complete as possible (Elwyn, 1980), bearing in mind existing depletion (Table

Table 76.12 The American Society of Anesthesiologist's nutritional classification

Class I	Excludes patients with malnutrition
Class II	Those under 10% weight loss, partial starvation
Class III	Hypermetabolic, requiring vigorous nutritional support
Class IV	Complex, extreme catabolism, sepsis, multiple pathologies

76.13). Energy needs are based as far as possible on expenditure rather than intake. Basal metabolic rate or REE is the largest component of energy expenditure, hence the value of calculating other components as multiples of this. Irrespective of height, the BMR per kg body weight varies inversely with body weight. The basis for estimating protein requirement remains the nitrogen balance which presents difficulties as it is extremely sensitive to energy intake. Resting metabolic rate of normal-weight individuals and the obese is higher on a high carbohydrate diet than on an isoenergetic high fat diet. The lower limit of intake for some nutrients is defined often by nutrient balance measuring intake and excretion of nutrients. An estimate of variability of requirements is then added to the average requirement to provide a safety margin. The upper limit of nutritional intakes appropriate to health are more difficult to define. There is obviously

Table 76.13 Recommended allowances of nutritional substances

Nutritional substance	Daily allowances to adults (per kg body weight)
Water	30 ml
Energy	30 kcal (0.13 MJ)
Amino acid nitrogen	90 mg (0.7 g amino acids)
Glucose	2 g
Fat	2 g
Sodium	1–1.4 mmol
Potassium	0.7–0.9 mmol
Calcium	0.11 mmol
Magnesium	0.04 mmol
Iron	1 μmol
Manganese	0.6 μmol
Zinc	0.3 μmol
Copper	0.07 μmol
Chlorine	1.3–1.9 mmol
Phosphorus	0.15 mmol
Fluorine	0.7 μmol
Iodine	0.015 μmol
Thiamine	0.02 mg
Riboflavine	0.03 mg
Nicotinamide	0.2 mg
Pyridoxine	0.03 mg
Folic acid	3 μg
Cyanocobalamin	0.03 μg
Pantothenic acid	0.2 mg
Biotin	5 μg
Ascorbic acid	0.5 mg
Retinol	10 μg
Ergocalciferol or cholecalciferol	004 mg
Phytylmenaquinone	2 μg
α-Tocopherol	1.5 mg

a wide range of susceptibility to a given intake. It must be remembered that published requirements relate to normal individuals, whereas considerable variation may occur in acute illness. Recommendations for electrolyte, vitamin and trace-element content of a TPN regimen are given below.

Wherever possible, the gastrointestinal tract should be used for feeding, as metabolic effects of nutrients given by this route are probably better than by the intravenous route (Yeung *et al.*, 1979); visceral protein synthesis may improve, and it is associated with far fewer complications than the intravenous route.

Enteral feeding

Enteral feeds and delivery systems were reviewed by Brown (1981). Characteristics of the currently available feeds are shown in Table 76.14.

Liquid diets prepared in hospitals become contaminated readily with yeasts and staphylococci and are inclined to block fine-bore nasogastric tubes. Commercially available liquid diets are safer and easier to handle.

Palatability is important where these feeds are used without a nasogastric tube. Administration is ideally by fine-bore nasogastric tube, but these carry a risk of displacement and pulmonary aspiration of feeds. The presence of an endotracheal tube, impaired cough reflex and the impossibility of retrograde withdrawal of feed, combined with the ready acceptability of these tubes, predispose to such pulmonary aspiration (Boscoe & Rosin, 1984). Fine-bore tubes may deliver 3–5/litre of nutrient solution in 24 hr without a pump.

Where gastric emptying is impaired but the intestine is functional otherwise, jejunostomy is invaluable. It is a very simple procedure and either wide- or fine-bore tubes may be used. Enteral feeding may take the form of nutritional supplementation, complete oral diets or elemental diets.

There is very little to choose between the many commercially available feeds. The author prefers Nutrauxil which is a whole-protein feed. Two litres (four bottles) provide 2000 kcal and 12 g nitrogen. The calorie:nitrogen ratio is 143:1, and additional carbohydrate may be added. Two litres contain 68 g of fat as sunflower oil, 15% of which is essential FA. The zinc content has been increased recently to good effect, but some electrolytes and trace elements are still rather low.

Long-term feeding requires supplementation with vitamin D. Nutrauxil is gluten- and lactose-free with

Table 76.14 Characteristics of some of the available enteral feeds

Products	Package size	Daily amount to supply approx. 2000 kcal	Dilution needed	Lactose free	Problems/features	Flavoured/unflavoured	Protein (g)	Fat (g)	CHO (g)	Calories	Osmolarity (mosmol/litre)	Price per 2000 kcal
Clinifeed Iso (Roussel)	375 ml can	× 6	No	No	Low sodium	Vanilla	63	92.4	294	2250	270	£6.00
Clinifeed 400 (Roussel) (Also available Clinifeed Protein Rich Vanilla)	375 ml can	× 5	Yes	No		Vanilla	75	67	275	2000	306 (dil.) 307 (undil.)	£4.75
Clinifeed Favour (Roussel)	375 ml can	× 6	No	Yes		Neutral or coffee	85	74	315	2250	365	£5.10
Triosorbon MCI (BDH)	85 g sachet	× 5	Yes	Watch contains carragenan	Minimal sodium	No	81	81	240	2000	238	£5.00
Ensure (Abbot) (Also available Ensure Plus)	240 ml cans or bottles	× 8	No	Yes		Vanilla	70	70	275	1930	380	£7.90 (bottles) £7.30 (tins)
Isocal (Mead Johnson)	250 ml can	× 8	No	Yes		No	64.1	83.2	252	2008	300 (osmolality)	£4.80
Nutrauxil (Kabi-Vitrum) (Also available Nutrauxil Sip Feed)	500 ml bottles × 4	No	Trace		Vanilla	76	68	276	2000	350 (osmolality)	£4.60
Flexical (Mead Johnson)	454 g can	× 1	Yes	Yes	Elemental	Unflavoured. orange, vanilla. fruit punch	45	68	308	2000	500 (osmolality) (normal dil.)	£9.36
Vivonex (Eaton Labs) (Also available Vivonex HN)	80 g sachet	× 6	Yes	Yes	Elemental preparation	No	38	2.6	408	1800	500	£7.82
Fortison Standard (Cow & Gate) (Also available 'Energy Plus', 'Low sodium' versions. 'Fortisip', 'Fortimel', suitable for 'sip' drinks)	500 ml	× 4	No	Trace		No	80	80	240	2000	260	£4.80
Fortison Soya	500 ml	× 4	No	Trace		No	80	80	240	2000	260	£5.00

an osmolality of 300 mosmol/kg. Diarrhoea is uncommon and related most frequently to antibiotic administration or uneven administration of nutrients. Lactose intolerance as a cause has been overstated.

The vitamin K content of Nutrauxil is rather high (0.1 mg phytomenadione per 100 ml feed) and the cost in 1988 was 38 p per g nitrogen. The requirement for warfarin is known to be increased with use of Isocal because of its vitamin K content (Watson *et al.*, 1984). High nitrogen Vivonex results in an increase in blood urea nitrogen compared with solid food and predigested protein in patients with malabsorption (Smith *et al.*, 1982). Elemental diets are effective in Crohn's disease in uncontrolled studies (O'Morian *et al.*, 1980).

Pump-assisted enteral feeding to ensure a better regulated delivery of the feed is indicated in a few patients with persistent diarrhoea and may obviate the need for TPN (Jones *et al.*, 1980). Whilst continuous feeding may be more comfortable for the patient and easier for nursing staff, it is metabolically less efficient than bolus feeding. Resting oxygen consumption is higher and nitrogen retention lower with continuous compared to bolus feeding. An undiluted hypertonic feed gives rise to better nitrogen balance for similar side-effects compared with an isotonic feed (Keohane *et al.*, 1984). Starter regimens may be abandoned also when elemental diets are administered nasogastrically over 24 hr (Rees *et al.*, 1985).

Recent intestinal perfusion studies suggest that small peptides are absorbed faster from the small intestine than equivalent AAs. There is some evidence that antacids in combination with enteral feeds precipitate, forming plugs which may lead to oesophageal obstruction. Similarly, Osmolite suspension solidifies at low pH (below 4) and had caused complete lower oesophageal obstruction which was very difficult to remove (Myo *et al.*, 1986). The trace element content of commercial enteral feeds may show a large discrepancy between levels stated by the manufacturers and those actually measured by analysis (Bunker & Clayton, 1983). Elemental diets consisting of free FAs, glucose, minerals and vitamins may result in essential FA deficiency with prolonged use, probably because of the low (1.3%) fat content.

Total parenteral nutrition (TPN)

Indications for TPN include: acute hypercatabolism (multiple trauma, burns, septicaemia), pyloric stenosis, pancreatitis, cardiac surgery, gastrointestinal cutaneous fistulae, imflammatory bowel disease, severe intra-abdominal sepsis after surgery, cancer surgery, cachexia. Figure 76.2 represents a guide to indications for TPN.

It should be remembered that if the gastrointestinal tract is functioning, oral or nasogastric supplements or full feeding is the nutritional method of choice. Many of the conditions requiring preoperative TPN need continued feeding into the postoperative period.

Pancreatitis

Where pancreatitis is prolonged, TPN keeps patients alive until pseudocysts can be drained surgically and oral nutrition commenced (Goodgame & Fischer, 1977).

Fistulae

In the presence of gastrointestinal cutaneous fistulae, TPN increases the spontaneous closure rate and reduces mortality (Sitges-Serra *et al.*, 1982). The output of the fistula probably decreases more rapidly with TPN compared with enteral nutrition. Long-term TPN results in closure of gastrointestinal fistulae in 70–80% of cases. There is preliminary evidence that somatostatin facilitates closure of persistent fistulae where TPN alone has failed (Costanzo *et al.*, 1982), although this is still contentious.

Inflammatory bowel disease

In the presence of inflammatory bowel disease there may be fewer postoperative complications and less extensive surgery may be required when preoperative TPN is used, and where disease extends beyond the superficial mucosal cells (Rombeau *et al.*, 1982). The benefits of TPN depend on the site of the disease. Where this is in the colon, intravenous feeding has little effect on the disease, but there are some advantages of TPN in acute exacerbations of Crohn's disease of the small gut (Dickinson *et al.*, 1980). 'Resting the gut' by the use of TPN, although it may maintain positive nitrogen balance, has an adverse effect on the gut, producing profound disuse atrophy (Williamson, 1983). Higher albumin concentrations lead to better healing of anastomoses (Daly *et al.*, 1972).

Total parenteral nutrition was used by Main *et al.* (1981) for 9 weeks to sustain pregnancy in a patient with Crohn's disease. Despite evidence of placental insufficiency at 36 weeks, the baby was normal.

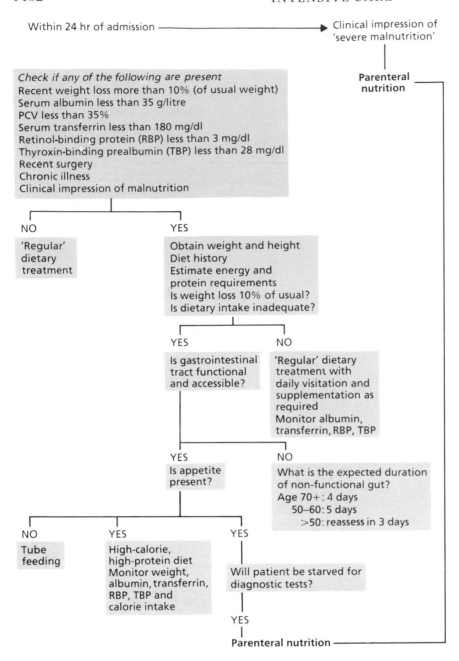

Within 24 hr of admission ⟶ Clinical impression of 'severe malnutrition'

Parenteral nutrition

Check if any of the following are present
Recent weight loss more than 10% (of usual weight)
Serum albumin less than 35 g/litre
PCV less than 35%
Serum transferrin less than 180 mg/dl
Retinol-binding protein (RBP) less than 3 mg/dl
Thyroxin-binding prealbumin (TBP) less than 28 mg/dl
Recent surgery
Chronic illness
Clinical impression of malnutrition

NO
'Regular' dietary treatment

YES
Obtain weight and height
Diet history
Estimate energy and protein requirements
Is weight loss 10% of usual?
Is dietary intake inadequate?

YES
Is gastrointestinal tract functional and accessible?

NO
'Regular' dietary treatment with daily visitation and supplementation as required
Monitor albumin, transferrin, RBP, TBP

YES
Is appetite present?

NO
What is the expected duration of non-functional gut?
Age 70+: 4 days
50–60: 5 days
>50: reassess in 3 days

NO
Tube feeding

YES
High-calorie, high-protein diet
Monitor weight, albumin, transferrin, RBP, TBP and calorie intake

YES
Will patient be starved for diagnostic tests?

YES
Parenteral nutrition

Fig. 76.2 Indications for total parenteral nutrition. (Redrawn from Matarese, 1973.)

Cardiac cachexia

Cardiac cachexia probably requires a prolonged period of preoperative nutritional support if postoperative mortality is to be improved.

Cancer

Many patients with cancer, especially those with gastrointestinal malignancies, are malnourished. Nutrition in the cancer patient has been reviewed by Dickerson (1984). Some patients show elevated resting energy expenditure, disturbances of carbohydrate metabolism and a failure to adapt to reduced food intake which is characteristic of cachexia. There is no firm evidence that preoperative TPN in cancer patients is of benefit. It may not prolong life although it may improve the quality of life, place patients in a satisfactory condition for specific antitumour therapy and reduce major postoperative complications although there is the concern that TPN stimulates tumour growth (Popp et al., 1983).

Muller et al. (1982) examined the influence of 10 days preoperative TPN in patients with gastrointestinal cancer. They found fewer major complications and reduced mortality in the TPN group compared with controls fed a regular ward diet. They attributed this to improvement of humoral and cellular immunocompetence and the protein status in the TPN group deterioration in the control group. The design of this study has been criticized; treated and control groups were matched badly, malnutrition ill-defined and no distinction was made between the malnourished and those with normal nutrition or between tumours at different sites. In a study of patients with gastric or oesophageal carcinoma, there was no reduction in the incidence of anastomotic leakage or death in patients receiving TPN preoperatively, except in those with a low albumin who had reduced incidence of wound infection and who would be expected to have poor healing and immunocompromise (Geefuysen et al., 1971). Meanwhile, pending further clarification, it is probably wise to reserve preoperative TPN for patients with oesophageal, gastric and pancreatic cancer only.

Other indications

Recent evidence suggests that nasogastric nutritional supplementation may accelerate growth and reduce the incidence and severity of complications in growth-retarded children with sickle-cell disease (Heyman et al., 1985). Nutritional support improves antibody response to influenza virus vaccine in the elderly (Chandra & Puri, 1985). Very thin patients with fractured neck of femur and a poor oral intake benefited from overnight supplementation by nasogastric tube in addition to daily normal ward diet. This manoeuvre reduced rehabilitation time and hospital stay without reducing voluntary oral food intake during the day (Bastow et al., 1983). The impact of preoperative nutritional support on perioperative mortality and morbidity remains controversial. Starker et al. (1986), seeking appropriate criteria for effective TPN, found that patients who failed to increase serum albumin after 1 week of TPN had a high morbidity and mortality. Their data suggested that TPN should not be given for a fixed time interval but instead the patient's response should be the indication for proceeding with elective surgery.

ASSESSMENT OF REQUIREMENTS FOR TOTAL PARENTERAL NUTRITION

A variety of techniques exist for investigating substrate metabolism in patients. These include indirect calori-

metry (Dauncey et al., 1978), substrate load tests, measurements of arteriovenous differences (Fick principle) and isotope infusions (Royle et al., 1981; Rennie, 1985).

The measurement of gas exchange, although seldom available clinically, can be useful for evaluation of the nutritional needs of hospitalized patients. If the resting respiratory quotient (RQ) is known, together with nitrogen excretion, the proportion of calorie requirements to nitrogen can be calculated.

Kinney developed a closed system with a rigid transparent head canopy and neck seal for determination of the metabolic state. This has proved a practical, non-invasive means of measuring gas exchange over a prolonged period in sick patients, but is less reliable in patients breathing high concentrations of oxygen (Gump et al., 1970b). This technique has been used by Askanazi et al., (1980) to determine the metabolic state in septic, injured and nutritionally depleted patients but it cannot be adapted readily to the patient with mechanically ventilated lungs. A fully automated instrument for measurement of oxygen consumption, carbon dioxide production and RQ in ventilated patients has been used for routine clinical evaluation of nutritional needs.

In critically ill, sedated patients with artificially ventilated lungs, total energy expenditure is only approximately 5% above REE, although this may increase to 18% during stressful procedures with a commensurate increase in carbon dioxide production (Weissman et al., 1986). Mann et al. (1985) pointed out that predicted metabolic requirements based on ideal body weight (1.75 REE) averaged 59% greater than metabolic expenditure measured by indirect calorimetry.

The recent development of the Siemens–Elema Servo Ventilator 900 series with attached carbon dioxide and oxygen analysers has been shown by Damask et al. (1982) to be accurate enough under a variety of conditions for continuous measurement of oxygen consumption and carbon dioxide production. However, such a system is clearly prone to error because of leakage. Measurement of energy requirements must be expressed as a function of body size. Measurement of total body energy expenditure in healthy subjects at rest represents a BMR of total cell mass of the body, which varies with age, sex and existing pathology. Body cell mass (BCM) is difficult to derive but correlates best with isotope measurements of potassium. Certain physiological states such as lactation seem to enhance metabolic efficiency (Illingworth *et al.*, 1986). In malnutrition, there is a loss of protein and BCM with water retention which expands extracellular volume. Smoking seems to increase total 24-hr energy expenditure by 10% without change in physical activity and mean BMR. This is associated with increased urinary excretion of noradrenaline and the effect is probably mediated therefore by the sympathetic nervous system (Hofsteller *et al.*, 1986). It may be that a reduction in energy expenditure occurs on stopping smoking with subsequent weight gain although other adaptive influences on body weight and variation in calorie intake have not been explored.

Our views of energy supply to patients requiring TPN have been modified greatly by the measurements made by MacFie (1984) who found the REE in uncomplicated convalescents to be only 10% greater than the preoperative state. More recent techniques using water double-labelled with deuterium and oxygen-18 and improved instrumentation for measuring isotope mass ratio gives accurate energy expenditure in normal mobile individuals and also gives carbon dioxide production. In patients with multiple injuries, REE increases to 10–30% over 2 weeks which correlates with a period of nitrogen excretion. The highest levels of nitrogen excretion are associated often with fever. The effect of various conditions on REE has been described by Elia *et al.* (1984) (Fig. 76.3).

In depleted and normal adults, nitrogen balance may be increased by increasing either nitrogen or energy intake, but depleted patients can only achieve a positive nitrogen balance at zero energy balance (Elwyn *et at.*, 1979). Where REE can be measured and repletion is required, the patient may be given 1.25–1.75 of daily REE for calorie requirements. Normal REE is approximately 115.5 kJ (27.5 kcal)/kg

daily. Measurements of REE do bear a relationship to free living conditions.

A nomogram is available for rapid measurement of metabolic requirements of patients with endotracheal tubes *in situ* (Smith *et al.*, 1984). This is accomplished by indirect calorimetry measuring mixed expired carbon dioxide tension, assuming an RQ of 0.8 and a leak-free circuit and that each litre of oxygen consumed by the body products 4.83 kcal at RQ 0.8.

Despite the limited evidence of reduced mortality and morbidity (Mullen *et al.*, 1980), nutritional support is used widely for patients in intensive therapy units (ITUs) (Woolfson, 1983). The aim is to give all nutrients required by the body in the appropriate proportion. A major dilemma at present is what is the most suitable energy substrate for which patient, the glucose versus fat controversy. The value of protein-sparing regimens in the postoperative period or specific AA therapy in various disease processes is unconfirmed.

Minimal technical detail is given here except where it is relevant to the complications.

Disturbances of water and electrolytes and severe hypoalbuminaemia should be corrected prior to starting TPN. Analgesia should be adequate and where it is considered appropriate the stress response obtunded. Peripheral vein infusion is possible if isotonic nutrients are used but usually this method cannot provide for the requirements of the critically ill. The author prefers a central line placed by the infraclavicular approach to the subclavian vein but interal jugular vein cannulation is associated with the highest rate of correct placement. LaSala *et al.* (1983) describe cannulation of the inferior vena cava via the saphenous system, tunnelling to mid-thigh level. Whichever route is used, the catheter should be inert and flexible, the best currently available being silicone coated.

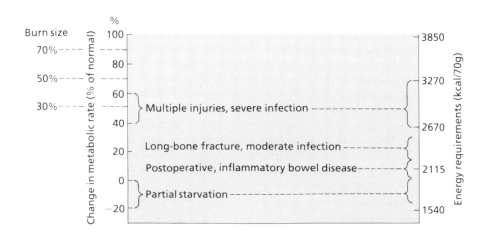

Fig. 76.3 Effects of various diseases on metabolic rate.

Administration of fluid requires either a volumetric infusion pump or less reliably a drop-rate counter. Volumetric infusion pumps, flow controllers or proportionating valves help to ensure continuous regulated flow rates. The Isoflux administration device includes an integral 15 μm filter to protect against plastic debris in TPN bags. A reduction in flow rate up to 22% occurs with addition of Multibionta and divalent cations.

GLUCOSE OR FAT AS ENERGY SUBSTRATE

Glucose is the most advantageous sugar for TPN although others may induce less hyperglycaemia. Most of the early work on the use of glucose as a calorie source was undertaken in the USA where at the time all fat emulsions were banned. Dudrick et al. (1969) showed that normal growth and nutrition could be maintained with glucose as the major calorie source. In Europe, Wretlind successfully introduced Intralipid as an energy substrate at an early stage (Hallberg et al., 1966). There are, however, still those who feel that Intralipid is useful solely to prevent FA deficiency and to replete fat stores, although this is done best by glucose. The main objections to the use of fat in the critically ill arose from the evidence of impaired fat utilization in this group of patients (Parodis et al., 1977). The increased insulin concentrations suppress fat mobilization. Some studies in humans, however, show increased fat clearance (Long et al., 1977) especially in hypermetabolic patients, and Askanazi et al. (1981, 1982) have shown that these patients can oxidize fat in spite of intravenous glucose administration.

Nitrogen balance is influenced by the amount of nitrogen in the diet, the metabolic rate and the quantity and source of non-protein energy. Elwyn et al. (1980) and others believe that glucose and Intralipid are equally effective in maintaining positive nitrogen balance. The relative advantages of each of these substrates depends in part on the patients. In depleted, non-catabolic patients, where protein intake is low or absent, fat administration has no effect on nitrogen excretion but carbohydrate reduces nitrogen loss. One hundred grams of carbohydrate are sufficient to replace gluconeogenesis from endogenous protein. When diet is adequate, isocaloric amounts of fat or glucose have equal nitrogen retention ability, although adaptation to the utilization of fat takes several days (Jeejeebuoy et al., 1976). In catabolic patients, carbohydrate is the main protein-sparing substrate (Long

et al., 1977), although 80% of energy requirements are derived from endogenous fat. Ketosis does not develop and endogenous protein continues to be broken down for gluconeogenesis. Under these circumstances, infused fat spares endogenous fat stores but not muscle protein. Addition of insulin to the glucose infusion improves protein sparing (Woolfson et al., 1979) and nitrogen balance although hypoalbuminaemia may result. A further advantage is that insulin enhances sodium-pump activity.

Administration of glucose in excess of an optimal $4 \text{ mg} \cdot \text{kg}^{-1} \cdot \text{min}^{-1}$, however, is harmful as it leads to increased carbon dioxide production and fat deposition in the liver (Burke et al., 1979). Energy cannot be lost from a biological system, so that where carbohydrate is given in excess of requirements, approximately 20% increases REE and 80% is converted to fat with RQ increasing to 7–9 (Elwyn et al., 1981). This is associated with an increase in plasma noradrenaline concentration suggesting that the increase in sympathetic response in the cause of the increased REE (Nordenstrom et al., 1981). Sympathetic-induced thermogeneis occurs also, constituting a further stress to the hypercatabolic injured patient. Increased carbon dioxide production leads to respiratory distress or failure in patients with compromised lung function. Oxygen consumption increases, particularly in hypercatabolic patients, and waste oxidation of FA occurs. This topic has been reviewed admirably by Robin et al. (1981) and Askanazi et al. (1982).

On balance, a mixed energy source which combines the advantages of each and obviates the disadvantages is recommended. An energy source of 50% Intralipid, 50% glucose is suitable for the majority of patients requiring TPN. Catabolic patients require at least 60% glucose. The hormonal profile of insulin suppression and elevation of the counteracting hormones glucagon, catecholamines and cortisol forms a strong theoretical basis for use of fat emulsion in the seriously ill population.

Glucose

Administration of the highly concentrated solutions required for TPN results in local venous complications and systemic problems due to hyperglycaemia and the hypertonic solution.

Fat

Intralipid is the most widely used fat source in this country. The particle size of this emulsion is in the same range as CMs but its structure differs as it contains no apoproteins or cholesterol. It is probably metabolized similarly to CMs or VLDLs by lipoprotein lipase and is removed by the reticuloendothelial system (RES).

No significant changes were detected in respiratory mechanics, oxygen consumption, carbon dioxide production, REE, liver function or nitrogen balance following the addition of 550 kcal lipid emulsion to glucose calories sufficient for energy requirements (Abbott et al., 1984).

Lipid emulsions in neonates and some adults can reduce Pao_2 and diffusing capacity. Pulmonary fat has been shown to accumulate in the lungs of preterm infants fed Intralipid in less than the recommended maximum dose (Levene et al., 1980). Intralipid may enhance also the risk of bacterial sepsis. The serum of some acutely ill patients agglutinates Intralipid. This reaction is thought to be produced by C-reactive protein in the presence of calcium ions. At postmortem, such patients showed evidence of microemboli which could have been a result of this agglutination. Intralipid should not therefore be given to such acutely ill patients. In rabbits with oleic acid-damaged lungs, Intralipid infusion increased pulmonary production of vasodilating prostaglandins and hypoxaemia. This effect was thought to be due to inhibition of pulmonary hypoxic vasoconstriction and the resultant increase in intrapulmonary right–left shunt.

In injured adult patients, an alternative, Lipofundin, did not produce any change in alveolar–arterial gradient. Lipofundin contains medium-chain triglycerides and when given to severely ill, malnourished patients receiving controlled mechanical ventilation of the lungs, it does not change arterial oxygen or carbon dioxide tensions, platelet or white cell count and does not activate complement.

Critically ill patients may have reduced intracellular carnitine content which might impair oxidation of long-chain FA. Further investigation is required to determine if carnitine should be added to the regimen or medium-chain FA substituted. Patients with carnitine deficiency are largely dependent on glucose for energy production.

Maintenance of nitrogen balance

Protein sparing

The effect of AA solutions after elective surgery has been found to prevent the malnutrition that develops in control patients (Shizgal et al., 1981). This effect is a result of AAs themselves and not avoidance of glucose (Greenberg et al., 1976). Some authorities recommend use of AA solutions in those patients who require nutritional support but may be expected to return to oral intake after a few days or in traumatized patients who may fail to absorb from the gastrointestinal tract for some time. Others believe this to be an expensive way of giving water or that this nitrogen sparing is no better than infusing an isocalorie amount of carbohydrate. Where nutrient intake must be limited, 10 g nitrogen and 1000 kcal total energy intake daily may provide optimal sparing of body cell mass. The minimal nitrogen requirement in normal people receiving adequate non-protein energy to achieve zero nitrogen balance is 0.1 g/kg daily.

Amino acid solutions

Total parenteral nutrition regimens require crystalline L-AA solutions as a nitrogen source. There is considerable controversy regarding the value of specific AAs in the synthetic crystalline AA mixtures available commercially, particularly those which contain high concentrations of glycine. Jackson and Golden (1980) suggest that glycine is catabolized to free ammonia rather than contributing useful nitrogen for transamination reactions. The limits of glycine turnover of 200 mg/kg daily are exceeded easily in some high nitrogen solutions available. Drug and Therapeutics Bulletin (1980) suggests the recosting of AA solutions excluding glycine. These solutions must contain sufficient concentrations of all essential AA. The optimal non-essential AA content of the diet is unknown but egg protein is taken as the standard (51% essential AAs).

There is a relationship between nitrogen intake and balance (Fig. 76.4) up to a certain point beyond which no further effect is seen, and this relationship holds whatever the amount of energy supplied, although a more positive nitrogen balance may be achieved by supplying energy in excess of metabolic requirements together with adequate nitrogen intake (Woolfson, 1979). Urinary nitrogen excretion in starvation depends also on the preceding nitrogen intake. Starved patients have a greater capacity for nitrogen retention than normal patients. Very few patients can tolerate more than 20 g nitrogen daily as such levels saturate the hepatic metabolic pathways resulting in deamination of AAs and increased urea production. Amino acid infusions increase minute ventilation, oxygen

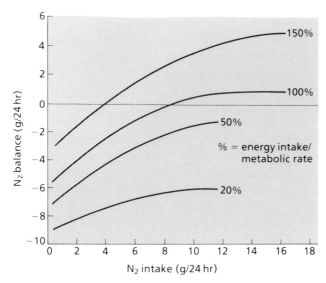

Fig. 76.4 Relationship between nitrogen balance and energy intake.

consumption and the response to hypoxia and hypercapnia. Increased ventilatory drive produced by increased protein intake may result in dyspnoea with increased rate and work of breathing (Burki, 1980).

LIVER DISEASE

In patients with cirrhosis, infusion of BCAAs may be beneficial (Vinnars, 1982), inducing a more positive nitrogen balance in the postoperative period than would a complete AA mixture. Patients with alcoholic hepatitis given 70–85 g of AA daily had an improvement in ascites, encephalopathy, plasma bilirubin and albumin compared with controls who were not given this supplement. Where this therapy was continued for 4 weeks, mortality rate decreased. In liver disease, aromatic AAs are not metabolized effectively and act as precursors for false neurotransmitters such as octopamine. Branched-chain amino acids are low. In encephalopathic patients, therapy to reduce gut uptake of glutamine or its conversion to ammonia may be useful.

RENAL DISEASE

Impending renal failure should not be a reason for withholding TPN. Instead, early dialysis should be used to control the metabolic state and allow room for feeding.

Nitrogen balance

Several means of improving nitrogen balance have been attempted. Remobilization is the best of these

(Booth & Gollnick, 1983). However, malnutrition produces an increase in intracellular calcium, and exercise, including physiotherapy, may further increase intracellular calcium and produce more ultrastructural damage unless accompanied by adequate nutritional repletion (Jeejeebuoy, 1985).

There is evidence in elderly patients that prevention of heat loss during and after surgery causes a significant decrease in muscle-protein degradation and nitrogen loss as measured by 3-methyl histidine excretion and urea nitrogen loss (Carli & Itiaba, 1986).

Leucine has some stimulatory effect on protein synthesis *in vitro*, and BCAAs were found by Cerra *et al.* (1983) to increase nitrogen retention in postoperative and multiple trauma patients. Freund and Fischer (1985) reported improved nitrogen balance in severely catabolic intensive-therapy patients with use of BCAA. Some visceral proteins improved, and insulin requirements decreased. A metabolite of leucine, α-ketoisocaproate, can reduce negative nitrogen balance and 3-methylhistidine excretion (Sapir *et al.*, 1983), although the usefulness of this latter parameter has been questioned (see above). This nitrogen sparing may be related to:

1 The increased ketosis, as KBs inhibit oxidation of BCAAs in muscle and their concentration is increased.
2 Decreased protein degradation, as plasma prealbumin and retinol-binding protein were lower;
3 An effect on liver protein turnover. The effect is unlikely to be a result of change in carbohydrate metabolism.

Prostaglandins are concerned with intracellular protein metabolism; it may therefore prove possible to reduce muscle protein breakdown with inhibitors of prostaglandin synthesis such as indomethacin (Rennie, 1984). Naftidrofuryl (Byrnes *et al.*, 1981; Jackson *et al.*, 1984), anabolic steroids, somatomedin and possibly proteinase inhibitors (Stracher, 1982) may also find a role in improving nitrogen balance.

Whole-body AA metabolism may be controlled by a carrier for glutamine isolated recently in rat muscle (Rennie *et al.*, 1986). These workers demonstrated a link between the size of the muscle glutamine pool and the rate of glutamine synthesis.

Complications of total parenteral nutrition

The complications associated with TPN may be summarized as: infective, metabolic and biochemical deficiencies, disorders of water, sodium and acid–base balance, jaundice, hypoalbuminaemia and technical complications. Many of these may occur also during enteral feeding.

INFECTION

Infection is a serious hazard of TPN, especially in the presence of invasive catheters, steroids and antibiotic-resistant, opportunistic organisms, and ranges from infusion phlebitis to suppurative mediastinitis and septicaemia. There is some evidence that surveillance skin cultures can identify those patients at high risk of infection, although this is controversial and stricter criteria for culture are required. The distinction between true infection and contamination is difficult (Collins et al., 1968). Catheter-associated infection may be reduced by the introduction of a 'control-of-infection team' giving proper education, advice and care, and filtration of the fluids may reduce infection also. Techniques and evaluation of tunnelling for this purpose have been reviewed by Peters (1982). Keohane et al. (1983) believe that tunnelling can reduce sepsis where nursing care is less than optimal, although these findings have been criticized on the basis of diagnosis of sepsis.

Broviac and Hickman catheters are useful for long-term TPN because of the low incidence of catheter blockage by fibrin and lipid. These catheters have a Dacron cuff at the catheter exit site. Fibrous tissue grows into this with fixation of the catheter. Indwelling intravascular catheters such as the Hickman become colonized with organisms readily giving rise to a positive blood culture with Gram-positive organisms. This is especially so in the immunocompromised patient, and whilst these organisms give rise to fever, they may produce no other clinical sequelae (Donnelly et al., 1985). Further confirmation and evaluation of this situation is required.

Some strains of coagulase-negative staphylococci seem able to survive cidal concentrations of certain antibiotics whilst adherent to polyvinyl chloride (PVC) catheters (Sheth et al., 1985).

HYPERGLYCAEMIA

Insulin therapy is required, ideally by continuous infusion using a dynamic scale. Insulin requirements vary throughout the day; the 'dawn phenomenon' of requirements increasing towards dawn is likely to be caused by a surge of GH at that time (Campbell et al., 1985). Haemodynamic effects of infusion of hyperos-molar glucose include expansion of blood volume, increase in stroke volume and reduction in pulmonary vascular resistance and wedge pressure.

METABOLIC BONE DISEASE

Severe bone pain may occur with marked disability in the presence of normal calcium, phosphate 25-hydroxyvitamin D_3 and parathyroid hormone. Bone biopsy may show osteomalacia, and hypercalciuria may occur, both of which resolved on discontinuing TPN. Hypercalcaemia may be precipitated by oliguria. The possibility remains that this is produced by administration of excessive phosphate (Allam et al., 1981).

DEFICIENCIES

Deficiency of any and every dietary component has been described; only a few important ones are included here.

Zinc deficiency

This may be overt or subclinical, and results partly from the low concentration of zinc in some TPN solutions and partly from the formation of Zn–AA complexes with histidine and cysteine which are excreted in the urine. The effects are delayed wound-healing and susceptibility to infection, diarrhoea, scaly rash and alopecia (Mozzillo et al., 1982). Zinc requirement is increased by diarrhoea and high fistula outputs (zinc concentration 12–17 mg/litre).

Phosphate depletion

This is common in postoperative patients especially when little blood has been transfused with phosphate in the anticoagulant solution. Hypophosphataemia is associated with diaphragmatic weakness and pulmonary insufficiency (Aubier et al., 1985) and CNS dysfunction resembling Guillain–Barré syndrome. In animals, acute hypophosphataemia occurring after weight loss and nutritional depletion produces rhabdomyolysis. Analysis of peripheral muscle shows accumulation of salt and water, loss of potassium and magnesium loss of and severe phosphorus loss with accumulation of calcium. Profound hypophosphataemia can mimic Wernicke's encephalopathy in alcoholics and simulate the clinical signs of brainstem death. Hypophosphataemic collapse has occurred after marathon running (0.32 mmol/litre) but appears to be transient (Dale et al., 1986).

Current replacement solutions are reviewed by Kingston et al. (1985). Iatrogenic hyperphosphataemia may occur (Chernow et al., 1981) accompanied by hypocalcaemia and hypomagnesiaemia; hence the importance of biochemical monitoring. Deficiency of magnesium alone is not uncommon.

Fatty acid depletion

Unless a fat emulsion is included in the regimen, essential FA deficiency is likely. This is most common in infants and presents as scaly dermatitis, alopecia, hepatomegaly, diminished skin pigmentation and fatty liver. Linoleic acid cannot be synthesized, and it is therefore recommended that 5–10% of calorie intake should be in the form of this essential FA. Deficiency cannot be prevented by topical application of corn oil. Stewart and Hensley (1981) describe four cases of acute polymyopathy associated with TPN which responded to discontinuation of the feeding regimen or intravenous lipid supplementation. In these cases, the aetiology was thought to be essential FA deficiency. Recent evidence has shown beneficial effects of polyunsaturated FAs found in fish. A diet rich in these FAs increased eicosapentaenoic acid content of neutrophils and monocytes and inhibited 5-lipo oxygenase pathways of arachidonic acid metabolism and leukotriene B_4-mediated inflammatory reactions (Lee et al., 1985). Dietary fish oils rich in $\Omega 3$-FAs reduced plasma lipid levels in normal patients and in those with hyperglyceridaemia. The negative association between fish consumption and mortality from coronary heart disease is still controversial. However $\Omega 3$-FAs are found in high concentration in purslane, a vegetable often used in soups and salads in Greece and Lebanon where such mortality is low. Fish oil contains the polyunsaturated FA eicosapentaenoate, and biosynthesis of thromboxanes (A_3) and prostacyclins (PGI_2) from this rather than the usual arachidonate may help to reduce the risk of atherosclerosis (Knapp et al., 1986). Fish oil may also reduce mild systolic hypertension (Norris et al., 1986). It seems likely that modification of fat supply will take place in future.

Taurine deficiency

Total parenteral nutrition does not contain taurine normally, and lack of this AA results in low blood concentrations and retinal dysfunction in children, which is reversed by adding taurine.

Vitamin E deficiency

Vitamin E deficiency presenting as spinocerebellar syndromes is a possibility.

INTRAHEPATIC CHOLESTASIS

This is not uncommon and may be related to intestinal overgrowth of anaerobic bacteria. The raised serum enzyme levels may be prevented by metronidazole (Capron et al., 1983).

THROMBOSIS AND EMBOLISM

Subclavian vein thrombosis occurs in an estimated 5–35% of catheters used for TPN. Heparin and filtration may reduce the incidence of phlebitis in peripheral infusions therefore, inclusion of heparin in the TPN solution is logical (Falchuk et al., 1985). A dose of 1000 unit/litre is recommended. This has the added advantage of activating lipoprotein lipase and enhancing fat clearance by speeding the hydrolysis of triglycerides. In patients receiving TPN, levels of antithrombin III are reduced. Intralipid has been incriminated in blockage of Hickman and Broviac catheters when mixed with all other nutrients for a prolonged period. This remains to be confirmed.

Catheter embolus is a serious complication which can occur also with tunnelled lines. Major complications such as cardiac perforation, pulmonary thrombosis and arrhythmia are likely if catheter emboli are not removed. Transvenous, non-surgical retrieval techniques are described. Paradoxical air embolus has been described also associated with a cracked filter attached to the central TPN feeding catheter. Cardiac tamponade produced by the central catheter is a potentially fatal complication.

Air embolus may be prevented by use of certain intravenous filters, although these do reduce the flow rate and cannot be used with fat emulsions.

Total parenteral nutrition in respiratory failure

The effects of TPN on oxygen consumption and carbon dioxide production have been discussed already. Diaphragmatic muscle fatigue occurs in malnutrition with onset of ventilatory failure (Rochester & Arora, 1983). The aim of feeding in respiratory failure is to improve respiratory muscle function and sensitivity of hypoxic drive, and TPN may allow earlier weaning (Bassili & Dietal, 1981). Ventilator-dependent patients who respond to nutritional support by increasing protein synthesis are more likely to wean from mechanical ventilation than those who do not (Larca & Greenbaum, 1982). Early in ventilatory failure, intercostal muscles may be depleted of high-energy phosphates with increase in lactate, whilst skeletal muscle values remain normal. Phosphate-binding antacids worsen the situation. Acute respiratory acidosis depresses glycolytic activity with an increase in plasma phosphate which is excreted subsequently in the urine. When pH is restored, hypophosphataemia occurs as phosphate shifts from blood into cells when glycolytic activity increases.

Total parenteral nutrition and drug administration

Antitumour drugs may have an effect on specific nutrients. Five-fluorouracil, perhaps in combination with other drugs, may produce thiamine deficiency. There is some evidence that this drug is tolerated better in patients receiving TPN.

A reduction in dietary protein is known to depress renal plasma flow and creatinine clearance. In normal subjects given oxypurinol, renal clearance of the drug was reduced by 64% after changing from high- to low-protein diet. This was produced by a large increase in net renal tubular reabsorption (Berlinger et al., 1985).

The effect of TPN regimens on oxidative drug metabolism has been highlighted recently by Vesell and Biebuyck (1984). It is known that diet can influence drug metabolism markedly (Pantuck et al., 1979). In a study of volunteers, a change from intravenous dextrose to AAs resulted in an increase in antipyrine metabolism. Patients receiving TPN may have a variety of other disturbances of organ blood flow and drug interaction to complicate the issue. However, it is wise to be cautious with administration of drugs to patients receiving TPN.

Planning the regimen

MacFie (1986) proposes that the cost of TPN may be reduced without compromising efficiency if we first ask: is TPN really necessary? What are the patient's actual requirements? What is the best way to administer them? Have we discussed it with the pharmacist?

There is little to choose between currently available TPN solutions, and it is not the intention to specify one regimen here. It is better for the prescriber to be familiar with a few regimens and understand the principles involved.

Some centres prefer a standard feeding regimen (Harper et al., 1983) which is very cost-effective and in this context, nutrition teams are valuable. However, most patients, and especially the critically ill, benefit

Table 76.15 Optimal calorie: nitrogen requirements. (From Woolfson, 1979)

	Starving	Catabolic	Hyper-catabolic
Nitrogen (g/24 hr) requirements for equilibrium	7.5	14	25
kcal (total including protein)	2000	3000	4000
Non-protein calorie: nitrogen ratio	250	200	135

Table 76.16 The composition of one ampoule of Solivito, Vitlipid and Addamel

Product	Ingredient	Quantity
Solivito	Vitamin B_1	1.2 mg
	Vitamin B_2	2.47 mg
	Nicotinamide	10 mg
	Vitamin B_6	2.46 mg
	Pantothenic acid	11 mg
	Biotin	0.3 mg
	Folic acid	0.2 mg
	Vitamin B_{12}	2 µg
	Vitamin C	34 mg
Vitlipid + glycine, Sodium Edetate and methyl hydroxy-benzoate	Retinol	75 µg (250 IU)
	Calciferol	3 µg (12 IU)
	Phytomenadione	150
	Fract. soybean oil	1000 mg
	Fract. egg phospholipids	120 mg
	Glycerol	225 mg
	NaOH to pH	8
Addamel	Calcium	5 mmol
	Magnesium	1.5 mmol
	Ferric iron	50 µmol
	Zinc	20 µmol
	Manganese	40 µmol
	Copper	5 µmol
	Fluoride	50 µmol
	Iodide	1 µmol
	Chloride	13.3 mmol

from an individually planned regimen (Kirkpatrick *et al.*, 1981). Computer programs exist which can be used at the bedside to predict individual nutritional requirements, facilitating appropriate treatment and often producing financial savings compared with administration of a standard feeding regimen to all patients (Colley *et al.*, 1985).

The factors determining design of an optimal regimen are considered elsewhere (Willatts, 1984). Although carbohydrate infusion has a progressive nitrogen-sparing effect, and nitrogen balance is related directly to calorie intake (Elwyn *et al.*, 1979), the increased negative nitrogen balance associated with severe surgical stress cannot be prevented completely (Radcliffe *et al.*, 1980).

The ideal non-protein:calorie ratio varies from 300:1 in starvation to 150:1 in hypercatabolic patients (Peters & Fischer, 1980). A scheme of optimal requirements is presented in Table 76.15.

Where fluid intake is restricted, a reasonable approach is to give as much protein as possible with a calorie:nitrogen ratio as low as possible with a mixed-fuel energy supply (Echenique *et al.*, 1982) as glucose alone is inclined to lead to more fluid retention than other energy substrates (Yeung *et al.*, 1979; MacFie *et al.*, 1981). Insulin is given by a separate

Table 76.17 Electrolyte, vitamin and trace element recommendations for patients receiving TPN

	Average patient	
Sodium	100–120 mmol/day (50–60 mmol/day in elderly and/or cardiopulmonary disease)	↑ with gastrointestinal losses by
Potassium	80–120 mmol/day	↓ with renal failure
Magnesium	12–15 mmol/day	↑ with gastrointestinal losses
Phosphorus	14–16 mmol/day	↓ when glucose alone is give ↓ with renal failure
Calcium	6.8–10 mmol/day	
Vitamin A	2500 IU/day	
Vitamin D	400 IU/day	
Vitamin E	50 IU/day (α-Tocopherol)	
Vitamin K	10 mg/week	
Thiamine	5 mg/day	
Riboflavin	5 mg/day	
Niacin	50 mg/day	
Pantothenic acid	15 mg/day	
Pyridoxine	5 mg/day	
Folic acid	5 mg/day	
Vitamin B_{12}	12 μg/day	
Vitamic C	300–500 mg/day	
Biotin	60 μg/day	
Iron	Men: 1 mg/day Women Premenopausal 2 mg/day Postmenopausal 1 mg/day	
Zinc	1 mg/day 2.5 mg/day when infusing amino acids + 12 mg/litre of small intestinal fluid loss + 17 mg/litre of stool loss	
Copper	0.3 mg/day 0.5 mg/day with diarrhoea None with abnormal liver function	
Chromium	10–20 μg/day	
Selenium	120 μg/day	
Iodine	120 μg/day	
Manganese*	0.2–0.8 mg/day None with abnormal liver function	

* No deficiency during TPN administration has been described in humans:

infusion at a rate determined by regular blood glucose estimation.

Ethanol is no longer included in TPN regimens as a result of adverse metabolic effects which include hypoglycaemia, increased blood concentrations of lactate, 3-hydroxybutyrate and free FAs, and reduced GH despite hypoglycaemia and raised cortisol.

The introduction of a 3-litre bag for infusion of a mixture of 24-hr nutritional requirement has proved popular. There seems to be no deterioration of AAs and glucose in this system nor changes in concentration of major electrolytes for up to 72 hr if the bags are refridgerated.

Vitamins and trace elements are less stable. Calcium may be precipitated if magnesium is low or pH high. If Intralipid is included in these mixtures, it causes a significant reduction in drop size of up to 40% depending on the concentration of the Intralipid or divalent cations, the amino acid solution and the presence of certain vitamin additives. Catheter occlusion with lipid material is beginning to be reported with the use of ethylvinyl acetate bags containing Intralipid and other nutrients, and there is a risk of leaching of plasticizers from PVC containers by fat emulsions.

The stability of parentrovite is limited in the presence of light to 6 hr.

The content of vitamin and trace element additives in common use is given in Table 76.16. Solivito contains insufficient folic acid so that supplementation (15 mg weekly) is required. Hypervitaminosis A may occur with exfoliative dermatitis and ectopic calcium deposition. The thiamine content of solivito seems inadequate to prevent deficiency (Anderson & Charles, 1985).

Recommended values for trace elements bear little relationship to clinical demands in the critically ill which are higher than in health. Table 76.17 gives electrolyte, vitamin and trace element recommendations for patients receiving TPN (Lemoyne & Jeejeebuoy, 1986).

If surgery is required in a patient receiving TPN, great care must be taken with the lines, to reduce the risk of sepsis. Different intravenous lines should be established for the perioperative period. The importance of perioperative maintenance of glucose homeostasis cannot be overemphasized.

Home parenteral nutrition is commonplace in the USA and practised by several centres in the UK. A register of cases has been set up and the service is likely to develop in a similar way to home dialysis. The main indications in the UK and Ireland are Crohn's disease, mesenteric vascular disease and extensive small bowel resection (Mughal & Irving, 1986). A dedicated unit with strict protocols is essential for success.

As malnutrition is corrected by feeding, the rate of restoration of body cell mass falls to zero at normal nutritional state. At this point, nitrogen balance never exceeds zero unless the individual is 'body building'. Planning individual TPN regimens and their cost-effectiveness may be aided by the use of computers.

Rational prescription of TPN in the critically ill must take into account multi-system dysfunction encountered in these circumstances. Knowledge of metabolic derangements in severe illness and attention to detail are outstandingly important.

References

Aarimaa M., Gyvalahati E., Viikari J. & Ovaska J. (1978) Insulin, growth hormone and catecholamines as regulators of energy metabolism in the course of surgery. *Acta Chirurgica Scandinavica* **144**, 411–22.

Abbott W.C., Grakauskas A.M., Bistrian B.R., Rose R. & Blackburn G.L. (1984) Metabolic and respiratory effects of continuous and discontinuous lipid infusions. *Archives of Surgery* **119**, 1367–71.

Allam B.F., Dryburgh F.J. & Shenkin A. (1981) Metabolic bone disease during parenteral nutrition. *Lancet* **1**, 385.

Allison S.P., Tomlin P.J. & Chamberlain M.J. (1969) Some effects of anaesthesia and surgery on carbohydrate and fat metabolism. *British Journal of Anaesthesia* **41**, 588–93.

Anderson S.H. & Charles T.J. (1985) Parenteral nutrition. *British Medical Journal* **291**, 1723–4.

Apelgren K.N., Rombeau J.L., Twomey P.L. & Miller R.A. (1982) Comparison of nutritional indices and outcome in critically ill patients. *Critical Care Medicine* **10**, 305–7.

Askanazi J., Carpentier Y.A., Elwyn D.H., Nordenstrom J., Jeejeevandam M., Rosenbaum S.H., Gump F.E. & Kinney J.M. (1980) Influence of total parenteral nutrition on fuel utilisation in injury and sepsis. *Annals of Surgery* **191**, 40–6.

Askanazi J., Nordenstrom J., Rosenbaum S.H., Elwyn D.H., Carpentier Y. & Kinney J.M. (1981) Nutrition for the patient with respiratory failure. *Anesthesiology* **54**, 373–7.

Askanazi J., Weissman C., Rosenbaum S.H., Hyman A.I., Milic-Emili J. & Kinney J.M. (1982) Nutrition and the respiratory system. *Critical Care Medicine* **10**, 163–72.

Aubier M., Murciano D., Lecoguic Y., Vüres N., Jaqueas Y., Squara P. & Pariente R. (1985) Effect of hypophosphataemia on diaphragmatic contractility in patients with acute respiratory failure. *New England Journal of Medicine* **313**, 420–4.

Baker J.P., Detsky A.S., Wesson D.E., Wolman S.J., Stewart S., Whitewell J., Langer B. & Jeejeebuoy K.N. (1982) Nutritional assessment. A comparison of clinical judgement and objective measurements. *New England Journal of Medicine* **306**, 969–72.

Baracos V., Rodemann P., Dinarello C.A. & Goldberg A.L. (1983) Stimulation of muscle protein degradation and prostaglandin E_2 release by leucocyte pyrogen (Interleukin-I). *New England Journal of Medicine* **308**, 553–8.

Bardosi L. & Tekeres M. (1985) Impaired metabolic activity of phagocytic cells after anaesthesia and surgery. *British Journal of Anaesthesia* 57, 520–3.

Bassili H.R. & Dietal M. (1981) Effect of nutritional support on weaning patients off mechanical ventilators. *Journal of Parenteral and Enteral Nutrition* 5, 161.

Bastow M.D., Raowlongs J. & Allison S.P. (1983) Benefits of supplementary tube feeding after fractured neck of femur: a randomised controlled trial. *British Medical Journal* 287, 1589–92.

Berlinger W.G., Park G.D. & Spector R. (1985) The effect of dietary protein on the clearance of allopurinol and oxypurinol. *New England Journal of Medicine* 313, 771–6.

Biebuyck J.L. (1981) Total parenteral nutrition in the perioperative period—a time for caution? *Anesthesiology* 54, 360–3.

Biebuyck J.L. (1983) Nutritional aspects of anaesthesia. *Clinics in Anesthesiology*. W.B. Saunders, London.

Birkhahn R.H., Long C.L., Fitkin D., Dyger J.W. & Blakemore W.S. (1980) Effects of major skeletal trauma on whole body protein turnover in man measured by L-^{14}C-leucine. *Surgery* 88, 294–9.

Bistrian B.R., Blackburn G.L., Hallowell E. & Heddle R. (1974) Protein status of general surgical patients. *Journal of the American Medical Association* 230, 858–60.

Boles J.M., Garre M.A., Youinou P.Y., Mialon P., Menez J.F., Jouquan J., Moissec P.J., Pennec Y. & LeMenn G. (1984) Nutritional status in intensive care patients: evaluation in 84 unselected patients. *Critical Care medicine* 11, 87–90.

Booth F.W. & Gollnick P.D. (1983) Effects of disuse on the structure and function of skeletal muscle. *Medicine and Science in Sports Exercise* 15, 415–20.

Boscoe M.J. & Rosin M.D. (1984) Fine bore enteral feeding and pulmonary aspiration. *British Medical Journal* 289, 1421–2.

Brandt M.R., Kehlet H., Skovsted L. & Hansen J.M. (1976) Rapid decrease in plasma tri-iodothyronine during surgery and epidural anaesthesia independent of afferent neurogenic stimuli and of cortisol. *Lancet* 2, 1333–6.

Briend A., Dykewicz C., Graven K. & Mazumder R.N. (1986) Usefulness of nutritional indices and classification in predicting death of malnourished children. *British Medical Journal* 293, 373–5.

Brough W., Horne E., Blount A., Irving M. & Jeejeebuoy K.N. (1986) Effects of nutrient intake, surgery, sepsis and long term administration of steroids on muscle function. *British Medical Journal* 293, 983–8.

Brown J. (1981) Enteral feeds and delivery systems. *British Journal of Hospital Medicine* 26, 168–75.

Brown R., Bancewicz J., Hamid J., Patel N.J. *et al.* (1982) Failure of delayed hypersensitivity skin testing to predict postoperative sepsis and mortality. *British Medical Journal* 284, 851–3.

Bunker V.W. & Clayton B.E. (1983) Trace element content of commercial enteral feeds. *Lancet* 2, 426–8.

Burke J.F., Wolfe R.R., Mullany C.J., Mathews D.E. & Bier D.M. (1979) Glucose requirements following burn injury. Parameters of optimal glucose infusion and possible hepatic and respiratory abnormalities following excessive glucose intake. *Annals of Surgery* 190, 274–85.

Burki N.K. (1980) Dyspnea in chronic airway obstruction. *Chest* 77 (Suppl.), 298.

Byrnes H.G.J., Galloway D.J. & Ledingham I.McA. (1981) Effect of naftidrofuryl on the metabolic response to surgery. *British Medical Journal* 283, 7–8.

Cahill G.F. jr. (1970) Starvation in man. *New England Journal of Medicine* 282, 668–75.

Campbell P.J., Bolli G.B., Cryer P.E. & Gerich J.E. (1985) Pathogenesis of the dawn phenomenon in patients with insulin dependent diabetes mellitus. *New England Journal of Medicine* 312, 1473–9.

Capron J-P., Gineston J-L., Herve M-A. & Braillon A. (1983) Metronidazole in prevention of cholestasis associated with parenteral nutrition. *Lancet* 1, 446–7.

Carli F. & Itiaba K. (1986) Effect of heat conservation during and after major abdominal surgery on muscle breakdown in elderly patients. *British Journal of Anaesthesia* 58, 502–7.

Cerra F.B., Mazuski J., Teasley K., Nuwer N. *et al.* (1983) Nitrogen retention in critically ill patients is proportional to the branched chain amino acid load. *Critical Care Medicine* 11, 775–8.

Chan S.T.F., McLaughlin S.J., Ponting G.A., Biglin J. & Dudley H.A.F. (1986) Muscle power after glucose–potassium loading in undernourished patients. *British Medical Journal* 293, 1055–6.

Chandra R.K. & Puri S. (1985) Nutritional support improves antibody response to influenza virus vaccine in the elderly. *British Medical Journal* 291, 705–6.

Chang R.W.S., Jacobs S. & Lee B. (1986) Use of Apache II severity of disease classification to identify intensive-care-unit patients who would not benefit from total parenteral nutrition. *Lancet* 1, 1483–7.

Chernow B., Rainey T.G., Georges L.P. & O'Brian J.T. (1981) Iatrogenic hyperphosphataemia: a metabolic consideration in critical care medicine. *Critical Care Medicine* 9, 772–4.

Colley C.M., Fleck A. & Howard J.P. (1985) Pocket computers; a new aid to nutritional support. *British Medical Journal* 290, 1403–6.

Collins R.N., Braun P.A., Zinner S.H. & Kass E.H. (1968) Risk of local and systemic infection with polythylene intravenous catheters: a prospective study of 1213 catheterisations. *New England Journal of Medicine* 279, 340–3.

Costanzo J.Di., Cano N. & Martin J. (1982) Somatostatin in persistent gastrointestinal fistula treated by total parenteral nutrition. *Lancet* 2, 338–9.

Cuthbertson D.P. & Tilstone W.J. (1969) metabolism during the post-injury period. *Advances in Clinical Chemistry* 12, 1.

Dale D., Fleetwood J.A., Inkster J.S. & Sainsbury J.R.C. (1986) Profound hyposphosphataemia in patients collapsing after a 'fun run'. *British Medical Journal* 292, 447–8.

Daly J.M., Dudrick S.J. & Copeland E.M. III (1979) Evaluation of nutritional indices and prognostic indicators in the cancer patient. *Cancer* 43, 925–31.

Daly J.M., Vars H.M. & Dudrick S.J. (1972) Effects of protein depletion on strength of colonic anastomoses. *Surgery, Gynecology and Obstetrics* 134, 15–21.

Damask M.C., Weissman C., Askanazi J., Hyman A.I., Rosenbaum S.H. & Kinney J.M. (1982) A systematic method for validation of gas exchange measurements. *Anesthesiology* 57, 213–18.

Dauncey M.J., Murgatroyd P.R. & Cole T.J. (1978) A human calorimeter for the direct and indirect measurement of 24 hour energy expenditure. *British Journal of Nutrition* 39, 587.

Dawson D. & Sear J.W. (1986) Influence of induction of anaesthesia with midazolam on the neuroendocrine response to surgery. *Anaesthesia* 41, 268–71.

Dickerson J.W.T. (1984) Nutrition in the cancer patient. *Journal of the Royal Society of Medicine* 77, 309–15.

Dickinson R.J., Ashton M.G. Axon A.T.R., Smith R.C., Yeung C.K. & Hill G.K., (1980) Controlled trial of intravenous hyperalimentation and total bowel rest as an adjunct to the routine therapy of acute colitis. *Gastroenterology* 79, 1199–204.

Donnelly J.P., Cohen J., Marcus R. & Guest J. (1985) Bacteraemia and Hickman catheters. *Lancet* 2, 48.

Drug and Therapeutics Bulletin (1980) 18, 85.

Dudrick S.J., Wilmore D.W., Vars H.M. & Rhoads J.E. (1969) Can intravenous feeding as the sole means of nutrition, support growth in a child and restore weight loss in an adult? *Annals of Surgery* **169**, 974.

Echenique M.M., Bistrian B.R. & Blackburn G.L. (1982) Theory and techniques of nutritional support in the ICU. *Critical Care Medicine* **10**, 546–9.

Elia M., Martin S. & Neale G. (1984) Effect of non-nutritional factors on muscle function tests. *Archives of Emergency Medicine* **1**, 175.

Elliott M.J. & Alberti K.G.M.M. (1983) The hormonal and metabolic response to surgery and trauma. In *New Aspects of Clinical Nutrition* (Eds Kleinberger G. & Deutsch E.) pp. 247–70. Karger, Basel.

Elwyn D.H. (1980) Nutritional requirements of adult surgical patients. *Critical Care Medicine* **8**, 9–20.

Elwyn D.H., Gump F.E., Munro H.M., Iles M. & Kinney J.M. (1979) Changes in nitrogen balance of depleted patients with increasing infusions of glucose. *Journal of Clinical Nutrition* **32**, 1597–1611.

Elwyn D.H., Kinney J.M. & Askanazi J. (1981) Energy expenditure in surgical patients. *Surgical Clinics of North America* **61**, 545–56.

Elwyn D.H., Kinney J.M., Gump F.E., Askanzi J., Rosenbaum M.H. & Carpentier Y.A. (1980) Some metabolic effects of fat infusions in depleted patients. *Metabolism* **29**, 125.

Engquist A., Brandt M.R., Fernandes A. & Kehlet H. (1977) The blocking effect of epidural analgesia on the adrenocortical and hyperglycaemia responses to surgery. *Acta Anaesthesiologica Scandinavica* **21**, 330–3.

Falchuk K.H., Peterson L. & McNeil B.J. (1985) Microparticulate-induced phlebitis: its prevention by in-line filtration. *New England Journal of Medicine* **312**, 78–82.

Forse R.A. & Shizgal H.M. (1980) The assessment of malnutrition. *Surgery* **88**, 17–24.

Freund H.R. & Fischer J.E. (1985) The use of branched chain amino acids in injury and sepsis. In *Proceedings of the 4th World Congress on Intensive and Critical Care Medicine* pp. 177–80. King & Winth Publishing Co., London.

Geefuysen J., Rosen E.V., Katz J., Ipp T. Metz J. (1971) Impaired cellular immunity in kwashiorkor with improvement after therapy. *British Medical Journal* **iv**, 527–9.

Geggel H.S., Ament M.E., Heckenlively J.R., Martin D.A. *et al.* (1985) Nutritional requirements for taurine in patients receiving long term parenteral nutrition. *New England Journal of Medicine* **312**, 142–6.

Glaeser B.S., Maher T.J. & Wurtman R.J. (1983) Changes in brain levels of acidic, basic and neutral amino acids after consumption of single meals containing various proportions of protein. *Journal of Neurochemistry* **41**, 1001.

Goode A.W., Herring A.N., Orr J.S. Ratcliffe W.A. & Dudley H.A.F. (1981) The effect of surgery with carbohydrate infusion on circulating tri-iodothyronine and reverse tri-iodothyronine. *Annals of the Royal College of Surgeons* **63**, 168–72.

Goodgame J.T. & Fischer J.E. (1977) Parenteral nutrition in the treatment of acute pancreatitis: effect on complications and mortality. *Annals of Surgery* **186**, 651–8.

Greenberg G.R., Marliss E.B., Anderson G.H., Langer B., Spence W., Tovee E.B. & Jeejeebuoy K.N. (1976) Protein sparing therapy in post-operative patients. *New England Journal of Medicine* **294**, 1141–6.

Gump F.E., Kinney J.M. & Price J.B. (1970a) Energy metabolism in surgical patients: oxygen consumption and blood flow. *Journal of Surgical Research* **10**, 613–27.

Gump F.E., Price J.B. & Kinney J.M. (1970b) Whole body and splanchnic blood flow and oxygen consumption measurements in patients with intraperitoneal infection. *Annals of Surgery* **171**, 321.

Hallberg D., Schubert O. & Wretlind A. (1966) Experimental and clinical studies with fat emulsion for intravenous nutrition. *Nutritio Dieta* **8**, 245.

Harper P.H., Royle G.T., Michell A., Greenall M.J., Grant A., Winsley B., Atkins S.M., Todd E.M. & Kettlewell M.G.W. (1983) Total parenteral nutrition: value of standard regime. *British Medical Journal* **286**, 1323–7.

Heyman M.B., Vichinsky, E., Katz R., Gaffield B., Castillo R., Kleman K., Thaler M.M., Lubin B., Hurst D., Chin D. & Ammann A.J. (1985) Growth retardation in sickle cell disease treated by nutritional support. *Lancet* **1**, 903–6.

Himms-Hagen J. (1984) Thermogenesis in brown adipose tissue as an energy buffer: implications for obesity. *New England Journal of Medicine* **311**, 1549–58.

Hjortso N-C., Christensen N.J., Andersen J. & Kehlet H. (1985) Effects of the extradural administration of local anaesthetic agents and morphine on the urinary excretion of cortisol, catecholamines and nitrogen following abdominal surgery. *British Journal of Anaesthesia* **57**, 400–6.

Hofsteller A., Schutz Y., Jequier E. & Wahren J. (1986) Increased 24 hour energy expenditure in cigarette smokers. *New England Journal of Medicine* **314**, 79–82.

Hulton N., Johnson D.J., Smith R.J. & Wilmore D.W. (1985) Hormonal blockade modifies post-trauma protein catabolism. *Journal of Surgical Research* **39**, 310–5.

Illingworth P.J., Jung R.T., Howie P.W., Leslie P. & Isles T.E. (1986) Diminution of energy expenditure during lactation. *British Medical Journal* **292**, 437–41.

Irvin T.T. (1978) Effects of malnutrition and hyperalimentation on wound healing. *Surgery, Gynecology and Obstetrics* **146**, 33–7.

Jackson A.A. & Golden M.H.N. (1980) N;s15;t glycine metabolism in normal man: the metabolic beta-amino nitrogen pool. *Clinical Science* **58**, 517–22.

Jackson J.M., Khawaja H.T., Weaver P.C., Talbot S.T. & Lee H.A. (1984) Naftidrofuryl on the metabolic response to surgery. *British Medical Journal* **289**, 581–4.

Jeejeebuoy K.N. (1985) Changes in body composition and muscle function and effect of nutritional support. *Proceedings of 4th World Congress on Intensive and Critical Care Medicine* pp. 161–4. King & Winth Publishing Co., London.

JeeJeebuoy K.N., Anderson G.H., Nakhooda A.F., Greenberg G.R., Sanderson I. & Marliss E.B. (1976) Metabolic studies in total parenteral nutrition. *Journal of Clinical Investigation* **57**, 125.

JeeJeebuoy K.N., Baker J.P., Wolman S.L., Wesson D.E., Langer B., Harrison J.E. & McNeill K.G. (1982) Critical evaluation of the role of clinical assessment and body composition studies in patients with malnutrition and after total parenteral nutrition. *American Journal of Clinical Nutrition* **35**, 1117–27.

Jones B.J.M., Payne S. & Silk D.B.A. (1980) Indications for pump-assisted enteral feeding. *Lancet* **i**, 1057–8.

Keohane P.P., Attrill H., Love M., Frost P. & Silk D.B.A. (1984) Relation between osmolality of diet and gastrointestinal side effects in enteral nutrition. *British Medical Journal* **288**, 678–80.

Keohane P.P., Jones B.J.M., Attrill H., Cribb A., Northover J., Frost P. & Silk D.B.A. (1983) Effect of catheter tunnelling and a nutrition nurse on catheter sepsis during parenteral nutrition. *Lancet* **2**, 1388–90.

Kingston M.R., Badawi Al. & Siba M. (1985) Treatment of severe hypophosphataemia. *Critical Care Medicine* **13**, 16–18.

Kinney J.M. & Hessov I.B. (1981) Protein energy malnutrition. In *Nutrition and the Surgical Patient* (Ed. Hill G.L) pp. 12–25. Churchill Livingstone, Edinburgh.

Kirkpatrick J.R., Dahn M.S. & Lewis L. (1981) Selective versus standard hyperalimentation, a randomised prospective study. *American Journal of Surgery* **141**, 116.

Klidjian A.M., Foster K.J., Kammerling R.M., Cooper A. & Karran S.J. (1980) Relation of anthropometric and dynamometric variables to serious postoperative complications. *British Medical Journal* **281**, 899–901.

Knapp H.R., Reilly I.A.G., Alessandrini P. & Fitzgerald G.A. (1986) *In vivo* indices of platelet and vascular function during fish oil administration in patients with atherosclerosis. *New England Journal of Medicine* **314**, 937–42.

Knaus W.A., Draper E.A., Wagner D.P. & Zimmerman J.E. (1985) A severity of disease classification system. *Critical Care Medicine* **13**, 818–29.

Larca I. & Greenbaum D.M. (1982) Effectiveness of intensive nutritional regimes in patients who fail to wean from mechanical ventilation. *Critical Care Medicine* **10**, 297–300.

LaSala P.A., Starker P.M. & Askanazi J. (1983) The saphenous system for long-term parenteral nutrition. *Critical Care Medicine* **11**, 378–80.

Lawson L.J. (1965) Parenteral nutrition in surgery. *British Journal of Surgery* **52**, 795–800.

Lee T.H., Hoover R.L., Williams J.D., Sperling R.I., Revalese J. III, Spur B.W., Robinson D.R., Corey E.J., Lems R.A. & Austen K.F. (1985) Effect of dietary enrichment with eicosapentaenoic and docosahexanenoic acids on *in vitro* neutrophil and monocyte leukotriene generation and neutrophil function. *New England Journal of Medicine* **312**, 1217–24.

Lemoyne M. & Jeejeebuoy K.N. (1986) Total parenteral nutrition in the critically ill patient. *Chest* **89**, 568–75.

Levene M.I., Wigglesworth J.S. & Desai R. (1980) Pulmonary fat accumulation in the preterm infant. *Lancet* **2**, 815–9.

Long J.M., Wilmore D.W., Mason A.D. & Pruitt B.A. (1977) Effect of carbohydrate and fat intake on nitrogen excretion during total intravenous feeding. *Annals of Surgery* **185**, 417.

Lowry S.F., Horowitz G.D., Jeevanandam M., Legaspi A. & Brennan M.F. (1985) Whole body protein breakdown and 3-methylhistidine excretion during brief fasting, starvation and intravenous repletion in man. *Annals of Surgery* **202**, 21–7.

MacFie J. (1984) Energy requirements of surgical patients during intravenous nutrition. *Annals of the Royal College of Surgeons of England* **66**, 39–42.

MacFie J. (1986) Towards cheaper intravenous nutrition. *British Medical Journal* **292**, 107–10.

MacFie J., Smith R.C. & Hill G.L. (1981) Glucose or fat as non-protein energy source? A controlled clinical trial in gastroenterologic patients receiving intravenous nutrition. *Gastroenterology* **80**, 103–7.

Main A.N.H., Shenkin A., Black W.P. & Russell R.I. (1981) Intravenous feeding to sustain pregnancy in patient with Crohn's disease. *British Medical Journal* **283**, 1221–2

Mann S., Westenstow D.R. & Houtchens B.A. (1985) Measured and predicted calorie expenditure in the acutely ill. *Critical Care Medicine* **13**, 173–7.

Marton K.I., Sox H.C. jr. & Krupp J.R. (1981) Involuntary weight loss: diagnostic and prognostic significance. *Annals of Internal Medicine* **95**, 568–74

Matarese L. (1973) Algorithm for nutritional support. In *Clinics in Anesthesiology*, vol.1, number 3, p. 583. W.B. Saunders, London.

Mozzillo N., Ayala F. & Federici G. (1982) Zinc deficiency syndrome in patient on long term total parenteral nutrition. *Lancet* **1**, 744.

Mughal M. & Irvin M. (1986) Home parenteral nutrition in the United Kingdom and Ireland. *Lancet* **2**, 383–7.

Mullen J.L., Busby G.P., Matthews D.C., Small R.F. & Risarto E.G. (1980) Reduction of operative mortality by combined preoperative and post-operative nutritional support. *British Journal of Surgery* **66**, 893–6.

Müller J.M., Dienst C., Brenner U. & Pichlmaier H. (1982) Preoperative parenteral nutrition in patients with gastrointestinal carcinoma. *Lancet* **1**, 68–71.

Myo A., Nichols P., Rosin M., Bryant G.D.R. & Peterson L.M. (1986) An unusual oesophageal obstruction during nasogastric feeding. *British Medical Journal* **293**, 596–7.

Nakao K. & Miyata M. (1977) The influence of phentolamine, an alpha-adrenergic blocking agent, on insulin secretion during surgery. *European Journal of Clinical Investigation* **7**, 41–5.

Newham D.J. (1986) Nutritional status and skeletal muscle activity. *British Journal of Parenteral Therapy* **7**, 93–6.

Nordenstrom J., Jeevanandam M., Elwyn D.H., Carpentier Y.A., Astanazi J., Robin A. & Kinney J.M. (1981) Increasing glucose intake during total parenteral nutrition increases norepinephrine excretion in trauma and sepsis. *Clinical Physiology* **1**, 525–84.

Norris P.G., Jones C.J-H. & Weston M.J. (1986) Effect of dietary supplementation with fish oil on systolic blood pressure in mild essential hypertension. *British Medical Journal* **293**, 104–6.

O'Morian C., Segal A.W. & Levi A.J. (1980) Elemental diets in the treatment of Crohn's disease. *British Medical Journal* **281**, 1173–5.

Pantuck E.J., Pantuck C.B., Garland W.A., Min B.H. & Conney A.H. (1979) Stimulatory effects of brussel sprouts and cabbage on human drug metabolism. *Clinical Pharmacology and Therapeutics* **25**, 88–95.

Pantuck E.J., Pantuck C.B., Weissman C., Askanazi J. *et al.* (1984) Effects of parenteral nutrition regimes on oxidative drug metabolism. *Anesthesiology* **60**, 534–6.

Pardridge W.M. (1983) Brain metabolism: a perspective from the blood brain barrier. *Physiological Reviews* **63**, 1481.

Parodis C., Spanies A.H., Calder M. & Shizgal H.M. (1977) Total parenteral nutrition with lipid. *American Journal of Surgery* **135**, 164.

Peters C.P. & Fischer J.E. (1980) Studies in calorie to nitrogen ratio for total parenteral nutrition. *Surgery, Gynecology and Obstetrics* **151**, 1–8.

Peters J.L. (1982) The evolution of tunnelling techniques for central venous catheters. *British Journal of Parenteral Therapy* **3**, 21–30.

Pettigrew R.A. & Hill G.L. (1986) Indicators of surgical risk and clinical judgement. *British Journal of Surgery* **73**, 47–51.

Phillipson B.E., Rothrock D.W., Connor W.E., Harris W.S. & Illingworth D.R. (1985) Reduction of plasma lipids, lipoproteins and apoproteins by dietary fish oils in patients with hypertriglyceridemia. *New England Journal of Medicine* **312**, 1210–6.

Popp M.B., Wagner S. & Brito O.J. (1983) Host and tumour responses to increasing levels of intravenous nutritional support. *Surgery* **94**, 300–8.

Porte D. & Robertson R.P. (1975) Control of insulin secretion by catecholamines, stress and the sympathetic nervous system. *Federation Proceedings* **32**, 1792.

Prentice A.M., Black A.E., Coward W.A., Davies H.L., Goldberg G.R., Murgatroyd P.R., Ashford J., Sawyer M. & Whitehead D.G. (1986) High level of energy expenditure in obese women. *British Medical Journal* **292**, 983–7.

Radcliffe A., Johnson A. & Dudley H.A.F. (1980) The effect of different calorific doses of carbohydrate on nitrogen excretion after surgery. *British Journal of Surgery* 67, 462–3.

Reeds P.J. & James W.P.T. (1983) Protein turnover. *Lancet* 1, 571–4.

Rees R.G.P., Keohane P.P., Grimble G.K., Frost P.G., Attrill & Silk D.B. (1985) Tolerance of elemental diet administered without starter regimen. *British Medical Journal* 290, 1869–70.

Rennie M.J. (1984) The role of prostaglandins in the control of lean tissue mass. *British Journal of Parenteral Therapy* 5, 51–4.

Rennie M.J. (1985) The doubly labelled water method. *British Journal of Parenteral Therapy* 6, 90–4.

Rennie M.J., Babij P., Taylor P.M., Hindal H.S., Jepson M.M., MacLellan P., Uatt D.W. & Millward D.J. (1986) Characteristics of a glutamine carrier in skeletal muscle have important consequences for nitrogen loss in injury, infection and chronic disease. *Lancet* 2, 1008–12.

Rennie M.J. & Harrison R. (1984) Effects of injury, disease and malnutrition on protein metabolism in man. *Lancet* 1, 323–5.

Rennie M.J. & Millward D.J. (1983) 3-Methylhistidine excretion and the urinary 3-methylhistidine/creatinine ratio are poor indicators of skeletal muscle protein breakdown. *Clinical Science* 65, 217–25.

Robin A.P., Askanazi J., Cooperman A., Carpentier Y.A., Elwyn D.H. & Kinney J.M. (1981) Influence of hypercalorie glucose infusions on fuel economy in surgical patients. *Critical Care Medicine* 9, 680–6.

Rochester D.F. & Arora N.S. (1983) Respiratory muscle failure. *Medical Clinics of North America* 67, 573–97.

Rombeau J.L., Barot R.L., Williamson C.E. & Mullen J.L. (1982) Preoperative total parenteral nutrition and surgical outcome in patients with inflammatory bowel disease. *American Journal of Surgery* 143, 139–43.

Royle G.T., Wolfe R.R. & Burke J.F. (1981) Techniques of investigating substrate metabolism in man. *Annals of the Royal College of Surgeons of England* 63, 413–9.

Russel D.M., Leiter L.A., Whitwell J., Marliss E.B. & Jeejeebuoy K.N. (1983) Skeletal muscle function during hypocalorie diets and fasting: a comparison with standard nutritional assessment parameters. *American Journal of Clinical Nutrition* 37, 133–8.

Ryan N.T. (1976) Metabolic adaptations for energy production during trauma and sepsis. *Surgical Clinics of North America* 56, 1073.

Ryan J.A. jr. & Taft D.A. (1980) Preoperative nutritional assessment does not predict morbidity and mortality in abdominal operations. *Surgical Forum* 31, 96–8.

Sapir D.G., Stewart P.M., Walser M., Moreadith C., Moyer E.D., Imbembo A.L., Rosenstein M.B. & Munoz S. (1983) Effects of alpha ketoisocaproate and of leucine on nitrogen metabolism in postoperative patients. *Lancet* 1, 1010–14.

Shakir A. & Morley D. (1974) Measuring malnutrition. *Lancet* 1, 758–9.

Sheth N.K., Franson T.R. & Sohnle P.G. (1985) Influence of bacterial adherence to intravascular catheters on *in vitro* antibiotic sensitivity. *Lancet* 2, 1266–8.

Shizgal H.M. (1981) Nutrition and the immune function. *Surgery Annual* 12, 15–29.

Sibbald W.J., Short A., Cohen M.P. & Wilson R.F. (1977) Variations in adrenocortical responsiveness during severe bacterial infections. *Annals of Surgery* 186, 29–33.

Sitges-Serra A., Jaurrieta E. & Sitges-Creus A. (1982) Management of postoperative enterocutaneous fistulas: the roles of parenteral nutrition and surgery. *British Journal of Surgery* 69, 147–50.

Smith J.L., Arteaga C. & Heymsfield S.B. (1982) Increased ureagenesis and impaired nitrogen use during infusion of a synthetic aminoacid formula. *New England Journal of Medicine* 306, 1013–8.

Smith H.S., Kennedy D.J. & Park G.R. (1984) A nomogram for rapid measurement of metabolic requirements of intubated patients. *Intensive Care Medicine* 10, 147–8.

Starker P.M., LaSala P.A., Askanazi J., Todd G. *et al.* (1986) The influence of total parenteral nutrition upon morbidity and mortality. *Surgery, Gynecology and Obstetrics* 162, 569–74.

Stewart P.M. & Hensley W.J. (1981) Acute polymyopathy during total parenteral nutrition. *British Medical Journal* 283, 1578.

Stoner H.B., Frayn K.N., Barton R.N., Thretfall C.I. & Little R.A. (1979) The relationship between plasma substrates and hormones and the severity of injury in 277 recently injured patients. *Clinical Science* 56, 563–73.

Stracher A. (1982) Proteinase inhibitors and muscle degradation. *Muscle and Nerve* 5, 494.

Studley H.O. (1936) Percentage of weight loss. A basic indicator of surgical risk in patients with chronic peptic ulcer. *Journal of the American Medical Association* 106, 458–60.

Thomas R., Aihawa N. & Burke J.F. (1979) Insulin resistance in peripheral tissues after burn injury. *Surgery* 86, 742.

Vessell E.S. & Biebuyck J.F. (1984) New approaches to assessment of drug disposition in the surgical patient. *Anesthesiology* 60, 529–32.

Vinnars E. (1982) Surgical trauma: conventional or special amino-acid solutions for parenteral nutrition. In *New Aspects of Clinical Nutrition* (Ed. Kleinberger G. & Deutsch E.) pp. 422–7. Karger, Basel.

Watson A.J.M., Pegg M & Green J.R.B. (1984) Enteral feeds may antagonise warfarin. *British Medical Journal* 288, 557.

Weissman C., Kemper M., Elwyn D.H., Askanazi J., Hyman A.I. & Kinney J.M. (1986) The energy expenditure of the mechanically ventilated critically ill patient. An analysis. *Chest* 89, 254–9.

Willatts S.M. (1984) Design of an optimal parenteral nutrition regime. *British Journal of Parenteral Therapy* 5, 117–23.

Williamson R.C.N. (1983) Effect of nutrition on the gut. *British Journal of Parenteral Therapy* 4, 35–8.

Wilmore D.W., Goodwin C.W., Aulick L.H., Powanda M.C., Mason A.D. & Pruitt B.A. (1980) Effect of injury on infection metabolism and circulation. *Annals of Surgery* 192, 492–504. visceral metabolism and circulation. *Annals of Surgery* 192,

Woolfe, B.M., Culebras J.M., Aoki T.T., O'Connor N.E., Finley R.J., Kaczowka A. & Moore F.D. (1979) The effects of glucagon on protein metabolism in normal man. *Surgery* 86, 248.

Woolfson A.M.J. (1979) Metabolic considerations in nutritional support. *Research and Clinical Forums* 1, 35–47.

Woolfson A.M.J. (1983) Artificial nutrition in hospital. *British Medical Journal* 287, 1004–6.

Woolfson A.M.J., Heatley R.V. & Allison S.P. (1979) Insulin to inhibit protein catabolism after injury. *New England Journal of Medicine* 300, 14.

Yeung C.K., Smith R.C. & Hill G.L. (1979) Effect of an elemental diet on body composition. *Gastroenterology* 77, 652–7.

77

Neurological Disease

L. LOH

Although there are numerous neurological diseases which may require intensive therapy management, the clinical problems which they present are often similar and fall generally into two main groups:

1 Patients in coma or with disorders of consciousness needing special nursing care, monitoring and protection of the airways.

2 Patients with impending or established ventilatory failure requiring close observation and perhaps artificial ventilation. Ventilatory failure may be an acute or chronic condition and may be central, arising from damage to the neural control of breathing, or peripheral as a result of respiratory muscle weakness.

Before specific neurological disorders are discussed, some preliminary comments are necessary on the anatomy of coma and the neural control of respiration. It is hoped that this will help in the assessment and management of disorders similar to those few illustrated in this chapter.

Coma

Consciousness is a state of awareness, both of self and the environment and this is demonstrated usually by voluntary and purposeful behaviour and speech in response to both internal and external stimuli. Coma is a sleep-like state in which the subject lies with eyes closed but it is distinguished from sleep as the subject cannot be roused by strong external stimulation. Coma is the converse of consciousness and may be defined in its simplest terms as an absence of awareness of self and environment.

The causes of coma generally involve either widespread dysfunction of both the cerebral hemispheres, as occurs in metabolic brain disease and hypoxic brain damage, or localized disruption of the ascending reticular activating system (ARAS) in the upper mid-brain by external compression or an intrinsic lesion of the brainstem (Plum & Posner, 1980). It is important to stress the key role of the ARAS in the maintenance of consciousness.

The ARAS is composed of a diffuse core of neurons extending from the medulla to the upper mid-brain. The main ascending pathway is the central tegmental tract which receives afferent signals from all areas of the brainstem and thalamus and projects to all areas of the cerebral cortex. A lesion of the upper mid-brain which disconnects the ARAS from the cortex, produces a state of coma; in experimental preparations it may be shown that such a lesion causes an EEG (electro-encephalogram) pattern similar to that of coma, whereas stimulation of this area may produce an awake-looking EEG (Bremer, 1937; Moruzzi & Magoun, 1949). A functioning ARAS is essential for awareness, and presumably anaesthetics act primarily on the ARAS to produce unconsciousness.

The ARAS is related very closely anatomically to the brainstem nuclei. Brainstem death is essentially death of the ARAS and recognized indirectly by the cessation of function of the cranial nerve nuclei with which it is intimately connected.

Coma is not a disease in itself but the expression of an underlying disorder of the nervous system. Table 77.1 classifies the causes of coma into three main groups:

1 Diseases which involve a widespread disorder of both cerebral hemispheres but where the brainstem function remains intact and there are no signs of focal neural damage. With intoxication, metabolic disturbance or hypothermia, there is usually extensive reduction of neuronal activity and cerebral metabolic rate. Epilepsy produces unconsciousness if it has spread to both hemispheres or has involved the diencephalon and interrupted transmission from the ARAS. In this

Table 77.1 Causes of coma

Disorders of cortical function with no focal signs
Intoxications
Alcohol, barbiturates, opioids, etc.
Metabolic disturbances
Anoxia, uraemia, hepatic coma, hypo- and
hyperglycaemia
Severe systemic infection
Pneumonia, typhoid, malaria, septicaemia
Cerebral ischaemia
Epilepsy
Hypo- and hyperthermia
Hypertensive encephalopathy
Concussion

Diseases with meningeal irritation
Subarachnoid haemorrhage, ruptured aneurysm,
arteriovenous malformation, trauma
Acute bacterial meningitis
Aseptic meningitis, viral meningitis

*Diseases causing focal brainstem or lateralizing cerebral
signs*
Brain haemorrhage
Brain infarction
Brain abscess
Brain tumour
Encephalitis
Cerebral thrombophlebitis

group of disorders, the computerized tomography (CT) scan is often normal and so is the cerebrospinal fluid (CSF). Often, the patients pass through various states of altered consciousness with drowsiness, confusion and stupor, both as the disease develops and during recovery. Sometimes the disease progresses to involve mid-brain and more caudal structures either by direct extension of the disease process or through cerebral swelling causing tentorial herniation and brainstem compression. The clinical picture then changes to one with focal brainstem signs, and coma is likely to be compounded by disruption of the ARAS.

2 Disorders with signs of meningeal irritation either from blood in the CSF or meningeal inflammation usually of bacterial origin. The CSF is abnormal, containing blood or an excess of white cells, and there are signs of meningism such as neck stiffness and photophobia, headache and vomiting, before coma develops. There may or may not be focal neurological signs, and the CT scan may be helpful in the diagnosis.

3 Diseases which demonstrate focal brainstem signs or lateralizing cerebral signs as a result of lesions which arise supra- or infratentorially and cause disruption of the ARAS by compression or destruction of the brainstem. Supratentorial lesions arise frequently from

one side and produce lateral compression of the brainstem, and there is a progression of signs which indicate, not necessarily with any great precision, the rostal to caudal involvement of the brainstem. These signs also indicate approximately the prognosis and response to treatment.

Of the many focal brainstem signs, probably the most useful clinically are those concerning the pupillary response, eye movements (oculocephalic and oculovestibular responses), motor responses to painful stimuli (extensor or flexor) and the pattern of respiration.

Pupillary responses

Pupil size and reactivity is determined not only by light falling on the retina but also by the continuity of the parasympathetic (constrictor) and sympathetic (dilator) pathways to the pupil. The parasympathetic fibres are carried by the third nerve. The sympathetic pathway is tortuous from the hypothalmus down the brainstem to the first thoracic segment of the spinal cord. From there, sympathetic fibres pass out into the stellate ganglion and back via the carotid arteries or the fifth nerve and reach the orbit via the nasociliary branch of V as the long ciliary nerves to the dilator muscles of the pupil.

Pupil size is determined by the balance between parasympathetic and sympathetic activity. If the third nerve is compressed, parasympathetic fibres are interrupted and the pupil becomes dilated and unreactive. If the sympathetic fibres from the hypothalamus and onwards are interrupted unilaterally, the pupil constricts but may still show some reaction to light (Horner's syndrome). Bilateral pupillary constriction may occur if the descending sympathetic pathway is interrupted in the diencephalon and pontine tegmental region of the upper mid-brain. If both parasympathetic and sympathetic supplies are interrupted by mid-brain and pontine compression, the pupils are mid-dilated and unreactive. The fixed dilated pupils of acute cerebral ischaemia are thought to be the result of circulating hormonal factors induced by ischaemia.

Eye movements

In the awake state, eye movements are controlled by voluntary or behavioural cortical responses, and if the head is turned rapidly from side to side, the eye movement reponse is variable depending on what the subject is observing. In the unconscious state, this behavioural factor is abolished and turning the head from side to side reveals the basic reflex movements determined by the vestibular apparatus. These are the oculocephalic (or 'dolls eye') movements. Similarly, in the unconscious state, cooling or warming the tympanic membrane and the fluid in the semicircular canals produces reflex tonic deviation of the eyes, as demonstrated by the oculovestibular or caloric tests. These reflexes depend on the integrity of the vestibular nuclei in the pontine–medullary region and also on the III, IV and VI nerve nuclei which control eye movements. Absence of these reflex eye movements indicate severe brainstem injury.

Damage to the nulclei concerned with eye movements and their connecting tracts may produce also divergent or convergent squints or asymmetrical eye movements (internuclear opthalmoplegia) indicative of localized brainstem damage.

Motor responses

Comatose subjects, although not aware, may still respond reflexly to a painful stimulus, and reflex withdrawal of a limb (a flexion response) to a painful stimulus is seen frequently in disorders involving just the cerebral hemispheres. However, if the lesion spreads to involve the diencephalon, the pattern of response may change to that of flexion of the upper limb and extension of the lower limb. This is often termed the decorticate response and is in effect a bilateral spastic hemiplegia. Further disruption of the upper mid-brain gives rise to an extensor response in both upper and lower limbs which is termed the decerebrate response. Pontine–medullary involvement produces no motor response (flaccid response) and holds a grave prognosis.

Provided the subject is not under the influence of drugs which alter the brainstem responses, and having taken into account also the nature of the primary lesion, the above clinical signs may be used to assess the depth of coma, determine the site of the lesion, chart the progress of the disease and arrive at a prognosis. In a clinical setting, the picture is often not as definite as might be supposed from the above description, and additional information may be derived from the study of the breathing pattern. In order to understand this, some knowledge of the anatomical organization of the neural control of breathing is necessary.

The neural control of breathing

Even after many years of investigation, the neural mechanisms which control breathing are still fairly obscure and the respiratory centres are regarded by the majority of anaesthesists as vague collections of neurons situated in the 'black box' of the pontine and medullary regions of the brainstem. Local trauma and disease of the brainstem and certain drugs acting on the brainstem have an effect on 'ventilation', which is the final result of the output of the breathing mechanism, but seldom are careful observations made of those changes in the pattern of breathing which may reflect the particular part of the system which is at fault.

An important point often forgotten is that there are two independent respiratory control mechanisms. One relates to the voluntary control of breathing and may be termed the behavioural system, and the other, the metabolic or automatic system, is devoid of conscious control, and responds to metabolic and other afferent stimuli. It is of clinical importance to appreciate that there are two systems when interpreting the various patterns of breathing seen in neurological disorders.

The behavioural system

Voluntary movements are subserved by the corticospinal tracts, the signals arising from the motor cortex and passing down the fibres of the internal capsule to decussate in the pons and thence, via corticospinal tracts in the lateral part of the spinal cord, to synapse with the anterior horn cells of the motor neurons supplying voluntary muscle. Voluntary control of breathing movements uses these same corticospinal pathways (Fig 77.1). In general, it overrides the respiratory drive from the metabolic system. It should be noted that the respiratory function tests requiring voluntary manoeuvres e.g. vital capacity, peak expiratory flow, maximum breathing capacity and voluntary cough, are only tests of the behavioural system and do not provide information on the integrity of the metabolic system.

The metabolic system

Groups of neurons forming longitudinal columns of cells in the medulla, concentrated in the regions of nucleus tractus solitarii (NTS) just beneath the floor

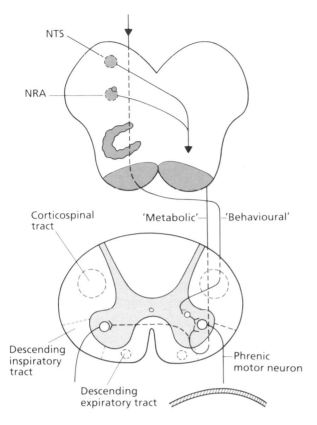

Fig 77.1 Diagrammatic section through the medulla and mid-cervical cord showing the pathway of the corticospinal tract of the 'behavioural' system and the medullary nuclei and projections of the descending inspiratory and expiratory tracts of the 'metabolic' system. NTS = nucleus tractus solitarii; NRA = nucleus retroambigualis. (Redrawn from Loh, 1986.)

of the fourth ventricle, and also nucleus retroambigualis (NRA) deeper in the medulla, cross in the medulla and project down the anterolateral part of the spinal cord to synapse with the anterior horn cells of respiratory muscles, probably via an internuncial neuron. The neurons of NTS and NRA project to both inspiratory and expiratory muscles, although those of NTS are largely inspiratory to the diaphragm. They also receive projections from various other neurons in the pons and medulla.

The generation of a rhythmical pattern of breathing is a highly complex interaction between the pontine and medullary respiratory nuclei and has not been defined clearly in experimental animals, let alone in man. There is probably a pontine rhythm generator which inhibits tonic inspiratory and expiratory medullary neuron activity, which are themselves mutually inhibitory (Sears et al., 1982). These neurons may form the fundamental basis of a rhythmic breathing

pattern which is modulated further by central and peripheral chemoreceptor drives, afferents from the lungs and chest-wall receptors and muscle spindles, in addition to pharyngeal, laryngeal and tracheal receptors. Body temperature and the general level of activity in the reticular activating system modify also the firing thresholds of neurons, not only centrally, but also at the spinal level.

Figure 77.2 illustrates the breathing pattern of a man who has had the corticospinal tracts interrupted as a result of infarction of the ventral pontine region. He was unable to move any muscle voluntarily which was innervated below the level of the lesion and, although completely aware, was able to communicate only with eye movements—an example of the 'locked-in' syndrome. The breathing pattern is extremely regular, showing the metabolic system driving respiration in isolation, uninfluenced by the behavioural system. When asked to take a deep breath or stop breathing, the patient was unable to do either, and yet he could augment his breathing reflexly following an increase in inspired carbon dioxide.

Figure 77.3 shows the irregular breathing pattern of a man who had a tumour invading the floor of the fourth ventricle with destruction of NTS bilaterally. He was unable to sleep because he feared, quite correctly, that he would stop breathing if he did not voluntarily drive his breathing. He required artificial ventilation in order that he could sleep. The irregular pattern of breathing correlates with changes in EEG when lower-voltage activity, indicating short lapses in attention, is associated with slow respiration. This is an example of disruption of the metabolic system of respiratory control, a true 'Ondine's Curse'. The patient could perform various voluntary respiratory manoeuvres but, when drowsy, would hypoventilate and show a slow irregular pattern of respiration with apnoeic periods.

Patients with a defect in the metabolic system may appear normal in the awake state, and may be able to perform various voluntary respiratory tests satisfactorily, but, if left alone, they may hypoventilate severely and even succumb through a failure by medical staff to recognize the abnormality in the metabolic system. Patients with medullary lesions should be observed very carefully for signs of hypoventilation, apnoeic episodes or slow irregular respiration, a situation not unlike an overdose of fentanyl, which is in effect a pharmacological disruption of the metabolic or automatic control system with preservation of the behavioural mechanism.

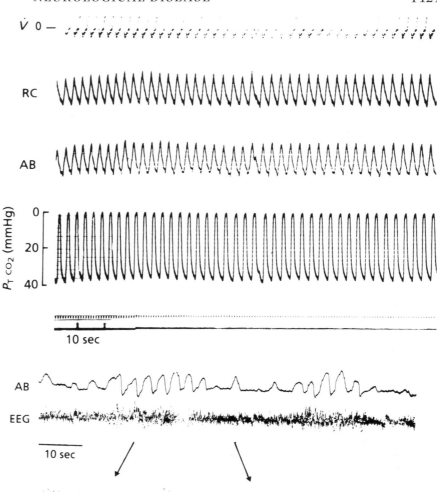

Fig. 72.2 Breathing pattern of a patient with 'locked-in' syndrome. V = airflow by pneumotachograph; RC = rib cage anteroposterior movement by magnetometers AB = abdominal anteroposterior movement by magnetometers; AB = abdominal regular pattern of breathing. In mid-trace the patient was asked to stop breathing, but no voluntary control was possible, the breathing being driven by the metabolic system in isolation. (Reproduced from Loh, 1986.)

Fig. 77.3 Irregular breathing pattern in a patient with disruption of the metabolic control system of breathing. AB = abdominal anteroposterior movement by magnetometer; EEG = simultaneous electroencephalogram. Below: expanded portions of EEG. Note low-voltage activity associated with slow respiratory rate. (Reproduced from Loh, 1986.)

The efferent and afferent neurons of the glossopharyngeal and vagal nuclei are situated close to NTS and NRA, and any lesion affecting one is likely to affect the other. Thus, patients who have loss of sensation of the pharynx and trachea or difficulty with swallowing, or who develop hiccup resulting from damage to the medulla, are likely to have respiratory disturbances of the metabolic system is addition.

The descending tracts of NTS and NRA, which carry the respiratory drive to the anterior horn cells of respiratory muscles, lie in the anterolateral part of the cord in what may be termed the reticulospinal tracts (Nathan, 1963). When a high cervical cordotomy is performed for pain relief, a unilateral lesion of the spinothalamic tracts also cuts the descending reticulospinal tract frequently, giving rise to a temporary disturbance of automatic breathing. Bilateral lesions lead to death from total failure of the metabolic system, an irremediable Ondine's Curse. Similar high cervical lesions from other causes have the same effects.

Whilst tests of the behavioural system involve tests of voluntary function, tests of a metabolic system should include observation of the breathing pattern during quiet breathing or sleep. Frequent sighs, hiccups, slow irregular breathing and apnoeic periods are indicative of disturbance of the metabolic system. Specific tests of ventilatory respone to hypoxia and carbon dioxide may be useful, although difficult to interpret.

The management of a deficiency of the metabolic system depends on the prognosis, but tracheostomy with artificial ventilation, especially during sleep, are necessary in the first instance. If the patient has a reasonable prognosis, this type of central respiratory failure is one of the few indications for phrenic nerve pacing (Glen *et al.*, 1972).

Disturbances of respiratory pattern

During normal quiet breathing in the awake subject, the pattern of breathing is reasonably regular, but the variations in tidal volume and inspiratory and expiratory time are greater than during slow-wave sleep, because the thinking individual alters his pattern of breathing e.g. reading, listening or thinking. During sleep, breathing is more regular and less variable except during REM (rapid eye movement) sleep when possibly dreaming may influence breathing patterns. Several disturbances of the normal pattern of breathing have been described which are related to the part of the respiratory control mechanism which is at fault.

Cortical disturbances

Cheyne–Stokes respiration is a characteristic pattern of breathing occurring in patients with cortical damage or ischaemia and a slow circulation time. It is seen in the presence of an intact respiratory control mechanism. Breathing increases progressively in depth to a peak and then wanes, the cycle often ending with a period of apnoea before commencing again. The pattern of change is smooth and regular. Cherniack and Longobardo (1973) suggested that cortical damage reduced a central inhibition of carbon dioxide sensitivity and that the combination of an increase in carbon dioxide sensitivity and a slow circulation, causing unusual delays between blood–gas exchange in the lungs and the sensing of such changes by the chemoreceptors, caused a type of hunting or instability in the control mechanism which gave rise to the Cheyne–Stokes respiratory pattern.

Afferent stimulation from lung and chest wall

Tachypnoea which is a regular and persistent increase of breath frequency, is almost always the result of lung complications such as pneumothorax, pulmonary oedema, lobar collapse or consolidation. Again, the neural control mechanism is intact but the afferent discharge from the lungs and chest-wall receptors is altered by disease to produce a shortening of inspira-

tion, a decrease in tidal volume and an increase in respiratory rate.

Mid-brain and pontine lesions

Cluster breathing describes an abrupt increase in respiratory frequency for short periods which is quite unlike Cheyne–Stokes respiration. It is seen in patients with encephalitis and brainstem lesions and probably results from a disturbance of rhythm generation by a pontine tegmental lesion.

Apneustic breathing, when there is an involuntary breath-hold in inspiration and *ratchet breathing*, when inspiration occurs in a series of steps, have been described also in pontine lesions.

Neurogenic hyperventilation is again a manifestation of a pontine lesion, following head injury occasionally. The hyperventilation is difficlut to control. In order to minimize respiratory work and prevent severe respiratory alkalosis, muscle paralysis and controlled ventilation may be necessary.

Medullary lesions

Irregular breathing with apnoeic periods is seen in lesions of NTS and NRA as illustrated in the case above, or when the descending reticulospinal pathway is interrupted. The subject may be reluctant to sleep, and careful examination may reveal damage to other cranial nerves arising from the medulla.

Hiccups may result from lesions in the region of NTS which remove an inhibitory influence which normally suppresses hiccups (Newsom-Davis, 1970). This periodic, massive inspiratory discharge is usually followed closely by glottic closure to produce the 'hic'. However, in patients in whom the trachea is intubated, limitation of inspiration by glottic closure cannot occur and the inspiratory activity produces large tidal volumes and gross hyperventilation. It appears that hypocapnia perpetuates the situation. Hiccups may sometimes be improved by carbon dioxide rebreathing. Strong vagal stimulation may also inhibit hiccups on occasion. It is important that hiccups in the patient with an intubated trachea are recognized and not mistaken for some other form of hyperventilation. It may be detected by the regular periodicity of inspiration, often interspersed with a few normal breaths.

Epilepsy

This is an intermittent derangement of the nervous system where sudden disorderly discharges of cerebral neurons produce disturbance in sensation, alterations in psychic function, convulsive movements and often loss of consciousness. Such an episode is often termed a seizure and is a manifestation of disease of the nervous system. Seizures may be idiopathic, when the nature of the original disease is unknown or secondary to a known cause.

Seizures may take several forms which can be allocated into generalized or partial or focal seizures. Grand mal seizures are the most dramatic of the generalized seizures. They may sometimes start with an aura or may occur unexpectedly. There is first a tonic phase with generalized muscle spasm, loss of consciousness, incontinence, absent respiration and the pupils are usually dilated and unreactive. This then passes on to a clonic phase when a mild generalized trembling gives way to violent, rhymthmic muscular contractions. Cyanosis, sweating, biting of the tongue and frothing of the lips are part of the picture. After 1–2 min the episode subsides, respiration resumes and for a minute the subject remains in a deep coma. The subject then regains consciousness but may remain drowsy for some hours. During the intense electrical activity there is an increase in local cerebral oxygen consumption and the possibility of severe local hypoxia

Table 77.2 Secondary causes of epilepsy

Cerebral trauma
Head injury
Postneurosurgical

Intracranial mass
Tumour
Abscess

Primary disease of the brain
Viral encephalitis
Parasitic disease
Creutzfeltd–Jakob disease
Bacterial meningitis

Hypoxic encephalopathy
Cardiac arrest
Carbon monoxide poisoning

Complications of acute illness
Water intoxication
Hypertensive encephalopathy
Hyperglycaemia
Uraemia

Withdrawal of drugs
Alcohol
Addictive drugs
Anticonvulsants

Table 77.3 Some details of common anticonvulsants

Anticonvulsant	Daily adult dosage (mg)	Half-life (hr)	Effective blood concentration (μg/ml)
Phenobarbitone	60–200	96	15–35
Phenytoin	200–400	24	10–20
Carbamazepine	600–1200	12	6–10
Sodium valproate	1000–2500	8	5–100

and permanent neuronal damage is always present, although cardiac output and cerebral blood flow are increased during the episode in compensation.

There are numerous precipitating factors which result in epileptic episodes and some of these are outlined in Table 77.2 and the common anticonvulsants used in the treatment of grand mal seizures is shown in Table 77.3.

Status epilepticus

This occurs when recurrent generalized seizures occur sufficiently frequently that there is no recovery of consciousness. Approximately 8–10% of grand mal seizures result in status epilepticus in which there is a 10% mortality. This condition is therefore not benign, and prolonged convulsions also carry a high risk of permanent neurological damage. It is important to suppress the seizure activity as soon as possible. Many anticonvulsants may be tried but in the first instance oxygen should be administered. A benzodiazepine such as diazepam may be given intravenously in a dose of 2 mg/min up to a total dose of 20 mg. If this has no benefit, it is probably most wise to intubate the airway and give a continuous infusion of diazepam at a dose of 40 mg/hr and to ventilate the lungs if necessary. Meanwhile it is essential to increase the maintenance anticonvulsant therapy with drugs such as phenytoin, phenobarbitone, carbamazepine and sodium valproate (which has a high therapeutic ratio). It is also important to check that these drugs are being given in sufficient dosage to achieve therapeutic plasma concentrations. If diazepam does not control the seizures chlormethizole is a reasonable second choice. It is administered by intravenous infusion preferably into a central vein as it may cause thrombophlebitis. It also has a tendency to produce a pyrexia if administered through PVC infusion tubing

(Lingam *et al.*, 1980), but despite these drawbacks it remains a useful drug, able often to control status epilepticus with relatively little suppression of respiration or cardiac function. The third intravenous anticonvulsant of choice is thiopentone, and this may be given first as a bolus of up to 500 mg followed by a continuous infusion of up to 25 mg/hr. Failing this, paraldehyde 4% or lignocaine may be tried, but thiopentone is usually successful in controlling the convulsions, but at the cost of cardiovascular and respiratory depression. There is little indication for muscle paralysis as this masks seizure activity which in turn may be causing cerebral damage.

It is useful to monitor the EEG to determine if seizure activity has been suppressed satisfactorily. The raw EEG signal is useful if it can be interpreted satisfactorily, but some intensive therapy units (ITUs) may find some form of cerebral function monitoring more useful. As a general rule, in severe epilepticus, it is best to maintain suppression of seizures for approximately 24 hr before starting to discontinue treatment, and if high doses of anticonvulsants are used, this period of elimination may be several days. A slow reduction of anticonvulsant over this period may be necessary with step-wise increases again if seizure activity recurs. It is wise to check the plasma concentrations of anticonvulsant frequently as drug interactions may alter these levels dramatically during the dynamic phases of control of seizures and the withdrawal of medication.

It is essential also to treat the precipitating cause of the convulsion and to arrange adequate supervision of the medical, physical and mental welfare of the patient after discharge from the ITU.

Herpes simplex encephalitis

Herpes simplex encephalitis is caused usually by the Type 1 virus and is the most common of the acute viral encephalitis' in the UK. In about 50% of cases it is fatal, and those who survive are often severely damaged. The presentation is similar to other forms of acute viral encephalitis often starting with fever, headache and progressing to confusion, stupor and finally coma. The virus spreads possibly from the branches of the fifth nerve and fifth nerve ganglion to involve characteristically the temporal lobes, and early temporal lobe seizures with gustatory and olfactory hallucinations and bizarre behaviour is sometimes observed.

There is an increase in lymphocytes and sometimes red cells and the protein is raised in CSF. The intracranial pressure is raised as a result of the marked haemorrhagic necrosis and oedema is found characteristically in the inferior and medial parts of the frontal and temporal lobes. It is the distribution of the lesion around the temporal lobes which enables a reasonably confident diagnosis to be made on CT scan. However, the virus is seldom isolated from CSF and confirmation of the diagnosis can be made only through brain biopsy using a fluorescent antibody technique or viral culture. Viral titres in blood are raised at a later stage and are not helpful in the initial diagnosis.

Oedema of the brain tissue increases intracranial pressure, and if tentorial herniation occurs, coma ensues then further brainstem compression results in respiratory arrest. This carries a grave prognosis.

Treatment is directed towards early elimination of the virus before the onset of brainstem compression. Acyclovir is the antiviral agent of choice and is administered as a slow intravenous infusion over 1 hr. The recommended dose is 10 mg/kg every 8 hr for 10 days. Corticosteroids, osmotic diuretics and renal loop diuretics are used to reduce cerebral oedema and prevent tentorial herniation. Early decisions are required on the need to control ventilation and seizures. The mortality and morbidity is increased considerably once brainstem disturbances have developed.

Acute inflammatory polyradiculoneuropathy or Guillain–Barré syndrome

The Guillain–Barré syndrome, noted first by Landry in 1859 and subsequently by Guillain, Barré and Strohl in 1916, may be described best as an acute inflammatory polyradiculoneuropathy (AIP) (Hughes, 1978), with a prevalence of approximately 1.5 per 100 000 of the population. It may affect individuals at any age, but the peak incidence is in the fifth decade (Lesser *et al.*, 1973). The disease is characterized by a progressive motor weakness, usually symmetrical, with areflexia and also some sensory symptoms (Asbury *et al.*, 1978). In approximately 60% of patients, the onset of motor weakness is preceded by a mild non-specific viral infection, commonly of the upper respiratory tract. In approximately 30% of patients, high titres of antibody to cytomegalovirus have been found (Dowling *et al.*, 1977), but several other viruses have been implicated, as have inoculations, mycoplasma, bacterial infections and pre-existing illness such as Hodgkin's disease and lymphoma. The motor weakness may progress rapidly over a few days, or the deterioration may occur more gradually, and in 90% of patients the weakness is maximum by 4 weeks. The weakness develops usually in the limbs, but may progress to involve the respiratory muscles and cranial nerves.

Sensory changes are typically paraesthesia of the glove and stocking type. In addition, there is frequently autonomic dysfunction. The pathological changes are predominantly lymphocyte infiltration of the peripheral nerves up to the spinal roots, resulting in segmental demyelination. In severe cases, there is also secondary axonal degeneration. There is marked slowing or blockade of nerve conduction as a result of demyelination and denervation; muscle fibrillation indicates axonal degeneration. An increase in CSF protein concentration is seen usually by the second week, but only a few cells are present. The disorder should be distinguished from porphyria, lead neuropathy, volatile solvent abuse, toxic neuropathy (e.g. from organophosphorus compounds), poliomyelitis, botulism and diphtheria.

As AIP is likely to be the result of a sensitivity reaction to Schwann cell myelin or other peripheral nerve protein, various forms of immunosuppressive treatment have neen tried. On the whole, steroids are not felt to be beneficial. There is some evidence of delayed recovery and a higher incidence of complication following steroid treatment (Hughes et al., 1978). Early use of plasma exchange may be useful in limiting the deterioration and demyelination (Editorial, 1984; Greenwood et al., 1984; Osterman, 1984). After studying 245 patients, The Guillain–Barré Syndrome Study Group (1985) came to the conclusion that plasma exchange was beneficial in inducing a quicker recovery and shortening hospital stay if introduced within 7 days of onset of symptoms.

The disease is very variable in severity and is self-limiting. The signs of recovery of neuronal function are seen usually within 4 weeks of the onset of symptoms. The majority of patients make a full recovery over several months to a year, but approximately 10% are left with residual disability. Mortality is approximately 10%. The prognosis, therefore, is good, and the aim of management is to prevent complications and thus keep the patient in good condition while awaiting spontaneous recovery.

Management

The main life-threatening problem in AIP is acute respiratory failure resulting from respiratory muscle weakness. This is likely to occur within the first 2

weeks of the illness and there is usually a progressive deterioration of respiratory muscle power over a few days. Vital capacity is a reasonable clinical test of respiratory muscle power, and if this shows a progressive decrease to less than 1 litre in an adult, it is likely that artificial ventilation is required.

A decreasing vital capacity together with bulbar weakness (with difficulty in swallowing and coughing) is a very dangerous combination, as such patients may be precipitated into acute respiratory failure by the aspiration of small quantities of saliva. Under these circumstances, it is best to intubate the trachea, and perhaps the best guides to the need for tracheal intubation are if the patient begins to look anxious and is restless, and if the respiratory rate increases and the accessory muscles of respiration are being used. Arterial blood gas tensions are not helpful in making an early decision to intubate the trachea.

The function of the diaphragm may be an important determinant of the need for tracheal intubation and ventilation, as it is the prime muscle of inspiration. Severe weakness or total paralysis of the diaphragm may be recognized by observation of the anterior abdominal wall during quiet respiration in the supine posture, when paradoxical inward movement of the upper abdominal wall occurs during inspiration. Such patients are likely to be distressed by the supine position and prefer to sit upright, and it is these patients who are most likely to require tracheal intubation and ventilation. It is also likely that satisfactory respiration will occur only after some diaphragm function has returned.

When tracheal intubation is necessary, early tracheostomy should be considered as it usually takes at least 2, and often several, weeks before extubation can take place satisfactorily. Patients accept artificial ventilation easily and there is no need for sedation or paralysis. The management of ventilation and care of the tracheostomy is straightforward and are not discussed further.

Vital capacity is a reasonable guide to recovery of respiratory muscle function. A vital capacity of 1–1.5 litre is often required before satisfactory spontaneous respiration can occur, and this is commonly obtained when abdominal paradoxical movement disappears, signifying the return of diaphragm activity. It is probably unwise to decannulate the tracheostomy until it has been well established that bulbar function is adequate and the return of a satisfactory gag reflex and swallowing have been demonstrated. In some patients it is wise to change to an uncuffed silver tracheostomy tube with speaking attachment as an intermediate step before decannulation.

Autonomic disturbances

Second to respiratory failure, the most common cause of death in AIP is cardiac arrhythmia (Lichtenfeld, 1971). Arrhythmias are associated frequently with autonomic abnormalities. Sinus tachycardia and persistent fluctuating hypertension are observed frequently early in the disease. Bradycardia and hypotension also occur, particularly following vagal stimulation from tracheal suction. Prolonged episodes of hypotension may occur with pallor and bouts of excessive sweating as a result of parasympathetic overactivity. Bladder and bowel function are seldom affected, although catheterization of the bladder may be needed for other reasons. Paralytic ileus lasting a few days, with failure to absorb feeds, may be the result of autonomic dysfunction also. Postural hypotension should be suspected, particularly when patients are being mobilized during the recovery phase of the illness.

Several studies have recorded sudden death in patients with autonomic disturbances, and our policy is currently to attempt to stabilize the cardiovascular system by partial β-blockade with propranolol to prevent tachycardia and hypertension, and also to give atropine 0.6 mg three to four times a day to avoid episodes of bradycardia during tracheal toilet and physiotherapy. Marked hypertension may be treated with a hypotensive drugs such as hydralazine. If episodes of marked bradycardia are noted, the insertion of a transvenous pacemaker should be considered.

Patients with profound muscle weakness are at risk from deep vein thrombosis and pulmonary embolus. Good nursing care, physiotherapy and hydration may help to prevent this complication. However, we prescribe a subcutaneous heparin regimen routinely (5000 IU twice daily).

Many patients complain of pain, which may last several days. It is often severe and persistent and felt usually in the back or calves. This pain is not relieved easily by analgesics and it may be most distressing.

The aim of management is to prevent complications and permit the natural recovery process to take place. Medical interference is secondary to good nursing care and physiotherapy. Attention must be paid to adequate nutrition and the prevention of muscle wasting. One of the most distressing problems is the inability of patients to communicate. Patients may be unable to signal with their hands or write, and in some cases the facial weakness is such that they cannot even signal with their eyes. Frequent reassurance is required. Television, radio and cassette tapes help to occupy the time and provide mental stimulation. Most important is the attitude and atmosphere created by the nursing staff and also the physiotherapy and occupational therapy staff who are involved throughout.

The milestones to recovery are return of respiratory muscle function and spontaneous breathing, recovery of speech, oral intake of food, decannulation of the tracheostomy, sitting up and supporting first the head and then torso, standing and walking with aid, and finally walking unaided.

Myasthenia gravis

In recent years it has become clear that myasthenia gravis (MG) is an autoimmune disease (Newsom-Davis, 1982). In the majority (85%) of individuals with the disease, it is possible to demonstrate an antibody in the IgG fraction which, through complement-mediated lysis, causes an increase in the rate of breakdown of acetylcholine receptors (AchR) on the postjunctional membrane of the neuromuscular junction (NMJ). This antibody, the anti-AchR antibody, eventually depletes the NMJ of AchRs, giving rise to a characteristic fatiguable muscle weakness. The weakness may affect some muscle groups more than others, so that some patients complain only of ptosis and diplopia, others may have proximal limb weakness and the most severely affected may develop bulbar and respiratory muscle weakness which may require intensive therapy management.

The diagnosis is suggested on the history of muscle weakness which is worsened by exercise and improved by rest. An improvement in muscle power following the administration of an anticholinesterase drug such as edrophonium and a characteristic decrement of the electromyograph (EMG) on repetitive stimulation of peripheral nerves add weight to the diagnosis, but MG is confirmed by the demonstration of the anti-AchR antibody in the patient's plasma, although the disease cannot be excluded if no antibody is detected.

The prevalence of MG is approximately one in 20 000 of the population and affects all age groups. There is a female preponderance, particularly in the group younger than 40 yr of age. Compston et al. (1980) showed an increased frequency of certain HLA antigens in non-thymoma patients, indicating that genetic factors probably have a role in the aetiology of the disease. This has been confirmed by Kerzin-Storrar et al. (1988). Occasionally, MG is associated with other autoimmune disorders such as rheumatoid arthritis, thyrotoxicosis and pernicious anaemia.

Thymoma occurs in approximately 10% of patients with MG and, although usually benign, the tumour may show malignant change and locally invade important mediastinal structures such as phrenic nerve and aorta.

Other forms of myasthenia

There are some rarer disorders of neuromuscular transmission which should be distinguished from the usual acquired form of MG. Neonatal myasthina occurs in one in eight babies born of mothers with MG and results from placental transfer of anti-AchR antibody from the mother (Morel et al., 1988). In the baby, this causes a transient muscle weakness which responds to anticholinesterases and which lasts usually for only 4–6 weeks. Following this, the baby is normal. A congential form of myasthenia has been described, in which the abnormality is in the AchR itself, and no immunological abnormality is found; these patients do not respond to immunosuppression.

The Lambert–Eaton myasthenic syndrome is an immunological disorder which produces a presynaptic defect in the release of acetylcholine from the nerve terminal. It is associated frequently with an oat-cell carcinoma of the bronchus, although in some cases no malignancy is found. Muscle power is improved transiently with exercise and the neurophysiological characteristics are different from those of MG. No antibody has been identified yet, but the condition may be improved with plasma exchange and immunosuppression. Freeze-fracture electron-microscopy indicated that there is a disorganization of calcium channels on the presynaptic membrane which may affect the liberation of the quanta of acetylcholine (Fukuoka et al., 1987).

Treatment of myasthenia gravis

ANTICHOLINESTERASE DRUGS

These drugs delay the breakdown of acetylcholine by cholinesterase at the NMJ and therefore presumably allow the more efficient transfer of acetylcholine to be depleted by AchRs on the postjunctional membrane.

They produce symptomatic improvement, but do not alter the underlying pathology. In fact, there is some evidence that prolonged, high-dose anticholinesterase drugs may themselves produce undesirable changes at the NMJ. Too much anticholinesterase produces a cholinergic muscle weakness in addition to excessive salivation, colic, diarrhoea and other symptoms of parasympathetic overactivity. It is best to keep the patient suboptimally dosed i.e. slightly myasthenic, rather than run the risk of cholinergic problems. Pyridostigmine bromide is the drug of choice, 30–120 mg 3-hourly, taken by mouth in tablet form or as an elixir via nasogastric tube. Atropine may be given to reduce the parasympathetic side-effects, but if the side-effects are troublesome, reduction in anticholinesterase therapy would be wise since the patient may be cholinergic, and alternative methods of management should be considered. Edrophonium (Tensilon) may be used as a test of the myasthenic or cholinergic state. After prior treatment with atropine 0.3–0.6 mg i.v., usually not more than 5 mg of edrophonium i.v. is required to produce a satisfactory response. If the patient is myasthenic then, within 30 sec there should be a marked improvement in muscle power which lasts for 2–3 min. The useful bedside tests of improved muscle power are loss of ptosis, recovery of facial muscle power, speech and voice, increased arm or leg outstretched time and improvement in vital capacity. If the improvement is marked, it would be reasonable to increase anticholinesterase therapy. However, if the response is marginal, one should contemplate a reduction in medication, bearing in mind that not all muscle groups behave equally and that some muscles may show a cholinergic response at the same time as others are myasthenic.

THYMECTOMY

Thymectomy alone produces an improvement in MG in approximately 60–70% of patients. The precise role of the thymus gland in MG is not clear, but it may be that some antigenic stimulus in the gland perpetuates the anti-AchR antibody production (Whiting et al., 1986). It has been demonstrated that, over a period of months, anti-AchR antibody concentrations decrease following thymectomy. Thymectomy is the treatment of choice in patients younger than 50 yr, when the thymus usually shows hyperplasia. Thymectomy is indicated in cases of thymoma.

The thymus gland is removed most satisfactorily

through a median sternotomy incision. The hazards of thymectomy are reduced considerably if patients come to operation in a good clinical state. Prior treatment with steroids or plasma exchange may improve the preoperative situation. The postoperative management is simplified by maintaining complete control of the airway with nasotracheal intubation for the first day or so after operation. Anticholinesterases are often discontinued before operation and re-introduced when indicated, usually at a lower dose, but guided by clinical state and testing with edrophonium. If comfortable, patients are allowed to breathe spontaneously through the nasotracheal tube, but at the first sign of respiratory distress, artifical ventilation is instituted easily. Extubation occurs when vital capacity is satisfactory and it is judged that respiratory assistance is unlikely to be required.

IMMUNOSUPPRESSION

Immunosuppression with steroids may produce a remission of symptoms in approximately 80% of patients. This may be achieved using an alternate day regimen of prednisolone, starting at a low dose of 10 mg and slowly increasing over a period of weeks up to a maximum of 120 mg on alternate days. Thereafter, the dose may be reduced very slowly to a minimum dose which maintains the improvement. If steroids are introduced too rapidly at high dose, temporary deterioration in muscle power can occur which may require tracheal intubation and ventilation of the lungs for a few days, but in this way, remission can be attained sooner. Thus, it may be justified to use a high-dose steroid regimen in those patients already in a poor clinical state and requiring artificial ventilation. Azathioprine may be used also for immunosuppression with a starting dose of 2.5 mg/kg body weight. Improvement is slow and may take up to 1 yr, but the side-effects are probably less than with steroids. Regular checks of haematology and liver function are required.

Quite frequently, steroids and azathioprine are used in combination; steroids being used to produce a more rapid improvement and azathioprine for long-term immunosuppression. It seems that immunosuppression needs to be continued indefinitely. Because of the side-effects of steroids and azathioprine, there is a reluctance to use these drugs in the younger age group, especially in women of child-bearing age. Thymectomy is still the treatment of choice in this younger age group because, if thymectomy alone produces a good

remission, the problems of immunosuppression can be avoided.

PLASMA EXCHANGE

Plasma exchange can reduce the anti-AchR antibody concentrations in blood very effectively and produce a remission of MG within a few days by allowing the effective regeneration of acetylcholine receptors. A series of approximately five daily exchanges removing approximately 50 ml/kg body weight of plasma each time can produce a marked clinical improvement, but it is relatively short-lived, lasting only 3–4 weeks. As the technique is very costly, it should be reserved for patients with severe disease who are awaiting the benefits of immunosuppression.

Intensive therapy unit problems

To the anaesthetist, the most significant fact regarding MG is the severe reduction in the number of AchRs, so that these patients are exceptionally sensitive to non-depolarizing muscle relaxants, but from the point of view of the intensive care specialist, the main problems are those of acute respiratory failure. Respiratory failure results usually from either a myasthenic or cholinergic crisis, but may be steroid-induced or the result of thymectomy. The majority are cholinergic crisis.

MYASTHENIC CRISIS

This occurs in patients with severe myasthenia who suddenly deteriorate as a result of an acute infection or stress of some other type and in whom the anticholinesterase requirements increase. However, recovery may not be achieved by an increase in anticholinesterase alone. It is also necessary to deal with the precipitating factor (such as infection). The safest course is to ensure an adequate airway by tracheal intubation and to ventilate the lungs until an improvement is achieved. Plasma exchange may be performed for a rapid improvement and the opportunity to introduce more effective immunosuppression should be considered.

CHOLINERGIC CRISIS

This occurs frequently from overdose with anticholinesterase drugs. The situation commonly arises following a myasthenic crisis in which only partial improvement with anticholinesterases occurs and more drug is administered progressively. This results in a cholinergic weakness which is not recognized as such. Eventually, the patient develops respiratory and bulbar muscle weakness, excessive salivation and abdominal cramps. Dangerous and acute respiratory failure may rapidly follow aspiration of secretions. Intubation of the trachea and ventilation of the lungs should be performed early and the anticholinesterase drugs withdrawn. In time, the patient returns to a myasthenic state and anticholinesterases may be re-introduced and the process of weaning from the ventilator started. It is unwise to expedite tracheal extubation early, and, in general, patients should be able to breathe without assistance for at least 24 hr before extubation. As with myasthenic crisis, plasma exchange and more effective immunosuppression should be considered.

It is worth noting that myasthenic patients may be made weaker by antibiotics of the aminoglycoside group such as streptomycin, gentamicin and neomycin, which reduce release of acetylcholine at the nerve terminal. Similarly, procainamide causes a reduction in release of acetylcholine, and quinine and quinidine reduce the speed of excitation along a muscle fibre, also making myasthenics weaker. In addition, a low serum potassium concentration should be avoided, as this potentiates muscle weakness.

Chronic neuromuscular respiratory failure

There are a number of neuromuscular disorders, the result of either neuronal damage such as poliomyelitis, or primary muscle disease as in the various myopathies and muscular dystrophies, which give rise to respiratory muscle weakness. Sometimes, the muscle weakness is such that a state of chronic respiratory failure develops in which the lungs are relatively normal, but the bellows function of the chest wall is impaired. If the condition is allowed to progress unrecognized, the patient may present in an ITU with unexplained respiratory failure. Occasionally, such patients are admitted having failed to breathe following anaesthesia or as difficult weaning problems, and some are admitted in congestive heart failure from chronic pulmonary hypertension. These neuromuscular problems may be diagnosed also as outpatients, provided one is attuned to the characteristic history. Patients often complain of breathlessness on exercise and often on assuming the supine posture, so that they sleep either propped up or in the lateral posture. A common feature is hypersomnolence with excessive sleepiness during the day, and yet disturbed sleep at night with frequent arousal and sometimes with nightmares. They are often difficult to rouse in the morning and wake up with a headache which clears shortly after getting up. These are symptoms of marked nocturnal hypoventilation with severe hypoxia and hypercapnia. On examination, there is evidence of neuromuscular weakness frequently affecting the shoulder girdle and neck muscles in addition to other muscle groups. In the majority of patients who suffer from this problem, there is evidence of marked diaphragm weakness (Newsom-Davis et al., 1976).

As mentioned earlier, weakness of the diaphragm may be seen best in the supine posture during quiet breathing, when the upper anterior abdominal wall moves paradoxically inwards during inspiration (Loh et al., 1977). This paradoxical movement is the result of the diaphragm failing to develop sufficient tension to prevent the abdominal contents moving up into the chest in the face of the more negative intrapleural pressure generated during inspiration. Awake, resting blood gas tensions reveal hypoxia and hypercapnia which may be corrected to a degree by voluntary hyperventilation, and there is normally an increased bicarbonate concentration, indicating long-standing respiratory acidosis.

Lung function tests may reveal a reduced vital capacity which may decrease further in the supine position. Ventilatory responses to hypoxia and hypercapnia are blunted, and exercise tolerance is poor. Pulmonary hypertension is a feature, and signs of congestive heart failure may be present. One of the problems in making a correct diagnosis is that the patients often appear relatively normal when upright and awake, and the problem reveals itself only during sleep. During sleep, the patient is at a gross disadvantage, both from a mechanical point of view because of the recumbent posture and from the respiratory drive to the breathing muscles.

In the upright posture, patients with weakness of the diaphragm may use abdominal muscle contraction to drive the abdominal contents up into the chest at end-expiration and then augment the inspiratory tidal volume by relaxing the abdominal muscles and allowing passive descent of the diaphragm and abdominal contents out of the chest in early inspiration. This mechanism is largely lost in the horizontal position. In addition, in the supine position the inspiratory muscles tend to be shorter and the mechanical advantage of extending the spine in the upright position is lost.

During sleep, the central drive to the breathing muscles is normally directed largely to the diaphragm, and if this muscle is non-functional, hypoventilation is to be expected. Also, because the ventilatory responses to hypoxia and hypercapnia are obtunded, there is a change in the threshold for arousal, and severe hypoxia and hypercapnia are allowed to persist. For these reasons, patients with diaphragm weakness are at risk during sleep and the correct diagnosis can be made only with certainty by observing what happens during sleep and making the relevant measurements.

Once the diagnosis is made, appropriate treatment may be attempted in the way of assisted ventilation during sleep with the aim of permanent use by the patient at home. This type of management should be undertaken by respiratory specialists and may be initiated in an ITU. The aims of treatment are to:

1 Prevent hypoxia and hypercapnia during sleep.
2 Reduce pulmonary hypertension.
3 Allow satisfactory sleep.
4 Rest fatigued respiratory muscles.

The results of satisfactory treatment are:

1 Abolition of hypersomnolence.
2 Reversal of congestive heart failure.
3 Induction of more normal blood gas tensions.
4 Improved quality of life.
5 Prolonged survival.

Treatment

NOCTURNAL ASSISTED VENTILATION

There are several ways of augmenting respiration during sleep. Rocking beds, which tip the patient head-up and then head-down regularly, assist ventilation by moving the abdominal contents in and out of the thorax, causing the diaphragm to act passively as a piston. Not all patients can tolerate the motion and, in some, ventilation is inadequate.

Positive-pressure ventilation via a tracheostomy or negative-pressure ventilation with a cuirass-type device are used more commonly for long-term home ventilation (Dunkin, 1983).

POSITIVE-PRESSURE VENTILATION

Positive-pressure ventilation is suitable particularly for the severely disabled patient who might find difficulty using a negative-pressure device, for patients for whom there is minimal assistance at night, and if there is need for a tracheostomy to overcome the problem of upper airways obstruction during sleep. Small, reliable, relatively inexpensive positive-pressure ventilators suitable for home use are available. The disadvantage of positive-pressure ventilation is that it does require a tracheostomy and, if an uncuffed tracheostomy tube is used, the leakage of air into the pharynx during the inspiratory phase may not be tolerated well. However, with perseverance this problem can usually be overcome.

NEGATIVE-PRESSURE VENTILATION

Negative-pressure ventilation is suitable provided the patient has a competent larynx, is able to breathe reasonably well on his own and is not entirely dependent on the device, and has adequate help at home. The advantage of negative-pressure devices is that tracheostomy may be avoided. Unfortunately, most of the devices are cumbersome, some may not be very efficient at ventilating and they may encourage upper airway obstruction during sleep.

Most of the apparatus available for home ventilation is of ancient design and, because of the small demand, commercial companies are reluctant to invest finance in the research and development of such apparatus. Specially tailored cuirass shells are available. It is possible to provide a patient with such equipment and a respiratory pump for approximately £3000.

More recently, it has been demonstrated that intermittent positive-pressure ventilation (IPPV) delivered via a nasal-mask is a realistic proposition for domicilliary ventilation (Ellis *et al.*, 1987). This method has the advantage of being simple and easy to apply, efficient in ventilation, overcomes the problems of upper airway obstruction and avoids tracheostomy. The possible problems of aspiration of oral secretions into the trachea or distension of the abdomen by ventilating gas seldom arise and leakage of ventilating gas out of the mouth during sleep and pressure sores from the nasal-mask are the main problems. These can be usually overcome with perseverance. This method of assisted ventilation may prove to be more satisfactory than negative-pressure respiration.

In order to pursue this type of therapy, one requires adequate medical expertise, adequate finance, good engineering back-up and interested and understanding nursing staff, so that the patient feels confident relying on the support of the hospital.

Many of the neuromuscular disorders which may be helped by assisted ventilation are only very slowly progressive, and often the condition affects young adults who have dependants. It can be extremely worthwhile and rewarding to assist these patients to lead happier, more productive and longer lives (Loh, 1983).

References

Asbury A.K., Arnason B.G.W., Karp H.R. & McFarlin D.E. (1978) Criteria for diagnosis of Guillain–Barré syndrome. *Annals of Neurology* 2, 565.

Bremer R. (1937) L'activité cérébrale au cours du sommeil et de la narcose: contribution a l'étude de mechanisme de sommeil. *Bulletin de l'Académie Royale de Medicine de Belgique* 2, 68–86.

Cherniack N.S. & Longobardo G.S. (1973) Cheyne–Stokes breathing. *New England Journal of Medicine* 288, 952.

Compston D.A.S. VIncent A., Newsom-Davis J. & Batchelor J.R. (1980) Clinical, pathological, HLA antigen and immunological evidence for disease heterogeneity in myasthenia gravis. *Brain* 103, 579.

Dowling P.C., Mendonna J.P. & Cook S.D. (1977) Cytomegalovirus complement fixation antibody in Guillain–Barré syndrome. *Neurology* 27, 1153.

Dunkin L.J. (1983) Home ventilatory assistance. *Anaesthesia* 38, 644.

Editorial 91984) Plasma exchange in Guillain–Barré syndrome. *Lancet* 2, 1312.

Ellis E.R. Bye P.T.P., Bruderer J.W. & Sullivan C.E. (1987) Treatment of respiratory failure during sleep in patients with neuro-muscular disease. Positive-pressure ventilation through a nose mask. *American Review of Respiratory Disease* 135, 148–52.

Fukuoka T., Engel A.G., Lang B., Newsom-Davis J., Prior C. & Wray D.W. (1987) Lambert–Eaton myasthenic syndrome: 1. Early morphological effects of IgG on the presynaptic membrane active zones. *Annals of Neurology* 22, 193–9.

Glen W.W.L., Holcomb W.G., McLaughlin A.J., O'Hare J.M., Hogan J.F. & Yasuda R. (1972) Total ventilatory support in a quadri-plegic patient with radiofrequency electrophrenic respiration. *New England Journal of Medicine* 286, 513.

Greenwood R.J., Newsom-Davis J., Hughes R.A., Aslan S., Bowden A.W., Chadwick D.W., Gordon N.S., McLellan D.L., Millac P., Stott R.B. & Armitage P. (1984) Controlled trial of plasma exchange in acute inflammatory polyradiculopathy. *Lancet* 1, 877.

Guillain–Barré Syndrome Study Group (1985) plasmapheresis and acute Guillain–Barré syndrome. *Neurology* 35, 109.

Hughes R.A. (1978) Acute inflammatory polyneuropathy. *British Journal of Hospital Medicine* 20, 688.

Hughes R.A., Newsom-Davis J., Perkin G.D. & Pierce J.M. (1978) Controlled trial prednisolone in acute polyneuropathy. *Lancet* 2, 750.

Kerzin-Storrar L., Metcalfe R.A., Dyer P.A., Kowalska G., Ferguson I. & Harris R. (1988) Genetic factors in myasthenia gravis: a family study. *Neurology* 38, 38–42.

Lesser R.P., Hauser W.A., Kurland L.T. & Mulder D.W. (1973) Epidemiologic features of the Guillain–Barré syndrome. Experience in Olmsted County, Minnesota. *Neurolgy* 23, 1269.

Lichtenfield P. (1971) Autonomic dysfunction in the Guillain–Barre syndrome. *American Journal of Medicine* 50, 772.

Lingam S., Bertwistle H., Elliston H.E. & Wilson J. (1980) Problems with intravenous chlormethiazole (Heminevrin) in status epilepticus. *British Medical Journal* 1, 155.

Loh L. (1983) Editorial—home ventilation. Anaesthesia, 38, 621.

Loh L. (1986) Neurological and neuromuscular disease. *British Journal of Anaesthesia* 58, 190–200.

Loh L., Goldman M. & Newsom-Davis J. (1977) The assessment of diaphragm function. *Medicine* 56, 165.

Morel E., Eymard B., Vernet-der-Garabedian B., Pannier C., Dulac O. & Bach J.F. (1988) Neonatal myasthenia gravis, a new clinical and immunological appraisal on 30 cases. *Neurology* 38, 138–42.

Moruzzi G. & Magoun H.W. (1949) Brainstem reticular formation and activation of the EEG. *Electroencephalography and Clinical Neuophysiology* 1, 455–473.

Nathan P.W. (1963) The descending inspiratory pathway in man. *Journal of Neurology, Neurosurgery and Psychiatry* 26, 487.

Newsom-Davis J. (1970) An experimental study of hiccup. *Brain* 93, 851.

Newsom-Davis J. (1982) Myasthenia. In *Advanced Medicine*, vol.18 (Ed. Sarner M.) p.149. Pitman, London.

Newsom-Davis J. (1985) The neural control of respiratory function. In *Neurosurgery: The Scientific Basis of Clinical Practice* (Eds Crockard H.A., Hayward R.D. & Hofff J.) p. 200. Blackwell Scientific Publications, Oxford.

Newsom-Davis J. Goldman M., Loh L. & Cassan M. (1976) Diaphragm function and alveolar hypoventilation. *Quarterly Journal of Medicine* 45, 87.

Osterman P.O., Fagius J., Lundemo G., Philstedt P., Pirskanen R., Siden A. & Safwenberg J. (1984) Beneficial effects of plasma exchange in acute inflammatory polyradiculoneuropathy. *Lancet* 2, 1296.

Plum F. & Posner J.B. (1980) *The Diagnosis of Stupor and Coma* 3rd edn., pp. 11–14. F.A. Davis Company, Philadelphia.

Sears T.A., Berger A.J. & Philipson E.A. (1982) Reciprocal tonic activation of inspiratory and expiratory motoneurones by chemical drives. *Nature* 299, 728.

Whiting P.J., Vincent A. & Newsom-Davis J. (1986) Myasthenia gravis: monoclonal antihuman acetylcholine receptor antibodies used to analyse specificities and responses to treatment. *Neurology* 36, 612–17.

78

Head Injury

W. FITCH

Head injury is common but the overall incidence is not known with any degree of precision. For example, estimates of the frequency of trauma to the head in the USA vary from 180 to 673 per 100 000 of the population per annum. Each year, in the UK, one person in 50 sustains an injury to the head of sufficient severity to require hospital attendance. In all probability, however, many others seek no medical advice unless complications develop. Fortunately, the majority of the injuries are minor: only 20–25% of those attending accident and emergency departments require admission to hospital. Nevertheless, the number of patients *admitted* to hospital as a consequence of an injury to the head has increased progressively (at least in Scotland) since the early 1960s. Of those admitted, most (approximately 60%) have comparatively trivial injuries, remain in hospital for less than 2 days and recover completely from their injury — with or without specific treatment.

At the other end of the spectrum, the *mortality* from head injury, although decreasing, is still substantial (nine deaths per 100 000 of the population of the UK in 1981). Head injury accounts for approximately 1% of all deaths in Western Europe (including the UK), 25% of all deaths from trauma and almost 50% of those associated with road traffic accidents. There are no national statistics on the mortality from head injury in the USA. However, annual death rates of 24–32 per 100 000 of the population have been reported in studies of selected regions.

The frequency of head injury is greatest in young males (motor vehicle accidents, violence) and the elderly (falls). Not surprisingly, the proportion of deaths from head injury is much greater in young males than in females of equivalent age or in the general population. Head injury accounts for 15% of all fatalities in males between the ages of 15 and 40 yr.

Sixty percent of all deaths from head injury occur *before* admission to hospital; 40% at the scene of the accident and 20% during transport to the nearest accident and emergency department, or before formal admission to the primary receiving unit. Even in hospital, the prognosis of the severely head-injured patient is poor: 30–50% dying despite a better understanding of the pathophysiology of head injury on the part of the clinician and the institution of apparently appropriate treatment.

This chapter considers principally the management of those patients with moderate to severe head injury (Glasgow coma score 13–3) (p. 1440) who reach hospital alive. In such patients, the primary injury has been of insufficient severity to cause death at the time of initial accident or in the period preceding admission to hospital. In theory at least, death should be preventable in such patients, as the sequelae of the secondary injury may be controlled by appropriate therapeutic interventions. This should not be taken to indicate that recovery is assured. The extent of the primary brain damage may be such that full recovery is 'out of the question': the patient remains severely disabled or vegetative. Nevertheless, it is this group of patients in whom good management may improve outcome materially and in whom inappropriate or inadequate treatment may decrease the chance of making a 'good' recovery. This chapter highlights certain fundamental *principles* relevant to the management of such patients, establishes a number of *priorities* in their management and, finally, details some current considerations on the *practicalities* of management.

Principles relevant to management

Brain damage never occurs in isolation

Although it is usual to place the emphasis on the damage to the brain *per se* as being the determinant of death or disability, injury to the *brain* never occurs in isolation. Although it is true that many of the most minor injuries require no more than the debridement and suturing of lacerations of the scalp, trauma of sufficient severity to injure the brain itself must, inevitably, damage other structures. Injury is inflicted on the scalp, skull and dura, perhaps on the spine and spinal cord and, especially in accidents involving motor vehicles, on the trunk, limbs and abdomen (30–40% of head-injured patients admitted to hospital have another significant injury elsewhere in the body). Such additional injuries may have devastating consequences as far as the traumatized brain is concerned. For example, a decrease in cerebral perfusion to critical values may be associated with haemorrhage from a ruptured spleen and the consequent decrease in systemic arterial pressure. Because arterial hypotension is a comparatively unusual feature of head injury *per se*, its presence should alert the clinician to the possibility of occult blood loss. If the dura is torn, meningitis may follow a depressed skull fracture or fracture of the anterior fossa and lead to severe disability—or even death—in a patient who should have recovered fully from a relatively trivial injury.

Brain damage may be primary or secondary

PRIMARY BRAIN DAMAGE

Following a severe insult to the brain—ischaemic, haemorrhagic or traumatic—a certain population of neurons is damaged irremediably. Function cannot be regained no matter how immediate or skilled the treatment. This primary injury is the result of the physical forces applied to the skull and the brain at the moment of the initial insult.

It is customary to characterize primary brain damage as being either focal (localized) or diffuse. Focal damage is the result of direct injury to the brain (as when associated with a depressed fracture or penetrating wound) or of the movement of the brain in relation to the skull. As a consequence of acceleration/deceleration forces, there may be obvious local bruising or more severe damage to the surface of the brain (contusions) localized to those areas of brain which have come into contact with the irregular bony prominences on the interior surface of the skull. If severe, contusions may be associated with actual lacerations of the cortex and haemorrhage from ruptured blood vessels.

Less obvious, but more significant, are small neuronal lesions which are scattered diffusely through-

out the brain. These are the result of the movement of one part of the brain in relation to another part of the brain. For example, the degree of acceleration (or deceleration) imparted to the cortical mantle by a given force differs from that affecting the deeper structures such as white matter or corpus callosum. This results in a 'shearing' injury which stretches and tears nerve fibres (and blood vessels), particularly in the white matter. This form of primary brain damage is now recognized widely and has been referred to by a variety of names; 'diffuse degeneration of white matter', 'shearing injury', 'diffuse white matter shearing injury', 'inner cerebral trauma'. Histological studies show evidence of diffuse damage to the axons of the nerve cells: hence, the current preference for the term 'diffuse axonal injury'.

Unless it is severe and widespread (under which circumstance, of course, the patient may not reach hospital alive) primary *focal* damage to supratentorial structures does not, of itself, affect consciousness. The initial severity of a head injury is determined by the number and extent of the *diffuse* lesions. If few in number and limited in extent, the patient is 'concussed': when they are more numerous and widespread, coma is irreversible.

SECONDARY BRAIN DAMAGE

Clearly, if the patient reaches hospital alive, it may be assumed that the primary mechanical insult has been of insufficient severity to cause death. Likewise, if the patient has had a 'lucid interval' or has 'talked coherently', it can be accepted that the primary brain damage *per se* has not been severe enough to cause prolonged (or irreversible) unconsciousness. Thus, if death, or coma, occur later, it can be argued with some justification that the deterioration in neurological function must have resulted from a second series of events which, although initiated possibly at the time of the primary insult, have progressed to cause secondary brain damage. Secondary brain damage, therefore, occurs some time *after* the primary injury. Essentially, it is the result of cerebral ischaemia/ hypoxia and is the sequel to the development of certain *intracranial* complications (haematoma, infection, cerebral oedema, brain shift and herniation, seizures) and/or the presence of one or more *extracranial* (systemic) factors (hypoxia, hypercapnia, anaemia, decrease in arterial pressure, pyrexia, coughing, straining, inappropriate anaesthesia).

At present, there is no treatment for primary brain damage. The role of the definitive management of the head-injured patient is to detect and treat (or better still prevent) secondary brain damage and so permit the greatest possible recovery of neuronal function consistent with the extent of the primary impact damage.

Secondary brain damage is preventable

Because secondary brain damage becomes evident after the initial insult, all the factors responsible for this second injury are treatable potentially. In theory, secondary brain damage is preventable. However, the clinical realities of the situation are less encouraging (Rose *et al.* 1977; Jennett & Carlin, 1978; Gentleman & Jennett, 1981). For example, these workers found that, after admission to hospital, one or more potentially avoidable factors were present in 74% of a group of patients who died subsequently having been sufficiently conscious to talk coherently some time after admission. In 54% of these patients it was concluded that one avoidable factor had contributed significantly to their eventual demise. Of those avoidable incidents which certainly contributed to mortality, 70% were intracranial and 30% extracranial (Table 78.1). Space does not permit a consideration of each factor individually: however, it is worth highlighting three.

AIRWAY OBSTRUCTION

Although airway obstruction was common, only approximately one in four of the incidents was regarded as having contributed definately to the eventual death of the patient. What is of interest, however, was the finding that 50% of the incidents of airway obstruction occurred during the movement or transport of the patient *within* the hospital, or during transfer *between* hospitals. For example, in one cohort of comatose patients, being transferred from a primary receiving unit to the regional neurosurgical centre, it was found that 55% did not have a nasogastric tube in place, 36% had no form of artificial airway whatsoever and 61% had been transported lying supine on a non-tilting stretcher.

SYSTEMIC ARTERIAL HYPOTENSION

The frequency of arterial hypotension [defined as a systolic arterial pressure of less than 12 kPa (90 mmHg)] is always underestimated. Decreases (or increases) in arterial pressure can be recognized only during those periods in which arterial pressure is measured accurately and recorded conscientiously. However, the significance of even minor decreases in arterial pressure is not in doubt (Table 78.2). When present, the combination of arterial hypotension and hypoxaemia was lethal in 100% of the patients studied by Gentleman and Jennett (1981).

INTRACRANIAL HAEMATOMA

The development of an intracranial haematoma may convert rapidly a relatively minor injury into a life-threatening emergency. Therefore, a high degree of suspicion is required by all those dealing with the head-injured patient. Although computerized tomographic (CT) scanning has proved to be a reliable, and usually non-invasive, means of diagnosing haematoma, not all hospitals are so equipped. Even in those hospitals with the facilities for CT scanning, it may be difficult to obtain repeated scans—particularly in the patient with multiple trauma receiving mechanical

Table 78.1 Avoidable incidents (as % of total preventable incidents) in a group of 166 patients who died after head injury. (From Jennett & Carlin, 1978)

Avoidable Factors	Certain effect (%)	Total (%)
Intracranial		
Delay in treating haematoma	48	36
Inadequate control of epilepsy	8	10
Meningitis	7	4
Other	7	7
Total	**70**	**57**
Extracranial		
Airway obstruction	9	15
Hypotension	8	14
Other	13	14
Total	**30**	**43**

Table 78.2 Effect of hypoxia and arterial hypotension on outcome after head injury. (From Gentleman & Jennett, 1981)

	No.	Dead (%)	Good recovery (%)
Hypotension alone	12	75	8
Hypoxia alone	29	59	17
Hypoxia or hypotension	46	67	13
Hypoxia and hypotension	5	100	0
Neither Factor	104	34	34

ventilation, cardiovascular support, etc. Moreover, several studies have shown that the availability of CT scanning does not, of itself, improve outcome because, ideally, the haematoma must be detected *before* secondary brain damage occurs.

Neurological deterioration should be predicted and prevented

Delay in recognition (and hence in eventual evacuation) of an intracranial haematoma occurs because it is usual to become suspicious only when the patient's level of responsiveness has begun to deteriorate. However, it is recognized now that this policy of 'wait and see' implies that definitive action is taken too late: secondary brain damage is well-established. In an attempt to pre-empt the development of secondary brain damage, series of guidelines (Appendix 1) have been drawn up which should enable the clinician to manage the patient appropriately *before* neurological deterioration has become evident clinically. For example, the likelihood of a patient having a haematoma —even though he or she has not (as yet) shown signs of deteriorating neurological function—may be deduced from simple critria (Teasdale & Galbraith, 1981) and suitable guidelines devised (Table 78.3).

Priorities in management

Resuscitation

If one accepts the principles outlined previously it is obvious that the patient with a moderate to severe head injury must receive—from the moment of injury if possible—appropriate care and aggressive resuscita-

tion. It was noted above that 60 % of all deaths from head injury occur before the patient is admitted to hospital. Although the majority of these patients die from overwhelming primary brain damage sustained at the time of the initial insult, there is a body of opinion which believes that more active treatment sooner might improve outcome in specific instances. Certainly, because the events precipitating secondary brain damage are triggered by the impact, one could argue logically that clinical management should begin at this time also. This view is supported by the results of a study in San Diego in which it was demonstrated that, after the introduction of 'advanced paramedic services', there was a significant decrease (25 to 14 %) in the number of patients with uncontrollable intracranial hypertension [an intracranial pressure greater than 5.32 kPa (40 mmHg) despite standard aggressive therapy] on arrival at the hospital.

Wherever resuscitation is initiated, it should follow the classic pattern: airway, breathing, circulation (p. 954). An adequate airway is essential: more patients die of hypoxia than from extradural haematoma. If necessary, the trachea should be intubated to secure the airway. The point at issue is not 'does this patient require intubation of the trachea?' but 'does this patient *not* require intubation of the trachea' (in patients with protective reflexes it may be adequate to make use of the lateral position and an oropharyngeal airway). Intubation of the trachea does not require necessarily the administration of drugs or the institution of artificial ventilation. However, the head-injured patient must not be allowed to strain or cough on the tracheal tube and many advise that the patient be given thiopentone (even if unconscious) and/or neuromuscular blocking drugs before intubation to ensure that he does not. Nasotracheal intubation is not indicated usually at this stage and is contra-indicated if there is any suspicion that the patient may have a fracture of the base of the skull. As far as the actual technique of intubation is concerned, one should assume that, until proven otherwise, there is a facture of the cervical spine and take appropriate precautions.

Supplementary oxygen is always necessary, even if ventilation and colour appear adequate on clinical examination. Any improvement (or otherwise) in oxygenation can be assessed readily by the measurement of arterial oxygen tension which should be maintained at greater than 9.3 kPa (70 mmHg). If this value cannot be achieved with spontaneous ventilation (plus appropriate oxygen therapy) one should consider the use of artificial ventilation.

Table 78.3 Criteria for the transfer of patients with head injuries to the Institute of Neurological Sciences, Glasgow. (From Teasdale, 1985)

Indications
Deterioration in neurological status
Skull fracture, unless alert, orientated and asymptomatic
Focal neurological signs
Any impairment of consciousness greater than confusion
Confusion that persists for 6 hr after injury

Contra-indications
Major multiple injuries until resuscitated
Patients over 70 yr of age in coma from time of injury
Patients of any age who are flaccid, with no motor response and apnoeic

Pre-eminently, the adequacy of breathing must be assessed objectively (blood gas analysis) and any evidence of underventilation treated. The indications for the urgent institution of artificial ventilation in the accident and emergency department are:

1 Pao_2 less than 9.3 kPa (70 mmHg) with air, or 13.3 kPa (100 mmHg) with an F_Io_2 of 0.4.

2 Underventilation ($Paco_2$ greater than 6.0 kPa (45 mmHg)) in association with spontaneous ventilation.

3 Hyperventilation [$Paco_2$ less than 3.5 kPa (25 mmHg)] in association with spontaneous respiration. (Note that not all units accept this criterion as an indication for the urgent institution of artificial ventilation.) (See Table 78.8 for additional indications for the use of artificial ventilation in the head-injured patient.)

The frequency of associated injuries in the patient with head injury has been emphasized previously: an intercostal drain (or drains) should be inserted if there is radiological evidence (or clinical suspicion) of the presence of a pneumothorax or haemothorax, before artificial ventilation is instituted.

The haemodynamic status of the patient is of great importance (p. 1441) and must be monitored accurately and frequently. Intravenous access should be secured, and cannulation of a central vein is advantageous [measurement of central venous pressure (CVP), infusion of fluids, infusion of mannitol] and is recommended in the patient with multiple trauma. However, cannulation of the basilic, median cephalic or subclavian vein is to be preferred to cannulation of the internal jugular vein in the head-injured patient. As far as possible, hypovolaemia should be corrected and arterial pressure restored to the 'normal' for that individual using physiological saline, colloids and/or blood as appropriate. Occult blood loss is dangerous and the control of intrathoracic or intra-abdominal haemorrhage must take precedence over the more definitive management of the head injury. If there is any doubt, diagnostic pleural tap or peritoneal lavage should be considered.

At this point, certain other aspects of the early management of the patient with a head injury should be considered, although they are not specifically part of the initial resuscitation.

1 Mannitol (1 g/kg) should be administered normally, if required, once the advice of a neurosurgeon has been obtained. However, its administration is urgent if an intracranial haematoma is found on CT scanning and/or if there is clinical evidence of a dilating

Table 78.4   Drugs (and doses) suitable for the management of seizures in the head-injured patient

Phenytoin
Slow injection i.v. (up to 1 mg·kg^{-1}·min^{-1})
Maximum loading dose: adults, 15 mg/kg; children, 5 mg/kg

Phenobarbitone
Slow injection i.v. (up to 1 mg·kg^{-1}·min^{-1})
Maximum loading dose 4 mg/kg

Tiopentone
Slow injection i.v. 2.5% (25 mg/ml) (up to 5 mg·kg^{-1}·min^{-1})
Maximum loading dose 20 mg/kg

Chlormethiazole
Infusion i.v. 0.8% (8 mg/ml) (up to 7 ml/min)
Maximum loading dose 10 mg/kg

pupil or progressive deterioration in conscious level.

2 Convulsions should be controlled by the intravenous administration of an anticonvulsant (Table 78.4). Ventilatory support may be required if respiratory depression occurs in association with the administration of a barbiturate or benzodiazepine. Clearly, convulsive motor activity should not be controlled by the use of a neuromuscular blocking drug alone.

3 It has now been shown that steroids are of no value in the management of the head injury itself (Dearden et al., 1986). Thus, they should be given only if there is a separate indication for their use.

4 Pain is not only unpleasant for the patient: it also increases cerebral blood volume and intracranial pressure. Analgesia (morphine, up to 0.1 mg/kg; papaveretum, up to 0.2 mg/kg; fentanyl up to 3 μg/kg) should not be withheld just because the patient has a head injury. Indeed, they may do more than relieve pain; they may also suppress acute increases in systemic arterial pressure and surges in intracranial pressure.

Assessment

The definitive neurological assessment of any patient with a head injury i.e. the initial assessment of the severity of the brain damage, must be undertaken *after* the institution of appropriate resuscitative measures, and once time has been allowed for any improvement in the patient's general condition to become manifest. Attempts to assess the severity of the head injury before correction of hypoxaemia or replacement of blood loss lead to erroneous conclusions and may militate against the rational choice of the most appropriate definitive management. For example, fixed and dilated pupils and/or apnoea at the moment of entry to hospital may be the result of an obstructed airway, or arterial hypotension or drugs rather than head injury itself. Likewise, measures to select those head-injured patients in whom prognosis is hopeless before the effects of resuscitation have become evident could lead to the loss of a number of patients who would recover otherwise.

The most effective way to assess the integrity of central and peripheral neurological function has been and continues to be the *clinical* neurological examination. This requires that the patient *responds to* auditory, visual and tactile stimuli in a defined way. Until 1965, the neurological examination of the *comatose* (unresponsive) patient was limited to those aspects of the traditional neurological examination which could be carried out—pupillary response to light, assessment of tendon reflexes and plantar response. In general terms, these provided little useful information. Once the role of the brainstem in the genesis of coma had become accepted, various measures were introduced by which the function of the brainstem could be assessed at the bedside. Subsequently, a number of 'coma' charts and 'coma' scales were designed and evaluated. The most widely used of these, the Glasgow coma scale (Table 78.5), is based on the assessment of three separate sets of function: eye opening, best verbal response and best motor response. Simple addition of the values on the right in Table 78.5 provides a coma 'score'. This is most useful as a means of classifying the severity of the brain damage: minor 14–15, moderate 9–13, severe 3–8. Use of the Glasgow coma scale alone does not ensure assessment of lower brainstem reflexes nor of changes in physiological variables such as heart rate, arterial pressure, or respiratory rate or pattern. Nevertheless, numerous studies have shown that it can serve as an adequate indicator of changing neurological state. However, in the individual patient, more information on overall neurological function may be obtained by the additional assessment of other physiological variables (arterial pressure, intracranial pressure).

What is assessed and how it is assessed varies from patient to patient. At one extreme there is the conscious patient who can talk, give an account of his injury and respond verbally to the various facets of the clinical examination of his neurological function. At the other extreme is the head-injured patient in an intensive care environment in whom the lungs are ventilated mechanically (either as an elective procedure or as a sequel to respiratory insufficiency) and who may be receiving neuromuscular blocking drugs, hypnotics or opioids to permit compliance with artificial ventilation. In this latter group, the majority (or possibly all) of the *clinical* features relied upon normally to monitor neurological status are lost. Although it is customary to allow such patients to 'lighten' intermittently so that a neurological assessment may be obtained, this is not satisfactory, and it must be accepted that the ability of the clinician to detect changes in neurological state is impaired. Despite this, there should be no hesitation in administering anticonvulsants, analgesics or neuromuscular blocking drugs, when indicated, as most of the initial decisions in regard to treatment are based on the findings of the CT scan and/or measurements of intracranial pressure. Before concluding the initial assessment of the patient, it is important to exclude other causes of depression of consciousness (diabetes, alcohol, hypothermia, epilepsy, cerebrovascular accident, drugs, hypoxia).

The initial neurological assessment of the head-injured patient (at the correct point in time) is of fundamental importance. It acts as a baseline on which progress (or deterioration) can be judged, prognosis can be predicted and treatment can be evaluated. *Repeated* neurological assessment is the cornerstone of

Table 78.5 Glasgow coma scale. Numbers on the right may be added (one number for each index of neurological function) to produce the Glasgow coma score

Eye opening	
Spontaneous	4
To speech	3
To pain	2
None	1
Best verbal response	
Orientated	5
Confused	4
Inappropriate words	3
Incomprehensible sounds	2
None	1
Best motor response	
Obey commands	6
Localize pain	5
Normal flexion to pain	4
Abnormal flexion to pain	3
Extension to pain	2
None	1

the management of this group of patients. Because this is so, this brief account should be augmented by a review of more comprehensive texts (Teasdale, 1976; Jennett & Teasdale, 1981; Teasdale, 1985; Miller 1987).

Diagnosis

Definitive management of the patient with a head injury requires a definitive diagnosis. Nowadays, this is obtained almost exclusively by CT scanning which should be performed as soon as possible when the patient's cardiovascular and respiratory variables have been stabilized and when injury to the spine has been excluded (for indications for CT scanning see Appendix 2). An anaesthetic may be required, especially if the patient is restless, to abolish movement artifacts and so optimize the acquisition of reliable information. If so, a technique of anaesthesia described in Chapter 32 should be employed. If CT scanning is unavailable, the search for a diagnosis should be pursued by the use of ultrasound, angiography and, possibly, burr hole exploration—*if equipment and expertise are available*. A good quality CT scan shows the location and extent of focal lesions but shows little in patients with diffuse axonal injury. Patients who have a focal lesion with evidence of midline displacement require surgery and, normally, go directly to the operating theatre. In situations in which surgery is not indicated, it is usual to transfer the patient to an intensive therapy unit (ITU) either in the centre to which the patient has been referred, or in the primary receiving unit.

The performance of CT scanning (and, indeed, of other radiological investigations: skull, cervical spine, chest, abdomen, pelvis, limbs and any other area of clinical suspicion) requires that the patient be moved either within the accident and emergency department or the primary receiving unit or between hospitals. Clearly, this is a time of increased risk as far as the patient is concerned although, of course, the information sought is crucial to any further management. It is important that the basic care of the patient (supplementary oxygen, intravenous fluids, control of pain, monitoring of arterial pressure and neurological function, etc.) be established before, and continued throughout, such manoeuvres. As an aside, it is worth noting that one of the purposes of the continuous monitoring of intracranial pressure is to aid in the definition of those occasions when a radiological study is indicated and so decrease the number of unnecessary movements undertaken by an individual patient.

Maintenance of cerebral perfusion

Evidence of cerebral ischaemia is present in more than 90% of patients who die following a head injury and, when present in a patient who survives, is associated with a poorer outcome. The fact that ischaemia is present implies that the delivery of substrate to the brain was inadequate to meet its metabolic requirements.

The supply of oxygen to the brain is dependent on the amount of blood reaching brain tissue (cerebral blood flow) and the amount of oxygen carried per unit of blood (arterial oxygen content). Thus, the delivery of oxygen may be optimized by ensuring an adequate flow of fully oxygenated blood to the brain (ideally, to the most threatened regions). In the head-injured patient, cerebral blood flow (especially the blood flow to the damaged or potentially ischaemic regions) is dependent largely on systemic arterial pressure. Thus, it is mandatory that arterial pressure be controlled adequately. However, care is necessary to prevent arterial pressure increasing significantly above the patient's pre-injury value. As parts of the cerebral vasculature cannot constrict in response to such increases in arterial pressure (Chapter 32), there is a high probability of marked swelling of the brain and, consequently, of increases in intracranial pressure. Many devices are now available which permit non-invasive monitoring of arterial pressure from the arm, leg or finger, and one of these may suffice in the majority of patients with a pure head injury. In the patient with multiple trauma, however, there are advantages in monitoring arterial pressure directly.

Mean cerebral perfusion pressure is equal to mean arterial pressure minus mean intracranial pressure, therefore any increase in intracranial pressure decreases perfusion of the brain and increases the likelihood of ischaemic damage (unless arterial pressure increases concomitantly). Although the decision to institute measurement of intracranial pressure is made normally by the neurosurgeon, it is relevant to note that one of the cardinal indications for the use of the technique is the patient with a head injury undergoing artificial ventilation of the lungs.

The importance of considering values of arterial pressure *and* intracranial pressure when making therapeutic decisions cannot be overemphasized. In the patient with a head injury a marked increase in arterial pressure is frequently a sequel to a shift of brain and/or an increase in intracranial pressure. The correct management in this situation is to decrease intracranial pressure (p. 1443). Any decrease in arterial pressure alone increases the likelihood of cerebral ischaemia.

Practicalities of management

This section considers the practical clinical management of the head-injured patient in an ITU. It is assumed that the patient's cardiovascular system is stable, and the remit of this chapter is to consider those modalities of management relevant to the head injury *per se* (management of other aspects of multiple trauma is detailed in Chapter 32).

Currently, the intensive care of such patients involves a 'package' of measures designed to maximize the delivery of oxygen to the brain and, hence, prevent, or ameliorate, the effects of secondary brain damage.

Basic care of the head-injured patient

Good general care of the patient is vital. This includes nursing the patient with a 20–30° head-up tilt, regular changes of position and physiotherapy. Although it has been argued that the use of the physiotherapy and the frequency of tracheal suction should be limited because of the associated surges in intracranial pressure, the prevention of a chest infection (and of pressure sores) is of greater importance. In any case, if required, the acute increases in intracranial pressure associated with physiotherapy and other stimulating procedures can be obtunded by the prior administration of etomidate, 2–6 mg, thiopentone, 100–200 mg, γ-hydroxybutyric acid, 1 g, or propofol, 100 mg. The eyes should be protected and examined regularly for corneal abrasions/ulceration. Analgesics should be given as required to provide continuing relief of pain.

The optimum body temperature for the head-injured patient is 35 °C. On no account should the patient be allowed to become pyrexial: tepid sponging, fanning and chlorpromazine, 0.1–0.2 mg/kg, may be helpful. Although routine prophylactic antibiotics should not be used (unless there is evidence of a fracture of the base of the skull) infection requires energetic and, preferably, specific therapy.

An anticonvulsant (for example, phenytoin 15 mg/kg in divided doses on day 1, 10 mg/kg in divided doses on day 2, thereafter 5 mg/kg) should be given prophylactically to all patients with an intracerebral haematoma or history of multiple post-traumatic seizures. If phenytoin is used, blood concentrations should be monitored from day 3 (therapeutic range 40–80 μmol/litre).

It is likely that a gastric tube will have been inserted at the accident and emergency department in order to decompress the stomach. Unless contra-indicated, nasogastric drainage should be maintained until enteral feeding is commenced (usually around 48–72 hr after the injury). Parenteral nutrition should be considered if enteral feeding is contra-indicated or fails. It is customary to give ranitidine (50 mg 8-hourly) in an attempt to prevent ulceration of and bleeding from the mucosa of the stomach.

Fluid balance and electrolyte concentrations should be monitored, particularly as trauma to the brain may disturb physiological regulating mechanisms and lead to diabetes insipidus, the inappropriate secretion of antidiuretic hormone, water overload/retention (the most common cause of low serum sodium concentration in head injury) and water depletion (increased serum sodium concentration). Diagnosis of these various problems requires measurement of urine volume, serum concentrations of sodium, potassium and urea, urinary content of sodium and potassium and serum, and urine osmolality.

Recent studies have highlighted the detrimental effects of increases in blood glucose concentration on neurological function after ischaemia (Fitch, 1988). Hence it is necessary to monitor blood glucose concentrations repeatedly and maintain these within the physiological range (hypoglycaemia has, of course, been known for some time to cause brain damage).

In adults, hourly fluid input should equal the previous hour's output of urine + 30 ml (to replace insensible losses) up to a maximum input of 150 ml/hr. Customarily, it has been recommended that dextrose 5% in saline 0.45% (with 20 mmol potassium chloride per 500 ml) be used initially, and that appropriate adjustments to the nature of the fluid(s) and the additives be made in the light of the results of the biochemical investigations. Concern over the role of hyperglycaemia in the augmentation of ischaemic damage has prompted several groups of workers to argue that 'glucose-containing solutions be avoided in patients undergoing operations that may have a significant risk of intraoperative ischaemia'.

A reasonable compromise would be the use of colloid (salt-poor if indicated) to maintain circulating blood volume and cardiac filling pressure, saline 0.9% solution whilst monitoring repeatedly the serum sodium concentration, and dextrose 5% solution as required to maintain normal blood glucose concentrations.

Specific treatment in the management of the head-injured patient

Specific treatment in the context of head injury aims to maximize the delivery of oxygen to the brain by optimizing the oxygen content of arterial blood and balancing cerebral metabolic demands and cerebral perfusion. This chapter has emphasized the importance of the former and the means by which the optimal carriage of oxygen may be realized (supplementary oxygen, correction of anaemia, management of chest injury, prevention of the aspiration of gastric contents, artificial ventilation). The latter can be achieved either by suppressing cerebral metabolism and so decreasing the demand for oxygen or by improving the supply. Although theoretically attractive, the use of barbiturates to decrease electively metabolic requirements of the damaged brain has not survived detailed prospective investigation (Schwartz et al., 1984; Ward et al., 1985). Likewise, the elective use of hypothermia to temperatures of 32–33 °C, as a means of decreasing cerebral metabolism deliberately, has fallen into disuse. Nevertheless, there are good theoretical arguments for attempting to achieve and maintain a core temperature of 35 °C. This can be obtained often by controlling the heat generated by muscle activity and allowing the patient to 'find his own value of temperature' in relation to the environment. However, current interest centres on the means by which cerebral perfusion may be increased. It is evident from the arguments put forward above that this may be achieved by increasing systemic arterial pressure, by decreasing intracranial pressure, or by a combination of both. In practice, this implies normalization of systemic arterial pressure (correction of blood loss, optimization of cardiac filling pressures and myocardial performance, relief of pain) and control of intracranial hypertension.

MANAGEMENT OF INCREASES IN INTRACRANIAL PRESSURE

Before discussing the specific modalities which may be employed to control intracranial pressure, it is important to consider two general points. First, it would seem logical intuitively to accept that a high intracranial pressure must be bad for the patient and, hence, any attempt to decrease it, beneficial. This presupposes that the increase in intracranial pressure is an aetiological *mechanism* in the development of cerebral ischaemia. The other side of this particular 'coin' is that the change in intracranial pressure is a *measure* of the damage to the brain with the proviso that one should treat, if possible, the cause of the brain swelling and not the measurement of its severity. Second, it must be stressed that, although we are about to consider the means by which increases in intracranial pressure may be attenuated or decreased, the ideal management would be to prevent any increase *ab initio*.

With a patient lying supine, the normal range of intracranial pressure is 0–2 kPa (0–15 mmHg) (Chapter 32). In those units which treat increases in intracranial pressure aggressively, specific therapy is introduced when intracranial pressure (measured with the zero reference at the external auditory meatus) exceeds 3.3 kPa (25 mmHg) for more than 5 min, *provided* there is no obvious, easily remediable cause (hypoxaemia, hypercapnia, pyrexia, compression of the jugular veins, 'fighting the ventilator', seizure activity).

The next stage in management is to validate the measurement and then to select one or more of the three measures (Miller, 1985) which are known to be effective in most patients and which carry a low risk of worsening the patient's condition (Table 78.6): hyperventilation, drainage of cerebrospinal fluid (CSF),

Table 78.6 Proven methods of controlling increases in intracranial pressure. (From Miller, 1985)

Treatment	Limitations	Risks
Hyperventilation	Blood vessels must be responsive to changes in P_{CO_2}	Vasoconstriction may produce brain ischaemia (although structural damage has never been shown to occur)
CSF drainage	From ventricular catheter only	Leakage of CSF may interfere with intracranial pressure recording. Haemorrhage in track of cannula through brain
Mannitol	Serum osmolality must be less than 320 mosmol/litre	Fluid and electrolyte disturbance and renal failure

CSF = cerebrospinal fluid.

administration of mannitol 20% solution. Mannitol 20% (0.5 g/kg) over 15–20 min is the first drug of choice for the rapid control of intracranial hypertension. Usually, an infusion of mannitol is required early in the management of the patient to control intracranial pressure initially. Thereafter, it may not be necessary to give mannitol on more than one further occasion, provided controlled hyperventilation is continued. However, if necessary, the above dose may be repeated 4-hourly: indeed, a 'closed-loop' system is in use in at least one unit. Mannitol has very few disadvantages but may produce acidosis and renal failure if the plasma osmolality exceeds 320 mosmol/litre. Although the use of loop diuretics in the treatment of intracranial hypertension is controversial, frusemide, 0.4–0.6 mg/kg, in addition to the mannitol (frusemide given 15 min after the start of the mannitol) is often beneficial. Central venous pressure should be measured during and following the administration of mannitol as arterial hypotension may occur as a result of a decrease in circulating blood volume.

Drainage of CSF may be a useful means of decreasing intracranial pressure, although it is less effective if the ventricles are small (as in patients with diffuse axonal injury). To prevent the collapse of the ventricles in other patients, the CSF should be drained against a positive pressure [approximately 3 kPa (22 mmHg)].

In many units, controlled ventilation is the most widely practised specific measure in the management of the head-injured patient because, in theory at least, it helps to maximize the oxygen content of blood and control intracranial pressure (McDowall, 1985).

Advocates of the elective use of controlled ventilation decrease Pa_{CO_2} to 3.5–4 kPa (26–30 mmHg) in all patients liable to develop intracranial hypertension. More pronounced hyperventilation [Pa_{CO_2} 2.6 kPa (20 mmHg)] may be employed in the treatment of an increasing intracranial pressure. By inducing hypocapnia (Table 78.7), hyperventilation produces cerebral vasoconstriction, a decrease in cerebral blood volume and a decrease in intracranial pressure. Because it is important that the head-injured patient does not cough, strain or 'fight the ventilator', neuromuscular blockade and sedation if indicated should be used to aid compliance with mechanical ventilation. If possible, the tidal volume should be adjusted so as to produce an inflation pressure of 20 cmH$_2$O or less. Ideally, Pa_{O_2} should be greater than 16 kPa (120 mmHg): certainly, it should not be allowed to decrease to less than 8 kPa (60 mmHg). If

Table 78.7 Advantages and disadvantages of induced hypocapnia in the management of the head-injured patient

Advantages
Induces vasoconstriction in cerebral blood vessels responsive to effects of carbon dioxide: decreases cerebral blood flow, cerebral blood volume and intracranial pressure.

May increase the perfusion to potentially ischaemic areas (inverse steal)

Improves autoregulation: protects against the effects of transient changes in arterial pressure

Helps to correct acidosis of brain tissue

Disadvantages
None—if patient is normovolaemic and if Pa_{CO_2} is not allowed to decrease below 2.7 kPa (20 mmHg)

adequate oxygenation proves difficult to achieve, even after an increase in F_1O_2 to greater than 0.5–0.6, positive end-expiratory pressure (PEEP) may be employed. However, a maximum value of +6 cmH$_2$O should not be exceeded (in the uncomplicated head injury), and cerebral perfusion pressure should be monitored closely.

The duration of mechanical ventilation is usually determined electively as 48–72 hr in the first instance. It would then be customary to permit the return of neuromuscular transmission and assess the patient neurologically. If the indications for artificial ventilation in the ITU (Table 78.8) remain, or if intracranial pressure increases again, hyperventilation is main-

Table 78.8 Indications for the use of artificial ventilation in the management of the head-injured patient. Note that the decision to introduce artificial ventilation as an elective procedure (i.e. not urgently) should be taken once the patient has been resuscitated and stabilized

Inadequate spontaneous breathing
$Pa_{O_2} < 9.3$ kPa (70 mmHg) with F_1O_2 0.21
$Pa_{O_2} < 13.3$ kPa (100 mmHg) with F_1O_2 0.40
$Pa_{CO_2} > 6.0$ kPa (45 mmHg)

Poor neurological function
No response to pain (Glasgow coma score 3)
Spontaneous extensor posturing (Glasgow coma score 4)
Repeated convulsions
Spontaneous hyperventilation: $Pa_{CO_2} < 3.5$ kPa (25 mmHg)
Intracranial pressure 25 mmHg for more than 5 min (no obviously remediable cause)
After intracranial surgery (for 12–24 hr)

Associated pathology
Chest injury
Prolonged surgery
Inhalation of gastric contents

tained for a further 24–48 hr—provided intracranial pressure decreases.

Monitoring the head-injured patient

Monitoring of the basic neurological, haemodynamic and respiratory status of the head-injured patient, and of the changes in the various indices, is a means of guiding the clinician so that appropriate therapeutic steps may be taken. The various modalities of monitoring relevant to the management of the head-injured patient have been mentioned above and are summarized in Table 78.9.

The goals of medical treatment in the head-injured patient are to preserve neurological function and promote physical and social rehabilitation. In this chapter we have considered only those aspects related to the acute phase of the illness. However, it must not forgotten that this is but the beginning of a long and often difficult process of recovery. A proportion of these patients develop brain death and may serve as a source of organ donation. The criteria for diagnosis of brain death are given in Appendix 3.

Appendix 1

Guidelines in regard to the initial management of an adult patient with a head injury
(Group of Neurosurgeons, 1984)

Criteria for X-ray examination of skull after a recent head injury (the presence of one or more of the following indicates a need for a skull X-ray):

1 Loss of consciousness or amnesia at any time.
2 Symptoms or signs of neurological deficit.
3 Cerebrospinal fluid or blood from nose or ear.
4 Suspected penetrating injury, scalp bruising or swelling.
5 Laceration of scalp.

Criteria for admission to hospital after a recent head injury (one or more of the following):

1 Confusion or any other depression of the level of consciousness at the time of examination (as measured by the Glasgow coma scale).
2 Fracture of the skull.
3 Neurological symptoms or signs, headache or vomiting.
4 Difficulty in the neurological assessment of the patient because of e.g. alcohol, epilepsy, age (the very young).
5 Other associated medical conditions: diabetes mellitus, haemophilia, patient receiving anticoagulant therapy.
6 Social problems: in particular the lack of a responsible adult to supervise the patient.

NB: post-traumatic amnesia with full recovery is not itself an indication for admission to hospital. Relatives or friends of patients sent home should receive written instructions on possible complications and what to do (e.g. return to hospital).

Table 78.9 Possible modalities of monitoring in the patient with a head injury. Note that the selected techniques of monitoring would be supplemented routinely with repeated assessments of fluid balance, serum electrolyte concentrations, urine and serum osmolalities

	Routinely	Frequently	Occasionally
Cerebral function	Neurological examination Coma scale/score Blood glucose conc. Temperature		EEG Evoked potentials CFM/CFAM
Cerebral perfusion	Arterial pressure ICP Heart rate ECG Pa_{CO_2}	CBF CVP Expired CO_2 conc.	PCWP Arterial–jugular venous O_2 difference
Oxygen carriage	Haemoglobin conc. F_IO_2 Pa_{CO_2} Respiratory rate Expired minute volume	Sa_{O_2} Pulse oximetry	Oxygen content

ICP = intracranial pressure.   CVP = central venous pressure.
CBF = cerebral blood flow.   PCWP = pulmonary capillary wedge pressure.

Criteria for consultation with a regional neurosurgical unit (one or more of the following) (see also Table 78.3):

1 Coma continuing after resuscitation.

2 Neurological deterioration after admission.

3 Depressed skull fracture.

4 Linear fracture of the skull in combination with either:

(a) Confusion or other depression of the level of consciousness,

(b) Focal neurological signs, or

(c) Seizures.

5 Suspected open injury of the vault or the base of the skull.

6 Confusion or other neurological disturbances persisting for more than 12 hr even if there is no fracture of the skull

NB: although the above guidelines may be helpful, clinical judgement is always necessary.

Appendix 2

Guidelines for CT scanning in patients with head injury

Immediate CT scan

1 Patients in coma (Glasgow coma score 8 or less). (Chance of having an intracranial haematoma is greater than 40%.)

2 Patients in whom level of consciousness is depressed (Glasgow coma score 9–13) and who have a skull fracture. (Chance of haematoma or other significant intracranial lesion is around 20%.)

3 Patients who show neurological deterioration to coma (Glasgow coma score 8 or less).

Urgent CT scan (within 6 hr)

1 Patients who are drowsy and/or disorientated (Glasgow coma score 14–15)and have a skull fracture (Chance of haematoma 15%.)

2 Patients with abnormal neurological signs plus skull fracture. (Chance of haematoma 15%.)

3 Patients with depression of consciousness (Glasgow coma score 9–13) plus focal neurological deficit, irrespective of presence of skull fracture.

4 Patients with unexplained increase in intracranial pressure.

CT scan within 24 hr

1 Patients who show neurological deterioration (by 2 or more points on Glasgow coma score).

2 Patients with confusion or severe headache, persisting for more than 48 hr, but no skull fracture.

CT scan before surgery

Patients with multiple injuries which require surgery and general anaesthesia and who have a Glasgow coma score of 15. In such patients, it is important to exclude intracranial haematoma positively. However, scan should be undertaken only if airway is secure and haemodynamic status satisfactory. If not, surgery should be undertaken first and the scan performed afterwards.

Appendix 3

Diagnosis of brain death

Statement issued by the Honorary Secretary of the Conference of Medical Royal Colleges and their Faculties in the UK (1976)

Criteria for considering diagnosis of brain death (all of the following should co-exist):

1 The patient is deeply comatose.

(a) There should be no suspicion that this state is due to depressant drugs.

(b) Primary hypothermia as a cause of coma should have been excluded.

(c) Metabolic and endocrine disturbances which can cause coma should have been excluded.

2 The patient is being maintained on a ventilator because spontaneous respiration had previously become inadequate or had ceased altogether.

Relaxants (neuromuscular blocking agents) and other drugs should have been excluded as a cause of respiratory inadequacy or failure.

3 There should be no doubt that the patient's condition is due to irremediable structural brain damage. The diagnosis should have been established fully.

Criteria for confirming brain death (all brainstem reflexes should be absent):

1 The pupils are fixed in diameter and do not respond to sharp changes in the intensity of incident light.

2 There is no corneal reflex.

3 The vestibulo-ocular reflexes are absent. These are absent when no eye movement occurs during or after the slow injection of 20 ml of ice-cold water into

each external auditory meatus in turn, clear access to the tympanic membrane having been established by direct inspection. This test may be contra-indicated on one or other side because of local trauma.

4 No motor responses within the cranial nerve distribution can be elicited by adequate stimulation of any somatic area.

5 There is no gag reflex or reflex to bronchial stimulation by a suction catheter passed down the trachea.

6 No respiratory movements occur when the patient is disconnected from the mechanical ventilator for long enough to ensure that the arterial carbon dioxide tension rises above the threshold for stimulating respiration i.e. the Pa_{CO_2} must normally reach 6.7 kPa (50 mmHg). This is achieved best by measuring the blood gases; if this facility is available, the patient should be disconnected when the Pa_{CO_2} reaches 5.3–6.0 kPa (40–45 mmHg) after administration of 5% carbon dioxide in oxygen through the ventilator.

If blood gas analysis is not available to measure the Pa_{CO_2} and Pa_{O_2}, the alternative procedure is to supply the ventilator with pure oxygen for 10 min (preoxygenation), then with 5% carbon dioxide in oxygen for 5 min, and to disconnect the ventilator for 10 min whilst delivering oxygen at 6 litre/min by catheter into the trachea.

Other considerations

1 Repetition of testing. It is customary to repeat the tests to ensure that there has been no observer error.

2 The interval between tests depends on the progress of the patient and might be as long as 24 hr.

3 Integrity of spinal reflexes. Reflexes of spinal origin may persist or return after an initial absence in brain-dead patients.

4 Confirmatory investigations. It is now accepted widely that electroencephalography is not necessary for diagnosing brain death.

5 Body temperature. The body temperature in these patients may be low because of depression of central temperature regulation by drugs or by brainstem damage, and it is recommended that it should be not less than 35 °C before the diagnostic tests are carried out. A low-reading thermometer should be used.

6 Specialist opinion and status of doctors concerned. Experienced clinicians in ITUs, acute medical wards, and accident and emergency departments should not normally require specialist advice. Only when the primary diagnosis is in doubt is it necessary to consult with a neurologist or neurosurgeon. The decision to withdraw artificial support should be made after all the criteria presented above have been fulfilled and can be made by any one of the following combinations of doctors:

(a) A consultant who is in charge of the case and one other doctor.

(b) In the absence of a consultant, his deputy who should have been registered for 5 yr or more and who should have had adequate experience in the care of such cases, and one other doctor.

References

Dearden N.M., Gibson J.S., Gibson R.M., McDowall D.G. & Cameron M.M. (1986) Effects of high-dose dexamethasone on outcome from severe head injury. *Journal of Neurosurgery* 64, 81–8.

Fitch W. (1988) Hyperglycaemia and ischaemic brain damage. In *Anaesthesia Review*, number 5 (Ed. Kaufman L.) pp. 119–30. Churchill Livingstone, Edinburgh.

Gentleman D. & Jennett B. (1981) Hazards of inter-hospital transfer of comatose head-injured patients. *Lancet* ii, 853–5.

Group of Neurosurgeons (1984) Guidelines for initial management after head injury in adults. *British Medical Journal* 288, 983–5.

Jennett B. & Carlin J. (1978) Preventable mortality and morbidity after head-injury. *Injury* 10, 31–9.

Jennett B. & Teasdale G. (1981) Assessment of impared consciousness. In *Management of Head Injuries. Contemporary Neurology*, number 20, pp. 77–93. F.A. Davis, Philadelphia.

McDowall D.G. (1985) Artificial ventilation in the management of the head-injured patient. In *Head Injury and the Anaesthetist* (Eds Fitch W. & Barker J.) pp. 149–63. Elsevier, Amsterdam.

Miller J.D. (1987) Neurological evaluation of the unconscious patient. In *Intensive Care and Monitoring of the Neurosurgical Patient* (Ed. Landolt A.M.) pp. 1–14. Karger, Basel.

Miller J.D. (1985) Head injury and brain ischaemia — implications for therapy. *British Journal of Anaesthesia* 57, 120–30.

Rose J., Valtonen S. & Jennett B. (1977) Avoidable factors contributing to death after head injury. *British Medical Journal* ii, 615–18.

Schwartz M.L., Tator C.H., Rowed D.W., Reid, S.R. & Meguro K. (1984) The University of Toronto Head Injury Study: a prospective, randomised comparison of pentobarbital and mannitol. *Canadian Journal of Neurological Sciences* 11, 434–40.

Teasdale G. (1976) Assessment of head injuries. *British Journal of Anaesthesia* 48, 761–6.

Teasdale G. (1982) Management of head injuries. *The Practitioner* 226, 1667–73.

Teasdale G. (1985) The clinical assessment of the head-injured patient. In *Head Injury and the Anaesthetist* (Eds Fitch W. & Barker J.) pp. 83–101. Elsevier, Amsterdam.

Teasdale G. & Galbraith S. (1981) Acute traumatic intracranial haematomas. In *Progress in Neurological Surgery* (Eds Krayenbyhl H., Maspes P.E. & Sweet W.H.) pp. 252–90. Karger, Basel.

Ward J.D., Baker D.P., Miller D., Choi S.C., Marmarou A., Wood C, Newton P.G. & Keenan R. (1985) Failure of prophylactic barbiturate coma in the treatment of severe head injury. *Journal of Neurosurgery* 62, 383–8.

79

Acquired Haemostatic Failure

G. DOLAN AND C. D. FORBES

Disorders of blood coagulation may be congenital or acquired, and a detailed history and thorough clinical examination may often distinguish between the two. Although the majority of haemostatic problems which become manifest for the first time in adult life are acquired, it must be remembered that not all patients with a congenital coagulation disorder have a family history, and those with milder forms may not present until challenged by trauma or surgery e.g. mild haemophilia, Christmas disease or von Willebrand's disease.

Acquired haemostatic failure is the result of a disease process affecting the haemostatic mechanism through one of the following mechanisms:

1 Disorders of synthesis of coagulation factors e.g. malabsorption states, oral anticoagulants.
2 Increased loss of coagulation factors and platelets through consumption or blood loss e.g. disseminated intravascular coagulation, cardiopulmonary bypass.
3 Through the production of substances which interfere with the function of coagulation factors e.g. acquired inhibitors or drugs, or which interfere with platelet function e.g. fibrinogen degradation products, drugs. Often, a combination of these mechanisms operate.

Clinical history

1 Specific questions about any family history should be asked.
2 The patient should be questioned on any previous haemorrhagic episodes:
 (a) Any tendency to easy bruising or prolonged bleeding?
 (b) Any haemorrhagic problems after operations, particularly tonsillectomy or dental extractions?

 (c) Any episodes of gastrointestinal or genitourinary bleeding including menorrhagia and obstetric blood loss?
3 Systematic enquiry to uncover sypmtoms of underlying systemic disease such as neoplasms, connective tissue diseases or liver disease should be made.
4 A detailed drug history with specific reference to anticoagulants and antiplatelet drugs should be taken.

Clinical examination

A detailed clinical examination noting the following should be made:
1 Main sites of bleeding, including extent and distribution of skin lesions, mucous membrane bleeding, gastrointestinal bleeding, haematuria, haemoptysis and haemarthroses.
2 Any bleeding from wound sites or venepuncture sites should be noted.
3 If excessive bleeding is noted during surgery, a thorough search for a local bleeding point should be made to distinguish a primary surgical problem from diffuse bleeding.
4 Any evidence of systemic disease such as stigmata of liver disease, evidence of weight loss, abdominal masses, lymphadenopathy, splenomegaly suggestive of neoplasia or skin rashes and joint abnormalities which may suggest connective tissue disease.
5 There may be evidence also of sequelae of previous bleeding e.g. neurological signs from cerebral bleeds, joint deformity from haemarthroses and other physical signs suggestive of nerve entrapment from haematoma. After completing the initial clinical assessment the following basic screening investigations should be undertaken.

(a) Full blood count including platelet count and examination of blood film.

(b) Serum urea and creatinine measurements to assess renal function.

(c) Liver function tests.

(d) Further assessment of any abnormality noted during clinical assessment e.g. by radiological screening, antinuclear antibody testing or erythrocyte sedimentation rate (ESR) estimation.

COAGULATION SCREEN

The screening tests employed commonly in the investigation of coagulation disorders are the prothrombin time (PT), partial thromboplastin time (PTT) and the thrombin clotting time (TCT). These tests are designed to help localize any abnormality in the coagulation pathway into either the extrinsic pathway, intrinsic pathway or common pathway (Fig. 79.1).

Prothrombin time

This involves adding a source of thromboplastin

(animal brain usually) and calcium to plasma thus activating Factor VII which activates Factor X. The cascade process continues with Xa and Va converting prothrombin to thrombin which in turn converts fibrinogen to fibrin. Thus, the PT bypasses the intrinsic pathway and is abnormal only with deficiencies of Factors VII, X, V, prothrombin or fibrinogen or if a coagulation inhibitor is present.

Partial thromboplastin time [or kaolin cephalin clotting time (KCCT)]

In this test, the contact Factors XII and XI are activated by kaolin, and phospholipid accelerates the reactions involving VIII and V. Thus, factor X is activated and is followed by formation of thrombin and fibrin. From the diagram it may be seen that the only factor not involved in this pathway is VII and thus this test gives prolonged times with deficiencies of XII, XI, IX, X, V, prothrombin or fibrinogen or by inhibitors (e.g. heparin).

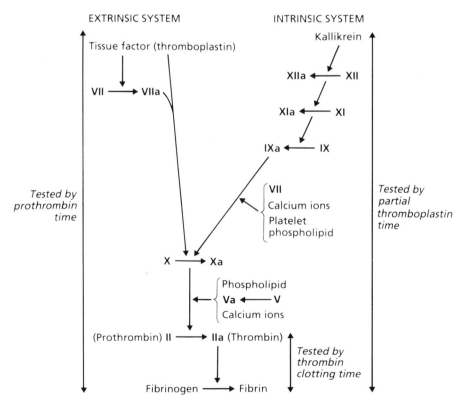

*The addition of the letter 'a' indicates the active form of the coagulation factor.

Fig. 79.1 The coagulation system.

Thrombin clotting time

This involves adding a source of thrombin to plasma, thus bypassing the extrinsic, intrinsic pathways and common pathways to the level of conversion of fibrinogen to fibrin. The TCT is prolonged with deficiency of fibrinogen or by inhibitors of the fibrinogen to fibrin conversion e.g. heparin or fibrin degradation products (FDPs).

Information obtained from these tests may help to localize a particular defect into one of the pathways and this may be followed by specific factor assays or inhibitor screens.

Classification of acquired haemostatic disorders

Classifications of the acquired haemostatic disorders is complex as, in most instances, several mechanisms are involved. The following discussion is based on the more common situations seen in clinical practice.

Acquired haemostatic disorders:

1 Disseminated intravascular coagulation.
2 Primary fibrinolytic bleeding.
3 Haemostatic abnormalities associated with vitamin K deficiency.
4 Haemostatic failure associated with liver disease.
5 Haemostatic problems with anticoagulant drugs.
6 Acquired inhibitors of coagulation.
7 Haemostatic defects associated with renal disease.
8 Haemostatic defects associated with massive transfusion.
9 Haemostatic defects associated with cardiopulmonary bypass.
10 Psychogenic bleeding.

Disseminated intravascular coagulation (DIC)

The haemostatic system is a dynamic one in which, under normal circumstances, there is a balance between intravascular coagulation and fibrinolysis. In DIC, a 'triggering' event occurs which disturbs this balance and leads to activation of the coagulation system with widespread deposition of fibrin and platelets and secondary activation of the fibrinolytic system.

Disseminated intravascular coagulation is not a disease or diagnosis in itself but occurs as part of the clinical picture of many diseases.

Pathogenesis

The initial event in the pathogenesis of DIC is activation of the coagulation sequence which may occur through three main triggering events (Muller-Berghaus, 1977).

RELEASE OF THROMBOPLASTIN

This causes activation of the extrinsic system and is a major component of DIC seen in tissue injury (including placental damage) (Page *et al.*, 1951), infection via the action of endotoxins (Cline *et al.*, 1968; Rivers *et al.*, 1975), released from leucocytes and also in disseminated malignancy (Gralnick & Abrell, 1973).

DIRECT ACTIVATION OF PROTHROMBIN AND FACTOR X

This is the probable mechanism in DIC seen after some cases of envenomation (Reid, 1984).

DAMAGE OF VASCULAR ENDOTHELIUM

Widespread vascular damage occurs in a variety of circumstances which result in activation of Factor XII (Hageman factor) and activation of the intrinsic system (Wilmer *et al.*, 1968). Exposed vascular endothelium also releases tissue thromboplastin and initiates platelet aggregation (Walsh, 1972).

Whatever the mechanism of activation of the coagulation sequence, the result is formation of thrombin. Once thrombin release has occurred, the pathophysiology follows a common pathway (Fig. 79.2).

Circulating thrombin cleaves fibrinopeptides from fibrinogen leaving behind fibrin monomers in the circulation. Most of these polymerize into fibrin in the microvascular circulation leading to microvascular and macrovascular thrombosis. The deposited fibrin in the microcirculation leads also to trapping of platelets and thrombocytopenia (Lasch *et al.*, 1967; Owen *et al.*, 1973).

Meanwhile, plasmin cleaves fibrinogen and fibrin into FDPs. These FDPs complex with fibrin monomers before they can polymerize, thus producing stable fibrin monomers which cannot polymerize (Fletcher *et al.*, 1966; Bang & Chang, 1974; Jakobsen *et al.*, 1974). Fibrin degradation products have also a high affinity for platelet membranes, and coat the surfaces of platelets to produce significant platelet dysfunction. Thus, in addition to a quantitative deficiency of platelets, there is also a qualitative one (Kopec *et al.*,

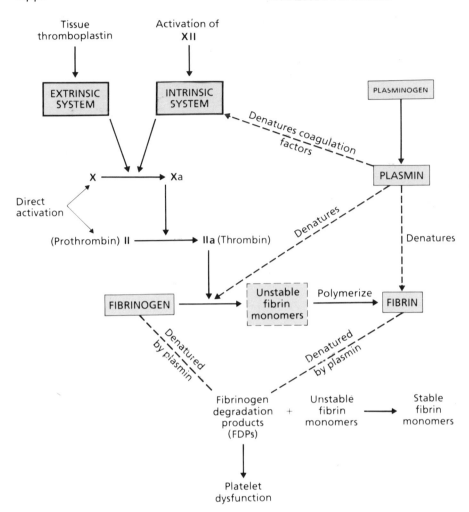

Fig. 79.2 Mechanisms involved in the pathogenesis of DIC.

1968; Niewiarowski *et al.*, 1972). Plasmin, in addition to degrading fibrin and fibrinogen, also degrades Factors V, VIII, IX and XI, contributing to deficiencies of these factors (Donaldson, 1960; Sharp, 1964; Pechet, 1965). Plasmin also activates the C_1 and C_3 complement sequence leading to red cell and platelet lysis, increased vascular permeability and shock. The liberation of kinins also contributes to development of shock (Schreiber *et al.*, 1973; Kaplan *et al.*, 1976).

Clinical aspects

Disseminated intravascular coagulation may manifest as a catastrophic illness with major haemorrhagic and thrombotic problems or as a chronic form with few clinical problems but which may progress to the acute form.

In the severely ill patient with DIC, general but non-specific signs of fever, hypotension, acidosis, hypoxia and proteinuria may be found. Often, it is not clear to what extent these signs result from the underlying clinical problem rather than to DIC.

More specific signs of coagulation upset such as petechiae and purpura, haemorrhagic bullae, acral cyanosis and occasionally frank gangrene may be found.

Any pattern of bleeding may be seen but bleeding from several sites is common, especially from wound and venepuncture sites. Haemorrhage into any organ may occur, leading to organ dysfunction. Organ dysfunction may occur also through microvascular and macrovascular thromboses which result in the high incidence of cardiac, pulmonary, renal and CNS dysfunction from ischaemia.

A microangiopathic haemolytic anaemia may result from fragmentation of red cells caused by the

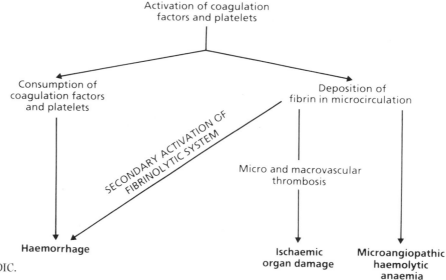

Fig. 79.3 Clinical manifestations of DIC.

fibrin network within the microvasculature (Fig. 79.3). Disorders associated with DIC:

1 Infection.
2 Obstetric complications.
3 Neoplasia.
4 Shock.
5 Hepatic disease.
6 Intravascular haemolysis.
7 Vasculitis.
8 Snake venom.
9 Burns.
10 Extracorporeal circulation.
11 Metabolic diseases e.g. severe diabetes mellitus hyperlipoproteinaemia.

INFECTION

Bacterial

Meningococcal septicaemia was the first infection in which DIC was described (McGehee *et al.*, 1967). Endotoxin from Gram-negative organisms can activate Factor XII directly, induce platelet aggregation, cause endothelial sloughing and initiate release of granulocyte procoagulant enzymes (McKay & Shapiro, 1958; Cline *et al.*, 1968). Studies on the mucopolysaccharide coating of Gram-positive organisms have shown similar properties (Cronberg, 1973). Many other generalized bacterial infections are associated with DIC.

Viral

Many acute viraemias have been associated with DIC. Those implicated most commonly are varicella, hepa-titis and cytomegalovirus. The mechanism is thought to involve antibody–antigen activation of XII, platelet release and endothelial sloughing (Wilmer *et al.*, 1968; Salmon *et al.*, 1971).

Others

Fungal infections e.g. aspergillosis and candidiasis, rickettsial infections (Lasch *et al.*, 1967) and protozoan infections e.g. malaria and schistosomiasis (Owen *et al.*, 1973; Bang & Chang, 1974) have all been associated with DIC.

OBSTETRIC COMPLICATIONS

Pregnancy may be considered to be a hypercoagulable state with increased concentrations of coagulation factors, depression of the fibrinolytic system and reduced reticulo-endothelial clearance of activated coagulation factors all making the mother particularly susceptible to DIC (Kleiner & Merskey, 1970; Muller-Berghaus, 1977; Talbert & Blatt, 1979). Obstetric problems have long been associated with DIC, and in experimental models, DIC appears to be particularly severe in pregnant animals (Muller-Berghaus, 1977).

Placental abruption

Hypofibrinogenaemia is reported to occur in 25% of abruptions, usually within 8 hr (Dieckman, 1936; Pritchard & Brekken, 1967). The full-blown picture of acute DIC with haemorrhage and thrombosis is much rarer, presumably from early delivery in such cases. From experimental work in animals, it seems likely that the mechanism involved is thromboplastins reaching the maternal circulation (Schneider, 1951; Cline et al., 1968).

Amniotic fluid embolus

It has been shown that through damage to the uterus and tears in the membranes, amniotic fluid gains access to the maternal circulation (Morgan, 1979; Rushton & Dowson, 1982). The coagulation abnormalities which may follow are ascribed to the thromboplastic activity of amniotic fluid. (Courtney & Allinton, 1972; Yaffe et al., 1977). Severe DIC may develop with hypofibrinogenaemia, reduced concentration of coagulation factors, thrombocytopenia and enchanced fibrinolysis (Bonnar, 1981). If the patient survives the initial cardiopulmonary collapse associated with embolism of amniotic fluid and fibrin thrombus in the pulmonary circulation, uncontrollable uterine haemorrhage may occur (Wiener & Reid, 1950).

Dead fetus syndrome

Evidence of DIC has been demonstrated in women in whom the fetus has died in utero, irrespective of the cause of death. It is thought that the triggering mechanism is the release of necrotic fetal tissues and enzymes acting as thromboplastins (Merskey et al., 1966; Merskey et al., 1967). If a woman retains a dead fetus in utero for more than 5 weeks, the incidence of DIC is approximately 30–40% (Pritchard, 1959; Pritchard, 1973), although in modern obstetric practice, this occurs rarely.

Abortion

Septic abortion, now a rarity because of legislative changes and availability or antibiotics, was a common cause of DIC. A combination of endotoxins and infected uterine tissue acting as thromboplastins were involved (Rubenberg et al., 1976).

Evidence of mild DIC has been shown to occur in some abortions using hypertonic saline and urea. Although there are usually no clinical problems, occasional reports of acute DIC have been made (Spivak et al., 1972; MacKenzie et al., 1975).

There have been occasional reports of DIC occurring in late dilatation and evacuation techniques in addition to use of prostaglandin and oxytocin. (Davis & Lin, 1972; Grundy & Graven, 1976; Savage, 1982).

Pre-eclampsia and eclampsia

Patients with severe pre-eclampsia and eclampsia have changes consistent with low grade DIC (Howie et al., 1976; Edgar et al., 1977; Douglas et al., 1982). Thrombocytopenia and decreased titres of clotting factors are present more commonly than elevation of soluble fibrin and FDPs. The exact mechanism of activation of coagulation is not known (Howie et al., 1975).

NEOPLASIA

Low grade DIC has long been associated with neoplastic disease, especially disseminated malignancy (Bick, 1978; Goldsmith, 1984). This, however, rarely constitutes a clinical problem unless surgery is contemplated. Nevertheless, the low grade nature may progress to an acute fulminating process when the disease progresses or with added stress such as infection. The pathogenesis is complex and is thought to involve the synthesis and release of thromboplastins and proteolytic enzymes which may activate coagulation factors and components accelerating the fibrinolytic pathway (Pitney, 1971; Mersky, 1973; Semararo & Donati, 1981). Acute promyelocytic leukaemia, prostatic carcinoma and carcinoma of lung, pancreas and ovary have the strongest associations with DIC.

SHOCK

Many cases of shock are associated with DIC especially if produced by trauma (Attar et al., 1966; Hardaway, 1966). It is thought that the main aetiological factor is widespread vascular damage from endotoxin, immune complexes, hypoxia or acidosis. The observations that in shock, thrombocytopenia is common and fibrinogen concentrations are often raised, had led to the postulation that platelet aggregation and microthrombus formation are major 'triggering events' (Hardaway, 1967).

HEPATIC DISEASE

Disseminated intravascular coagulation is one of the several processes involved in the haemostatic failure associated with liver disease. This is discussed later (p. 1460).

INTRAVASCULAR HAEMOLYSIS

Haemolysed red cells have been recognized as a stimulus for DIC since early experimental work began (Krevans et al., 1957). Severe DIC with marked hypofibrinogenaemia and thrombocytopenia has followed haemolytic reactions such as transfusion of incompatible blood (Muirhead, 1951; Langdell & Hedgpeth, 1959; Culpepper, 1975) and near drowning in fresh water (Mannucci et al., 1969). Some workers have postulated that shock accompanying such haemolytic reactions is an important part of the pathogenesis. (Crosby & Stefanini, 1952; Willoughby et al., 1972).

VASCULITIS

Collagen vascular diseases, haemolytic–uraemic syndrome and thrombotic thrombocytopenia purpura (Moskowitz syndrome) are among the vasculitic processes associated with DIC.

The haemolytic–uraemic syndrome is a disease of childhood in which renal impairment, thrombocytopenia and haemolytic anaemia occur (Brain, 1969; Willoughby et al., 1972; Lieberman, 1972). The aetiological agent is uncertain but is probably of an infective nature. It has been suggested that damage to the vascular endothelium is responsible, possibly causing failure of prostacyclin relase (Remuzzi et al., 1978).

Thrombotic thrombocytopenic purpura is a rare and fatal disorder of adults in which there is acute impairment of the CNS associated with microangiopathic haemolytic anaemia, renal impairment and a degree of disseminated intravascular coagulation (Pisciotta & Goltschall, 1980). The aetiological agent has not been identified and is thought to cause widespread vascular damage (Grain & Chardry, 1981). Treatment is empirical and usually unsuccessful.

SNAKE VENOM

Disturbance of the haemostatic system is a predominant effect of the venom of members of the Viperidae family. Most of these venoms are strongly procoagulant and may result in defibrination; in addition, increased fibrinolytic activity and thrombocytopenia produced by vascular damage may occur (Warrell et al., 1972; Lee, 1979; Reid, 1984).

Although encountered rarely in a clinical situation in the Western world, intravascular coagulation following snake bite is a major cause of morbidity and mortality from acquired haemostatic failure in a worldwide setting.

Laboratory diagnosis of DIC

In establishing the presence of DIC, one is aiming to demonstrate evidence of activation of the coagulation system and also of increased fibrinolytic activity. It is, however, important to realize that not all cases of DIC demonstrate the classical coagulation abnormalities.

Investigations may be classified into those that may be performed quickly and those that may provide additional information but which are either not practical or not required immediately (Table 79.1).

ADDITIONAL TESTS

Reptilase time

This test is based on the fact that the venom of certain snakes acts directly on fibrinogen to form fibrin. This action is not affected by heparin. As normal values are found in the presence of heparin, if a patient has been heparinized this test may help distinguish if the coagulation abnormality results from DIC or from heparin. Results are less reliable if the level of FDPs is very high.

Ethanol gelation test (EGT) and the protamine sulphate precipitin test

Both tests detect the presence of fibrin monomer complexes in the blood. The results are non-specific, as fibrin monomer complexes are found also in trauma and infection.

Other abnormalities described in DIC have been reported widely and some of these are included in Table 79.2. Most of these investigations are time consuming, many are provided only in specialist centres and in the majority of cases yield little additional information.

Treatment of DIC

Much controversy exists concerning some aspects of the treatment of DIC, and many reports based on anecdotal observations or reports on small numbers of patients are found in the literature. There are no reports on large controlled clinical trials.

Table 79.1 First-line coagulation investigations in DIC

Investigation	Abnormality	Comment
Hb estimation	↓	Bleeding ± haemolysis
Platelet count	↓	May be normal in chronic DIC
Prothrombin time	↑	Markedly prolonged in acute DIC May be less so or normal in chronic DIC
Partial thromboplastin time	↑	May be markedly prolonged in acute DIC, less so in chronic DIC
Thrombin clotting time	↑	May be normal, depending on level of fibrinogen
Fibrinogen concentration	↓	May be normal or even increased in some circumstances
Fibrinogen degradation products	↑	Usually increased

↑ Prolonged or increased.
↓ Shortened or decreased.

Table 79.2 Some of the abnormalities described in DIC

Assay of Factor V and VIII	Concentrations usually decreased
Factor VIII : C and VIII : RAg	There is often a discrepancy between these values with Factor VIII : C being diminished
Euglobulin lysis time	This is decreased reflecting enhanced fibrinolysis
Fibrinopeptide A Fibrinopeptide B	Levels are elevated and are a sensitive reflection of thrombin generation
B β15–42 fragments	Provide confirmatory evidence of fibrinolysis
Platelet aggregation studies	Almost always abnormal but as there is no classical abnormality in DIC, these are of little diagnostic value
β-thromoglobulin (BTG)	Evidence of platelet activation and release of granules
Antihrombin III levels	Decrease in level is a common finding in DIC but is also present in many stressful situations. May be of value in monitoring therapy (see later section)

The one point on which there is little disagreement is that the main aim should be to eradicate the underlying cause, as this is the only likely way in which resolution can occur (Cash 1977; Brozovic, 1981; Preston, 1982; Collen, 1983; Nyman, 1985). Thus, in patients in whom there is no evidence of infection, appropriate antibiotics should be administered immediately and in obsteric cases such as abruption, dead fetus syndrome and pre-eclampsia, evacuation of the uterus should be undertaken as soon as is feasible (Sharp *et al.*, 1958; Kleine & Merskey, 1970; Bailton & Letsky, 1985).

With this single most important point in mind,

other steps in management may be classified into:
1 Support of the patient.
2 Replacement therapy.
3 Controlling the haemostatic process.

SUPPORT OF THE PATIENT

Patients with acute DIC are often critically ill, either because of the underlying condition or because of the complications of DIC, and these patients are often to be found in an intensive therapy unit (ITU). The presence of DIC may make management very difficult e.g. haemorrhage and shock may necessitate transfusion of large volumes of fluid which may be made less feasible if there is impaired cardiac function as a result of ischaemia. Insertion of a central venous catheter and arterial catheter which is often required in such patients is made hazardous by the haemorrhagic tendency.

Adequate oxygenation may be difficult to achieve because of adult respiratory distress syndrome (ARDS) which has a strong but unclear association with DIC, and even if adequate arterial oxygenation is achieved, micro- and macrovascular thromboses may prevent adequate tissue oxygenation.

Attention to acid–base balance is also especially important because of the increased risk of thrombosis associated with acidosis (Beller, 1971; Bell, 1980).

REPLACEMENT THERAPY (see Chapter 22)

Most authors recommend that despite abnormal coagulation screen results, no attempt should be made to introduce coagulation factors unless uncontrolled bleeding occurs and the precipitating cause cannot be dealt with quickly (Bick et al., 1976; Collen, 1983).

The rationale behind this is that by introducing a concentrated source of coagulation factors, one may change the balance of the haemostatic system further and 'add fuel to the fire' (Preston, 1982; Prentice, 1985).

However, when heavy bleeding does occur, transfusion of blood and the following blood products may be required:

Platelets

Transfusions of platelets are given usually if the platelet count is below 30×10^9/litre. It may be helpful to recheck the platelet count 1 hr after transfusion to confirm that an increment has been achieved, as in some cases transfused platelets are consumed quickly and further therapy is likely to be useless unless the coagulation process is controlled.

Even when the platelet count remains above this value, there is likely to be significant platelet dysfunction as the concentration of FDPs is high and transfused platelets are also likely to be affected in this circumstance (Kopec et al., 1968; Niewiarowski et al., 1972).

Fresh frozen plasma (FFP)

Fresh frozen plasma contains all the non-cellular coagulation factors including fibrinogen at a concen-

tration which is less than that of normal plasma. Fresh frozen plasma is useful as replacement therapy and also as a plasma expander. However, as the volumes required to maintain adequate levels of coagulation factors can be large, the practical applications are limited because of the risk of circulatory overload.

Cryoprecipitate

Cryoprecipitate provides a more concentrated source of fibrinogen and also of Factor VIII. The actual concentrations vary (p. 382). Cryoprecipitate is more useful in situations where hypofibrinogenaemia is marked and the effectiveness of therapy should be monitored by transfusing approximately 10 units and rechecking the fibrinogen concentration shortly afterwards.

STOPPING THE COAGULATION PROCESS

Inhibitors of coagulation are used in some cases of DIC in the hope that the coagulation process can be halted, thus abolishing the stimulus to compensatory fibrinolysis and allowing resolution of the DIC process.

Heparin

The rationale for using heparin in DIC is that it augments the role of antithrombin III in inhibiting Factor Xa and thrombin, thus counteracting the acceleration of blood coagulation produced by thromboplastin release and thrombin formation in the circulation.

However, the use of heparin remains controversial (Brodsky & Siegel, 1970; Corrigan & Jordan, 1970; Deykin, 1970; Lawrence, 1971; Colman et al., 1972) because of the lack of consistent response, lack of controlled clinical trials (Prentice, 1976) and the risk that heparin merely adds to the bleeding risk (Kleine & Bell, 1974; Mant & King, 1979). Although used enthusiastically by earlier clinicians, its use is not standard practice nowadays, and at present the decision as to whether or not to use heparin should be based on each individual case and what one thinks the most likely triggering event is to the DIC process. Its use should be confined to those patients with no fresh wounds or raw surfaces from which haemorrhage may occur. Amniotic fluid embolus, some cases of shock including septicaemia, some cases of neoplasia and in patients in whom thrombosis is a major feature are conditions in which heparin is employed more commonly.

One recommended regimen is a bolus of 5000 units and 1000 unit/hr as a continuous infusion (Prentice, 1985) and serial measurements of fibrinogen and platelet count should be made to assess efficacy (Wilmer *et al.*, 1968; Gralnick & Abrell, 1973; Reid, 1984).

Antithrombin III

Considerable interest in using antithrombin III as a replacement therapy in DIC has been aroused following reports of successful treatment in small groups of patients.

Antithrombin concentrations are usually low in DIC and it is thought that by increasing these by infusion, deceleration of the coagulation process may be brought about by inhibition of Xa.

The attraction of this form of therapy is that it does not carry the same risk of bleeding as with heparin, and it is likely that it will be employed more as supplies become more available, although controlled clinical trials are required to justify widespread use (Schipper *et al.*, 1978; Laursen *et al.*, 1981; Blauhut *et al.*, 1982; Hellgren *et al.*, 1984).

Antiplatelet agents

Antiplatelet agents e.g. prostacyclin, have aroused some interest which has been encouraged by occasional reports of successful treatment in haemolytic–uraemic syndrome and thrombotic thrombocytopenic purpura, and it may be that in cases where platelet aggregation is thought to be the main triggering event this would be useful.

PRIMARY FIBRINOLYTIC BLEEDING

In DIC, increased fibrinolysis occurs secondary to the increased intravascular coagulation component. In some circumstances, fibrinolysis is increased by activation of plasminogen without evidence of intravascular coagulation (Fig. 79.4).

Primary fibrinolysis has been described in association with neoplastic disease (Davidson *et al.*, 1969), and some tumours are thought to produce plasminogen activator.

Conditions in which primary fibrinolysis may be found

1 Carcinoma of prostrate (Tagnon *et al.*, 1952).
2 Carcinoma of pancreas (Ratnoff, 1952).

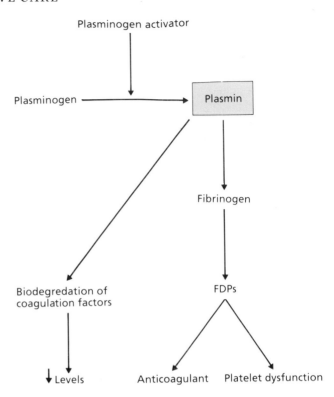

Fig. 79.4 Mechanisms involved in primary fibrinolysis.

3 Acute leukaemias (Pisciotta & Schultz, 1955).
4 Systemic lupus erythematosus (SLE) (Zwicka *et al.*, 1961).
5 Hepatic cirrhosis (Grossi *et al.*, 1961; Fletcher *et al.*, 1964).

Laboratory tests of coagulation may be very similar to those seen in DIC, and although a low platelet count does occur in primary fibrinolysis, it may be present as a complication of the underlying disorder e.g. cirrhosis, leukaemia. Time-consuming and elaborate tests measuring concentrations of coagulation factors and assessing fibrinolysis and its products may be required to distinguish between the two.

This is of some clinical relevance in that if there is strong evidence of primary fibrinolysis, fibrinolytic inhibitors such as ε-amino-caproic acid (EACA) and tranexamic acid (cyclocapron) may be of considerable benefit in controlling haemorrhage.

Epsilon amino-caproic acid acts as a competitive or non-competitive inhibitor of plasminogen, depending on the concentration. It is usually given orally at a dose of 3 g 6-hourly. Tranexamic acid has a similar action and may be given orally or intravenously. The use of these drugs may be hazardous in DIC, as unlysable thrombus may form in vessels or, in the presence of haematuria, unlysable fibrin clot may obstruct the urinary tract.

Haemostatic abnormalities associated with vitamin K deficiency

The vitamin K-dependent clotting Factors II, VII, IX and X undergo γ-carboxylation to form γ-carboxy-glutamic acid residue forms in order to develop calcium-binding properties which are essential for their normal activity (Hemker et al., 1963; Nelsestuen et al., 1974). Vitamin K acts as a co-factor in this carboxylation reaction (Fig. 79.5).

Vitamin K is not synthesized by the body but is obtained from green vegetables and vitamin K-producing intestinal bacteria, and, being lipid-soluble, requires the presence of bile salts in the small intestine for its absorption (Udall, 1956; Shearer et al., 1980).

Deficiencies of active vitamin K dependent clotting factors occur in the following circumstances.

1 Reduced availability of vitamin K e.g. reduced dietary intake or use of antibiotics interfering with intestinal supply.

2 Malabsorption of vitamin K as in complete biliary obstruction or intestinal disease.

3 Failure of utilization as in common anticoagulant therapy or hepatic disease.

4 Very rarely, congenitial deficiency from enzyme deficiency.

The following discussion considers the most common clinical examples:

Haemorrhagic disease of the newborn

The levels of the vitamin K-dependent clotting factors are decreased in the neonate and availability of vitamin K is low because human milk is a poor dietary source

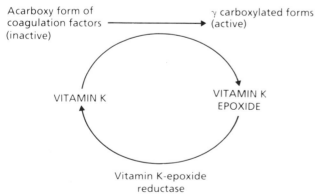

Fig. 79.5 Activation of vitamin K-dependent coagulation factors.

and the intestine has not been colonized by bacteria (Foley et al., 1977; Donaldson, 1984).

This may cause a haemorrhagic tendency with bleeding from the umbilicus, gastrointestinal tract or intracranial bleeding. The bleeding problem can be corrected by parenteral administration of vitamin K, 1 mg 8-hourly until coagulation returns to normal (Lucey & Dolan, 1958; Donaldson, 1984).

Malabsorption states

Malabsorption of vitamin K may result from:

Intestinal disease. Vitamin K deficiency may be part of a malabsorption syndrome with wide-ranging clinical features e.g. coeliac disease, inflammatory bowel disease, intestinal surgery.

Biliary disease. In obstructive jaundice, there is a lack of bile salts in the small intestine and consequent malabsorption of vitamin K.

Inadequate intake. Patients with a poor diet for a long period of time may become deficient in vitamin K though this is rare and is usually accompanied by either surgery or prolonged use of broad spectrum antibiotics.

Coumarin-like anticoagulants

These drugs, the most commonly used being warfarin, antagonize the action of vitamin K thus blocking the γ-carboxylation of the vitamin K-dependent clotting factors (see later section) (Muller-Berghaus, 1977).

Hepatic Disease

The titres of vitamin K-dependent clotting factors are reduced in parenchymal liver disease, and utilization of vitamin K in carboxylation reaction is also defective (Goodnight et al., 1971; Lechner, 1972).

CLINICAL FEATURES

There may be no bleeding problems despite an abnormal coagulation screen, or there may be multiple bruises and bleeding from mucous membranes, gastro-intestinal, genito-urinary tract or any other pattern of bleeding.

Of more immediate relevance is the need to treat any deficiency if contemplating surgery e.g. relief of biliary obstruction or intestinal surgery, or before liver biopsy.

LABORATORY FEATURES

The defect in coagulation from vitamin K deficiency affects both the extrinsic and intrinsic pathways but does not cause a prolongation of TCT nor does it affect the platelet count (Table 79.3).

TREATMENT

If no bleeding occurs, parenteral vitamin K, 10 mg, should be given. This increases the concentrations of clotting factors and corrects the PT within 8–12 hr.

If the patient is bleeding heavily and more rapid correction is required, transfusion of FFP beginning with approximately 500 ml should be given concomitantly with the vitamin K. Vitamin K is required also for the γ-carboxylation of Protein C and Protein S which both inhibit the active forms of V and VIII. The activity of both these decrease in vitamin K deficiency leading to a potential thrombotic state which may be important when considering the action of coumarins.

Haemostatic failure associated with liver disease

The liver is thought to be the main site of synthesis of fibrinogen, Factors II, VII, IX, X, V, XI, XII, XIII in addition to plasminogen, antithrombin III and inhibitors of fibrinolysis. It follows that hepatocellular disease may cause a significant haemostatic defect which may involve several mechanisms (Ratnoff, 1963; Walls & Lavarsky, 1971; Roberts & Lederbaum, 1972; Duckert, 1973; Bloom, 1977; Shaw et al., 1979; Flute, 1982).

Table 79.3 Coagulation test abnormalities in vitamin K deficiency

Investigation	Abnormality
Prothrombin time	↑
Partial thromboplastin time	↑
Thrombin clotting time	Normal
Fibrinogen	Normal
Platelet count	Normal

↑ Prolonged.

FAILURE OF SYNTHESIS OF COAGULATION FACTORS

Vitamin K-dependent clotting factor

As mentioned in the previous section, low titres of II, VII, IX and X are found as a result of decreased synthesis of protein precursors (Goodnight et al., 1971; Lechner, 1972). This may be associated with vitamin K deficiency and there may also be defective utilization of vitamin K (Mann, 1952; Spector & Corn, 1967; Blanchard et al., 1981).

Factor V deficiency

As with vitamin K-dependent clotting factors, low titres of V are found in a wide range of acute and chronic liver disorders (Owren, 1949; Rapaport et al., 1960; Giddings et al., 1975; Cederblad et al., 1976) but not in obstructive jaundice, primary biliary cirrhosis or metastatic liver disease (Quick et al., 1935; Owren, 1949; Rapaport et al., 1960). Factor V contributes to the prolonged PT and PTT but its contribution to the bleeding tendency is perhaps less important, as patients with congenital factor V deficiency have lower concentrations of Factor V usually and have only a mild bleeding tendency.

In addition defective synthesis, increased consumption in intravascular coagulation and plasmin degradation may occur.

Other factors

Deficiencies of XI, XII and XIII have been demonstrated in acute and chronic hepatic disorders but it is not thought that these are significant clinically (Hathaway & Alsever, 1970; Lechner et al., 1977; Saito et al., 1978).

Fibrinogen (Factor I)

The normal concentration of fibrinogen in plasma is 1.5–4.0 g/litre. This is synthesized by the liver and the concentration varies with stress (Miller et al., 1951; Miller & Bale, 1954; Ratnoff, 1980).

Plasma fibrinogen concentrations are not usually decreased in liver disease and are often normal or increased although the increase in fibrinogen in response to stress may be impaired in cirrhosis (Ratnoff, 1954; Volwiler et al., 1955; Bergstrom et al., 1960; von Felten et al., 1969; Green et al., 1977; Lipinski et *al.*, 1977; Higuchi *et al.*, 1980). Severe hypofibrinogenaemia is found usually as a near terminal phenomenon as in fulminant hepatitis when it may be a result of decreased synthesis, increased consumption in DIC, increased fibrinolysis or loss in massive haemorrhage.

Acquired dysfibrinogenaemia may be present at an early stage of a wide range of hepatic disorders including cirrhosis, hepatic carcinoma, severe acute hepatitis and chronic aggressive hepatitis but is reported to be rare in metastatic liver disease (Ham & Curtis, 1938; Hallen & Nilsson, 1964; Horder, 1969; Grun *et al.*, 1974; Hillenbrand *et al.*, 1974; Rubin *et al.*, 1978). The pathogenesis of this acquired defect is not clear but the end-result is reduced aggregation of fibrin monomers. This phenomenon may contribute to a bleeding tendency, although patients with congenital dysfibrinogenaemia tend to have a mild bleeding tendency.

DISSEMINATED INTRAVASCULAR COAGULATION

In liver disease, several factors may be present which may encourage DIC. These include:
1 Reduced hepatic or reticuloendothelial clearance of activated coagulation factors (Ratnoff, 1984).
2 Decreased clearance of plasminogen activator (Murray-Lyon *et al.*, 1972; Ratnoff, 1984).
3 Decreased titres of antithrombin III (Damus & Wallace, 1975).
4 Decreased synthesis of fibrinolytic system inhibitors (Aoki & Yamanaka, 1978).

The triggering event may be necrotic hepatocytes acting as thromboplastins (Verstraete *et al.*, 1974), endotoxins (Wardle, 1974) or some other factor.

Intravascular infusion of ascitic fluid as occurs in systems such as the Le Veen shunt is known to cause DIC also (Lerner *et al.*, 1978; Harmon *et al.*, 1979).

Despite the great interest in the role of DIC in liver disease, firm laboratory support for the presence of DIC is not found in many patients with acute or chronic liver disease (Gralnick & Abrell, 1973; Rivers *et al.*, 1975; Reid, 1984). Assessment is made more difficult because reduced titres of coagulation factors and thrombocytopenia may already be present in liver disease (Ratnoff, 1984).

DISORDERS OF PLATELETS

Thrombocytopenia is common in liver disease, and although the concentration is rarely low enough to cause spontaneous haemorrhage, bleeding from local lesions e.g. varices or erosions, may be made worse and surgical procedures made more hazardous (Lasch *et al.*, 1967; Walsh, 1972; Owen *et al.*, 1973; Bang & Chang, 1974).

Causes of thrombocytopenia include:
1 Splenic sequestration from portal hypertension (Tocantins, 1948; Aster, 1966).
2 Decreased production because of concurrent folic acid deficiency in alcoholics (Jandl & Lear, 1956).
3 Decreased production through marrow suppression by alcohol (Larkin & Watson-Williams, 1984).

In addition to the quantitative defect in platelets described, various qualitative defects have been reported, although the clinical significance is not clear (Thomas *et al.*, 1967; Ballard & Marcus, 1976; Rubin *et al.*, 1977).

The coagulation screen may become abnormal before any other liver function test result, as in paracetamol poisoning where the PT is used to detect early liver damage.

Prothrombin time is also the minimum investigation that should be undertaken prior to liver biopsy. If the PT is more than 1.5 times the control value, bleeding problems are likely after biopsy (Table 79.4).

Treatment

Vitamin K_1 should be administered, as deficiency may represent part of the defect. Ten mg each day for three days should be tried, although this is often at most only partially successful.

Management of patients with a haemostatic defect is aimed at supporting them until resolution of the underlying disease process. However, such patients have often a source of bleeding which may be aggravated by a haemostatic defect such as oesophageal varices, gastric erosions, peptic ulcers or require liver biopsy or surgery. In such circumstances, transfusion of FFP may be useful, although this may have to be repeated to maintain haemostasis.

Platelet transfusions may be beneficial because of thrombocytopenia and a qualitative defect, but the benefit may be short-lived if there is hypersplenism.

A prolonged TCT may indicate a qualitative or quantitative defect in fibrinogen and cryoprecipitate transfusion may be given.

If the patient is gravely ill, bleeding, and cannot tolerate large volumes of fluid as may occur in advanced liver failure, activated prothrombin complex

Table 79.4 Coagulation test abnormalities in liver disease

Investigation	Abnormality	Cause
Prothrombin time	↑	Reduced synthesis of factors Defective utilization of vitamin K
Partial thromboplastin time	↑	Consumption in DIC Plasmin degradation
Thrombin clotting time	↑	Dysfibrinogenaemia Hypofibrinogenaemia
Fibrinogen	May be low in advanced liver disease	Consumption in DIC
Platelets	↓	Splenic sequestration Decreased production

↑ Prolonged.
↓ Decreased.

(contains Factors II, IX and X concentrate) may be given, although the risk of precipitating DIC is high.

Haemostatic problems with anticoagulant drugs

Heparin

There are several ways in which heparin can influence the coagulation system. The most important of these is its potentiation of the inhibition of Factors XIIa, XIa, IXa, Xa and thrombin by the plasma co-factor antithrombin III (Fig. 79.6).

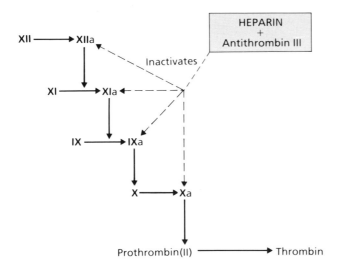

Fig. 79.6 The increased rate of inactivation of activated coagulation factors by the interaction of heparin and antithrombin III.

Heparin is used widely in the prophylaxis and treatment of venous thromboembolism and is used also in extracorporeal circulations.

The main side-effect of heparin is bleeding, the risk of which is dependent on the following:

Dose

When low doses of heparin are used, as in prophylaxis of venous thrombosis, the risk of bleeding is low unless some other risk factor is present. The risk of bleeding is higher with increased anticoagulant effect (American Heart Association, 1973; Norman & Provan, 1977; Wilson & Lampman, 1979).

Route of administration

The risk of bleeding is lowest with subcutaneous administration, and incidence of bleeding is higher when intravenous intermittent administration is used compared with intravenous continuous infusion. This may be related also to the total dose delivered (Salzman *et al.*, 1975; Glazier & Cravell, 1976; Mant *et al.*, 1977; Wilson & Lampman, 1979).

Patient's characteristics

1 Risk of bleeding is increased in elderly patients, especially women (Jick *et al.*, 1968; O'Sullivan *et al.*, 1968; Viweg *et al.*, 1970; Glazier & Cravell, 1976; Wilson & Lampman, 1979).
2 Risk is increased if there is recent trauma or surgery (Salzman *et al.*, 1975; Wilson & Lampman, 1979).

3 Risk is increased if there is any other haemostatic defect (Pitney et al., 1970).

4 Risk is increased if antiplatelet drugs are administered (Pitney et al., 1970).

5 As heparin is metabolized by both the liver and kidneys, any decrease in function may lead to prolonged half-life (Pitney et al., 1970).

To reduce the risk of bleeding, the effect of heparin should be monitored carefully.

MONITORING THERAPY

In the past, the whole-blood clotting time was used as the method of monitoring heparin. Nowadays, measuring the activated partial thromboplastin time (APTT) or heparin level by protamine titration are the preferred methods.

Using the APTT method, the result is often expressed as a ratio compared to a control sample. The therapeutic range should be 1.5–2.0.

If the protamine titration method is used, the heparin concentration should be 0.3–0.5 unit/ml (Hirsch, 1986).

TREATMENT OF BLEEDING

If any invasive procedure is contemplated on a patient who is heparinized fully by infusion, heparin should be discontinued for 1–2 hr before and after the procedure. As the half-life of heparin is 60 min, this should be sufficient to allow the coagulation system to return to normal. Also, if bleeding occurs during heparin administration and is mild and controlled easily, all that is required is to discontinue the heparin or reduce the dose.

With more severe bleeding, however, heparin should be neutralized by slow intravenous injection of protamine sulphate depending on the dose and time of administration of heparin. If protamine is given within minutes of an intravenous bolus of heparin, protamine sulphate 1 mg/100 unit heparin should be given; if 30 min after, protamine sulphate 0.5 mg/100 unit heparin should be given; if 2 hr after, protamine sulphate 0.25 mg/100 unit heparin should be given.

Protamine has anticoagulant properties in vitro (Ollendorff, 1962) but it is unlikely that enough would be administered in error to produce any clinical problem.

In the rare case of bleeding occurring after subcutaneous administration of heparin (usually associated with some other risk factor), repeated doses of protamine may be required, as heparin continues to be absorbed for 8–12 hr afterwards. In this circumstance, 50% of the calculated dose of protamine should be given and repeated 3-hourly.

If bleeding persists or is marked, a coagulation screen including PT, APTT, TCT, reptilase time and platelet count should be measured, as there may be another cause for bleeding.

Thrombocytopenia has been reported in 1–2% of all treatment episodes with heparin, and occurs usually after 1 week of heparin therapy. It has been shown to recur after rechallenge (Keltan & Levine, 1986).

Warfarin and related drugs

These drugs are derived from hydroxycoumarin and have a similar structure to vitamin K. Their anticoagulant action is complex and involves interfering with the cyclic interconversion of vitamin K and its 2,3-epoxide vitamin K form (Fig. 79.7).

The net result is that coagulation Factors II, VII, IX and X are not carboxylated and therefore not activated. The most widely used of these drugs is warfarin whose absorption, metabolism, excretion and bioavailability varies widely between individuals and is influenced greatly by drug therapy, disease and diet.

Its main uses are in the treatment and prophylaxis of venous thromboembolism, valvular and arterial thromboses and vascular disease.

Bleeding is the main risk during warfarin therapy and may result from overdose, potentiation by other drugs, change in patient's clinical condition such a liver disease or habits e.g. increased alcohol intake. Bleeding may be aggravated also in a pre-existing lesion such as peptic ulcer disease, even though the level of anticoagulation is well within the therapeutic range.

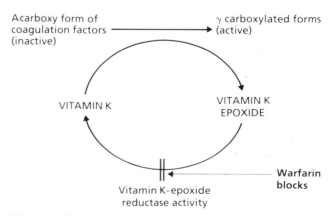

Fig. 79.7 Site of activation of warfarin.

Warfarin therapy is monitored by measuring the PT, comparing the result to an international standard and expressing the result as a ratio, the international normalized ratio (INR). Previous methods were British comparative ratios (BCR) and Thrombotest.

The therapeutic range for INR is 2.0–4.2 depending on the clinical indication (British Society of Haematology, 1984).

TREATMENT OF BLEEDING

When bleeding occurs, the aim is to restore the active vitamin K-dependent factors either immediately using FFP or, within 8 hr, using intravenous vitamin K_1. However, one has to take into account the possible risk of transmission of disease using blood products and the possible overcorrection of anticoagulation by vitamin K_1 which makes re-introduction of treatment very difficult for several days.

In patients who have a very long PT, reflected by an INR above the therapeutic range and who do not bleed, it is usually safe to stop warfarin for 24–48 hr and restart at a lower dose. If the INR is above 7.0, one would consider giving 1–2 mg of vitamin K_1 orally or intravenously.

If bleeding occurs but is not life-threatening and the patients need to remain on anticoagulants e.g. those patients with prosthetic heart valves, FFP should be given. This produces haemostatic levels of the vitamin K-dependent factors but this may have to be repeated.

In those who bleed and who do not require to remain on anticoagulants, vitamin K_1 20–30 mg should be given intravenously. This is effective within 8 hr, and FFP may be required to secure haemostasis in the intervening period. Patients who have taken a massive overdose of warfarin may require repeated injections.

Those patients who cannot tolerate the fluid load of FFP may be given activated prothrombin complexes. This produces haemostatic levels of II, IX and X but carries a risk of causing thrombosis and carries also a risk of DIC.

Thrombolytic drugs

At present, the two main drugs in clinical use are streptokinase, prepared from β-haemolytic streptococci, and urokinase which is prepared from cultures of human fetal kidney cells. It is probable that human

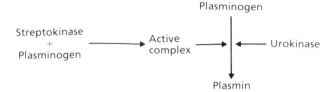

Fig. 79.8 Site of activation of thrombolytic drugs.

tissue plasminogen activator, produced by recombinant technology or from modified streptokinase, will become available in the near future. They have the advantage of being more fibrin specific but will be extremely expensive.

Streptokinase forms an active complex with plasminogen and this in turn converts plasminogen to plasmin (Kaplan *et al.*, 1978) (Fig. 79.8). Urokinase acts more directly. As streptokinase is antigenic, a loading dose has to be given to neutralize naturally occurring antibodies, the usual loading dose is 250 000 units. Steroids are often given to prevent anaphylaxis. The maintenance dose is usually around 100 000 unit/hr by infusion.

Treatment is continued usually for 3–7 days during which time antibodies will develop to streptokinase and limit its effectiveness. Urokinase is not usually antigenic and does not require a loading dose. However, it is more expensive. There is at present no consensus view as to how to monitor thrombolytic therapy, as there is poor correlation between the laboratory parameters of systemic fibrinolysis, and the incidence of bleeding or thrombus resolution (Marder *et al.*, 1977; Marder, 1979). The main aim of coagulation investigations is to establish that fibrinolysis is enhanced (Marder, 1979).

As may be seen from Table 79.5, shortened whole-blood or euglobulin clot lysis time occurs, and reduction in plasma fibrinogen and coagulation factors leads to prolongation of the PT, PTT and TCT. Elevated concentrations of FDPs may also contribute to test abnormalities. Reduced plasminogen and antiplasmin concentrations are contributory evidence of enhanced fibrinolysis.

BLEEDING PROBLEMS

Patients should be selected carefully for thrombolytic therapy and should have a strong clinical indication for its use (e.g. pulmonary embolism) and should have no lesion from which bleeding may occur (e.g. recent operation peptic ulcer).

The most common form of bleeding seen during

Table 79.5 Coagulation changes found during thrombolytic therapy with streptokinase and urokinase

Investigation	Result
Prothrombin time	↑
Partial thromboplastin time	↑
Thrombin clotting time	↑
Plasma fibrinogen	↓
Fribrin degradation products	↑
Euglobulin lysis time	Rapid
Whole-blood clot lysis time	Rapid
Plasminogen concentrations	↓
Antiplasmin concentrations	↓

↑ Prolonged or increased.
↓ Decreased.

therapy is oozing from venepuncture site or other small wound site. This may be controlled using local pressure. If more severe bleeding occurs or bleeding into any organ is suspected, therapy is stopped immediately and the patient is given transfusion of blood. Transfusion of cryopreciptate also raises the plasma fibrinogen concentrations, and haemostasis should be achieved within 1 hr. If this is not effective, intravenous administration of antifibrinolytic agents such as EACA or tranexamic acid reverses the fibrinolytic state more rapidly. However, this is required rarely.

The efficacy and safety of the newer thrombolytic agents such as tissue-type plasminogen activator (tPA), acylated streptokinase–plasminogen complex and single chain urokinase-type plasminogen activator or pro-urokinase (scuPA) are being evaluated in world-wide trials.

Antiplatelet agents

The most commonly used drug therapeutically is aspirin. The major effect of this drug is irreversible acetylation of platelet cyclo-oxygenase with inhibition of synthesis of thromboxane A_2. This impairs platelet aggregation and in turn impairs haemostasis (Roth & Majerus, 1975; O'Grady et al., 1980).

As acetylation is irreversible, this defect remains for the duration of platelet lifespan, approximately 7–11 days. With otherwise normal haemostasis, however, the clinical risk of bleeding is small, and even with wounds, prolonged oozing is the only usual problem.

However, where there is another defect of haemostasis e.g. heparin therapy, haemophilia or thrombocytopenia, bleeding may be severe, and treatment for the underlying disorder in addition to platelet transfusions may be required.

Prostacyclin infusions prevent platelets adhering to endothelial surfaces and may cause bleeding through this effect. If serious bleeding does occur, stopping the infusion should be sufficient, as prostacyclin has a very short half-life.

Acquired inhibitors of coagulation

Autoantibodies against coagulation factors may arise in patients with a congenital deficiency who have been treated with factor concentrates or may arise in individuals who have had no previous haemorrhagic problems (Shapiro, 1975; Green & Lechner; 1981).

Several specific inhibitors have been described, the most common and most clinically important being Factor VIII inhibitors.

Factor VIII inhibitors

Five to 10% of patients with haemophilia A develop factor VIII inhibitors (Barr et al., 1969; Shapiro, 1975). These inhibitors are usually IgG or IgM antibodies and tend to occur in severe haemophiliacs and also tend to persist. Haemophiliacs with inhibitors can be divided into:

1 *High responders.* In these patients, the inhibitor concentration is high and Factor VIII treatment tends to be unsuccessful and may produce an amnesic response. The titre may diminish if Factor VIII therapy is withheld but recurs after subsequent rechallenge.

2 *Low responders.* The concentration of inhibitor is low and does not tend to increase after exposure to Factor VIII. These patients may be treated with high doses of Factor VIII.

Low responders may be managed successfully through operations or injuries using high doses of Factor VIII and rechecking the plasma concentration regularly. However, high responders are a considerable problem, and high-dose Factor VIII is rarely enough to ensure haemostasis. Other options for these patients include plasmapheresis, high purity procine Factor VIII or prothrombin complex concentrates.

Factor VIII inhibitors have also been described in non-haemophiliac patients with a variety of clinical problems and in whom the pathogenesis is not clear:

1 Postpartum women (Voke & Letsky, 1977; Reece et al., 1982).

2 Drug reactions (particularly ampicillin and penicillin) (Allain *et al.*, 1981: Green & Lechner, 1981).

3 Autoimmune disorders e.g. SLE, rheumatoid arthritis (Shapiro, 1975; Green & Lechner 1981).

4 Neoplastic disease, particularly lymphoproliferative disorders (Green & Lechner 1981).

5 Apparently normal individuals (Shapiro, 1975; Allain *et al.*, 1981; Green & Lechner, 1981).

In almost all of these cases, the inhibitor is discovered during investigation of haemorrhagic problems. The cause is variable and the inhibition may disappear spontaneously or with immunosuppressive treatment. If bleeding occurs, treatment with Factor VIII concentrate or prothrombin complex concentrates may be successful (Voke & Letsky, 1977; Green & Lechner, 1981; Spero *et al.*, 1981).

Laboratory diagnosis

If a Factor VIII inhibitor is present, the PTT is prolonged and the clotting activity of Factor VIII (VII : C) is low. When normal plasma is added to the plasma of a patient with an VIII inhibitor, these tests do not correct whereas in a patient with a pure deficiency state, they do correct. Further specialized assays can then measure the titre of the inhibitor (Table 79.6).

Lupus anticoagulant

Lupus anticoagulants are inhibitors which are directed against phosholipids and inhibit the interaction between the complex of (Xa, V, phospholipid and calcium ions) and prothrombin.

Lupus anticoagulant may be found in SLE, other autoimmune disorders and some haematological malignancies but often no underlying disease state can be found (Schleider *et al.*, 1976; Shapiro & Thiagarjan, 1982).

In laboratory screening tests, the most common finding is a prolonged PTT which is not corrected by addition of normal plasma. However, despite this prolongation of the PTT, bleeding is a rare event unless some other haemostatic defect is present. The more common associated defects are thrombocytopenia and hypoprothrombinaemia.

Thrombotic events and recurrent abortions in pregnant patients are the more common clinical problems and these cases may be treated with immunosuppressants and anticoagulants (Carreras *et al.*, 1981; Scott, 1981; Shapiro & Thiagarjan, 1982).

Haemostatic defects associated with renal disease

Acute and chronic renal failure may be associated with haemostatic abnormalities which cause bleeding such as epistaxes and excess bruising, although occasionally more serious haemorrhage occurs. Even though clinical problems with bleeding are usually trivial, the problem assumes more importance when the patient with renal failure is faced with an operation or when

Table 79.6 Features of other acquired inhibitors

Inhibitor	Coag. abnormality	Features
IX	Partial thromboplastin time ↑	1–3% of patients with haemophilia B Acquired inhibitor in non-haemophiliac very rare
von Willebrand	Partial thromboplastin time ↑ Platelet dysfunction	Rare in patients with vW treated with cryoprecipitate Very rare in non affected individual
V	Prothrombin time ↑	Rare, usually occurs in previously normal individuals following surgery or antibiotics
	Partial thromboplastin time ↑	Usually mild bleeding problems
XII XI	Partial thromboplastin time ↑	Rare, may occur together Few bleeding problems
XIII	Unstable fibrin clot	Rare but may cause persistent and severe bleeding
Inhibitors directed at fibrinogen	May have Prothrombin time ↑ Partial thromboplastin time ↑ Thrombin clotting time ↑	Rare Usually only mild bleeding tendency

↑ Prolonged.

an ill patient develops renal failure and needs a biopsy for proper assessment.

The most important haemostatic defect in renal failure is acquired platelet abnormalities (Rabiner, 1972b). Other potential problems are coagulation factor deficiencies and DIC.

PLATELET ABNORMALITIES

Thrombocytopenia is a well-recognized finding in renal failure and may occur through several mechanisms.

1 Uraemia may lead to depression of megakaryocyte production, thus causing decreased platelet production.

2 Thrombocytopenia may occur as a prominent feature of the underlying condition causing renal failure e.g. thrombotic thrombocytopenic purpura, haemolytic–uraemic syndrome, pre-eclamptic toxaemia. In these examples, much attention has been directed to the role of prostacyclin in pathogenesis.

3 Consumption of platelets may occur if DIC supervenes when septicaemia or some other problem develops.

Thrombocytopenia may develop with the use of heparin in dialysis.

Although thrombocytopenia is a well-recognized finding in renal failure, platelet count is a poor predictor of the risk of bleeding in these patients, and serious haemorrhage may occur with normal platelet counts (Rabiner, 1972a).

Reversible abnormalities of platelet function are much more important in causation of bleeding problems. Most aspects of platelet function including adhesion, aggregation, secretion, procoagulant activity and clot retraction are abnormal (Rabiner, 1972b).

The cause of these abnormalities is the accumulation of products of metabolism such as guanidosuccinic acid, phenol compounds and urea which interfere with normal platelet function. These products are dialysable, and platelet function and bleeding time corrects temporarily with dialysis. Increased vascular prostacyclin levels may also contribute to the bleeding tendency (Eknoyan et al., 1969; Harowitz et al., 1970; Rabiner & Molinus, 1970; Remuzzi et al., 1978a).

Coagulation factors

Coagulation factor deficiency is uncommon in renal disease, indeed some factors e.g. Factor VIII, are commonly present at increased concentrations.

As with any ill patient, especially if food intake is reduced and long-term antibiotics have been administered, vitamin K deficiency may occur with the corresponding coagulation abnormalities.

In advanced renal disease, hepatic impairment may occur and the associated coagulopathy may develop.

Isolated deficiencies of Factor IX and XII have been reported in the nephrotic syndrome. The pathogenesis is not clear but appears to be related to proteinuria (Castaldi, 1984).

Factor XII deficiency has also been reported but its clinical relevance is doubtful (Losowsky & Walls, 1969).

DISSEMINATED INTRAVASCULAR COAGULATION

Evidence of localized DIC occurring in some cases of glomerular injury have been reported, and acute DIC may occur if some other factor such as septicaemia occurs. It has also been reported during rejection of renal transplant.

Laboratory diagnosis

A full blood and platelet count should be taken as well as a coagulation screen when any bleeding occurs or if an invasive procedure is contemplated. A reptilase time should be undertaken if the patient has been exposed to heparin.

Platelet function tests are abnormal, although these are performed rarely, as a bleeding time is an easier method of assessing this. The bleeding time is the best indicator of the risk of bleeding.

Treatment

Before surgical procedures, treatment should be aimed at improving renal function or removing accumulated metabolites by dialysis. Haemodialysis often reduces the severity of bleeding problems but the results are sometimes disappointing.

Reports of transient shortening of prolonged bleeding times (Rabiner, 1972a, b; Ellison et al., 1987) with cryoprecipitate (Janson et al., 1980) and deamino-8-D-arginine vasopressin (DDAVP) (Mannucci et al., 1983) allowing surgical procedures to be carried out without significant haemorrhagic problems have aroused great interest.

Vitamin K and blood products such as FFP and cryoprecipitate may be administered if there is evidence from coagulation studies that they are indicated, though patients with oliguria or anuria may not be able to tolerate the volumes unless dialysis or ultrafiltration techiques are used.

Heparin should be neutralized after dialysis and a reptile time should be performed if coagulation tests are abnormal in a patient who has been heparinized previously.

Haemostatic defect associated with massive transfusion

Patients who require large transfusions of stored blood, as in severe trauma, may develop haemostatic abnormalities because of loss of coagulation factors and platelets by haemorrhage and replacement by fluids containing greatly reduced concentrations (Miller *et al.*, 1971; Counts *et al.*, 1979).

Stored blood contains greatly reduced concentrations of Factors V, VIII and XI and virtually no platelets (Collins, 1976) (p. 380).

The amount of stored blood transfused before haemostatic abnormalities become apparent is variable. Some abnormality is usual after transfusion of 10 litre but as little as 2.5 litre may cause significant problems if there is underlying disease e.g. liver failure.

In addition to dilution, the other component contributing to the haemostatic defect is DIC (Collins, 1976). Patients who require massive transfusion have often been in shock which predisposes to DIC (Attar *et al.*, 1966; Hardaway, 1966).

Thrombocytopenia is a frequent occurence in massive transfusion, and although rarely falling below 50×10^9/litre, this concentration may cause serious surgical bleeding. If DIC occurs, profound thrombocytopenia with heavy bleeding may occur (Miller *et al.*, 1971; Counts *et al.*, 1979). Platelet function defects have also been noted.

Laboratory diagnosis

Standard coagulation screen, full blood count and platelet count are required. Hypofibrinogenaemia and resultant long TCT time does not occur in massive transfusion *per se*, as fibrinogen concentration is not reduced in stored blood. This may help distinguish this coagulation abnormality from that of DIC.

Replacement therapy consisting of platelets and FFP is indicated if bleeding occurs, and prophylactic transfusions of both during blood transfusion are often given where blood loss is expected to be very high (Table 79.7).

Table 79.7 Coagulation test abnormalities which may be found through haemodilution in massive transfusion

Investigation	Result
Prothrombin time	↑
Partial thromboplastin time	↑
Thrombin clotting time	Normal
Platelet count	↓
Fibrinogen	Normal
Fibrin degradation products	Normal

↑Prolonged.
↓Decreased.

Haemostatic defects associated with cardiopulmonary bypass

Much information has been gathered on abnormalities of the haemostatic system associated with cardiopulmonary bypass (CPB). Despite this, the clinical significance of many of the individual abnormalities is not certain, and the complex interrelationships involved in CPB are not understood completely (Ionescu *et al.*, 1981).

The more common abnormalities are described below.

PLATELET ABNORMALITIES

Thrombocytopenia

This is a well-recognized finding following CPB (de Leval *et al.*, 1981), although there is a lower reported incidence in later studies probably reflecting differences in surgical and pumping techniques (Bick *et al.*, 1975; Bick, 1976).

There is a relationship between bypass time and the degree of thrombocytopenia, but a poor correlation between degree of thrombocytopenia and incidence of actual CPB haemorrhage (Kevy *et al.*, 1966; Porter & Silver, 1968; Signori *et al.*, 1969).

The aetiology of thrombocytopenia is not clear, although it is probable that damage to platelets during blood flow through the pump system is involved (Bick, 1985).

Platelet function defects

It has been shown that significant platelet function defect is induced in virtually all patients undergoing CPB (Bick, 1984).

A wide range of abnormalities of *in vitro* tests of Platelet function have been reported. The actual aetiology is not certain although it seems likely that platelet membrane damage from contact with artificial surfaces or the action of shear forces in the pumping system plays a major role (Bick & Fekete, 1979; Edmunds *et al.*, 1982).

Platelet function defects are regarded as the most significant haemostatic abnormality associated with some CPB systems, particularly those using bubble or membrane oxygenator systems (Longmore *et al.*, 1981).

The major change in platelets occurs immediately following contact with artificial surfaces of the extracorporeal circuit and oxygenator. There is inhibition of platelets during bypass and this persists for some hours after cessation of the procedure. It is not clear if restoration of platelet function after CPB results from recovery of previously inhibited platelets or from formation of new platelets.

The potential haemorrhagic risk is increased if the patient has taken drugs which interfere with platelet function e.g. aspirin (Bunting & Moncada, 1980).

Prostyacyclin (Woods *et al.*, 1978) and heparin (Kalter *et al.*, 1979; Harker *et al.*, 1980) given during bypass have been shown to be effective in preserving platelet function and number.

COAGULATION FACTOR ABNORMALITIES

Decreased concentrations of coagulation factors may be found during CPB (Kalter *et al.*, 1979; Bick, 1984). Again, the aetiology is not certain, although decreased concentrations of II, V, VII, VIII, IX and X have been attributed to dilution and adsorption onto artificial surfaces (Harker *et al.*, 1980).

Decreased concentrations of fibrinogen and other coagulation factors have also been reported as being a result of increased fibrinolysis (O'Neill *et al.*, 1966; Porter & Silver, 1968; Bick *et al.*, 1975).

There is no clear relationship between these reported abnormalities and the incidence of bleeding.

In theory, excess heparin or inadequate neutralization may cause haemorrhage following bypass but it is reported rarely as the cause of bleeding after CPB. This may reflect greater experience in the use of heparin with CPB (Bick, 1985).

Disseminated intravascular coagulation was once considered a relatively common occurrence in CPB. The diagnosis, however, was difficult to establish in the presence of primary hyperfibrinolysis and heparin.

More recent opinion suggests that DIC is in fact uncommon in CPB unless there is some other triggering factor such as sepis present (Bick, 1984).

INCREASED FIBRINOLYSIS

Fibrinolytic activity is decreased usually during and after surgery (Tsitouris *et al.*, 1961; Lackner & Javid, 1973) except in CPB where it is shown to be increased frequently. It has been reported that a primary hyperfibrinolytic state occurs in the majority of patients undergoing CPB (Bick, 1985).

The activation of the fibrinolytic system probably occurs in the pump/oxygenator systems.

The clinical significance of this increased fibrinolytic state is not clear. Controlled studies comparing patients in whom antifibrinolytic agents were used empirically with those in whom they were not given, show no difference in incidence of CPB haemorrhage (Tice & Worth, 1968; Verska *et al.*, 1972). Some studies showed an increased incidence of bleeding with their use (Gomes & McGoon, 1970).

OTHER FACTORS

Other factors known to be associated with increased risk of CPB haemorrhage although the mechanisms involved are incompletely understood) include: long perfusion times (Bick, 1985), prior ingestion of coumarins (Verska *et al.*, 1972), cyanotic congenital heart disease (Signori *et al.*, 1969; Gomes & McGoon, 1970), hypothermic perfusions (O'Neill *et al.*, 1966; Tice & Worth, 1968) and preoperative use of antiplatelet drugs (Bick & Fekete, 1979).

Investigation

A standard full blood count with platelet count and blood film should be taken. A coagulation screen consisting of PT, PTT, TCT and fibrinogen concentration should be performed.

In addition, if the TCT is prolonged, a reptilase time or heparin assay should be undertaken to assess if coagulation screen abnormalities are produced by heparin.

Increased FDPs may be found in association with primary hyperfibrinolysis or DIC.

Many coagulation laboratories do not have the facilities for measuring components of the fibrinolytic system such as plasminogen or plasmin, but if available, these investigations may help to decide whether antifibrinolytic agents are indicated.

Table 79.8 summarizes patterns of abnormalities which may be found in association with CPB.

Treatment

One may have to transfuse platelets, cryoprecipitate and FFP as an emergency in a patient who is bleeding excessively after CPB. One should have ensured that heparin neutralization has been adequate before this step.

It is important to send samples to the laboratory for coagulation screen before transfusion of these blood products as the results may decide the strategy to be adopted, should haemorrhage continue.

Platelet concentrates should be given, even if there is a normal platelet count because of the likely platelet dysfunction present. Fresh frozen plasma may be indicated to correct deficiencies occuring after adsorption of coagulation factors or dilution with stored blood and other fluids. Cryoprecipitate may be used as a source of fibrinogen if this is decreased from fibrinolysis.

Antifibrinolytic agents are indicated rarely and should be used only if there is clear evidence of primary hyperfibrinolysis without DIC and if previous measures have failed to control haemorrhage. Under these circumstances EACA 5–10 g should be slowly infused intravenously and followed by 1–2 g hourly until bleeding ceases (Bick, 1976).

Psychogenic bleeding

Rarely, a patient may present with a self-induced haemorrhagic state, and it is often only after exclusion of other potential causes that the diagnosis is made (Ratnoff, 1980b).

Warfarin ingestion and occasionally heparin administration in patients who have access to them e.g. health workers have been reported. In these instances the usual patterns with coagulation results

Table 79.8 Patterns of abnormal coagulation tests which may be seen in cardiopulmonary bypass

Test	Thrombocytopenia	Platelet dysfunction	DIC	Excess heparin	Primary hyperfibrinolysis
Platelet count	↓	Normal	↓	Normal	Normal
Prothrombin time	Normal	Normal	↑	↑	Normal
Partial thromboplastin time	Normal	Normal	↑	↑	May be ↑
Thrombin clotting time	Normal	Normal	↑	↑	↑
Fibrinogen	Normal	Normal	↓	Normal	May be ↓
Fibrin degradation products	Normal	Normal	↑	Normal	↑
Reptilase time (or equivalent)	—	—	↑	Normal	↑
Other relevant	—	Bleeding time	—	Protamine neutralization	Plasmin plasminogen studies

↑ Prolonged.
↓ Shortened or decreased.

and the diagnosis is clinical with assay of specific drugs (Agle *et al.*, 1970; Forbes *et al.*, 1974; O'Reilly & Aggeler, 1976).

Patients suffering from hysterical states are also reported to have haemorrhagic events, although these are almost always minor and do not cause bleeding problems during surgery.

Conclusion

The anaesthetist deals with patients in a wide variety of clinical settings, including pre- and postoperative general surgical patients, cardiothoracic surgery, intensive care and obstetric practice, and this chapter has attempted to cover the more likely acquired haemostatic disorders that may be encountered in these situations.

Consultation with the haematolgist or other specialist with an interest in coagulation is of great importance in planning investigation and management of patients with a haemostatic defect, as they are usually aware of the full resources of the local laboratory.

Most of the discussions in this chapter are up to date at the time of going to press but it is likely that future developments may significantly alter our thinking on some problems e.g. pathogenesis and treatment of DIC.

References

Agle D.P., Ratnoff O.D. & Spring G.K. (1970) The anticoagulant malingerer, psychiatric studies on 3 patients. *Annals of Internal Medicine* **73**, 67–72.

Allain J.P., Gaillandre A. & Frommel D. (1981) Acquired haemophilia: functional study of antibodies to factor VIII. *Thrombosis and Haemostasis* **45**, 285–9.

American Heart Association (1973) The Urokinase Pulmonary Embolism Trial. A National Co-operative Study. Monograph No. 39. *Circulation* **47** (Suppl. 2), 11–108.

Aoki N. & Yamanaka T. (1978) The alpha 2-plasmin inhibitor levels in liver diseases. *Clinica Chimica Acta* **84**, 99–105.

Aster, R.H. (1966) Pooling of platelets in the spleen : role of the pathogenesis of hypersplenic thrombocytopenia. *Journal of Clinical Investigation* **45**, 645–57.

Attar S., Mansberger A.R., Irani B., Kirby W., Masaitis C. & Cowley R.A. (1966) Coagulation changes in clinical shock II. Effect of septic shock on clotting times and fibrinogen in humans. *Annals of Surgery* **164**, 41–50.

Bailton F.E. & Letsky E.A. (1985) Obstetric haemorrhage: causes and management. In *Haematological Disorders in Pregnancy. Clinics in Haematology* (Ed. Letsky) pp. 683–728. W.B. Saunders, Philadelphia.

Ballard H.S. & Marcus A.J. (1976) Platelet aggregation in portal cirrhosis. *Archives of Internal Medicine* **136**, 316–19.

Bang N.U. & Chang M. (1974) Soluble fibrin complexes. *Seminars in Thrombosis and Hemostasis* **1**, 91–128.

Barr R.D., Forbes C.D. & McNicol G.P. (1969) Inhibitors of anti-haemophilic globulin (factor VIII) and various spontaneous anticoagulants. An account of six cases with review of the literature. *Coagulation* **2**, 323.

Bell W.R. (1980) Disseminated intravascular coagulation. *Johns Hopkins Medical Journal* **146**, 289–99.

Beller F.K. (1971) Experimental animal models for the production of disseminated intravascular coagulation. In *Thrombosis and Bleeding Disorders* (Eds Bang N.U., Beller F.K., Deutsch E. & Mammen E.F.) p. 514. Academic Press, New York.

Bergstrom K., Blomback B. & Kleen G. (1960) Studies on the plasma fibrinolytic activity in a case of liver cirrhosis. *Acta Medica Scandinavica* **168**, 291–305.

Bick R.L. (1976) Alteration of hemostasis associated with cardiopulmonary bypass: pathophysiology, prevention, diagnosis and management. *Seminars in Thrombosis and Hemostasis* **3**, 59–82.

Bick R.L. (1978) Alterations of hemostasis associated with malignancy: etiology, pathophysiology, diagnosis and management. *Seminars in Thrombosis and Hemostasis* **5**, 1–26.

Bick R.L. (1984) Alterations of hemostasis associated with surgery, cardiopulmonary bypass surgery and prosthetic devices. In *Disorders of Hemostasis* (Eds Ratnoff O.D. & Forbes C.D.) p. 379. Grune & Stratton, London.

Bick R.L. (1985) Hemostasis defects associated with cardiac surgery, prosthetic devices and other extracorporeal circuits. *Seminars in Thrombosis and Hemostasis* **11**, 249–80.

Bick R.L. & Fekete L.F. (1979) Cardiopulmonary bypass haemorrhage. Aggravation by pre-op ingestion of anti-platelet agents. *Vascular Surgery* **13**, 277.

Bick R.L., Schmalhorst W.R., Crawford L., Holtermann M. & Arbegast N.R. (1975) The haemorrhagic diathesis created by cardiopulmonary by pass. *American Journal of Clinical Pathology* **63**, 588.

Bick R.L., Schmalhorst W.R. & Fekete L.F. (1976) Disseminated intravascular coagulation and blood component therapy. *Transfusion* **16**, 361–5.

Blanchard R.A., Furie B.C., Jorgensen M., Kruger S.F. & Furie B. (1981) Acquired Vitamin K dependent carboxylation deficiency in liver disease. *New England Journal of Medicine* **305**, 242–8.

Blauhut B., Necek S., Vinazzer H. & Bergman H. (1982) Substitution therapy with an anti-thrombin III concentrate in shock and DIC. *Thrombosis Research* **27**, 271–8.

Bloom A.L. (1977) Intravascular coagulation in the liver. *British Journal of Haematology* **30**, 1–7.

Bonnar J. (1981) Haemostasis and coagulation disorders in pregnancy. In *Haemostasis and Thrombosis* (Eds Bloom A.L. & Thomas D.P.) p. 454. Churchill Livingstone, New York.

Brain M.C. (1969) The haemolytic uraemic syndrome. *Seminars in Hematology* **6**, 162–80.

British Society for Haematology (1982) *Guidelines on Oral Anticoagulantion.* BSCH Haemostasis and Thrombosis Task Force.

Brodsky I. & Siegel N.H. (1970) The diagnosis and treatment of disseminated intravascular coagulation. *Medical Clinics of North America* **54**, 555–65.

Brozovic M. (1981) Acquired disorders of blood coagulation. In *Haemostasis and Thrombosis* (Eds Bloom A.L. & Thomas D.P.) p. 411–38. Churchill Livingstone, Edinburgh.

Bunting S. & Moncada S. (1980) Prostacyclin, by preventing platelet activation, prolongs activated clotting time in blood and platelet rich plasma and potentiates the anticoagulant effect of heparin. *British Journal of Pharmacology* **69**, 268–9.

Carreras L.O., Vermylen J., Spitz B. & Assche A. (1981) 'Lupus' anticoagulant and inhibition of prostacyclin formation in patients with repeated abortion, intrauterine growth retardation and intrauterine death. *British Journal of Obstetrics and Gynecology* **88**, 890–4.

Cash J.D. (1977) Disseminated intravascular coagulation. In *Recent Advances in Blood Coagulation* (Ed. Polle L.) p. 293. Churchill Livingstone, Edinburgh.

Castaldi P.A. (1984) Haemostasis and the kidney. In *Disorders of Haemostasis* (Eds Ratnoff O. & Forbes C.D.) pp. 473–484. Grune & Stratton, London.

Cederblad G., Korstan-Bengstein K. & Olsson R. (1976) Observation of increased levels of blood coagulation factors and other plasma proteins in cholestatic liver disease. *Scandinavian Journal of Gastroenterology* **11**, 391–6.

Cline M.J., Melman K.L., Davis W.C. & Williams H.E. (1968) Mechanism of endotoxin interaction with human leucocytes. *British Journal of Haematology* **15**, 539–47.

Collen D. (1983) Treatment of DIC. *Bibliotheca Haematologica* **49**, 295–305.

Collins J.A. (1976) Massive blood transfusion. *Clinics in Haematology* **5**, 201–21.

Colman R.W., Robbay S.J. & Minna J.D. (1972) Disseminated intravascular coagulation (DIC): an approach. *American Journal of Medicine* **52**, 679–89.

Corrigan J.J. & Jordan C.M. (1970) Heparin therapy in septicaemia with disseminated intravascular coagulation. *New England Journal of Medicine* **283**, 778–82.

Counts R.B., Haisch C., Simon T.L., Maxwell N., Heinbach D.M. & Carrico C.J. (1979) Haemostasis in massively transfused trauma patients. *Annals of Surgery* **190**, 91–9.

Courtney L.D. & Allington M. (1972) Effect of amniotic fluid on blood coagulation. *British Journal of Haematology* **22**, 353–5.

Cronberg S., Skansberg P. & Nivenius-Larsson K. (1973) Disseminated intravascular coagulation in septicaemia caused by beta haemolytic streptococci. *Thrombosis Research* **3**, 405–11.

Crosby W.H. & Stefanini M. (1952) Pathogenesis of the plasma transfusion reaction with especial reference to the blood coagulation system. *Journal of Laboratory and Clinical Medicine* **40**, 374–86.

Culpepper R.M. (1975) Bleeding diathesis in fresh water drowning. *Annals of Internal Medicine* **83**, 675.

Damus P.S. & Wallace G.A. (1975) Immunologic measurement of antithrombin III—heparin co-factor and 2 macroglobulin in disseminated intrasvascular coagulation and hepatic failure coagulopathy. *Thrombosis Research* **6**, 27–38.

Davidson J.F., McNicol G.P., Frank G.L., Anderson T.J. & Douglas A.S. (1969) A plasminogen activator-producing tumour. *British Medical Journal* **1**, 88.

Davis G. & Liu D.T. (1972) Mid-trimester abortion. *Lancet* **ii**, 1026.

de Leval M.R., Hill J.D. & Mielke C.H. (1981) Haematological aspects of extracorporeal circulation. In *Techniques in Extracorporeal Circulation* 2nd edn. (Ed. Ionescu M.D.) p. 345. Butterworths, London.

Deykin D. (1970) The clinical challenge of disseminated intravascular coagulation. *New England Journal of Medicine* **283**, 636–44.

Dieckman W.J. (1936) Blood chemistry and renal function in abruptio placentae. *American Journal of Obstetrics and Gynecology* **31**, 734–5.

Donaldson V.H. (1960) Effect of plasmin *in vitro* on clotting factors in plasma. *Journal of Laboratory and Clinical Medicine* **56**, 644–51.

Donaldson V.H. (1984) Haemorrhagic disorders of neonates. In *Disorders of Haemostasis* (Eds Ratnoff O.D. & Forbes C.D.) p. 409. Grune & Stratton, London.

Douglas J.T., Shah M., Lowe G.D.O., Belch J.J.F., Forbes C.D. & Prentice C.R.M. (1982) Plasma fibrinopeptide A and β throm-boglobulin in pre-eclampsia and pregnancy hypertension. *Thrombosis and Haemostasis* **47**, 54.

Duckert F. (1973) Behaviour of antithrombin III in liver disease. *Scandinavian Journal of Gastroenterology* **8** (Suppl. 19), 109–12.

Edgar W., McKillop C., Howie P.W. & Prentice C.R.M., (1977) Composition of soluble fibrin complexes in pre-eclampsia. *Thrombosis Research* **10**, 567–74.

Edmunds L.H. jr., Ellison N., Colman R.W., Niewiarowski S., Rao A.K., Addonizio V.P., Stephenson L.W. & Edie R.N. (1982) Platelet function during cardiac operation. Comparison of membrane and bubble oxygenators. *Journal of Thoracic and Cardiovascular Surgery* **83**, 805–12.

Eknoyan G., Wacksman S.G., Glueck H.I. & Will J.J. (1969) Platelet function in renal failure. *New England Journal of Medicine* **280**, 677.

Ellison R.T., Corrao W.M., Fox M.J. & Braman S.S. (1987) Spontaneous mediastinal haemorrhage in patients on chronic haemodialysis. *Annals of Internal Medicine* **95**, 704–6.

Fletcher A.P., Alkjaersig N. & Fishers (1966) The proteolysis of fibrinogen by plasmin: the identification of thrombin-clottable fibrinogen derivatives which polymerize abnormally. *Journal of Laboratory and Clinical Medicine* **68**, 780–802.

Fletcher A.P., Biederman O. Moore D., Alkjaersig N. & Sherry S. (1964) Abnormal plasminogen–plasmin system activity (fibrinolysis) in patients with hepatic cirrhosis: its cause and consequences. *Journal of Clinical Investigation* **43**, 681–95.

Flute P.T. (1982) Acquired disorders of blood coagulation. In *Blood and its Disorders* 2nd edn. (Eds Hardisty & Weatherall D.J.) p. 1161. Blackwell Scientific Publications. Oxford.

Foley M.E., Clayton J.K. & McNicol G.P. (1977) Haemostatic mechanisms in maternal, umbilical vein and umbilical artery blood at time of delivery. *British Journal of Obstetrics Gynaecology* **84**, 81–7.

Forbes C.D., Prentice C.R.M. & Sclare A.B. (1974) Surreptitious ingestion of Warfarin. *British Journal of Psychiatry* **125**, 245.

Giddings J.C., Shaw E., Tuddenham E.G.D. & Bloom A.L. (1975) The synthesis of factor V in tissue culture and isolated organ perfusion. *Thrombosis et Diathesis Haemorrhagia* **34**, 321.

Glazier R.L. & Cravell E.B. (1976) Randomized prospective trial of continuous v intermittent heparin therapy. *Journal of the American Medical Association* **236**, 1365–7.

Goldsmith G.H. (1984) Haemostatic disorders associated with neoplasia. In *Disorders of Haemostasis* (Eds Ratnoff O.D. & Forbes C.D.) p. 351–66. Grune & Stratton, New York.

Gomes M.M. & McGoon D. (1970) Bleeding patterns after open heart surgery. *Journal of Thoracic and Cardiovascular Surgery* **60**, 87–97.

Goodnight S.H., Feinstein D.I., Osterud B. & Rapaport S.I. (1971) Factor VII antibody-neutralization material in hereditary and acquired factor VII deficiency. *Blood* **38**, 1–8.

Grain S.M. & Chardry A.M. (1981) Thrombotic thrombocytopenic purpura. A reappraisal. *Journal of the American Medical Association* **246**, 1243–6.

Gralnick H.R. & Abrell E. (1973) Studies on the procoagulant and fibrinolytic activity of promyelocytes in acute promyelocytic leukaemia. *British Journal of Haematology* **24**, 89–99.

Green D. & Lechner K. (1981) A survey of 215 non-hemophilic patients with inhibitors to Factor VIII. *Thrombosis and Haemostasis* **45**, 200–3.

Green G., Thomson J.M., Dymock I.W. & Poller L. (1977) Abnormal fibrin polymerization in liver disease. *British Journal of Haematology* **34**, 427–39.

Grossi C.E., Moreno A.H. & Rousselot L.M. (1961) Studies on spontaneous fibrinolytic activity in patients with cirrhosis of the liver and its inhibition by epsilon aminocapioic acid. *Annals of Surgery* **153**, 383–93.

Grun M., Liehr H., Brunsing D. *et al.* (1974) Regulation of fibrinogen synthesis is portal hypertension. *Thrombosis et Diathesis Haemorrhagia* **32**, 292–305.

Grundy M.F.B. & Graven E.R. (1976) Consumption coagulopathy after intra-amniotic urea. *British Medical Journal* **18**, 677.

Hallen A. & Nilsson I.M. (1964) Coagulation studies in liver disease. *Thrombosis et Diathesis Haemorrhagia* **11**, 51–63.

Ham T.H. & Curtis F.C. (1938) Plasma fibrinogen response in man. Influence of the nutritional state, induced hyperpyrexia, infectious disease and liver damage. *Medicine* **17**, 413–45.

Hardaway R.M. (1966) *Syndrome of Disseminated Intravascular Coagulation with Special Reference to Shock and Haemorrhage.* Charles C. Thomas, Springfield.

Hardaway R.M. (1967) Disseminated intravascular coagulation in experimental and clinical shock. *American Journal of Cardiology* **20**, 161–73.

Harker L.A., Malpass T.W., Branson H.E. *et al.* (1980) Mechanism of abnormal bleeding in patients undergoing cardiopulmonary bypass: acquired transient platelet dysfunction associated with selective and granule release. *Blood* **56**, 824–34.

Harmon D.C., Dermirjian Z., Ellman L. & Fischer J.E. (1979) DIC with peritovenous shunt. *Annals of Internal Medicine* **90**, 774–6.

Hathaway W.E. & Alsever J. (1970) The relation of 'Fletcher factor' to factor XI and XII. *British Journal of Haematology* **18**, 161.

Hellegren M., Javelin L., Hagnevik K. *et al.* (1984) Antithrombin III concentrate as adjuvant in DIC treatment. A pilot study in 9 severely ill patients. *Thrombosis Research* **35**, 459–66.

Hillenbrand P., Parboo S.P., Jedrychowski A. & Sherlock S. (1974) Significance of intravascular coagulation and fibrinolysis in acute hepatic failure. *Gut* **15**, 83.

Hemker H.C., Veltkamp J.J. Hensen A. (1963) Nature of prethrombinaemia in Vitamin K deficiency. *Nature* **200**, 589.

Higuchi A., Sakuruda R. & Miyazaki T. (1980) Acquired dysfibrinogenaemia associated with liver disease. *Proceedings of the 18th Congress of the International Society of Haematology* p. 247.

Hirsch J. (1986) Mechanisms of action and monitoring of anticoagulants. *Seminars in Thrombosis and Haemostasis* **12**, number 1.

Horder M.H. (1969) Consumption coagulopathy in liver cirrhosis. *Thromboses et Diathesis Haemorrhagia* **36** (Suppl.), 313.

Horowitz H.I., Stein I.M. & Cohen B.D. (1970) Further studies on the platelet-inhibitory effect of guanidosuccinic acid and its role in uremic bleeding. *American Journal of Medicine* **49**, 336–45.

Howie P.W., Prentice C.R.M. & Forbes C.D. (1975) Failure of heparin therapy to affect the clinical cause of severe pre-eclampsia. *British Journal of Obstetrics and Gynaecology* **82**, 711–17.

Howie P.W., Purdie D.W., Begg C.B. & Prentice C.R.M. (1976) Use of coagulation tests to predict the clinical progress of pre-eclampsia. *Lancet* **ii** 323–5.

Ionescu M.I., Tandon A.P. & Roesler M.F. (1981) Blood loss following extracorporeal circulation for heart valve surgery. In *Techniques in Extracorporeal Circulation* 2nd edn. (Ed. Ionescu M.I.) p. 345. Butterworths, London.

Jakobsen E., Ly B. & Kieulf P. (1974) Incorporation of fibrinogen with soluble fibrin complexes. *Thrombosis Research* **4**, 499.

Jandl J.H. & Lear A.A. (1956) The metabolism of folic acid in cirrhosis. *Annals of Internal Medicine* **45**, 1027–44.

Janson P.A., Jubelirer S.J., Weinstein M. & Deykin D. (1980) Treatment of bleeding tendency in uremia with cryoprecipitate. *New England Journal of Medicine* **303**, 1318–22.

Jick H., Slone D., Borda I.T. & Shapiro S. (1968) Efficacy and toxicity of heparin in relation to age and sex. *New England Journal of Medicine* **279**, 284–6.

Kalter R.D., Saul C.M., Wetstein L., Soriano C. & Reiss R.F. (1979) Cardiopulmonary bypass. Associated haemostatic abnormalities. *The Journal of Thoracic and Cardiovascular Surgery* **77**, 427–35.

Kaplan A.P., Castellino F.J., Collen D., Wiman B. & Taylor F.B. (1978) Molecular mechanisms of fibrinolysis in man. *Thrombosis and Haemostasis* **39**, 263–83.

Kaplan A., Meier H. & Mandle R. (1976) The Hageman factor dependent coagulation pathways of coagulation, fibrinolysis and kinin generation. *Seminars in Thrombosis and Hemostasis* **3**, 1–26.

Kelton J.G. & Levine M.N. (1986) Heparin-induced thrombocytopenia. *Seminars in Thrombosis and Hemostasis* **12**, 59–62.

Kevy S.V., Glickman R.M. & Bernhard W.F. (1966) The pathogenesis and control of the hemorrhagic defect in open heart surgery. *Surgery, Gynecology and Obstetrics* **123**, 313–18.

Klein H.G. & Bell W.R. (1974) Disseminated intravascular coagulation during heparin therapy. *Annal of Internal Medicine* **80**, 477.

Kleiner G.J., Merskey C., Johnson A.J. & Markus W.B. (1970) Defibrination in normal and abnormal parturition. *British Journal of Haematology* **19**, 159.

Kopec M., Wegrzynowiczy Z. & Budzykski A. (1968) Interaction of fibrinogen degradation products with platelets. *Experimental Biology and Medicine* **3**, 73.

Krevans J.R., Jackson D.P., Cowley C.L. & Hartmann R.C. (1957) The nature of the haemorrhagic disorder accompanying haemolytic transfusion reactions in man. *Blood* **12**, 834.

Lackner H. Javid J.P. (1973) The clinical significance of the plasminogen level. *American Journal of Clinical Pathology* **60**, 175–81.

Langdell R.D. & Hedgpeth E.M. jr. (1959) A study of the role of haemolysis in the haemostatic defects of transfusion reactions. *Thrombosis et Diathesis Haemorrhagia* **3**, 566–71.

Larkin E.C. Watson-Williams E.J. (1984) Alcohol and the Blood. *Medical Clinics of North America* **68**, 105–120.

Lasch H.G., Heene D.L., Huth K. & Sandritter W. (1967) Pathophysiology, clinical manifestations and therapy of consumption coagulopathy. *American Journal of Cardiology* **20**, 381–91.

Laursen B., Mortensen J.Z., Frost L. & Hansen K.B. (1981) Disseminated intravascular coagulation in hepatic failure treated with antithrombin III. *Thrombosis Research* **22**, 701–4.

Lawrence L. (1971) Lack of significant protection afforded by heparin during endotoxin shock. *American Journal of Physiology* **220**, 901–5.

Lechner K. (1972) Immune reactive factor IX in acquired factor IX deficiency. *Thrombosis et Diathesis Haemorrhagia* **27**, 19–24.

Lechner K., Niessner H. Thaler E. (1977) Coagulation abnormalities in liver disease. *Seminars in Thrombosis and Hemostasis* **4**, 40.

Lee C.Y. (1979) *Snake Venoms*, vol. 52. Springer-Verlag, New York.

Lerner R.G., Nelson J.C., Corines P. & del Guercio L.R.M. (1978) DIC—complication of peritovenous shunts. *Journal of the American Medical Association* **240**, 2064–6.

Lieberman E. (1972) Haemolytic–uraemic syndrome. *Journal of Paediatrics* **80**, 1–16.

Linder M., Muller-Berghaus G. & Lasch H.G. (1970) Virus infection and blood coagulation. *Thrombosis et Diathesis Haemorrhagia* **23**, 1.

Lipinski B., Lipinska I. & Nova A. (1977) Abnormal fibrinogen heterogeneity and fibrinolytic activity in advanced liver disease. *Journal of Laboratory & Clinical Medicine* **90**, 187–94.

Longmore D.B., Bennett, J.G., Hoyle P.M., Smith M.A., Gregory A., Osivand T. & Jones W.A. (1981) Prostacyclin administration during cardiopulmonary bypass in man. *Lancet* **i**, 800–4.

Losowsky M.S. & Walls W.D. (1969) Abnormal fibrin stabilization in renal failure. *Thrombosis et Diathesis Haemorrhagia* **22**, 216.

Lucey J.F. & Dolan R.G. (1958) Injections of a Vitamin K compound in mothers and hyperbilirubinaemia in the newborn. *Paediatrics* **221**, 605–6.

McGehee W.G., Rapaport S.I. & Hjort P.F. (1967) Intravascular coagulation in fulminant meningococcaemia. *Annals of Internal Medicine* **67**, 250–6.

McKay D.G. & Shapiro S.S. (1958) Alterations in the blood coagulation system induced by bacterial endotoxin. 1: in vitro (generalized Schwartzman reaction). *Journal of Experimental Medicine* **107**, 353–67.

MacKenzie I.Z., Sayers L., Bonnar J. & Hillier K. (1975) Coagulation changes during second trimester abortion induced by intra-amniotic prostaglandin E_2 and hypertonic solutions. *Lancet* **ii**, 1066–9.

Mann J.D. (1952) Plasmin prothrombin in viral hepatitis and hepatic cirrhosis. Evaluation of the two stage method in 75 cases. *Gastroenterology* **21**, 263–70.

Mannucci P.M., Lobina G.F., Caocci L. & Dioguardi N. (1969) Effect on blood coagulation of massive intravascular haemolysis. *Blood* **33**, 207–12.

Mannucci M.M., Remuzzi G., Pusineri F., Lombardi R., Valsecchi C., Mecca G. & Zimmerman T.S. (1983) Desamino-8-D-Arginine vasopressin shortens the bleeding time in uremia. *New England Journal of Medicine* **308**, 8.

Mant M.J. & King E.G. (1979) Severe, acute disseminated intravascular coagulation. *American Journal of Medicine* **67**, 557.

Mant M.J., O'Brien B.D., Thong K.L., Hammond G.W., Birtwhistle R.V. & Grace M.G. (1977) Haemorrhagic complications of heparin therapy. *Lancet* **i**, 1133.

Marder V.J. (1979) Use of Thrombolytic agents: choice of patients, drug administration, laboratory monitoring. *Annals of Internal Medicine* **90**, 802–8.

Marder V.J., Soulen R.L. & Artichartalcon V. (1977) Quantitative venographic assessment of deep vein thrombosis in the evaluation of streptokinase and heparin therapy. *Journal of Laboratory of Clinical Medicine* **89**, 1018–29.

Merskey C. (1973) Defibrination syndrome or .... *Blood* **41**, 599.

Merskey C., Johnson, A.J., Kleiner G.J. & Wohl H. (1967) The defibrination syndrome. Clinical features and laboratory diagnosis. *British Journal of Haemetology* **13**, 528–9.

Merskey C., Kleiner G.J., & Johnson A.J. (1966) Quantitative estimation of split products of fibrinogen in human series: relation to diagnosis and treatment. *Blood* **28**, 1–18.

Miller L.L. & Bale W.F. (1954) Synthesis of all plasma protein functions except gamma globulins by the liver. The use of zone electrophoresis and lysine C^{14} to define the plasma proteins synthesized by the isolated perfused liver. *Journal of Experimental Medicine* **99**, 125–32.

Miller L.L., Bly, G.G., Watson M.L. & Bale M.F. (1951) The dominant role of the liver in plasma protein synthesis. A direct study of the isolated perfused rat liver with the aid of lysine. *Journal of Experimental Medicine* **94**, 431–53.

Miller R.D., Robbins T.O., Tong M.J. & Barton S.L. (1971) Coagulation defects associated with massive blood transfusion. *Annals of Surgery* **174**, 794–801.

Morgan M. (1979) Amniotic fluid embolism. *Anaesthesia* **34**, 20.

Muirhead E.E. (1951) Incompatible blood transfusions with the emphasis on acute renal failure. *Surgery, Gynecology and Obstetrics* **42**, 734–46.

Muller-Berghaus G. (1977) Pathophysiology of generalized intravascular coagulation. *Seminars in Thrombosis and Hemostasis* **3**, 209–46.

Murray-Lyon, Minchin Clarke H.G.M., McPherson K. & Williams R. (1972) Quantitative immunoelectrophoresis of serum proteins in cryptogenic cirrhosis, alcoholic cirrhosis and active chronic hepatitis. *Clinica Chimica Acta* **39**, 215–20.

Nelsestuen G.L., Zytkovicz T.H. & Havard J.B. (1974) Mode of action of Vitamin K, identification of carboxyglutamic acid as component of prothrombin. *Journal of Biological Chemistry* **249**, 6357.

Niewiarowski S., Regoeczi E., Stewart G., Senyi A.F. & Mustard J.F. (1972) Platelet interactions with polymerizing fibrin. *Journal of Clinical Investigation* **51**, 685–700.

Norman C.S. & Provan J.L. (1977) Control and complications of intermittent heparin therapy. *Surgery, Gynecology and Obstetrics* **145**, 338–42.

Nyman D. (1985) Discussion and definition of DIC and its treatment. *Scandinavian Journal of Clinical and Laboratory Investigation* **45** (Suppl. 178), 31–3.

O'Grady J., Bunting S. & Moncada S. (1980) Antithrombotic drugs in relation to prostaglandin metabolism. *Clinics in Haematology* **9**, 535–55.

Ollendorff P. (1962) The nature of the anticoagulant effect of heparin, protamine, polybrene and toludene blue. *Scandinavian Journal of Clinical and Laboratory Investigation* **14**, 267–76.

O'Neill J.A., Ende N., Collins J.S. & Collins H.A. (1966) A quantitative determination of perfusion fibrinolysis. *Journal of Thoracic and Cardiovascular Surgery* **51**, 777–82.

O'Reilly R.A. & Aggeler P.M. (1976) Covert anticoagulant ingestion: study of 25 patients and review of world literature. *Medicine* **55**, 389–99.

O'Sullivan E.F., Hirsh J., McCarthy R.A. et al. (1968) Heparin in the treatment of venous thrombo embolic disease. Administration, control and results. *Medical Journal of Australia* **2**, 153.

Owen C.A., Bawie E.J.W. & Cooper H.A. (1973) Turnover of fibrinogen and platelets in dogs undergoing induced intravascular coagulation. *Thrombosis Research* **2**, 251–60.

Owren P.A. (1949) Diagnostic and prognostic significance of plasma prothrombin and factor V levels in parenchymatous hepatitis and obstructive jaundice. *Scandinavian Journal of Clinical and Laboratory Investigation* **1**, 131–40.

Page E.W., Fulton L.D. & Glendening M.B. (1951) The cause of the blood coagulation defect following abruptio placentae. *American Journal of Obstetrics and Gynecology* **61**, 1116–21.

Pechet L. (1965) Fibrinolysis. *New England Journal of Medicine* **273**, 966–73.

Pisciotta A.V. & Goltschall J.L. (1980) Clinical features of thrombotic thrombocytopenic purpura. *Seminars in Thrombosis and Hemostatis* **6**, 330–40.

Pisciotta A.V. & Schultz E.J. (1955) Fibrinolytic purpura in acute leukaemia. *American Journal of Medicine* **19**, 824–8.

Pitney W.R. (1971) Disseminated intravascular coagulation. *Seminars in Haematology* **8**, 65–82.

Pitney W.R., Pettit J.E. & Armstrong L. (1970) Control of heparin therapy. *British Medical Journal* **4**, 139–41.

Prentice C.R.M. (1976) Heparin and disseminated intravascular coagulation. In *Heparin: Clinical Chemistry and Usage* (Eds Kakkar W. & Thomas D.P.) pp. 219–22. Academic Press, London.

Prentice C.R.M. (1985) Acquired coagulation disorders. In *Clinics in Haematology: Coagulation Disorders* pp. 413–42. W.B. Saunder, Philadelphia.

Preston F.E. (1982) Disseminated intravascular coagulation. *British Journal of Hospital Medicine* **28**, 129–320.

Pritchard J.A. (1959) Fetal death in utero. *Obstetrics and Gynaecology* **14**, 573–80.

Pritchard J.A. (1973) Haematological problems associated with delivery, placental abruption, retained dead fetus and amniotic fluid embolism. *Clinics in Haematology* **2**, 563–86.

Pritchard J.A. & Brekken A.L. (1967) Clinical and laboratory studies on severe abruptio placentae. *American Journal of Obstetrics and Gynecology* **97**, 681–95.

Porter J.M. & Silver D. (1968) Alterations in fibrinolysis and coagulation associated with cardiopulmonary bypass. *Journal of Thoracic and Cardiovascular Surgery* **56**, 869–78.

Quick A.J., Stanley-Brown M. & Bancroft F.W. (1935) A study of the coagulation defect in haemophilia and in jaundice. *American Journal of the Medical Sciences* **190**, 501–11.

Rabiner S.F. (1972a) Uraemic Bleeding. *Progress in Hemostasis and Thrombosis* **1**, 233.

Rabiner S.F. (1972b) The effect of dialysis on platelet function of patients in renal failure. *Annals of the New York Academy of Sciences* **201**, 234.

Rabiner S.F. & Molinas F. (1970) The role of phenol and phenolic acids in the thromocytopathy and defective platelet aggregation of patients with renal failure. *American Journal of Medicine* **49**, 346–51.

Rapaport S.I., Ames S.B., Mikkelsen S. & Goodman J.R. (1960) Plasma clotting factors in chronic hepatocellular disease. *New England Journal of Medicine* **263**, 278–82.

Ratnoff O.D. (1952) Studies as a proteolytic enyzme in human plasma VII. A fatal haemorrhagic state associated with excessive proteolytic activity in a patient undergoing surgery for carcinoma of head of pancreas. *Journal of Clinical Investigation* **31**, 521–8.

Ratnoff O.D. (1954) An accelerative property of plasma for the coagulation of fibrinogen by thrombin. *Journal of Clinical Investigation* **33**, 1175–82.

Ratnoff O.D. (1963) Haemostatic mechanisms in liver disease. *Medical Clinics of North America* **47**, 721–36.

Ratnoff O.D. (1980a) Why do people bleed? In *Blood, Pure and Eloquent* (Ed. Wintrobe M.M.) p. 600. McGraw Hill, New York.

Ratnoff O.D. (1980b) The psychogenic purpuras: a review of autoerythorocyte sensitization, autosensitization to DNA, 'hysterical' and factitial bleeding, and the religious stigmata. *Seminars in Hematology* **17**, 192–213.

Ratnoff O. (1984) Haemostatic defects in liver and biliary tract disease and disorders of vitamin K metabolism. In *Disorders of Haemostasis* (Eds Ratnoff O. & Forbes C.D.). Grune & Stratton, New York.

Reece E.A., Fox H.E. & Rapaport F. (1982) Factor VIII inhibitor: a cause of severe post partum haemorrhage. *American Journal of Obstetrics and Gynecology* **144**, 985–7.

Reid A.H. (1984) Clinical Haemostatic Disorders Caused by Venoms. In *Disorders of Haemostasis* (Eds Ratnoff O. & Forbes C.D.) pp. 511–26. Grune & Stratton, New York.

Remuzzi G., Marchesi D., Mecca G., Misiani R., Livio M., de Gaetano G. & Donati M.B. (1978) Altered platelet and vascular prostaglandin-generation in patients with renal failure and prolonged bleeding time. *Thrombosis Research* **13**, 1007.

Remuzzi G., Marchesi D., Mecca G. *et al.* (1978) Haemolytic–uraemic syndrome: deficiency of plasma factors regulating prostacyclin activity? *Lancet* **ii**, 871–2.

Rivers R.P.A., Hathaway W.E. & Weston W.L. (1975) Endotoxin induced coagulant activity of human monocytes. *British Journal of Haematology* **30**, 311–6.

Roberts H.R. & Lederbaum A.I. (1972) The liver and blood coagulation: physiology and pathology. *Gastroenterolgy* **63**, 297–320.

Roth G.J. & Majevus P.W. (1975) The mechanism of the effect of aspirin on human platelets. 1. Acetylation of a particular fraction protein. *Journal of Clinical Investigation* **56**, 624–32.

Rubenberg M.J., Baker L.R., McBride J.A., Sevitt L.H. & Brain M.C. (1967) Intravascular coagulation in a case of C1 perfringeus septicaemia. *British Medical Journal* **4**, 271–4.

Rubin R.N., Kies M.S. & Posch J.J. (1978) Coagulation profiles with metastatic liver disease. *Blood* **52** (Suppl. 1), 193.

Rubin M.H., Weston M.L., Bullock G., Roberts J., Langley P.G., White Y.S. & Williams R. (1977) Abnormal platelet function and ultrastructure in fulminant hepatic failure. *Quarterly Journal of Medicine* **46**, 339–52.

Rushton D.I. & Dowson I.M.P. (1982) The maternal autopsy. *Journal of Clinical Pathology* **35**, 909–12.

Saito H., Poon M-C., Vicic W., Goldsmith G.H. & Menitove J.E. (1978) Human plasma prekallikrein (Fletcher factor) clotting activity and antigen in health and disease. *Journal of Laboratory and Clinical Medicine* **92**, 84–95.

Salinon S.J., Lambert P.H. & Louis J. (1971) Pathogenesis of intravascular coagulation induced by immunological reactions. *Thrombosis et Diathesis Haemorrhagia* **45**, 161.

Salzman E.W., Deykin D., Shapiro R.M. & Rosenberg R. (1975) Management of heparin therapy, controlled prospective trial. *New England Journal of Medicine* **292**, 1046–50.

Savage W. (1982) Abortion, methods and sequelae. *British Journal of Hospital Medicine* **27**, 364–84.

Schipper H.G., Kahle L.H., Jenkins C.S.P. *et al.* (1978) Antithrombin III transfusion in disseminated intravascular coagulation. *Lancet* **ii**, 854–6.

Schleider M.A., Nackman R.L., Jaffe E.A. & Coleman M. (1976) A clinical study of the lupus anticoagulant. *Blood* **48**, 499–509.

Schneider C.L. (1951) 'Fibrin embolism' (disseminated intravascular coagulation) with defibrination as one of the end results during placental abruption. *Surgery, Gynecology and Obstetrics* **92**, 27–34.

Schreiber A.D. & Austen K.F. (1973) Inter-relationships of the fibrinolytic, coagulation, kinin generation and complement systems. *Seminars in Hematology* **6**, 593–600.

Scott J.S. (1981) Connective tissue diseases antibodies and pregnancy. *American Journal of Reproductive Immunology* **6**, 19–24.

Semeraro N. & Donati M.B. (1981) Pathways of blood clotting initiation by cancer cells. In *Malignancy and the Haemostatic System* (Eds Donati M.B., Davidson J.F. & Garattini S.) pp. 65–81. Raven Press, New York.

Shapiro S.S. (1975) Acquired inhibitors to the blood coagulation factors. *Seminars in Thrombosis and Hemostasis* **1**, 336–85.

Shapiro S.S. & Thiagarjan P. (1982) Lupus anticoagulants. In *Progress in Haemostasis and Thrombosis*, vol. 6 (Ed. Spaed T.) p. 263. Grune & Stratton, New York.

Sharp A.A. (1964) Pathological Fibrinolysis. *British Medical Bulletin* **20**, 240–5.

Sharp A.A., Howie B., Biggs R. & Methuen D.T. (1958) Defibrination syndrome in pregnancy (value of various diagnostic tests). *Lancet* **ii**, 1309–12.

Shaw E., Giddings J.C., Peake I.R. *et al.* (1979) Synthesis of procoagulant factor VIII, factor VIII related antigen and other coagulation factors by the isolated perfused rat liver. *British Journal of Haematology* **41**, 585–91.

Shearer M.J., Allan V., Haroon Y. & Barlchan P. (1980) Nutritional aspects of Vitamin K in the human. In *Vitamin K Metabolism and Vitamin K Department Proteins* p. 317. University Park Press, Baltimore.

Signori E.E., Penner J.A. & Kahn D.R. (1969) Coagulation defects and bleeding in open heart surgery. *Annals of Thoracic Surgery* **8**, 521.

Spector I. & Corn M. (1967) Laboratory tests of haemostasis. The relation to haemorrhage in liver disease. *Archives of Internal Medicine* **119**, 577–82.

Spero J.A., Lewis J.H. & Hasiba U. (1981) Corticosteroid therapy for acquired factor VIII:C inhibitors. *British Journal of Haematology* **48**, 635–42.

Spivak J.L., Springler D.B. & Bell W.R. (1972) Defibrination after intra-amniotic injection of hypertonic saline. *New England Journal of Medicine* **287**, 321–3.

Tagnon H.J., Whitmore W.F. & Schulman N.R. (1952) Fibrinolysis in metastatic carcinoma of prostate. *Cancer* **5**, 9–12.

Talbert I.M. & Blatt P.M. (1979) Disseminated intravascular coagulation in obstetrics. *Clinical Obstetrics and Gynaecology* **22**, 889–90.

Thomas D.P., Ream V.J. & Stuart R.K. (1967) Platelet aggregation in patients with Laennec's cirrhosis of the liver. *New England Journal of Medicine* **276**, 1344–8.

Tice D.A. & Worth M.H. (1968) Recognition and treatment of post-operative bleeding associated with open heart surgery. *Annals of the New York Academy of Science* **146**, 745–53.

Tocantins L.M. (1948) The haemorrhagic tendency in congestive splenomeglay: its mechanism and management. *Journal of the American Medical Association* **136**, 616–25.

Tsitouris G., Bellet S., Eilberg R., Feinberg L. & Sandberg H. (1961) Effects of major surgery on plasmin–plasminogen systems. *Archives of Internal Medicine* **108**, 98–104.

Udall J.A. (1956) Human sources of absorption of Vitamin K in relation to anticoagulation stability. *Journal of the American Medical Association* **194**, 127–9.

Verska J.J., Lonser E.R. & Brewer L.A. (1972) Predisposing factors and management of hemorrhage following open heart surgery. *Journal of Cardiovascular Surgery* **13**, 361–8.

Verstraete M. & Collen D. (1986) Thrombolytic therapy in the Eighties. *Blood* **67**, 1529–41.

Verstraete M., Vermylen J. & Collen D. (1974) Intravascular coagulation in liver disease. *Annual Review of Medicine* **25**, 447.

Viweg W.V.R., Pistcatelli R.L., Hauser J.J. & Proulx R.A. (1970) Complications of intravenous administration of heparin in elderly women. *Journal of the American Medical Association* **213**, 1303–10.

Voke J. & Letsky E. (1977) Pregnancy and antibody to factor VIII. *Journal of Clinical Pathology* **30**, 928–32.

Volwiler W., Goldsworthy P.D., MacMartin P., Wood P.A., MacKay I.R. & Freemont-Smith K. (1955) Biosynthetic determination with radioactive sulphur of turnover rates of various plasma proteins in normal and cirrhotic man. *Journal of clinical Investigation* **34**, 1126–46.

von Felten A., Straub P.W. & Frick P.D. (1969) Dysfibrinogenaemia in a patient with primary haematoma. First observation of an acquired abnormality of fibrin monomer aggregation. *New England Journal of Medicine* **280**, 405–9.

Walls W.B. & Lavarsky M.S. (1971) The haemostatic defect of liver disease. *Gastroenterology* **60**, 108–11.

Walsh P.N. (1972) Evidence for an alternative pathway in intrinsic coagulation not requiring Factor XII. *British Journal of Haematology* **22**, 393–405.

Wardle E.N. (1974) Fibrinogen in liver disease. *Archives of Surgery* **109**, 741–6.

Warrell D.A., Davidson N. McD., Greenwood B.M., Ormerod L.D., Pope H.M., Watkins B.J. & Prentice C.R.M. (1977) Poisoning by bites of the saw scaled or carpet viper (*Echis carinatus*) in Nigeria. *Quarterly Journal of Medicine* **46**, 33–62.

Wiener A.E. & Reid D.E. (1950) Pathogenesis of amniotic fluid embolism III. Coagulant activity of amniotic fluid. *New England Journal of Medicine* **243**, 597–8.

Willoughby M.L.N., Murphy A.V., McMorris S. & Jewel F.G. (1972) Coagulation studies in haemolytic uraemic syndrome. *Archives of Diseases of Children* **47**, 766–71.

Wilmer G.D., Nossel H.D. & Le Roy E.C. (1968) Activation of Hageman Factor by Collagen. *Journal of Clinical Investigation* **47**, 2608–15.

Wilson J.R. & Lampman J. (1979) Heparin therapy: a randomized prospective study. *American Heart Journal* **97**, 155–8.

Woods H.F., Ash G., Weston M.J., Bunting S., Moncada S. & Yane J.R. (1978) Prostacyclin can replace heparin in hemodialysis in dogs. *Lancet* **ii**, 1075–7.

Yaffe H., Eldor A., Hornshslein E. & Sadovsky E. (1977) Thromboplastin activity in amniotic fluid during pregnancy. *Obstetrics and Gynaecology* **50**, 454–6.

Zwicka H., Kopec M., Latallo Z. *et al.* (1961) Anticoagulant circulant vessemblant a l'antithrombin IV au cairs d'un lupus erythemateux dissemine. *Thrombosis et Diathesis Haemorrhagia* **6**, 63–72.

80

The Burned Patient

D. A. B. TURNER

Although the first written documentation describing the treatment of thermal injury dates back almost four millenia (Bryan, 1931), it is only in the last half of this century, with the refinement of fluid resuscitation techniques, the introduction of effective antimicrobial agents and the development of specialized burns units that any significant improvement in survival has occurred (Thomsen, 1977). In the last two decades, the realization that invasive infection and protein–calorie malnutrition are major factors contributing to delayed mortality has resulted in increasing enthusiasm for prompt excision and grafting of the burn wound using either autografts and/or cultured or artificial skin together with the early use of enteral or parenteral nutrition. These strategies would appear to improve outcome further, especially in patients with extensive injury (Demling, 1983; Alexander, 1985).

In England and Wales, over 10 000 patients per annum sustain burns severe enough to warrant hospitalization, and of these, over 600 die as a result of their injuries. The overall mortality is related to the percentage of the body surface affected, the age of the patient and their premorbid physical status (Bull, 1971; Zawacki et al., 1979). Inhalation injury has a negative prognostic impact, being an important cause of death in patients with otherwise survivable cutaneous burns (Clarke et al., 1986).

Many complex physiological and metabolic adjustments accompany thermal injury and a clinical approach should be based logically on a thorough understanding of these associated pathophysiological events. Although thermal injury usually involves variable destruction of the skin and its appendages, severe burns are associated with alterations in virtually every organ system.

Pathophysiology of the burn injury

Cutaneous response

The skin is the largest organ of the body, constituting 15% of total body weight. It is usually the most severely affected organ in thermal injury and its destruction represents a breach in the body's protective shield allowing both uncontrolled evaporative water loss and bacterial colonization. Whilst the average insensible water loss through intact skin amounts to $15 \, \text{ml} \cdot \text{metre}^{-2} \cdot \text{hr}^{-1}$ (700–1000 ml/day), loss through areas of full thickness burn may reach $200 \, \text{ml} \cdot \text{metre}^{-2} \cdot \text{hr}^{-1}$. This is accompanied by loss of the latent heat of vaporization which approximates to 500 calories of heat for the evaporation of 1 litre of water. Thus, energy expenditure must be increased to maintain body temperature (Harrison et al., 1964). Bacterial proliferation of skin commensals occurs soon after cutaneous injury, and most wounds are colonized by Gram-negative organisms by the fifth day after burning.

Human skin can tolerate temperatures up to 40 °C for relatively long periods of time without apparent injury. However, temperatures above this level result in a logarithmic increase in the degree of tissue destruction which is dependent on both the temperature and the duration of exposure to the heat source (Moritz & Henriques, 1947). Histologically, the area of tissue injury consists of three concentric zones. A central 'zone of coagulation' characterized by irreversible coagulation necrosis is surrounded by a 'zone of stasis' in which cells are potentially recoverable if the deleterious effects of infection and desiccation can be prevented. Peripherally is a 'zone of hyperaemia' in which there is minimal tissue destruction and in which spontaneous healing may be expected (Jackson, 1983).

Vascular response

The extent and severity of damage to local vasculature is variable and ranges from total destruction of superficial capillaries with widespread endothelial swelling and disruption to partial occlusion of vessels with thrombus.

The liberation from burned tissue of a multitude of vasoactive substances such as histamine, 5-hydroxytryptamine and bradykinin, results in a profound transcapillary fluid exchange which, at least initially, may be generalized and extend beyond the area of injury. Plasma-like fluid is sequestered in the extravascular space resulting in oedema formation in the burn wound. The magnitude of the oedema caused by this increased microvascular permeability is compounded by a generalized cell membrane defect that results in intracellular swelling (Baxter, 1974). A complication of the albumin loss is a decrease in plasma colloid osmotic pressure which promotes further extravascular fluid retention (Demling et al., 1983). In addition, blood viscosity is increased as a result of haemoconcentration secondary to this fluid loss.

The overall effect of these derangements on the systemic circulation is a profound loss of intravascular volume which is proportional to the extent of burn injury. The result of this decrease in intravascular volume is an initial decrease in cardiac output and thus tissue perfusion. As in most cases of hypovolaemic shock, the maintenance of cerebral and myocardial perfusion is obtained at the expense of the kidneys, liver and small intestine but the resulting state of uneven tissue perfusion may be corrected by early, aggressive and adequate volume resuscitation. The functional integrity of the capillary is re-established gradually over the ensuing 48–72 hr; lymphatic drainage and the restoration of oncotic pressure gradients encourage re-entry of sequestered fluid into the intravascular space and the progressive reduction in intravascular volume slows. Red cell mass is decreased also following thermal injury (Muir, 1961). Red blood cells are destroyed directly by heat, but this is compounded by stasis and a reduced red blood cell half-life consequent upon increased fragility. The magnitude of loss of red cell mass is related to the size of full-thickness burn, and deficits of up to 40% may occur in severe injury.

Metabolic response

Extensive burns are associated with a rapid increase in metabolic rate which is greater than that seen with any other form of trauma or sepsis (Cope et al., 1953; Moncrief, 1973). This increase reaches a peak only a few days postburn and persists until effective wound closure has occurred. Oxygen consumption studies have demonstrated that the basal metabolic rate (BMR) of 35–40 $cal \cdot metre^{-2}$ body surface area (BSA) $\cdot hr^{-1}$ may double in patients whose burn affects more than 50% of their body surface and, in general, the degree of hyper-metabolism is proportional to the size of the burn. This endocrine response to burn injury is characterized by protein catabolism, nitrogen wasting, hyperthermia, hyperglycaemia and increased carbon dioxide production and oxygen utilization (Kien et al., 1978). Although this was attributed originally to the need to generate more heat because of the large evaporative water losses from the burn wound, evidence exists which suggests that thermal injury triggers greatly increased activity of the sympathetic nervous system and the hypothalamic–pituitary–adrenal axis. This results in persistently increased levels of circulating catecholamines, glucocorticoids and glucagon (Wilmore et al., 1974). It is thought that these hormones are directly responsible for the runaway catabolism and that their effects may be compounded by any need to generate heat to maintain body temperature (Zawacki et al., 1970; Neely et al., 1974).

Immediate care of the burn victim

An evaluation of the extent and severity of the injury is conducted simultaneously with the institution of volume resuscitation (Brown & Ward, 1984).

Initial evaluation

The priorities of treatment that are well established for any trauma patient apply equally to the burn victim, and attention to the burn wound should not take precedence over the assessment and treatment of life-threatening problems such as cardiovascular collapse or upper airway obstruction. A primary survey should be conducted to ensure the patency of the patient's airway, the adequacy of ventilation and the ability of the cardiovascular system to maintain acceptable cerebral and coronary perfusion.

Burn size

A visual inspection delineates those areas of the body involved, and a rapid assessment of the appropriate percentage of the body surface area affected (excluding non-blistering erythematous areas) should be performed. The 'rule of nine' is a widely accepted method for this purpose (Lund & Browder, 1944). This rule is based on the fact that various regions of the body represent 9% of the BSA or a multiple thereof (Fig. 80.1). For smaller areas, a good guide is that the area covered by the patient's hand and fingers represents approximately 1% of their body surface. In general, if the total percentage BSA involved exceeds 15% in an adult or 10% in a child, then volume resuscitation should be instituted as a matter of urgency.

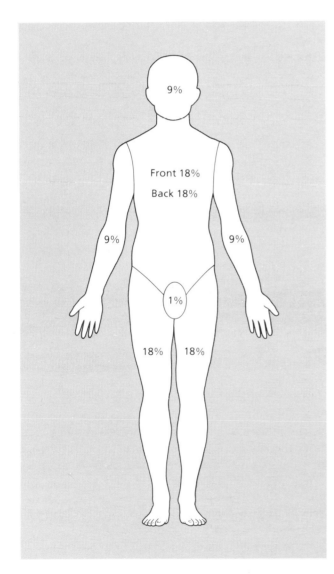

Fig. 80.1 'Rule of nine'.

Burn depth

The assessment of burn depth (Fig. 80.2) is more prone to error but should be attempted as it has important therapeutic and prognostic implications. Although burn wounds have been classified conventionally into three 'degrees' of depth, the imprecision and subjectivity of this method (particularly with regard to second-degree injury) has led to the adoption of a simplified classification based on the depth of tissue destruction (Fig. 80.1 and Table 80.1).

When erythema is present, the protective barrier of the skin is maintained, there is minimal fluid loss or chance of infection and it is therefore not included in the burn size calculations when estimating fluid requirements. Superficial, partial-thickness burns may be expected to heal in 7–10 days provided infection is prevented, but deep, partial-thickness burns require 4 weeks for epithelial regeneration to occur from the few remaining glands and hair follicles. In the case of full-thickness burns, healing may occur by wound contraction, and this requires skin grafting for definitive closure. Deep, partial-thickness burns may be

Table 80.1 Classification of burn depth

Erythema	Damage is limited to epidermis resulting in a non-blistered erythematous area Minimal oedema Painful Heal spontaneously in 48–72 hr
Partial thickness, superficial	Destruction of *outer* layers of dermis is also present, but hair follicles, sebaceous and sweat glands are spared Typically, vesicle formation occurs and erythema blanches with pressure Heal in 7–10 days if infection does not supervene
Partial thickness, deep	Only the deepest dermal appendages are spared Skin is blistered, oedematous and usually white Painless Hair can be pulled out easily
Full thickness	All epithelial elements and the full thickness of the dermis are destroyed The area is anaesthetic, dry and either charred or white

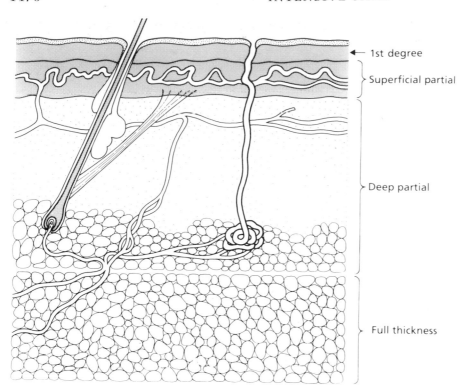

Fig. 80.2 Estimation of depth of burn.

converted to full-thickness by either infection or desiccation, and are treated often as full thickness.

Fluid resuscitation

Although the necessity for fluid resuscitation in patients with burns exceeding 15–20% BSA is not questioned, the actual composition and rate of fluid administration remains the subject of controversy (Monafo *et al.*, 1973; Arturson, 1985; Demling, 1985). Over the years, numerous formulae have been advocated and most involve multiplying the product of percentage BSA involved and body weight by some constant 'factor'. This calculation determines the quantity of fluid to be infused during the first 24 hr postburn. These formulae vary, depending on the value of this constant factor, and on the inclusion or exclusion of colloid-containing solution. Because of the marked increase in capillary microcirculatory permeability that occurs in burned tissue, most fluid resuscitation schemes produce some degree of burn tissue oedema. However, in patients with extensive burn injury, oedema occurs often in non-burned soft tissue. This appears to be attributable to the hypoproteinaemia consequent upon albumin loss in areas of injury rather than to some diffuse alteration in capillary protein permeability as was thought previously (Demling, 1985).

It is also difficult, in the absence of inhalation, to demonstrate any significant alteration in pulmonary capillary permeability. A number of studies have failed to demonstrate any early increase in extravascular lung water during controlled fluid administration after major burn injury (Tranbaugh *et al.*, 1980). This evidence would suggest that colloid infusion might minimize oedema in non-burned tissue and maintain plasma volume better than crystalloid solutions. This has resulted in the inclusion of colloid in the resuscitation regimens in many centres. The tendency, especially in North America, to avoid the use of colloid during the initial 24 hr is based on the supposition that any colloid given during this period is of little benefit in maintaining plasma albumin concentration (and, therefore, osmotic gradients) because it leaks out into the extravascular space and further encourages extravascular fluid retention. Although there is some logic in this argument, it should be emphasized that definitive studies demonstrating the superiority of one resuscitation regimen over another is lacking, and it is *early* and aggressive fluid resuscitation that is of paramount importance. Regardless of the regimen used, the goal is to maintain an effective plasma volume and optimize vital and non-vital organ perfusion in the face of massive loss of protein and fluid from the circulation.

Two commonly used 'formulae' are presented in Table 80.2. The Mount Vernon formula popularized by Muir and Barclay in the 1950s (Muir *et al.*, 1987) is popular in the UK and relies heavily on the infusion of plasma protein fraction. The Brooke and Modified Brooke (excludes colloid in the first 24 hr) formulae are popular in North America and favour a more balanced regimen.

The two most common errors made in the resuscitation of the burn victim are *delay* in initiating resuscitation and failure to *vary* from the calculated requirements when signs of vital organ perfusion are not achieved. It cannot be overstated that all formulae are only guidelines for planning fluid therapy and may need to be adjusted frequently depending on clinical response (Aikawa, 1982).

MONITORING RESUSCITATION

The response to resuscitation should be assessed frequently using conventional clinical criteria (mental status, vital signs, capillary refill, urine output, central venous pressure) and laboratory data (packed cell volume, electrolytes, osmolalities). An adequate urine output ($0.5-1 \text{ ml} \cdot \text{kg}^{-1} \cdot \text{hr}^{-1}$) is the most useful single guide to the adequacy of volume replacement (Settle, 1974). If urine output decreases below $0.5 \text{ ml} \cdot \text{kg}^{-1} \cdot \text{hr}^{-1}$, the rate of fluid administration may need to be increased. If urine output exceeds $1.5 \text{ ml} \cdot \text{kg}^{-1} \cdot \text{hr}^{-1}$, the patient should be re-evaluated to ascertain that fluid requirements have not been overestimated. The indications for the use of central venous or pulmonary artery flotation catheters are the same as for any trauma victim, and the burn injury itself does not contra-indicate their use. Any patient who remains oliguric despite a fluid challenge requires an immediate haemodynamic assessment. This would require some assessment of right ventricular or left ventricular filling pressure (Aikawa *et al.*, 1978). The need for transfusion of blood should be assessed at intervals, and most patients with extensive injury require transfusion if packed cell volume drops below 30%.

From the practical standpoint, vascular access may present difficult problems in the burn patient. Non-burned areas are preferred for all peripheral and central insertion sites because of the risk of infection (as well as the problem of securing lines to eschar). However, line placement through burned tissue is allowable if the catheter is needed and no suitable non-burned site is available. As a rule, 'cutdowns' should be avoided because of the prohibitively high infection rates associated with their use.

Inhalation injury

Once the primary survey has been completed and volume resuscitation is in progress, the possibility of inhalation injury must be considered because effective treatment may depend on early recognition.

Three separate entities may be encountered with inhalation injury (Fein *et al.*, 1976; Trunkey, 1978); notably, direct thermal injury to the upper airway, carbon monoxide poisoning and smoke inhalation. Inhalation injury is more likely if the conflagration occurred in a closed space. Although each pattern of injury may occur in isolation, it is not uncommon for two or all three to exist in combination.

DIRECT THERMAL INJURY

The clinical spectrum of direct heat injury ranges from asymptomatic supraglottic oedema to life-threatening upper airway obstruction. The upper airway possesses considerable heat-exchanging ability so that if hot air is inhaled, most of the heat energy is dissipated in the nose, pharynx and upper airway (Moritz *et al.*, 1945). This results in progressive mucosal oedema which is limited usually to the mouth, tongue and hypo-pharyngeal region. Heat injury below the level of the cords is rare but does occur if superheated steam is

Table 80.2 Fluid replacement formulae

Muir and Barclay	$0.5 \text{ ml} \cdot \text{kg}^{-1} \cdot \%$ BSA burn of colloid (as plasma protein fraction) is given every 4 hr for the initial 12 hr postburn and then every 6 hr for the succeeding 12 hr period
Brooke	$0.5 \text{ ml} \cdot \text{kg}^{-1} \cdot \%$ BSA burn of colloid *plus* $1.5 \text{ ml} \cdot \text{kg} \cdot \%$ BSA burn on crystalloid (to a maximum limit of 50% BSA) *plus* 2 litre of water as dextrose 5% is the *total volume* given over the first 24-hr period
	50% is given over the initial 8 hr and 25% in the second and third 8-hr periods

Time zero is the time of injury. All calculations are based from the time of injury inhaled. The speed of onset, severity and duration of the oedema varies, but is usually maximal within the first 24 hr. As mucosal burns are rarely full thickness, the oedema may be expected to subside in 3–5 days.

Suspicion of direct thermal injury should be aroused by any patient involved in a closed-space fire who has evidence of facial burns, particularly oedema of the lips, which is associated invariably with underlying pharyngeal oedema. If there is any clinical suggestion of upper airway obstruction, the presence of hypopharyngeal oedema should be assumed and the patient observed closely for evidence of increasing upper airway obstruction (Wanner, 1973). This allows complete obstruction to be pre-empted by tracheal intubation.

As fluid resuscitation might be expected to exacerbate oedema (and worsen airway obstruction), many authorities recommend an aggressive approach to diagnosis which involves direct visualization of the upper airway in any patient in whom direct thermal trauma is suspected. This may be achieved using a fibre-optic endoscope over which a nasotracheal tube may be passed should supraglottic oedema be present. As clinical experience with these instruments grows, it is likely that there will be an increasing tendency to perform early examination and intubation.

CARBON MONOXIDE POISONING

Carbon monoxide (CO) is a colourless, odourless gas produced by the incomplete combustion of many carbon-containing materials. The primary hazard with CO lies with its propensity to tie up oxygen binding sites in the haemoglobin molecule (Douglas et al., 1912). Although both gases bind to the α-chain, haemoglobin has an affinity for CO that is 230–270 times greater than its affinity for oxygen. Thus, CO fills oxygen binding sites at very low partial pressures. For example, a Pa_{CO} of 0.133 kPa (1 mmHg) may result in a carboxyhaemoglobin saturation of over 40%. In addition, the rate of dissociation of CO from haemoglobin is slow, and high levels of carboxyhaemoglobin cause a leftward shift of the oxygen dissociation curve. Thus, the major concern with CO poisoning is tissue hypoxia, particularly cerebral and myocardial hypoxia.

Although the symptoms of CO poisoning tend to be vague, they do correlate with the carboxyhaemoglobin level to some extent (Table 80.3). The classical description of cherry red facial discolouration is helpful but by no means always present, and the diagnosis depends on a history of smoke or exhaust fume

Table 80.3 Signs and symptoms of carbon monoxide poisoning

Percentage carboxyhaemoglobin	Clinical manifestations
0–10	None
10–20	Slight headache Angina may occur in patients with ischaemic heart disease
20–30	Throbbing headache Dyspnoea Dilatation of cutaneous blood vessels
30–40	*Above* plus nausea and vomiting Impairment of mental processes
40–50	Tachypnoea Tachycardia Syncope
60–70	Cardiovascular collapse and death

exposure in a closed space coupled with a direct measurement of CO saturation by CO-oximetry. A pitfall in the diagnosis of CO poisoning is to assume that a patient who is centrally pink with a normal arterial oxygen tension (Pa_{O_2}) is not hypoxic. Arterial oxygen partial pressure may be normal in the presence of CO poisoning, and if oxygen saturation is derived (as it is on many blood gas machines), instead of directly measured spectrophotometrically, the result may be misleading.

The treatment of CO poisoning involves facilitating the elimination of gas via the lungs. The rate of dissociation of CO from its oxygen binding sites is slow because there is usually only a small gradient in partial pressure at the alveolar interface. Alveolar CO partial pressure (P_{A}_{CO}) should approach zero and if Pa_{CO} is 0.266 kPa (2 mmHg) there is a gradient of only 0.266 kPa (2 mmHg) available to displace CO from the haemoglobin molecule. However, as CO competes with oxygen for the same sites in the α-chain, increasing Pa_{O_2} increases competition for the sites already occupied by CO. It has been demonstrated that the half-life of carboxyhaemoglobin is 5 hr breathing room air ($F_{I}_{O_2}$ 0.21), but this may be reduced to under 1 hr by breathing 100% oxygen ($F_{I}_{O_2}$ 1). Thus, increasing

Table 80.4 Delayed complications of carbon monoxide poisoning

Erythematous, bullous skin lesions
Rhabdomyolysis, myoglobinaemia, acute renal failure
Cerebral oedema (48 hr to 2 weeks postinsult)
Demyelination/anoxic leukoencephalopathy manifesting as persistent neuropsychiatric symptoms

Pao_2 is the single most useful manoeuvre to enhance CO elimination. Patients with suspected CO poisoning and/or those in whom a spectrophotometrically measured carboxyhaemoglobin level exceeds 20% should be given 100% oxygen by non-rebreathing mask if this is practicable. If the patient is obtunded sufficiently, tracheal intubation protects the airway and allows titrated oxygen therapy. This should be continued until carboxyhaemoglobin levels are below 15–20%. Also absolute rest and ECG monitoring would seem appropriate. Patients who survive the initial period are at risk from delayed complications (Table 80.4) which are treated on standard lines. Permanent disability is not unusual (Smith & Brandon, 1973).

SMOKE INHALATION

The composition of smoke depends on the composition of the material that is burning. It consists usually of irritant carbon particles (ash) suspended in a mixture of gases and vapours, the chemical components of which cause airway irritability, airway obstruction (by damage to the tracheobronchial mucosa) and, occasionally, damage to the alveolar air–blood interface. The heat-induced decomposition of manufactured petrochemical byproducts, such as plastics and synthetic fibres, produces a bewildering spectrum of toxic fumes and gases (Table 80.5).

Despite this, it is unusual for smoke inhalation to constitute the predominant aspect of inhalation injury, probably because most victims succumb to CO poisoning before a sufficient 'smoke dose' has been inhaled. In addition, conscious victims may be able to escape from smoke especially if it contains some of the more pungent, soluble toxic gases such as chlorine, ammonia or sulphur dioxide. Some of the less pungent, insoluble, toxic gases and vapours, however, are recognized less easily and therefore tolerated for longer periods of time. These gases are more likely to be associated with lower airway injury (nitrogen dioxide, phosgene). Acrolein is an aldehyde produced during the combustion of wood, cotton, acrylics and some plastics. It produces intense irritation and inflammation of mucous membranes and pulmonary oedema. It has been incriminated frequently as a cause of mortality in house fires (Zikria et al., 1972). The combustion of polyvinylchloride (PVC), another common houschold material, results in the production of phosgene and chlorine. These gases, on contact with moist mucous membranes result in the formation of hydrochloric acid. Likewise the thermal decomposition of nitrogen-containing polymers (polyurethane, nylon) result in the formation of hydrogen sulphide which, in addition to being a systematic poison, is hydrolysed to hydrocyanic acid. This causes an intense inflammatory reaction and cyanide toxicity.

Table 80.5 Toxic products of combustion

Substance/material	Toxic product
Polyvinyl chloride (PVC)	Hydrochloric acid phosgene, chlorine
Wood, cotton, paper	Acrolein, acetaldehyde, formaldehyde, acetic and formic acid
Polyurethane	Isocyanate, hydrogen cyanide
Nylon	Ammonia, hydrocyanic acid
Acrylics	Acrolein, carbon monoxide

TREATMENT OF INHALATION INJURY

Treatment of inhalation injury is mainly supportive. All patients need oxygen and this should be given in as high a concentration as possible until a carboxyhaemoglobin level has excluded CO poisoning. Early nasotracheal intubation may pre-empt complete airway obstruction in patients with supraglottic oedema. Patients who have been exposed to smoke or toxic fumes require meticulous respiratory care to prevent lethal complications. The importance of intensive physiotherapy and tracheobronchial toilet with efficient humidification of inspired gases cannot be overstated, and the fibre-optic bronchoscope is a useful aid to remove sloughed mucosa (Moylan et al., 1975). Minitracheostomy may be useful if this is a recurrent problem.

The use of continuous positive airway pressure (CPAP) or positive end-expiratory pressure (PEEP) in patients with alveolar injury who are hypoxaemic with poorly compliant lungs is logical but as airflow limitation with gas trapping is common after smoke inhalation, this modality of treatment should be applied with circumspection (Venus *et al.*, 1981).

Definitive care of the burn victim

The primary goal of this stage of care is surgical closure of the burn wound, before invasive bacteral infection supervenes. Bacterial infection of burned tissues delays healing and may possibly destroy remaining epithelial cells and convert a partial-thickness burn into a full-thickness burn. It is also likely to prevent successful skin grafting. Bacterial invasion of underlying tissues may result in fulminating septicaemia. Prevention of burn-wound infection is, therefore, of paramount importance. Wound closure is accomplished definitively by surgery, but requires adequate metabolic support and meticulous nursing care to prevent burn wound contamination.

Prevention of infection

Any large, open wound that contains devitalized tissue represents an ideal culture medium for bacterial colonization. The burn wound itself, followed by the lungs are the most common sites for serious infection to occur. Whilst virulent strains of *Pseudomonas* and methicillin-resistant *Staphylococcus aureus* (MRSA) are being incriminated increasingly, it appears that diminished host resistance is a more important factor in determining the severity of burn-wound infection than the virulence of the causative organisms. The burn victim is in a state of immunocompromise (Alexander *et al.*, 1978) and alterations in both the cellular and humoral components of the immune response have been identified. Impaired phagocyte function, reduced neutrophil chemotaxis and abnormalities in macrophage activity have all been demonstrated (Davies *et al.*, 1980). Derangements in lymphocyte function have also been reported. T-suppressor lymphocytes, which normally inhibit T-cell stimulation of antibody production are found in increased numbers in burn victims, and this may represent an indication of the risk of sepsis (McIrvine *et al.*, 1982). Reduced concentrations of both γ-globulin and the opsonic protein, fibronectin, occur also but the clinical significance of this is uncertain.

Protection of the patient against bacterial cross-infection involves strict attention to detail in all aspects of nursing care. More recently, many burns units have employed single-room isolation and barrier nursing techniques. The purpose of these units is to prevent bacterial contamination of the patient from staff and equipment, and from cross-contamination from other patients. In its simplest form, patients are placed in a single cubicle with reverse flow ventilation and strict barrier nursing, but more sophisticated laminar airflow units such as the bacteria-controlled nursing unit (BCNU) exist, which may reduce the chance of infection further. This provides a small (1.8 × 3 metre) area which, through the use of clear, plastic walls and a continuous downflow of filtered, bacteria-free air provides a non-contaminated environment (Burke *et al.*, 1977). With this unit, temperature and humidity may be controlled also.

Systemic antibiotics are unable to penetrate surface eschar, and control of bacterial growth over the burn wound is accomplished using topical antibiotics which continue to be the mainstay of wound-infection control. Numerous topical preparations are available and each has its inherent advantages and disadvantages (Moncrief, 1979).

Silver nitrate solution (0.5 %) is a bacteriostatic agent effective against a broad spectrum of organisms. It is applied in the form of saturated mesh gauze which serves the dual purpose of reducing bacterial growth and minimizing evaporative water loss. Application is painless and, although little systemic absorption occurs, leaching of sodium from the burn wound in addition to reduced evaporative loss may result in hyponatraemia. Dressings are saturated with the solution every 2 hr and the dressing changed once or twice a day.

Silver sulphadiazine cream (Flamazine) is also painless on application and is unable to penetrate eschar. It has broad antibacterial activity and side-effects are rare.

Mafenide acetate (Sulphamyalon cream) is a sulphonamide preparation that can penetrate surface eschar and control bacterial growth at the interface between eschar and granulation tissue. Proliferation of organisms at this site may progress to burn-wound invasion and infection in non-burned viable tissue. Application to partial-thickness burns is painful and it needs to be applied once or twice a day. Mafenide inhibits carbonic anhydrase activity leading to bicarbonaturia and metabolic acidosis. This is rarely a serious problem but has led to its use on an alternate day basis with one of the other preparations.

Surgical approaches

The conventional surgical approach involves the use of topical antibiotics combined with repeated cleansing and debridement of the burn wound which, in time, either heals or allows skin grafting to be performed.

This form of conservative treatment is suitable for partial-thickness injuries. In cases where the differentiation between partial-thickness and full-thickness burns cannot be made with any degree of certainty, this conservative approach is warranted (to prevent infection and desiccation of the wound) until the distinction can be made (usually 14–21 days). The treatment of choice for full-thickness injury is removal of slough and early grafting. Indeed, in the presence of extensive injury when the conservative approach is both uncomfortable for the patient and involves the inherent danger of preserving an open wound in an immunocompromised host, there is increasing enthusiasm for prompt excision of the burn wound followed by immediate wound closure, especially for full-thickness and deep, partial-thickness burns (Burke et al., 1974). If, as may be the case in patients with extensive injury, there is insufficient healthy skin for autografting, a skin substitute may be used and excision and grafting may proceed in a sequential manner (Burke et al., 1981). Materials which restore the important barrier function of the skin either temporarily or permanently have obvious positive metabolic and microbiological implications. It may be that there is some correlation between survival and rapidity of wound closure (Echinard et al., 1982).

Metabolic support

The increase in metabolic rate that occurs in the postresuscitation phase may approach 100% in patients with cutaneous burns exceeding 50% BSA. This hypermetabolism is associated with increased net protein breakdown, nitrogen loss, lipolysis and accelerated gluconeogenesis and may result rapidly in severe protein–calorie malnutrition. In association with this increased metabolism, there is often a slight increase in core temperature of 1–2 °C which appears to result from resetting of the hypothalamic temperature centre. Any attempt to reduce core temperature by changing ambient temperature results in an additional increase in energy expenditure in an attempt to maintain body temperature (Barr et al., 1968). Thus, a low ambient temperature may exaggerate the stress response and result in the production of wasted energy

Table 80.6 The Harris–Benedict formula

Male
Basal metabolic rate = 66 + (13.7 × W) + (5 × H) − (6.8 × A)

Female
Basal metabolic rate = 66 + (9.6 × W) + (1.7 × H) − 4.7 × A)

W = ideal body weight in kg.
H = height in cm.
A = age in yr.
Total daily caloric requirement = BMR × 1.5 − 2.

(Wilmore et al., 1975). Maintaining ambient temperature at approximately 30 °C has been found to reduce significantly the total energy expenditure, and this practice is standard in many burns units.

In addition to ambient temperature control, early and aggressive nutrition is necessary to prevent malnutrition (Wilmore, 1979). Oxygen consumption studies have demonstrated that if ambient temperature is maintained, BMR seldom exceeds twice the BMR as predicted from the Harris–Benedict formula and approximate energy require-ments may be obtained from this formula (Table 80.6).

The choice of substrate to provide this energy is more difficult to rationalize. The marked hepatic gluconeogenesis may be suppressed by the infusion of exogenous glucose, and this should constitute at least 50% of the total caloric intake. Fifteen to twenty percent of calories are given as protein and the remainder as fat. There is recent evidence (Alexander et al., 1980) to suggest that the use of high-protein nutrition (with a non-protein calorie : nitrogen ratio of 100 : 1) is associated with improved immuno-competence. It remains to be seen if this has any impact on outcome on the incidence of infection in adults.

Nutritional support should commence as soon as possible in the postresuscitation phase. Preference is for the enteral route but, as a paralytic ileus accompanies extensive burns frequently, enteral feeds should be withheld until peristalsis returns. If the ileus persists beyond 72 hr, consideration should be given to parenteral alimentation.

As a general rule, patients with burns exceeding 20–25% BSA benefit from nutritional support and control of ambient temperature.

Anaesthetic considerations

Following resuscitation, the severely burned patient faces the physiological and psychological trauma of burn-wound closure. Whether this is achieved by prompt excision and grafting or by multiple wound debridements and grafting with reconstructive procedures, it necessarily involves anaesthesia. Some anaesthetic problems are unique to the burn patient (de Campo & Aldrete, 1981).

Vascular access may be difficult, and as blood loss may be considerable (even with a minor debridement or wound excision), a large-bore, reliable intravenous line must be established prior to surgery.

Monitoring. Cutaneous or oesophageal ECG, non-invasive or invasive arterial pressure measurement, temperature and urine output monitoring should be standard for all but the most minor procedures. Central venous pressure measurement is useful if excessive blood loss is anticipated.

Temperaure control. The combination of low ambient temperature, large exposed areas of body surface, infusion of large volumes of cold fluid and lengthy operations sets the scene for hypothermia with deleterious metabolic consequences. The onset of postoperative shivering may result in severe arterial desaturation. As a rule, the ambient temperature should be as high as the theatre staff can tolerate comfortably, and attempts should be made to insulate exposed areas; all intravenous fluids and preparation solutions should be warmed to $37\,^\circ$C and inspired gases fully humidified.

Pharmacological considerations

Suxamethonium

It is well-known that suxamethonium is associated with ventricular arrhythmias and cardiac arrest in burn patients, and for this reason its use should be avoided (Tolmie *et al.*, 1967). This abnormal response is a result of hyperkalaemia although why burned patients should exhibit such an exaggerated response is uncertain (Bush *et al.*, 1962). The magnitude of the increase in plasma potassium concentration is related to the dose of suxamethonium administered, the time that has elapsed since injury and on the severity or extent of burn injury. It has been speculated that, as in the case of denervation injury, there is a proliferation of nicotinic acetylcholine receptors over the whole muscle membrane when they are limited normally to the area of the neuromuscular junction. The possibility

of a hyperkalaemic response to suxamethonium may persist for up to 2 yr after the injury.

Non-depolarizing, neuromuscular blocking drugs

The observation that burn patients are relatively resistant to the effects of non-depolarizing, neuromuscular blocking drugs has been confirmed by numerous recent studies (Martyn *et al.*, 1980; Martyn *et al.*, 1982). To achieve a given response, both the dose administered and the serum concentration required are increased by a factor of 2–3. Numerous hypotheses have been presented to explain this, but the increase in nicotinic acetylcholine receptor density secondary to disease atrophy and immobilization may best explain this altered response.

Miscellaneous drugs

The clinical impression that analgesics, anxiolytics and hypotensive agents need to be given in large doses to burned patients is not supported as yet by pharmacokinetic studies (Martyn, 1986).

Anaesthetic techniques

Many different anaesthetic techniques have been employed successfully in burn patients. All patients require a detailed airway assessment including the extent of mouth opening and neck movements. Anticipation of any difficulty is a resonable indication for awake, blind, nasal intubation preferably with the help of a fibre-optic instrument. This technique should be mastered by all anaesthetists involved with burn victims (Lamb, 1985). Ketamine has been used widely in burned patients and in low doses (1.5–2 mg/kg i.m.) may provide adequate analgesia and amnesia for minor wound debridements and cleansing. Its administration should be preceded by an antisialogogue, and in this dosage it allows rapid establishment of important activities such as eating.

Halothane remains a widely used volatile agent although its advantage over the available agents relate to its predictability and lack of pungency, which facilitates inhalation induction. The possibility of liver injury with repeated administration may be less important in the burned patient, as evidence for halothane hepatotoxicity is lacking in this group of patients (Martyn, 1986). If the hepatotoxic effects of halothane are mediated immunologically, it may be that the anergic state of the burn patient accounts for this anomaly. Despite this, repeated halothane exposure cannot be recommended.

Complications of thermal injury

Acute renal failure

Severe impairment of renal function is a serious complication of thermal injury and has negative prognostic implications (Cameron & Miller-Jones, 1967). Acute, oliguric renal failure results invariably from acute tubular necrosis representing one extreme of a spectrum of impaired renal function. Non-oliguric renal failure is a more common problem and implies loss of tubular concentrating ability. Causes of renal failure in the context of thermal injury include persistent hypovolaemia, the presence of urinary pigments (haemoglobin or myoglobin) and Gram-negative sepsis. Any patient with pre-existing renal impairment may be expected to be particularly susceptible to these abnormalities. Monitoring of hourly urine output together with frequent estimation of urine osmolality and sodium concentration allow assessment of glomerular filtration and tubular concentrating ability. Calculation of various derived indices, such as fractional excretion of sodium and osmolal clearance, aid in the differential diagnosis of oliguria.

Haemoglobinuria and myoglobinuria occur classically in patients suffering from high-voltage electrical injury, but any full-thickness burn may result in red blood cell and muscle breakdown with the release of haemoglobin and myoglobin into the circulation. It is probable that these pigments predispose the patient to renal injury especially in the presence of renal hypoperfusion. Treatment of renal failure should be instituted early; although peritoneal dialysis may be adequate to cope with mild fluid overload, it is likely that haemodialysis will be necessary in the hypermetabolic patient.

Hypertension

This is seen commonly after severe burns, especially in children (Faulker et al., 1978). It appears within 2 weeks of injury, and the clinical manifestations range from mild irritability to somnolence progressing to convulsions. It is associated with prolonged elevation of plasma catecholamines and increased plasma renin activity. Although reserpine has been advocated, an angiotensin-converting enzyme inhibitor may be more appropriate.

Burn encepalopathy

Acute CNS dysfunction in the absence of raised systemic arterial pressure may be a major problem in burn patients, and presents as an acute brain syndrome which may progress to seizures and coma (Anton et al., 1972). The exact cause is unclear but metabolic factors (hypoxia, hyponatraemia) or septicaemia may precipitate events.

Gastroduodenal ulceration

Described initially by Curling in 1842, acute erosions of the gastric and duodenal mucosa occur in 86% of patients with major burns, within 72 hr of injury (Czaja et al., 1976). Reduction in gastric mucosal blood flow and increased gastric acid output are thought to be aetiological factors. Erosions may be manifest as torrential life-threatening haemorrhage, or insidious, acute gastrointenstinal blood loss. The mainstay of treatment lies in prevention with early enteral nutrition and the routine use of H_2-receptor antagonists and antacids. In the hyperdynamic phase of injury, the dose requirement for cimetidine increases substantially as both the total and renal clearance of the drug are elevated. The magnitude of this change is proportional to the size of the burn. As this may result in subtherapeutic plasma concentrations, it has been suggested that after 24 hr the dose should be doubled. The pharmacokinetics of ranitidine have not been characterized yet.

Outcome

Survival after thermal injury has improved progressively over the past decade. The size of injury associated with a 50% survival has reached 65%, 66%, 47% and 30% in age groups 0–14 yr, 15–40 yr, 41–65 yr and over 65 yr respectively (Lutterman & Curreri, 1987). Such figures emanate from a centre of excellence and are quoted to illustrate the potential value of surgery and intensive care techniques to the burn victim. There remains, however, a small group of patients with severe cutaneous burns (over 90% BSA) combined with inhalation injury who have no reasonable chance of recovery (e.g. self-immolation). Medical technology should not be applied to prolong death and suffering and such patients should be given every measure of pain relief, comfort and hygiene. If upper airway obstruction develops, tracheal intubation is indicated to prevent the distress caused by asphyxia rather than as a life-saving manoeuvre. Such decisions should be taken by senior members of the unit team.

References

Aikawa N., Ishibiki K., Naito C. & Abe O. (1982) Individualised fluid resuscitation based on haemodynamic monitoring in the management of extensive burns. *Burns* **8**, 249–55.

Aikawa N., Martyn J.A.J. & Burke J.F. (1978) Pulmonary artery catheterisation and thermodilution cardiac output determination in the management of critically ill burned patients. *American Journal of Surgery* **135**, 811–19.

Alexander J.W. (1985) Burn care; a speciality in evolution. 1985 Presidential Address, American Burn Association. *Journal of Trauma* **26**, 1–6.

Alexander J.W., MacMillan B.G. & Stinnett J.D. (1980) Beneficial effects of aggressive protein feeding in severely burned children. *Annals of Surgery* **192**, 503–17.

Alexander J.W., Ogle C.K., Stinnett J.D. & MacMillan B.G. (1978). A sequential, prospective analysis of immunologic abnormalities and infection following thermal trauma. *Annals of Surgery* **188**, 809–16.

Anton A.Y., Volpe J.J. & Crawford J.D. (1972) Burn encephalopathy in children. *Pediatrics* **50**, 609–16.

Arturson G. (1985) Fluid therapy of thermal injury. *Acta Anaesthesiologica scandinavica* **29**, 55–9.

Barr P-O., Birke G., Liljedahl S.O. & Plantin L.O. (1968) Oxygen consumption studies and water losss during treatment of burns. *Lancet* **I**, 164–8.

Baxter C.R. (1974) Fluid volume and electrolyte changes in the early post burn period. *Clinics in Plastic Surgery* **1**, 693–703.

Brown J. & Ward D.J. (1984) Immediate management of burns in casualty. *British Journal of Hospital Medicine* **00**, 360–8.

Bryan C.P. (1931) Minor Surgery. In *The Papyrus Ebers*, Chapter 12. Appleton, New York.

Bull J.P. (1971) Revised analysis of mortality due to burns. *Lancet* **2**, 1133–4.

Burke J.F., Bondoc L.L. & Quinby W.C. (1974) Primary burn excision and immediate grafting — a method of shortening illness. *Journal of Trauma* **14**, 389.

Burke J.F., Quinby W.C., Bondoc L.L., Sheely F.M. & Moreno H.C. (1977) The contribution of a bacterially isolated environment to the prevention of infection in seriously burned patients. *Annals of Surgery* **186**, 377–87.

Burke J.F., Yannas I.V., Quinby W.C., Bondoc L.L. & Jung W.K. (1981) Successful use of a physiologically acceptable artificial skin in the treatment of extensive burn injury. *Annals of Surgery* **194**, 413–28.

Bush G.H, Graham H.A.P. & Littlewood A.H.M. (1962). Danger of suxamethonium and endotracheal intubation in anaesthesia for burns. *British Medical Journal* **2**, 1081–5.

Cameron J.S. & Miller-Jones C.M.H. (1967) Renal function and renal failure in badly burned childern. *British Journal of Surgery* **54**, 132–41.

Clarke C.J., Reid W.H., Gilmour W.H. & Campbell D. (1986) Mortality probability in victims of fire trauma; a revised equation to include inhalation injury. *British Medical Journal* **292**, 1303–5.

Cope O., Nardi G.L., Quijano M., Rovit R.L., Stanbury J.B. & Wight A. (1953) Metabolic rate and thyroid function following acute thermal trauma in man. *Annals of Surgery* **137**, 165–74.

Curling T.B. (1842) On accute ulceration of the duodenum in cases of burns. *Medic-chir Trans* **25**, 260–81.

Czaja A.J., McAlhamy J.L. & Pruitt B.A. (1976) Acute gastroduodenal disease after thermal injury; an endoscopic evaluation of invidence and natural history. *New England Journal of Medicine* **29**, 925–9.

Davies J.M., Dineen P. & Gallin J.Z. (1980) Neutrophil degranulation and abnormal chemotaxis after thermal injury. *Journal of Immunology* **124**, 1467–71.

de Campo T. & Aldrete J.A. (1981) The anaesthetic management of the severely burned patient. *Intensive Care Medicine* **7**, 55–62.

Demling R.H. (1983) Fluid resuscitation after major burns. *Journal of the American Medical Association* **260**, 1438–40.

Demling R.H. (1983) Improved survival after massive burns. *Journal of Trauma* **23**, 179–84.

Demling R.H. (1985) Burns. *New England Journal of Medicine* **313**, 1389–98.

Demling R.H., Kramer G. & Harris B. (1984) Role of thermal injury induced hypoproteinaemia on fluid flux and protein per-meability in burned and non burned tissue. *Surgery* **95**, 136–44.

Douglas C.G., Haldane J.S. & Haldane J.B.S. (1912) The laws of combination of haemoglobin with carbon monoxide and oxygen. *Journal of Physiology* **44**, 275.

Echinard C., Sajdel-Sulkowska E. & Burke P. (1982) The beneficial effects of early excicion on clinical response and thymic activity after burn injury. *Journal of Trauma* **22**, 560–565.

Faulkner B., Roven S. & De Clement F.A. (1978) Hypertension in children with burns. *Journal of Trauma* **8**, 213–17.

Fein A., Leff A., & Hopewell P. L. (1976) Pathophysiology and management of the complications resulting from fire and the inhaled products of combustion. *Critical Care Medicine* **4**, 144–150.

Harrison H.N., Moncrief J.A. & Duckett J.W. (1964) The relationship between energy metabolism and water loss from vapourisation in severely burned patients. *Surgery* **56**, 203.

Jackson D. MacG. (1983) The William Gissane Lecture 1982. The burn wound; its character, closure and complications. *Burns* **10**, 1–8.

Kien C.L., Young V.R., Rohrbaugh D.K. & Burke J.F (1978) Increased rates of whole body protein synthesis and breakdown in children recovering from burns. *Annals of Surgery* **187**, 383–91.

Lamb J.D. (1985) Anaesthetic considerations for major thermal injury. *Canadian Anaesthetists' Society Journal* **32**, 84–92.

Lund C.C. & Browder N.C. (1944) Estimation of area of burns. *Surgery, Gynecology and Obstetrics* **79**, 352.

Lutterman A. & Curreri P. W. (1987) Burns and electrical injuries. In *Current Therapy in Critical Care Medicine* (Ed. Parillo J.E.) p. 314–18. B.C. Decker Inc., Toronto.

Martyn J.A.J. (1986) Clinical pharmacology and drug therapy in the burned patient. *Anesthesiology* **65**, 67–75.

Martyn J.A.J., Matteo R.S., Szyfelbein S.K. & Kaplan R.F. (1982) Unprecendented resistance to the neuromuscular blocking effects of metocurine with persistence of complete recovery in a burned patient. *Anesthesia and Analgesia* **61**, 614–17.

Martyn J.A.J. Szyfelbein S.K., Matteo R.S., Ali H.H. & Savarese J. J. (1980) Increased d-tubocurarine requirement following major thermal injury. *Anesthesiology* **52**, 352–5.

McIrvine A.J., O'Mahony J.B., Saporoschetz I. & Memmick J.A. (1982) Depressed immune response in burn patients; use of monoclonal antibodies and functional assays to define the role of suppressor cells. *Annals of Surgery* **196**, 297–301.

Monafo W.W., Chuntrasakul C. & Agvazian V.H. (1973) Hypertonic sodium solutions in the treatment of burn shock. *American Journal of Surgery* 126, 778–83.

Moncrief J.A. (1979) Topical antibacterial treatment of the burn wound. In *Burns; A Team Approach* (Eds Artz C.P., Moncrief J.A. & Pruitt B.A.) pp. 250–69. W.B. Saunders, Philadelphia.

Moncrief J.A. (1973) Burns. *New England Journal of Medicine* 288, 444–54.

Moritz A.R. & Henriques F.C. (1947) Studies of thermal injury II. The relative importance of time and surface temperature in the causation of cutaneous burns. *American Journal of Pathology* 23, 695–720.

Moritz A..R., Henriques F.C. & McLean R. (1945) The effects of inhaled heat of the air passages and lung. *American Journal of Pathology* 21, 311–31.

Moylan J.A., Adib K. & Birnbaum M. (1975) Fibreoptic bronchoscopy following thermal injury. *Surgery, Gynecology and Obstetrics* 140, 541–3.

Muir I.F.K., Barclay T.L. & Settle J.A.D. (1987) The practical management of burns shock. In *Burns and their Management* 3rd edn. p. 30–5. Butterworths, London.

Muir I.F.K. (1961) Red cell destruction in burns. *British Journal of Plastic Surgery* 4, 273.

Neely W.A., Petro A.B., Holloman G.H., Rushton F.W., Turner D.M. & Hardy J.D. (1974) Researches on the cause of burn hypermetabolism. *Annals of Surgery* 179, 291–4.

Settle J.A.D. (1974) Urine output following severe burns. *Burns* 1, 23–42.

Smith J.S. & Brandon S. (1973) Morbidity from carbon monoxide poisoning at a 3 year follow-up. *British Medical Journal* 1, 319–21.

Thomsen M. (1977) Historical landmarks in the treatment of burns. *British Journal of Plastic Surgery* 30, 212–17.

Tolmie J.D., Joyce J.H. & Mitchell G.D. (1967) Succinylcholine danger in the burned patient. *Anesthesiology* 28, 467–70.

Tranbaugh R.F., Lewis F.R., Christensen J.M. & Elings V.B. (1980) Lung water changes after thermal injury; the effects of crystalloid administration and sepsis. *Annals of Surgery* 192, 479–88.

Trunkey J.D. (1978) Inhalation injury. *Surgical Clinics of North America* 58, 1133–40.

Venus B., Matsuda T., Copiozo J.B. & Mathru M. (1981) Prophylactic intubation and continuous positive airway pressure in the management of inhalation injury in burn victims. *Critical Care Medicine* 9, 519.

Wanner A. & Cutchavaree A. (1973) Early recognition of upper airway obstruction following smoke inhalation. *American Review of Respiratory Diseases* 108, 1421–3.

Wilmore D.W. (1979) Nutrition. In *Burns; A Team Approach* (Eds Artz C.P., Moncrief J.A. & Prutt B.A.) pp. 453–60. W.B. Saunders, Philadelphia.

Wilmore D.W., Long J.M., Mason A.D., Skreen R.W. & Pruitt B. A. (1974) Catecholamines—mediator of the hypermetabloic response to thermal injury. *Annals of Surgery* 180, 653–69.

Wilmore D.W., Mason A.D., Johnson D. & Pruitt B.A. (1975) Effect of ambient temperature on heat production and heat loss in burn patients. *Journal of Applied Physiology* 39, 593.

Zawacki B.E., Azen S.P., Imbus S.H. & Chang Y.T.C. (1979) Multifactorial probit analysis of mortality in burned patients. *Annals of Surgery* 189, 1–5.

Zawacki B.E., Spitzer I.C.W., Mason A.D. & Johns L.A. (1970) Does increased evaporative water loss cause hypermetabolism in burn patients? *Annals of Surgery* 171, 236–40.

Zikria B.A., Ferrer J.M. & Floch H.F. (1972) The chemical factor contributing to pulmonary damage in 'smoke poisoning'. *Surgery* 71, 704–9.

81

Drug Use in the Intensive Therapy Unit

M. WOOD

On average, a patient receives between 5 and 10 different medications per hospital admission, and adverse responses develop in approximately 5% of patients. Multiple drug therapy is almost always required in the intensive therapy unit (ITU) and therefore the potential is great for adverse drug interactions or effects to occur. Drugs should be administered to patients in a critical care setting only after considering both current drug therapy and the patients physiological state, as impairment of renal, hepatic or cardiovascular function may alter patient response to drug therapy. Changes in drug therapy should be kept to a minimum, and dosage adjustments made on the basis of titration to effect or the plasma concentration with the careful observation of response over a period of time.

Pharmacokinetics in the ITU
(see Chapter 15)

Continuous intravenous infusion regimens

Many drugs are given in the ITU by continuous intravenous infusion or by multiple doses. Obviously, it is important that plasma concentrations are maintained within the therapeutic range to maximize optimal drug effect. The plasma concentration at steady state (C_{SS}) achieved by continuous infusion may be calculated from a knowledge of clearance (Cl) and rate of administration. At steady state:

$$\text{Rate of administration} = \text{rate of elimination}$$
$$\text{Rate of elimination} = Cl \times C_{SS}.$$

Thus:

$$Rate\ of\ administration = Cl \times C_{SS}.$$

Thus, if we know the desired plasma concentration (C_{SS}) and the drug clearance, we can calculate the rate of administration required. However, it is usual to administer a loading dose before starting the infusion in order to achieve the therapeutic concentration more rapidly.

The loading dose of a drug is that dose required to raise the plasma drug concentration to the therapeutic range and is equal to the amount of drug in the body at therapeutic plasma concentration. Thus:

$$\text{Amount of drug in the body} = \text{plasma concentration} \times \text{volume of distribution.}$$

The loading dose required to achieve a plasma concentration of C_{SS} is therefore dependent on the volume of distribution, and

$$Loading\ dose = \text{volume of distribution} \times C_{SS}.$$

Alternatively, loading dose may be expressed in terms of the usual maintenance dosage regimen

$$Loading\ dose = \frac{\text{usual maintenance dose}}{\text{usual dosing interval}} \times \frac{t_{\frac{1}{2}}}{0.693}.$$

These equations allow the clinician to approximate drug administration for an individual patient, and dosage refinements based on the actual plasma concentration or patient response are required as treatment progresses.

EFFECT OF DISEASE ON PHARMACOKINETICS

Patients in the ITU may exhibit marked alterations in drug pharmacokinetics as a result of the abnormal physiological states that exist in these patients. Such alterations are important to recognize in order that appropriate dosage adjustments can be made before the development of drug toxicity is produced by inappropriately high plasma drug concentrations. These disease-induced changes in drug disposition are a result often of reduced drug excretion produced by either alteration in drug metabolism or renal excretion of either the drug itself or its metabolites.

Renal disease

The kidneys are the primary route of excretion for a number of water-soluble drugs and also for the water-soluble metabolites of less polar compounds. Excretion of such compounds (e.g. pancuronium) is reduced in patients with impaired renal function. Impaired renal function may be a result of chronic renal disease or the acute reduction in glomerular filtration seen frequently in the ITU. Administration of the customary dose of renally excreted drug to such patients results in drug accumulation and toxicity. To prevent such toxicity, appropriate dosage adjustments are required. Changes in drug binding in renal disease have been shown for a small number of drugs and may lead to alterations in volume of distrubution and therefore an adjustment in the loading dose. However, in the absence of a change in volume of distribution in renal disease, no change is required in the loading dose of drug. As stated previously, the maintenance dose of drug required to achieve a therapeutic concentration of drug in plasma at steady state (C_{SS}) is dependent on the rate of drug clearance. Thus, a dosage reduction is required to maintain the same plasma drug concentration when drug excretion decreases e.g. in patients with renal failure. Many drugs which are excreted in the kidney are excreted also by other routes, so that:

Total clearance = renal clearance
+ non-renal clearance.

In renal failure, only the renal clearance is altered predictably, so that adjustment of dosage needs to take into account the proportion of drug which is excreted non-renally (Table 81.1). The renal clearance of a drug excreted by glomerular filtration falls in proportion to the change in the patient's creatinine clearance. If the normal creatinine clearance is taken as 100 ml/min in a patient with renal disease:

Patient's renal drug clearance =

$$\text{normal renal} \atop \text{drug clearance} \times \frac{\text{patient's creatinine clearance}}{100}.$$

Table 81.1 Renal and non-renal clearance of some important drugs used in the ITU. (From Wilkinson & Oates, 1987)

Drug	Renal clearance* (ml/min)	Non-renal clearance (ml/min)
Ampicillin	340	12
Carbenicillin	68	10
Digoxin	110	36
Gentamicin	78	3
Kanamycin	60	0
Penicillin G	340	36

*Renal clearance when creatinine clearance = 100 ml/min.

Thus,

Patient's total drug clearance =

$$\text{normal renal} \atop \text{drug clearance} \times \frac{\text{patient's creatinine clearance}}{100}$$

+ non-renal clearance.

Although measurement of creatinine clearance is optimal, this is not always possible and the creatinine clearance (Cl_{cr}) may be calculated from a knowledge of the serum creatinine:

$$Cl_{cr} = \frac{(140 - \text{age}) \times \text{wt (kg)}}{72 \times \text{serum creatinine (mg/100 ml)}}.$$

Or:

$$Cl_{cr} = \frac{(140 - \text{age}) \times \text{wt (kg)} \times 1.23}{\text{serum creatinine (}\mu\text{mole)}}.$$

The calculated value should be reduced to 85% of this value in females.

Having calculated the appropriate total dose, there are two approaches to making the dosage adjustment. First, the dosage interval may be maintained at that used in patients with normal renal function and the amount of each dose reduced appropriately. Second, the normal dose may be given less frequently. This results in considerable variation between peak and trough plasma concentrations. It should be emphasized that both methods result in the same *average* plasma concentrations.

In addition to the effect of renal disease on the clearance of renally excreted drugs, the effects of diminished renal function on the clearance of drug metabolites needs to be considered also e.g. the principal route of excretion for pethidine is normally by metabolism in the liver. N-demethylation of pethidine yields norpethidine which is then excreted renally. Norpethidine accumulates in renal failure so that the ratio of metabolite:parent drug is approximately four-fold higher in renal failure than in patients with normal renal function. Norpethidine is active pharmacologically with approximately 50% of the potency of pethidine as an analgesic and two times the potency of pethidine as a convulsant. In patients with renal insufficiency, the accumulation of norpethidine after chronic pethidine dosing may cause excitability, twitching and seizures.

The pharmacologically active metabolites of the antiarrhythmic drug encainide also accumulate in renal failure. Because of the accumulation of these active metabolites during chronic encainide administration, the dose of encainide should be reduced in patients with renal disease. Thus, drugs that should be used with dosage adjustments in renal disease include digoxin, pancuronium, pethidine, morphine,

Table 81.2 Therapeutic concentrations of some drugs

Drug	Therapeutic range
Carbamazepine	3–10 μg/ml
Clonazepam	20–70 ng/ml
Diazepam	600–1200 ng/ml
Digitoxin	10–20 ng/ml
Digoxin	0.5–2 ng/ml
Ethosuximide	60–100 μg/ml
Lignocaine	4–6 μg/ml
Lithium	0.5–1.3 mmol/litre
Phenobarbitone	10–25 μg/ml
Phenytoin	10–25 μg/ml
Primidone	< 10 μg/ml
Procainamide	4–8 μg/ml
Propranolol	50–100 ng/ml
Quinidine	2–5 μg/ml
Theophylline	10–20 μg/ml
Thiocyanate	< 100 μg/ml
Valproic acid	50–100 μg/ml

gentamicin, kanamycin, cimetidine and lithium, and for many of these drugs monitoring of plasma concentrations is indicated (Table 81.2).

Liver disease
Hepatic disease might be expected to decrease the metabolism and clearance of drugs whose major route of excretion is by hepatic metabolism. Unfortunately, there is no measure of liver function which may be used to predict the decline in hepatic drug metabolism in the same way as creatinine clearance may be used to predict the decrease in drug excretion by the kidney. The situation is complicated further by the fact that the effects of hepatic disease on drug metabolism appear to be dependent on the metabolic pathway by which the drug is metabolized, so that drugs whose principal route of metabolism is by oxidation are affected more than those which are metabolized by glucuronidation. This has been demonstrated well for the benzodiazepines. The clearances of diazepam and chlordiazepoxide, which undergo oxidation, are decreased in liver disease whilst the clearances of lorazepam and oxazepam which are glucuronidated are unaffected (Table 81.3).

In addition to alterations in drug-metabolizing ability in liver disease, haemodynamic alterations occur also and result from both intra- and extrahepatic shunting of blood. Therefore, following oral administration and entry of drug into the portal circulation, some of the drug bypasses functioning liver tissue to enter the systemic circulation directly. For drugs which are normally highly extracted by the liver, such as propranolol or lignocaine, this portacaval shunting results in a substantial increase in plasma drug concentrations.

Shock, reduced cardiac output and cardiac failure
Drug delivery both to the organs of excretion, the liver and kidney, and to the tissues in which the drug is distributed is dependent on adequate tissue perfusion.

Drug	Initial route of metabolism	Cirrhosis	Hepatitis
Diazepam	Oxidation	Decrease	Decrease
Chlordiazepoxide	Oxidation	Decrease	Decrease
Lorazepam	Glucuronidation	No change	No change
Oxazepam	Glucuronidation	No change	No change

Table 81.3 Effects of route of metabolism on the clearance of benzodiazepines in liver disease.

In shock or states of low cardiac output, perfusion of certain tissues is reduced in order to maintain perfusion of vital organs. The reduction in liver and hepatic blood flow may result in reduced drug clearance with elevation of drug concentrations during multiple-dose therapy. In addition, because drug concentrations following an initial loading dose are dependent on drug distribution and hence perfusion of the tissues to which drug is distributed, reduced tissue perfusion such as is seen in shock, cardiac failure or other low cardiac output states may be associated with elevated drug concentrations if the usual loading dose of drug is given. In patients with reduced cardiac output or reduced tissue perfusion, a reduced loading dose of drug should be administered followed by appropriate dosage adjustment to take account of impaired drug excretion.

The multiple mechanisms altering drug disposition in cardiac failure are illustrated well by lignocaine. Lignocaine is excreted primarily by hepatic metabolism and, being a high-clearance drug, its clearance is influenced principally by hepatic blood flow. The reduction in hepatic blood flow together with reduced hepatic drug metabolizing ability in patients with cardiac failure contributes to reduced drug clearance; if usual doses of lignocaine are administered, increased and potentially toxic plasma lignocaine concentrations are produced. The active and potentially toxic metabolites of lignocaine undergo renal excretion, and because of the reduced glomerular filtration may accumulate to toxic concentrations. Finally, the reduced tissue perfusion results in a reduction in both the initial and steady-state volumes of distribution of lignocaine so that the initial loading dose must be reduced if toxicity is to be avoided. Thus, patients with low cardiac output should receive both a lower loading dose and a reduced maintenance dose of lignocaine. Other drugs are affected in the same way so that appropriate caution needs to be exercised in administering drugs to patients with reduced tissue perfusion in the ITU.

Plasma drug concentration monitoring

For some drugs, dosage may be assessed and monitored by direct measurement of the clinical pharmacological response; for example, reduction in arterial pressure following institution of antihypertensive therapy. However, for many drugs, this is not possible, and the measurement of plasma drug concentrations plays an important role in the individualization of patient drug management; particularly for patients in the ITU with acute and chronic disease states. By titrating drug dosage to maintain plasma concentrations within the 'therapeutic window', we may maximize therapeutic effects and reduce toxicity and unwanted pharmacokinetic drug interactions. The monitoring of therapeutic plasma concentrations is useful especially for drugs that have a narrow therapeutic window and exhibit a large interindividual variation in drug dosage. It is important that drug effect should correlate closely with drug concentration and not a metabolite. In addition, a suitable assay should be available for routine use. Table 81.2 lists the therapeutic drug concentrations for a number of drugs used commonly in the ITU.

Respiratory pharmacology in the ITU

Three major groups of drugs are used to treat patients with reversible obstructive airway disease; methylxanthine derivatives such as aminophylline, sympathomimetic bronchodilators such as β_2-agonists, and adrenocorticosteriods.

Pharmacology of bronchodilator drugs

In 1948, Ahlquist suggested that adrenergic receptors should be classified into two types; α and β. Lands subdivided further the β-receptors into β_1- and β_2-receptors: stimulation of β_1-receptors leads to chronotropic and inotropic stimulation and stimulation of β_2-receptors leads to smooth muscle relaxation with peripheral vasodilatation, bronchodilatation and inhibition of histamine or mast-cell mediator release. Thus, for bronchospastic patients in the ITU, bronchodilator drugs with minimal α or β_1 effects would be beneficial. The role of the β_2-receptor in the production of bronchodilatation is shown in Fig. 81.1. Sympathomimetic β_2-agonists stimulate the β_2-adrenergic receptor causing an increase in cyclic AMP which acts as the second messenger and initiates a series of events resulting in bronchial smooth muscle relaxation. Decreased concentrations of cyclic adenosine monophosphate (AMP) lead to bronchoconstriction. Cyclic AMP is then broken down to the inactive 5'-adenosine monophosphate by the enzyme phosphodiesterase. Prostaglandins E_1 and E_2 increase cyclic AMP concentrations but prostaglandin $F_{2\alpha}$ decreases cyclic AMP and causes bronchoconstriction.

Cyclic guanosine monophosphate cyclic (GMP) is another second messenger which is under the control

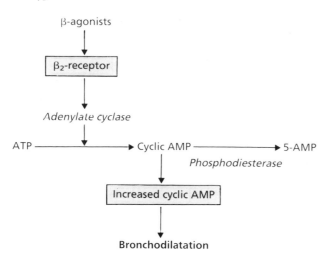

Fig. 81.1 Sympathetic nervous system and control of bronchomotor tone.

ATP = adenosine triphosphate.
Cyclic AMP = cyclic adenosine monophosphate.
5 AMP = 5-adenosine monophosphate.

of the parasympathetic nervous system and causes bronchoconstriction. Stimulation of cholinergic receptors increased cyclic GMP concentrations and increases bronchomotor tone.

The allergic response is a major factor in the production of an asthmatic attack, and mast-cell chemical mediators such as histamine, kinins and slow releasing substance of anaphylaxis (SRSA) cause bronchial smooth muscle constriction. Cyclic AMP prevents the release of chemical mediators; thus β-agonists and methylxanthines inhibit mediator induced bronchospasm.

Table 81.4 lists the smooth muscle receptors of the respiratory tract and the effects resulting from receptor stimulation.

AMINOPHYLLINE

The solubility of the xanthine compounds is low but is increased by formation of compounds with a

Table 81.4 Airway smooth muscle receptors

Type	Effect
Adrenergic	
α_1 and α_2	Contraction, bronchoconstriction
β_2	Relaxation, bronchodilatation
Cholinergic	Contraction
Histamine	
H_1	Contraction
H_2	Relaxation

wide range of salts; aminophylline is the ethylenediamine salt of theophylline. Theophylline is known to inhibit the enzyme phosphodiesterase, leading to increased concentrations of cyclic AMP which then initiate the physiological response, such as bronchodilatation. However, this effect is produced only at high concentrations, and it is believed now that inhibition of phosphodiesterase may not be the major factor in producing the pharmacological effects of aminophylline. Other mechanisms, such as theophylline-mediated catecholamine release, alterations in intracellular calcium and prostaglandin antagonism may contribute to the clinical effects produced by aminophylline.

The major therapeutic effect of aminophylline is bronchodilatation. Aminophylline is effective optimally in producing bronchodilatation at plasma concentrations of 10–20 mg/litre. Bronchodilatation increases progressively as the serum aminophylline concentration increases, and the use of aminophylline in the ITU is limited by the toxicity rather than plateau or ceiling effects. At levels above 25 mg/litre, 75% of patients exhibit signs of toxicity. The most frequent side-effects include gastrointestinal (anorexia, nausea, vomiting and abdominal discomfort) and CNS (headache, nervousness, anxiety) symptoms. At concentrations of 20–40 mg/litre, cardiac arrhythmias may occur, and at concentrations above 40 mg/litre, seizures or cardiorespiratory arrest may result. The monitoring of serum aminophylline concentrations is the only reliable method of assessing the risk of toxicity and should be undertaken whenever patients with asthma or bronchospastic disease require aminophylline therapy in the ITU. Xanthine derivatives may be given orally and intravenously. Extreme caution should be exercised in patients entering the ITU who have been taking oral theophylline already and in whom systemic therapy is considered. Rapid injection intravenously may cause hypotension. Table 81.5 outlines an infusion regimen for aminophylline.

Table 81.5 Aminophylline dosage regimen in the ITU

	Loading dose (mg/kg over 20 min)	Maintenance intravenous infusion ($mg \cdot kg^{-1} \cdot hr^{-1}$)
Children	6.0	1.10
Adults	6.0	0.90

Theophylline has a mean plasma elimination half-life of approximately 4.5 hr in adults and 3.6 hr in children. The elimination of theophylline is reduced in premature infants and increases dramatically in childhood. In the late teens, clearance values approach those in adults. Thus, as can be seen in Table 81.5, the loading dose is the same for adults and children but the maintenance infusion rate is increased in children. These are starting point dosage regimens, and the dose should be titrated to clinical effect and toxicity, together with monitoring plasma theophylline concentrations. The half-life of theophylline is increased in patients with severe liver disease and pulmonary oedema, and maintenance doses should be reduced for these patients.

BETA$_2$-RECEPTOR AGONIST

Sympathomimetic bronchodilators stimulate β_2-adrenergic receptors which leads to an increase in cyclic AMP concentrations and finally bronchodilatation. The endogenous adrenergic agonists, adrenaline and noradrenaline, are potent β-receptor agonists but produce unwanted α-induced haemodynamic effects also. Isoprenaline, a non-selective β_1 and β_2 stimulant, produces bronchodilatation but also stimulation of β_1-receptors, causing positive chronotropic and inotropic effects. More selective β_2 stimulants have replaced isoprenaline in the treatment of bronchospastic disease. However, selective β_2-agonists act also on β_1-receptors to some extent and elicit tachycardia and cardiac arrhythmias if given in high enough doses. Prolonged use of β-receptor agonists leads to 'down-regulation' and a reduction in β-receptor number or activity so that desensitization or tolerance develops. This can occur over a period of 1–2 weeks and requires the same period of restoration of normal β-receptor function following termination of drug therapy. When patients are admitted to the ITU for therapy of bronchospasm, they have frequently self-administered large doses of β-sympathomimetic agents, and termination of β-receptor agonist therapy with other supportive measures such as steriods and mechanical ventilation may allow the re-introduction of sympathomimetic bronchodilator therapy at a later date. Most of the selective β_2-agonists may be administered orally, parenterally or via the respiratory tract as inhaled aerosols or nebulized solutions. Administration by inhalation allows lower doses to be used for the same degree of bronchodilatation and thus minimizes β_1 side-effects. Table 81.6 lists guidelines for drug dosages of the β_2-adrenergic agonists, salbutamol, terbutaline and rimiterol.

Terbutaline is a selective β_2-agonist which may be administered orally, intravenously or by nebulization to treat reversible airway obstruction. Side-effects include β_1 cardiac effects (tachycardia, cardiac arrhythmias), hypokalemia and tachyphylaxis with chronic administration. The hypokalemia results from β_2-receptor stimulation, which causes potassium to be driven into the cells. Duration of action is 4–6 hr.

Salbutamol is a selective β_2-agonist which reduces airway resistance for 4–6 hr. It may be administered by aerosol, nebulizer or intravenously. Cardiac effects are said to be low when the aerosol dose is kept below 400 μg. Side-effects are similar to other selective β_2-agonists and include β_1 cardiac effects and hypokalaemia.

Rimiterol is another selective β_2-agonist that is also effective in reversible airway obstruction. Side-effects and indications are similar to those stated previously. Duration of effect is similar to isoprenaline.

Steroids. The mechanism by which steroids act in bronchospastic disease is unknown. They may have multiple actions in reversing asthmatic obstruction (reduction of inflammatory mucosal swelling, direct effects on airway vasculature causing vasoconstriction and reduced capillary permeability). Also, they are useful agents in restoring the responsiveness of asthmatic patients to sympathomimetic agents. Intravenous hydrocortisone may be administered to the patient in status asthmaticus in the ITU in doses of 4 mg/kg 6-hourly which achieves plasma concentrations around 100–150 mg/100 ml; a concentration considered to be within the therapeutic range. Steroids are useful in improving airflow in patients with chronic obstructive pulmonary disease with acute exacerbations.

Ipratropium is a derivative of atropine that is used to treat chronic obstructive pulmonary disease and asthma. Atropine and other anticholinergic drugs cause bronchodilatation by antagonizing the action of acetylcholine at the cholinergic receptor (Table 81.4) and by inhibiting the release of cyclic GMP. Side-effects of ipratropium are those of other anticholinergic drugs, such as dry mouth, blurred vision, palpitations, urinary retention and glaucoma. Ipratropium is a

Table 81.6 Drug dosage for selective β-agonists in reversible airway obstructive disease

Drug	Drug dosage and route of administration			Duration of action (hr)
	Subcutaneous	Intravenous	Nebulizer	
Terbutaline	0.25–0.5 mg s.c., i.m.	Loading = 250–500 μg maintenance = 1.5–5.0 μg/min	2–10 mg up to a maximum of 6-hourly (dilute in 2 ml normal saline)	4–6
Salbutamol	8 μg/kg s.c., i.m.	Loading = 250 μg maintenance = 5–20 μg/min	2.5–5.0 mg up to a maximum of 6-hourly (dilute in 2 ml normal saline)	4–6
Rimiterol			0.6 mg, repeated after 30 min. Maximum of 24 doses in 24 hr	1·5–3

quaternary ammonium compound with low lipid-solubility; thus, it is absorbed poorly across cell membranes and when given via the inhalational route, effects are limited to the cholinergic receptors within the lung. Systemic absorption is limited. Ipratropium bromide may be given via a metered-dose inhaler (36 mg per two inhalations) up to four times daily. It may also be given as a nebulized solution 500 μg to 1.0 mg 6-hourly if available.

Cardiovascular pharmacology in the ITU

Inotropes

SYMPATHOMIMETICS

Sympathomimetic drugs mimic the effects of stimulation of the sympathetic nervous system. Noradrenaline, adrenaline and dopamine are endogenous sym-

Table 81.7 Important effects of adrenergic stimulation

α-receptor stimulation	β-receptor stimulation
	Heart; predominantly β₁ Contractility ↑ Rate (sinoatrial node) ↑ Atrioventricular conduction velocity ↑ Refractory period ↓
Vasoconstriction Skin, viscera, gut	*Vasodilatation; β₂* Skeletal muscle
Mydriasis	*Bronchial relaxation; β₂*
	Uterine relaxation; β₂

↑ Increase
↓ Decrease.

pathomimetics, whilst isoprenaline is a synthetic catecholamine. Table 81.7 shows the important effects of adrenergic stimulation.

Adrenaline has α and β effects, noradrenaline has predominantly α effects and isoprenaline has predominantly β₁ and β₂ effects. Dopamine has α and β effects depending on dosage and also dopaminergic effects on receptors in the renal and mesenteric beds. Dobutamine has predominantly β₁ effects. Table 81.8 describes the effects of the inotropes, noradrenaline, adrenaline, isoprenaline, dopamine and dobutamine, while Table 81.9 gives infusion regimens for these drugs.

OTHER INOTROPIC DRUGS

Amrinone represents a new class of cardiac inotropic agents, distinct from the catecholamines and cardiac glycosides. It acts by increasing myocardial cellular concentrations of cyclic AMP by stimulation of adenylate cyclase or inhibition of phosphodiesterase (Fig. 81.1). The increased cyclic AMP concentrations lead to activation of myocardial contractile proteins, thereby increasing myocardial contractility and cardiac output. Amrinone also reduces afterload and preload, as a result probably of direct relaxant effects on vascular smooth muscle. Therefore, amrinone, when given to patients with congestive heart failure, increases cardiac output because of both its inotropic and vasodilatory effects. Pulmonary capillary wedge pressure and total peripheral resistance decrease. Heart rate is unchanged generally or it may increase slightly. Amrinone has an elimination half-life of approximately 3.6 hr. The drug may be given as a loading dose of

Table 81.8 Comparison of the effects of noradrenaline, adrenaline, isoprenaline, dopamine and dobutamine

Effect	Noradrenaline	Adrenaline	Isoprenaline	Dopamine	Dobutamine
Heart					
Rate	Slowed (reflex AP increase)	Increased	Increased	Little change or increased	Little change or increased slightly
Myocardial contractility	Little effect	Increased	Increased	Increased	Increased
Cardiac output	Little effect or reduced	Increased	Increased	Increased	Increased
Automaticity	Increased	Much increased	Much increased	Increased	Increased slightly
Arterial pressure					
Systolic	Rises	Rises	Little change or may fall	Little change or slightly decreased at lower doses	Slightly increased
Diastolic	Rises	Falls	Falls	—	Little changed or increased
Mean	Rises	Rises	Falls	—	
Vascular beds					
Muscle	Constricted	Dilated	Dilated	Dilated or constricted	Dilated
Skin/viscera	Constricted	Constricted	Dilated	Dilated*	Dilated
Kidney	Constricted	Constricted	Constricted	Dilated	Dilated
Coronary blood flow	Increased	Increased	Increased	Increased	Increased
Total peripheral resistance	Greatly increased	Increased	Decreased	Small increase	Small increase
Bronchi	Little effect	Relaxed	Relaxed	—	Relaxed
Uterus (pregnant)	Stimulated	Inhibited	Inhibited	—	Inhibited

*Dopamine can cause both relaxation or contraction of vascular smooth muscle, depending on the degree of α- or β- adrenergic receptor stimulation which is dose related. In addition, dopamine stimulates specific dopaminergic receptors causing vasodilatation of renal, mesenteric, and coronary vascular beds.

AP = arterial pressure.

Table 81.9 Inotrope dosage in the ITU

Drug	Dosage ($\mu g \cdot kg^{-1} \cdot min^{-1}$)
Adrenaline	0.01–0.2
Noradrenaline	0.01–0.1
Dopamine	2.0–30.0
Isoprenaline	0.01–0.1
Dobutamine	2.0–30.0
Phenylephrine	0.15–0.7

0.75 mg/kg followed by a maintenance infusion of between 5 and 10 $\mu g \cdot kg^{-1} \cdot min$. Side-effects include thrombocytopenia and gastrointestinal symptoms such as nausea, vomiting and abdominal pain.

Milrinone does not appear to cause thrombocytopenia.

Prenalterol is a selective β_1-agonist which may be used as an inotropic agent. The drug increases heart rate slightly. Other haemodynamic effects are predictable; an increase in cardiac output, myocardial contractility, tachyarrhythmias and an increase in total peripheral resistance. Prenalterol may be administered intravenously with doses of 1–5.0 mg given slowly.

Vasodilator therapy in the ITU

Vasodilators are used commonly in the ITU to: (1) control arterial pressure; (2) enhance myocardial function in acute ventricular failure by reducing afterload and thereby decreasing the pressure work of the ventricle; and (3) for unstable angina and myocardial ischaemia by affecting the factors that determine myocardial oxygen consumption i.e. heart rate, myocardial contractility and myocardial wall tension.

Table 81.10 Classification of hypotensive and vasodilator drugs according to site of action

Decreased central sympathetic activity
Central α_2-receptor agonists
e.g. clonidine, methyldopa
β-receptor antagonists
e.g. propranolol, labetalol

Adrenergic receptor antagonists
e.g. phentolamine (α_1 and α_2), prazosin (α_1)

Vasodilators
Arteriolar vasodilators
e.g. hydralazine, minoxidil, diazoxide, pinacidil
Arteriolar and venodilators
e.g. nitroprusside, nitroglycerin

Serotonin antagonists
e.g. ketanserin

Angiotensin-converting enzyme inhibitors
e.g. captopril, enalapril

Calcium antagonists
e.g. nicardipine, nifedipine

Ganglion-blocking agents
e.g. trimetaphan

Table 81.10 gives a classification of the hypotensive and vasodilator drugs. Nitroprusside and nitroglycerin are the vasodilators used commonly in the ITU, although other agents may be used in special circumstances.

The mechanism of action of nitroglycerin and other nitrates and nitroprusside has been understood only recently. The nitrate vasodilators act through the production of nitric acid. Nitric oxide formation activates the soluble guanylate cyclase present in the cytosol of smooth muscle cells which results in cyclic GMP production, activation of a cyclic GMP-dependent protein kinase and eventually, dephosphoryation of myosin light chains. This causes smooth muscle relaxation. Other vasodilators such as histamine appear to act through the same final common pathway.

Arteriolar vasodilators such as hydralazine reduce peripheral resistance by a direct vasodilator effect on the arterioles without affecting the venous capacitance vessels to any great extent. The reduction in afterload and absence of effect on venous capacitance vessels result in increased venous return, increased preload and reflex increase in cardiac output. The reduction in arterial pressure activates the baroreceptor reflex and results in increased sympathetic activity, with reflex tachycardia, increased myocardial contractility, increased cardiac output, increased myocardial work and hence increased myocardial oxygen demand. This may precipitate angina or myocardial infarction in patients with ischaemic heart disease. Thus, hydralazine is an unsuitable vasodilator for many patients in the ITU. Nitroprusside and nitroglycerin are arteriolar and venodilators, but the organic nitrates (nitroglycerin) produce predominantly venous dilatation. Therefore, the degree of afterload reduction is greater with nitroprusside than nitroglycerin. Nitroprusside has variable effects on myocardial oxygen balance. In the patient with severe hypertension, reduction in arterial and venous blood pressure reduces myocardial oxygen demand. However, there is evidence from the laboratory and also from clinical studies that suggests that nitroprusside may shunt coronary blood flow though collaterals away from ischaemic zones. Nitroglycerin may thus be the vasodilator of choice in patients with ischaemic heart disease.

The calcium antagonists nicardipine and nifedipine, which have pronounced vasodilator effects, have been administered as a continuous intravenous infusion to control hypertension in the ITU effectively. Labetalol, an α- and β-blocking agent, may be used to control hypertension also in the ITU when it can be administered intravenously in doses up to 20 mg given slowly over a 2-min period or as a continuous infusion (Table 81.11). The dosage should be reduced initially in the treatment of postoperative hypertension when the residual effects of anaesthetic agents and other drugs may be present.

Phentolamine, an α_1- and α_2-adrenergic blocking agent may be useful occasionally in the ITU, especially for the treatment of pulmonary hypertension. A compensatory reflex increase in heart rate is common. It has a rapid onset of action of 1–2 min and a duration of action of 20 min. Prostaglandin E_1 or alprostadil is a potent vasodilator that is used widely in the medical management of congenital heart disease to maintain the patency of the ductus arteriosus. However, it may

Table 81.11 Vasodilator therapy dosage in the ITU

Drug	Dosage ($\mu g \cdot kg^{-1} \cdot min^{-1}$)
Nitroprusside	0.25–5.0
Nitroglycerin	0.25–5.0
Isosorbide	0.8–2.0
Trimetaphan	5.0–30.0
Labetalol	0.03 (2 mg/min)
Diazoxide	3–5 mg/kg i.v. bolus
Phentolamine	0.5–20 (0.5 mg i.v. bolus)

be beneficial as a pulmonary (and systemic) vasodilator in adults. Other drugs that have been used as vasodilators in pulmonary hypertension include hydralazine and diazoxide.

It is important that, whenever vasodilator drugs are used in the ITU, alone or in combination with an inotropic agent, invasive haemodynamic monitoring is carried out and that these drugs are titrated carefully to a clinical effect. Cardiac output, cardiac filling pressures, pulmonary and vascular resistances should be calculated to aid in the selection of particular vasodilator drug acccording to the site of action and physiological effects pertaining to that agent.

Table 81.11 gives a summary of dosage administration for common vasodilators in the ITU.

Central nervous system pharmacology in the ITU

Status epilepticus

Monitoring of drug concentrations in plasma or serum is important to maximize therapeutic benefit while minimizing adverse effects (Table 81.2). It is important to recognize that plasma concentrations are usually measures of total drug in plasma. Many drugs used in the treatment of epilepsy are highly protein bound, and factors that decrease protein binding may cause unexpected toxicity if only total concentrations and not free unbound (pharmacologically active) concentrations are considered when making dosage adjustments.

Diazepam is a valuable agent in the management of status epilepticus. Plasma concentrations of 600–1200 ng/ml are required to suppress seizure discharge. Diazepam should be administered as an intravenous bolus in doses of 0.15–0.25 mg/kg and by infusion of up to 3.0 mg/kg over a 24 hr period. Clonazepam, another benzodiazepine, is useful also in the treatment of status epilepticus in doses of 1–3 mg by slow

intravenous infusion. Adverse effects for both of these drugs include severe cardiovascular and respiratory depression. In addition, CNS toxicity such as drowsiness, ataxia, dysarthria and sedation occur. Phenytoin may be used also in the treatment of status epilepticus. The recommended dose is 150–250 mg by slow intravenous injection, and then 100–150 mg after 30 min if required.

Status epilepticus is a medical emergency and requires immediate treatment. Anticonvulsants should be given and maintenance anticonvulsant therapy started immediately. However, in addition, to prevent the risk of cerebral hypoxia, an adequate airway and oxygenation should also be established quickly. This requires tracheal intubation, neuromuscular paralysis and ventilation if oxygenation is obviously impaired or the patient is unconscious for more than 15–30 min.

Sedation in the ITU (p. 1294)

Many patients in the ITU require sedation not only to perform mechanical ventilation more easily but also to decrease anxiety. Table 81.12 gives a summary of dosage regimens for some of the drugs used. Etomidate is no longer recommended for intravenous use in the ITU because of the adrenocortical suppression that it produces.

References

Wilkinson G.R. & Branch R.A. (1984) Effects of hepatic disease on clinical pharmacokinetics. In Pharmacokinetic Basis for Drug Treatment (Eds Benet L.Z. et al.). Raven Press, New York.

Wilkinson G.R. & Oates (1987) In Harrison's Principles of Internal Medicine 11th edn. McGraw Hill, New York.

Further reading

Armstrong P.W., Walker D.C., Burton J.R. & Parker J.O. (1975) Vasodilator therapy in acute myocardial infarction: a comparison of sodium nitroprusside and nitroglycerin. Circulation 52, 1118–22.

Bennet W.M., Aronoff G.R., Morrison G., Golper T.A., Pulliam J., Wolfson M. & Singer I. (1983) Drug prescribing in renal failure: dosing guidelines for adults. American Journal of Kidney Disease 3, 155–93.

Benotti J.R., Grossman W., Braunwald E., Davolos D.D. & Alousi A.A. (1978) Hemodynamic assessment of amrinone: a new inotropic agent. New England Journal of Medicine 299, 1373–7.

Bjornsson T.D. (1986) Nomogram for drug dosage adjustment in patients with renal failure. Clinical Pharmacokinetics 11, 164–70.

Braunwald E. (1977) Vasodilator therapy: a physiologic approach to the treatment of heart failure. New England Journal of Medicine 297, 331–2.

Cohen A.T. & Kelly D.R. (1987) Assessment of alfentanil by

Table 81.12 Dosage regimen of drugs which used to provide sedation in the ITU

Drug	Dosage
Pethidine	$0.3 \text{ mg} \cdot \text{kg}^{-1} \cdot \text{hr}^{-1}$
Midazolam	$0.1–3.0 \ \mu\text{g} \cdot \text{kg}^{-1} \cdot \text{min}^{-1}$ (loading dose 0.1–0.2 mg/kg)
Propofol	$13.0 \ \mu\text{g} \cdot \text{kg}^{-1} \cdot \text{min}^{-1}$ (maximum $2.0 \ \mu\text{g} \cdot \text{kg}^{-1} \cdot \text{min}^{-1}$)
Alfentanil	$0.3–0.5 \ \mu\text{g} \cdot \text{kg}^{-1} \cdot \text{min}^{-1}$ (maximum $2.0 \ \mu\text{g} \cdot \text{kg}^{-1} \cdot \text{min}^{-1}$)

intravenous infusion as long-term sedation in intensive care. *Anaesthesia* **42**, 545–8.

Cohn J.N. & Franciosca J.A. (1977) Vasodilator therapy of cardiac failure. *New England Journal of Medicine* **297**, 27–31, 254–8.

Cottrell J.E. & Turndorf H. (1978) Intravenous nitroglycerin. *American Heart Journal* **96**, 550–3.

Fabre J. & Baland L. (1976) Renal failure, drug pharmacokinetics and drug action. *Clinical Pharmacokinetics* **1**, 99–120.

Grounds R.M., Lalor J.M., Lumley J., Royston D. & Morgan M. (1987) *British Medical Journal* **294**, 397–400.

Perucca E., Grimaldi R. & Crema A. (1985) Interpretation of drug levels in acute and chronic disease states. *Clinical Pharmacokinetics* **10**, 498–513.

Prescott L.F. (1972) Mechanisms of renal excretion of drugs with special reference to drugs used by anaesthetists. *British Journal of Anaesthesia* **44**, 246–50.

Roberts R.K., Desmond P.V. & Schenker S. (1979) Drug prescribing in hepatobiliary disease. *Drugs* **17**, 198–12.

Rockett B.A. (1985) Kidney function and drug action. *New England Journal of Medicine* **313**, 816–18.

Rutman H.I., LeJemetel T.H. & Sonnenblick E.H. (1987) New cardiotonic agents: implications for patients with heart failure and ischemic heart disease. *Journal of Cardiothoracic Anaesthesia* **1**, 59–70.

Schlueter D.P. (1986) Ipratropium bromide in asthma. *American Journal of Medicine* **81**, 55–60.

Sear J.W. (1983) General kinetic and dynamic principles and their application to continuous infusion anaesthesia. *Anaesthesia* **38**, 10–25.

Tatham M.E. & Gellert A.R. (1985) The management of acute severe asthma. *Postgraduate Medical Journal* **61**, 599–606.

Webb-Johnson D.C. & Andrews J.L. (1977) Bronchodilator therapy (first of two parts). *New England Journal of Medicine* **297**, 476–82.

Webb-Johnson D.C. & Andrews J.L. (1977) Bronchodilator therapy (second of two parts). *New England Journal of Medicine* **297**, 758–64.

Yate P.M., Thomas D., Short S.M., Sebel P.S., & Morton J. (1986) Comparison of infusions of alfentanil or pethidine for sedation of ventilated patients on the ITU. *British Journal of Anaesthesia* **58**, 11091–9.

Index